Maternal Critical Care

A Multidisciplinary Approach

Maternal Critical Care

A Multidisciplinary Approach

Marc Van de Velde
Professor of Anesthesiology and Chair of the Department of Anaesthesiology, Catholic University of Leuven and University Hospitals Leuven, Leuven, Belgium

Helen Scholefield
Consultant Obstetrician and Lead Obstetrician for Critical Care and Clinical Governance, Liverpool Women's Hospital, Liverpool, UK

Lauren A. Plante
Director of Maternal–Fetal Medicine and Associate Professor, Departments of Obstetrics & Gynecology and of Anesthesiology, Drexel University College of Medicine, Philadelphia, PA, USA

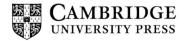

CAMBRIDGE UNIVERSITY PRESS

CAMBRIDGE UNIVERSITY PRESS
Cambridge, New York, Melbourne, Madrid, Cape Town,
Singapore, São Paulo, Delhi, Mexico City

Cambridge University Press
The Edinburgh Building, Cambridge CB2 8RU, UK

Published in the United States of America by Cambridge University Press, New York

www.cambridge.org
Information on this title: www.cambridge.org/9781107018495

First published 2013

Printed and bound by Grafos SA, Arte sobre papel, Barcelona, Spain

A catalogue record for this publication is available from the British Library

Library of Congress Cataloguing in Publication data
Maternal critical care : a multidisciplinary approach / [edited by] Marc van de Velde, Helen Scholefield, Lauren A. Plante.
    p. ; cm.
Includes index.
ISBN 978-1-107-01849-5 (hardback)
I. Velde, Marc van de, 1966–   II. Scholefield, Helen.   III. Plante, Lauren A.
[DNLM: 1. Critical Care – methods.   2. Pregnancy Complications – prevention & control.   3. Intensive Care
Units.   4. Maternal Health Services.   5. Pregnancy. WQ 240]
618.2′028–dc23

2012047376

ISBN 978-1-107-01849-5 Hardback

For Kieran and Aislinn, who have been amazingly patient with this process even if they would, all told, have actually preferred a baby brother.
Lauren A. Plante

To my Mother and Father, who are the most fabulous parents ever. You have been instrumental in all my achievements. Thank you.

To my marvelous children Sofie, Michiel, Bas, and Ella. Thank you for being so patient throughout my work. I do it all out of love for you.

To Eva, my wonderful, patient and loving wife. Thank you for supporting me every day. You are the best. You make me happy.
Marc Van de Velde

Contents

Contributors

Victoria M. Allen
Department of Obstetrics and Gynaecology, Dalhousie University, Halifax, NS, Canada

Frederic Amant
Division of Obstetrics and Gynaecology, University Hospital Leuven, Leuven, Belgium

Sarah Armstrong
University College London Hospital, London, UK

Thomas F. Baskett
Department of Obstetrics and Gynecology, Dalhousie University, Halifax, NS, Canada

Michael A. Belfort
Baylor College of Medicine and Texas Children's Hospital, Department of Obstetrics & Gynecology, Division of Maternal–Fetal Medicine, Houston, TX, USA

Meredith Birsner
Department of Gynecology and Obstetrics, Division of Maternal Fetal Medicine, Johns Hopkins Hospital, Baltimore, MD, USA

Renee D. Boss
Division of Neonatology, Department of Pediatrics, Johns Hopkins School of Medicine, Berman Institute of Bioethics, Baltimore, MD, USA

Leanne Bricker
Liverpool Women's NHS Foundation Trust, Liverpool, UK

Josaphat K. Byamugisha
Makerere University College of Health Sciences School of Medicine, Department of Obstetrics & Gynaecology, Kampala, Uganda

Giorgio Capogna
Department of Anesthesiology, Citta di Roma Hospital, Rome, Italy

Michael P. Casaer
Intensive Care Department and Burn Centre, Catholic University Hospitals Leuven, Leuven, Belgium

Frank A. Chervenak
Department of Obstetrics and Gynecology, Weill Medical College of Cornell University, New York, USA

Vicki Clark
Simpson Centre for Reproductive Health, Royal Infirmary, Edinburgh, UK

Filip Claus
Department of Radiology, Universital Hospitals Leuven, Leuven, Belgium

Malachy O. Columb
Acute Block Intensive Care Unit, University Hospital of South Manchester, Wythenshawe, UK

Charles Cox
The Royal Wolverhampton Hospitals NHS Trust, Wolverhampton, UK

Jean T. Cox
Department of Obstetrics and Gynecology. University of New Mexico School of Medicine, Albuquerque, NM, USA

Vegard Dahl
Department of Anaesthesia and Intensive Care, Baerum Hospital, Norway

John Davison
Newcastle upon Tyne Hospitals NHS Foundation Trust, Newcastle upon Tyne, UK

Jan Deprest
Department of Obstetrics and Gynecology, University Hospital Gasthuisberg and Research Unit of Fetus, Placenta, & Neonate, Academic Department of Development and Regeneration, Faculty of Medicine, KU Leuven, Leuven, Belgium

ix

Clifford S. Deutschman
Department of Anesthesiology and Critical Care, Hospital of the University of Pennsylvania, Philadelphia, PA, USA

Roland Devlieger
Department of Obstetrics and Gynaecology, University Hospitals Leuven, Leuven, Belgium

Karim Djekidel
Drexel University College of Medicine, Philadelphia, PA, USA

Steven Dymarkowski
University Hospitals Leuven, Leuven, Belgium

Roshan Fernando
University College London Hospital, London, UK

Clare Fitzpatrick
Liverpool Women's NHS Foundation Trust, Liverpool, UK

Sreedhar Gaddipati
Department of Obstetrics & Gynecology, Columbia University Medical Center, New York, USA

Thierry Girard
University Hospital of Basel, Basel, Switzerland

Emily Gordon
Department of Anesthesiology and Critical Care, Hospital of the University of Pennsylvania, Philadelphia, PA, USA

Ian A. Greer
Faculty of Health & Life Sciences, University of Liverpool, Liverpool, UK

David Grooms
Department of Respiratory Therapy, Sentara Norfolk General, Leigh, & Princess Anne Hospitals, VA, USA

Sina Haeri
Department of Obstetrics and Gynecology, Texas Children's Hospital, Houston, TX, USA

Katy Harrison
Specialist Registrar in Obstetrics and Gynaecology, Bradford Royal Infirmary, Bradford, UK

Edward J. Hayes
Division of Perinatology, Aurora Bay Care Medical Center, Green Bay, WI, USA

Michelle Hladunewich
Division of Nephrology, Sunnybrook Health Sciences Centre, and Division of Nephrology, University Health Network, Toronto, ON, Canada

Andra H. James
Division of Maternal–Fetal Medicine, Department of Obstetrics and Gynecology, Duke University Medical Center, Durham, NC, USA

Tracey Johnston
Birmingham Women's Hospital, Edgbaston, Birmingham, UK

Bellal Joseph
Department of Surgery, University of Arizona, Tucson, AZ, USA

Erin Keely
Division of Endocrinology and Metabolism, Ottawa Hospital and Departments of Medicine and Obstetrics/Gynecology, University of Ottawa, Ottawa, ON, Canada

Ruth Landau
Department of Anesthesiology and Pain Medicine, University of Washington Medical Center, Seattle, WA, USA

Stephen E. Lapinsky
Mount Sinai Hospital, University of Toronto, Toronto, ON, Canada

Susanna I. Lee
Department of Radiology, Massachusetts General Hospital, Harvard Medical School, Boston, MA, USA

Larry Leeman
Department of Family and Community Medicine and Department of Obstetrics and Gynecology, University of New Mexico School of Medicine, Albuquerque, NM, USA

Hennie Lombaard
Obstetrics Unit, Department of Obstetrics and Gynecology, Steve Biko Academic Hospital, University of Pretoria, Gezina, Pretoria, South Africa

Stephen Lu
Department of Surgery, University of New Mexico School of Medicine, Albuquerque, NM, USA

Alison MacArthur
Department of Anesthesia, Mount Sinai Hospital, University of Toronto, Toronto, ON, Canada

Laura A. Magee
Departments of Obstetrics and Gynaecology and Medicine, and the Child and Family Research Institute, University of British Columbia, Vancouver, BC, Canada

Paul E. Marik
Department of Medicine, Division of Pulmonary and Critical Care Medicine, Eastern Virginia Medical School, Norfolk, VA, USA

Laurence B. McCullough
Center for Medical Ethics and Health Policy, Baylor College of Medicine, Houston, TX, USA

Alexandre Mignon
Department Anesthesie Reanimation, Université Paris Descartes, Paris, France

Carlo Missant
Department of Anesthesiology, University Hospitals Leuven, Leuven, Belgium

Jack Moodley
University of Kwa-Zulu Natal, Durban, South Africa

Lisa E. Moore
Department of Obstetrics & Gynecology, University of New Mexico School of Medicine, Albuquerque, NM, USA

Kate Morse
Drexel University, College of Nursing and Health Professions, Philadelphia, PA, USA

Warwick D. Ngan Kee
Department of Anaesthesia and Intensive Care, Chinese University of Hong Kong, Prince of Wales Hospital, Hong Kong, China

Catherine Nelson-Piercy
Women's Health Academic Centre, London, UK

Clemens M. Ortner
Department of Anesthesiology and Pain Medicine, University of Washington Medical Center, Seattle, WA, USA

Geraldine O'Sullivan
Department of Anaesthesia, Guys and St Thomas' NHS Foundation Trust, London, UK

Luis D. Pacheco
Departments of Obstetrics/Gynecology and Anesthesiology, Divisions of Maternal–Fetal Medicine and Surgical Critical Care, University of Texas Medical Branch at Galveston, Galveston, TX, USA

Fathima Paruk
Cardio-Thoracic Surgical Intensive Care Unit, Department of Anesthesiology, University of Witwatersrand, Johannesburg, South Africa

Melina Pectasides
Department of Radiology, Massachusetts General Hospital, Harvard Medical School, Boston, MA, USA

Nigel Pereira
Department of Obstetrics and Gynecology, Drexel University College of Medicine, Philadelphia, PA, USA

Patricia Peticca
Division of Endocrinology and Metabolism, University of Ottawa, Ottawa, ON, Canada

Sharon T. Phelan
Department of Obstetrics and Gynecology. University of New Mexico School of Medicine, Albuquerque, NM, USA

Felicity Plaat
Queen Charlotte's Hospital, London, UK

Lauren A. Plante
Departments of Obstetrics & Gynecology and of Anesthesiology, Drexel University College of Medicine, Philadelphia, PA, USA

Michael P. Plevyak
Department of Obstetrics and Gynecology, Tufts University School of Medicine, Baystate Medical Center, Springfield, MA, USA

Dianne Plews
Department of Haematology, South Tees Hospitals NHS Foundation Trust, Middlesbrough, UK

Wendy Pollock
Faculty of Health Sciences, School of Nursing and Midwifery, Department of Midwifery, La Trobe University, Mercy Hospital for Women, Melbourne, Australia

Laura C. Price
Royal Brompton Hospital, London, UK

Peter Rhee
Division of Trauma, Critical Care and Emergency Surgery, University of Arizona, Tucson, AZ, USA

Leiv Arne Rosseland
Department of Anaesthesia, Division of Critical Care, University of Oslo, Oslo, Norway

Kathryn M. Rowan
ICNARC, London, UK

Helen Ryan
Departments of Obstetrics and Gynaecology, University of British Columbia, Vancouver, BC, Canada

Helen Scholefield
Liverpool Women's NHS Foundation Trust, Liverpool, UK

Neil S. Seligman
Department of Obstetrics and Gynecology, Division of Maternal–Fetal Medicine, University of Rochester Medical Center, Rochester, NY, USA

Nadir Sharawi
Department of Anaesthesia, Guys and St Thomas' NHS Foundation Trust, London, UK

Alex Sia
KK Women's and Children's Hospital, Singapore, Singapore

Bob Silver
Department of Maternal–Fetal Medicine, University of Utah, Salt Lake City, UT, USA

Mieke Soens
Department of Anesthesiology, Perioperative and Pain Medicine, Brigham and Women's Hospital, Boston, MA, USA

Ulrich J. Spreng
Department of Anaesthesia and Intensive Care, Baerum Hospital, Norway

Silvia Stirparo
Department of Anesthesiology, Citta di Roma Hospital, Rome, Italy

Nova Szoka
Department of Surgery, University of New Mexico School of Medicine, Albuquerque, NM, USA

Andrew Tang
Department of Surgery, The University of Arizona, Tucson, AZ, USA

Kha M. Tran
Department of Anesthesiology and Critical Care Medicine, Perelman School of Medicine at the University of Pennsylvania, Children's Hospital of Philadelphia, Philadelphia, PA, USA

Els Troost
Department of Congenial and Structural Cardiology, University Hospitals Leuven, Leuven, Belgium

Lawrence C. Tsen
Department of Anesthesiology, Perioperative and Pain Medicine, Brigham and Women's Hospital, Boston, MA, USA

Derek Tuffnell
Bradford Hospitals NHS Trust, Bradford, UK

Kristel Van Calsteren
Department of Obstetrics and Gynaecology, University Hospital Leuven, Leuven, Belgium

Marc Van de Velde
Department of Anaesthesiology, Catholic University of Leuven and University Hospitals Leuven, Belgium

Marcel Vercauteren
Department of Anesthesiology, Antwerp University, Antwerp, Belgium

Chris Verslype
Department of Hepatology, University of Leuven, Leuven, Belgium

Peter von Dadelszen
Department of Obstetrics and Gynaecology, and the Child and Family Research Institute, University of British Columbia, Vancouver, BC, Canada

Carl Waldman
Intensive Care Unit, Royal Berkshire Hospital, Reading, UK

Michelle Walters
Nuffield Department of Anaesthesia, John Radcliffe Hospital, Oxford University Hospitals NHS Trust, Oxford, UK

Linda Watkins
Liverpool Women's NHS Foundation Trust, Liverpool, UK

Paul Westhead
Obstetrics and Gynaecology, Mersey Deanery, Liverpool, UK

Cynthia A. Wong
Department of Anesthesiology, Northwestern University Feinberg School of Medicine, Chicago, IL, USA

Gerda G. Zeeman
Department of Obstetrics and Gynaecology, Division of Obstetrics & Prenatal Medicine, Erasmus MC, University Medical Centre Rotterdam, Rotterdam, the Netherlands

Joost J. Zwart
Department of Obstetrics/Gynaecology, Deventer Hospital, Deventer, the Netherlands

Preface

The border territory between normal obstetrics and critical care is little understood and lightly inhabited. Pregnancy is a normal event in the lives of most women, undertaken happily with the expectation of a joyful result.

Yet critical illness may afflict a pregnant woman. She may have a preexisting medical condition which complicates, or is complicated by, the fact of pregnancy, such as heart disease or renal failure. Or she may develop acute obstetric morbidity such as hemorrhage or eclampsia. Severe acute morbidity, even mortality, may plague a woman during this time, converting a joyous time to a tragedy.

Obstetricians and midwives, while accustomed to supervising the normal process, are well prepared for common obstetrical complications but not necessarily for the rare life-threatening event. Intensivists, well versed in the management of critical illness, are not generally prepared for either the usual physiological alterations brought about by pregnancy or for the complicating presence of a fetus. Anesthesiologists, perhaps better exposed to both sides, may nevertheless be more focused on the acute management of crisis in the operating room.

When a new mother, or mother-to-be, ends up in the intensive care unit, it is a shock to all concerned: to the woman herself, if she is aware; to her family; and to the physicians and nurses that care for her in that situation. Obstetricians are often intimidated by the staggering complexity of intensive care, while intensivists are often fetophobic. The balance of care requires input from an entire team of care providers with varying expertise.

Hence this book. We have made an attempt, in these pages, to review both the obstetric and critical care issues, and we have solicited input from a distinguished group of authors on both sides of the aisle. Wherever feasible, we have sought to have chapters collaboratively authored by experts in more than a single specialty: we wanted the most diverse set of viewpoints available. Understanding that practice may vary across regions, we have recruited those experts internationally.

It is our hope that the reader, whether novice or expert, will find something here to be useful or thought provoking, and that the team approach that drove this book will echo in the clinical hallways where our patients, and yours, are managed.

Chapter 1

The scope for maternal critical care: epidemiology

Victoria M. Allen, Thomas F. Baskett, and Kathryn M. Rowan

Definitions of maternal mortality and maternal near miss

Pregnancy-related death is defined by the World Health Organization (WHO) as the death of a woman while pregnant or within 42 days of termination of pregnancy despite the cause of death [1]. Although a relatively rare event in developed countries, accurate assessment and surveillance of maternal deaths is difficult in the absence of structured obstetric review [2]. While the Confidential Enquiries into Maternal Deaths and Child Health (CEMACH) in the UK is an established assessment of maternal mortality [3], evaluation of maternal mortality and significant maternal morbidity in North America has proven to be challenging. In the USA, surveillance is limited by poorly defined or inconsistent coding, or absence of documentation of pregnancy on death certificates [4]. In Canada, the Canadian Perinatal Surveillance System has identified variability in the detail and quality of data, under-reporting of maternal mortality by the Canadian Vital Statistics System, and discrepancies in rates of selected severe maternal morbidities, among both provincial and national data sources, as obstacles to the comprehensive determination of rates of maternal mortality and significant maternal morbidity [5]. In addition, information in Canada is not systematically shared across administrative health jurisdictions [5].

The study of maternal near miss, in addition to maternal mortality, evaluates the provision of obstetric care and allows for enhancement of such services with the identification of deficiencies. The WHO defines maternal near miss as a woman who nearly died but survived a complication that occurred during pregnancy, childbirth, or within 42 days of termination of pregnancy [1]. This definition resolves differences observed with previous near miss and severe acute maternal morbidity definitions and is also aligned with the definition of maternal death in the *International Statistical Classification of Diseases and Related Health Problems*, 10th edition (ICD-10 [1]).

Prevalence of maternal near miss

Maternal morbidity may be described as a continuum of adverse events, progressing from normal pregnancy to morbidity to severe morbidity to near miss to death [6]. An national evaluation of delivery hospitalizations in the USA utilized the *International Statistical Classification of Diseases and Related Health Problems*, 9th Revision, Clinical Modification (ICD-9-CM) [7] codes for severe maternal morbidity and showed 5 of every 1000 pregnant women had at least one indicator of severe morbidity during their delivery hospitalization [8]. They found a significant increase in coding for blood transfusion during the study period (1991–2003), an important indicator of severe obstetric hemorrhage. A similar study in Canada from 1991–2001 found a severe maternal morbidity rate of 4.4 per 1000 deliveries, and blood transfusion was a leading contributor of severe morbidity [9]. The presence of major pre-existing conditions increased the risk of severe maternal morbidity to six-fold [9].

Risk factors for maternal near miss

Extremes of age, pre-existing medical conditions, language barriers, ethnicity, and socioeconomic status are recognized risk factors for maternal and obstetric complications. Older maternal age, African-American race and Hispanic ethnicity, obesity, prior cesarean section, and gravidity in particular were identified as risk factors in a New York population of pregnant women [10]. In the USA, social, economic, and medical conditions were considered in an evaluation of maternal near miss in African-American, Hispanic, and white populations,

Maternal Critical Care: A Multidisciplinary Approach, ed. Marc Van de Velde, Helen Scholefield, and Lauren A. Plante.
Published by Cambridge University Press. © Cambridge University Press 2013.

which demonstrated significantly higher rates of maternal near miss among Hispanic, but not African-American, women compared with white women (relative risk 1.45; 95% confidence interval, 1.14–1.84) [11]. In Canada, universal availability of healthcare, through national and provincial funding programs, minimizes discrepancies in access to obstetric care. However, while specific information on vulnerable populations such as Aboriginal women is not routinely available in Canada, it is recognized that there are important differences in health and social indicators of Aboriginal women compared with non-Aboriginal women [12] that influence perinatal outcomes such as preterm birth, stillbirth, and infant death [13]. Challenges to providing safe obstetric care to Aboriginal communities include limited resources, large geographic distances, varying language groups, and differing cultural beliefs and traditions [12]. Recognition of risk factors modifiable through medical care, education, or social support systems is essential.

Preventability of maternal near miss

In the most recent CEMACH report, poor recognition of early warning signs of impending maternal collapse was highlighted as a primary contributor to maternal morbidity and maternal near miss [3]. The report provided an example of an obstetric early warning chart to assist in the timely recognition of women who have, or are developing, a critical illness [3]. Following an examination of maternal morbidity and mortality that showed an association between preventable determinants and progression from severe to near miss outcomes, a preventability model in maternal death and morbidity has been developed and validated in the USA to identify quality of care issues, and to apply this information in the development of appropriate interventions for change [14]. This analysis demonstrated that one third of all cases of maternal morbidity and mortality were preventable, and that the majority of the preventable events was influenced by provider-related factors such as delay or failure in diagnosis or recognition of high-risk patient conditions, inappropriate treatment, and inadequate documentation [14].

Classification of maternal near miss

An important challenge to the identification of maternal near miss outcomes has historically been varying definitions between local, national, and international institutions. The majority of definitions may be classified as clinically based, organ system based, or management/intervention based [15]. Clinical criteria related to disease-specific morbidities, such as severe obstetric hemorrhage, are easily interpretable and quantified and may be collected retrospectively. Organ-system dysfunction criteria are based on abnormalities detected by laboratory tests, such as platelet levels, and basic critical care monitoring. These criteria establish patterns of disease and may be collected prospectively, but they are influenced by the quality of care and access to laboratories and critical care monitoring. Management-based criteria, such as admissions to intensive care units, have been employed in North America to identify relevant patients; however, quality of data may vary with distance to care, level of care (intermediate versus intensive), and availability of intensive care beds [15]. Recent international reviews of obstetric admissions for critical care have demonstrated that the overall requirement for intensive care is low (mean incidence $\leq$ 5 per 1000 deliveries) [16,17]. While studies showing need for critical care in the USA alone was consistent with overall rates [16], a recent Canadian study demonstrated a rate of 0.5/1000 pregnant women requiring transfer to intensive care [18].

The WHO has recently proposed that signs of organ dysfunction following life-threatening conditions be used to identify maternal near miss, so that the classification of underlying causes is consistent for both maternal deaths and near misses. Comparability across institutions would be feasible with the uniform use of these definitions in international surveillance. With a collaboration of clinicians, epidemiologists, program implementers, and researchers, WHO established several principles guiding a classification system designed to optimize maternal near miss surveillance [1]; it was required to be practical and understood by its users, with underlying causes exclusive of all other conditions, and compatible with the 11th revision of ICD. The definition with identification criteria for maternal near miss was developed and tested in datasets in Brazil and Canada prior to review by the WHO Advisory Group [1].

The WHO definition proposed a standard terminology for cause of maternal death, including direct and indirect maternal deaths and unanticipated complications of management, categorized by disease category and individual underlying causes [1]. In addition, maternal near miss is identified by a set of markers that include basic laboratory tests, management-related markers, and clinical criteria based on clinical assessment (Table 1.1) [1]. Thresholds for these markers were

Table 1.1. World Health Organization identification and classification of maternal near miss

Criteria	Features
Clinical criteria	
Acute cyanosis	
Gasping	Terminal respiratory pattern where the breath is convulsively and audibly caught
Respiratory rate	>40 or <6/min
Shock	Persistent severe hypotension, defined by a systolic blood pressure <90 mmHg for ≥60 minutes with a pulse rate of at least 120 beats/min despite aggressive fluid replacement (>2 L)
Oliguria non-responsive to fluids or diuretics	Urinary output 30 mL/h for 4 hours or 400 mL/24 h
Clotting failure	Assessed by the bedside clotting test or absence of clotting from an intravenous site after 7–10 minutes
Loss of consciousness lasting ≥ 12 hours	A profound alteration of mental state that involves complete or near-complete lack of responsiveness to external stimuli; defined as a Coma Glasgow Scale <10 (moderate or severe coma)
Loss of consciousness *and* absence of pulse/heart beat	
Stroke	Neurological deficit of cerebrovascular cause that persists beyond 24 hours or is interrupted by death within 24 hours
Uncontrollable fit/total paralysis	Brain in a state of continuous seizure
Jaundice in the presence of pre-eclampsia	Pre-eclampsia is defined as the presence of hypertension associated with proteinuria. Hypertension is defined as a blood pressure of ≥140 mmHg (systolic) or ≥90 mmHg (diastolic) on at least two occasions and at least 4–6 hours apart after the 20th week of gestation in women known to be normotensive beforehand. Proteinuria is defined as excretion of ≥300 mg protein every 24 hours; if 24 hour urine samples are not available, proteinuria is defined as a protein concentration of 300 mg/L or more (≥1+ on dipstick) in at least two random urine samples taken at least 4–6 hours apart
Laboratory-based criteria	
Oxygen saturation reduced	90% for ≥60 minutes
Arterial oxygenation efficiency reduced	Ratio of partial pressure of arterial O_2 to the fraction of inspired O_2 of 200 mmHg
Creatinine increased	≥300 µmol/L (≥3.5 mg/dL)
Bilirubin increased	>100 mmol/L or >6.0 mg/dL
Severe acidosis	≤pH 7.1
Lactate increased	>5 mmol/L
Acute thrombocytopenia	Platelet count 50×10^9/L or less
Loss of consciousness *and* the presence of glucose and ketoacids in urine	
Management-based criteria	
Use of continuous vasoactive drugs	For example, continuous use of any dose of dopamine, epinephrine, or norepinephrine
Hysterectomy following infection or hemorrhage	
Transfusion required	≥5 units red cell transfusion
Intubation and ventilation	For ≥60 minutes not related to anesthesia
Dialysis	For acute renal failure
Cardiopulmonary resuscitation	

Source: Reprinted from *Best Practice & Research Clinical Obstetrics & Gynaecology*, **23**, Say L, Paulo Souza J, Pattinson RC, WHO working group on maternal mortality and morbidity classifications. Maternal near miss: towards a standard tool for monitoring quality of maternal healthcare, pp. 287–296, Copyright (2009), with permission from Elsevier [2].)

derived from the Sequential Organ Failure Assessment score [19].

Maternal near miss surveillance in the UK

In 2006, using management-based criteria of critical care unit admission for maternal near miss, the Intensive Care National Audit & Research Centre incorporated surveillance of maternal near miss into their national clinical audit, the Case Mix Programme, covering more than 90% of adult, general critical care units (intensive care or combined intensive care/high dependency units) in England, Wales, and Northern Ireland. Maternal near miss surveillance was incrementally adopted by the participating units during 2006–2007.

For the period April 2008 to March 2011, of 289 669 admissions to 205 adult, general critical care units (88% of all adult general critical care units), 127 804 (44.1%) admissions were women and 36 244 (28.4%) were aged between 16 and 50 years. Of these, 2.2% were currently pregnant and 9.8% were recently pregnant (within 42 days of admission to the critical care unit). On extrapolation, maternal near miss (critical care admissions of currently or recently pregnant women) represented approximately 15.0 admissions per 100 000 women aged 16 to 50 years, approximately 2.8/1000 live births, or approximately 2.8/1000 maternities.

For currently pregnant women, the primary reason for admission to critical care was non-obstetric for the majority (92%) while approximately two thirds of recently pregnant women had an obstetric-related primary reason for admission. For all women aged between 16 and 50 years admitted for critical care and either currently or recently pregnant, Table 1.2 presents age, trimester, acute severity, mortality, and length of stay. For currently pregnant women, median gestation at admission to critical care was 26 weeks (interquartile range (IQR), 19–32) and ranged from 2 to 40 weeks. For recently pregnant women, median gestation at delivery was 38 weeks (IQR, 33–40) and ranged from 2 to 45 weeks. Gestation (in weeks) by outcome of recent pregnancy is presented in Figure 1.1; 60% of recently pregnant women were admitted to critical care on the same day as delivery, a further 28% within 1 week, and 12% between 7 and 42 days following delivery. Delivery method is presented in Figure 1.2.

Future challenges for maternal near miss surveillance

In addition to standardizing the identification of cases of maternal near miss to allow improved data collection and comparability among institutions, it is important to recognize factors that alter the rates of maternal near miss and, therefore, influence a comparison of rates over time. Changing maternal characteristics, such as older maternal age and higher pre-pregnancy obesity [20], increase the effect of these risk factors on hypertension and diabetes in pregnancy. Demographics of obstetric populations are becoming more multiethnic and multicultural and, so far, data on the adequacy of prenatal care has been insufficiently collected [11]. Complications from pre-existing medical conditions such as chronic heart disease are emerging as an important cause of maternal near miss, as improvements in medical care allow more women to live to reproductive age [21]. Increasing numbers of multiple gestations linked to the use of assisted reproductive technologies alters the influence of twins and higher-order multiples on significant adverse maternal outcomes [18]. Increasing rates of cesarean delivery reflect these changing maternal and obstetric factors [20]. Developing maternal–fetal medicine interventions such fetal surgery for fetal structural abnormalities have been associated with maternal intensive care unit admissions after the procedures [22]. Contemporary North American data during pandemic influenza virus infection demonstrated significant maternal morbidity and critical care admission [23,24].

Conclusions

Complete and comprehensive surveillance of maternal mortality and maternal near miss should increase the consistency and accuracy of the data. Relevant factors should be determined to delineate the interactions between the healthcare system, the healthcare provider, and the woman's social and cultural determinants in contributing to maternal near miss events. Improved coding with comparable consistency between institutions, and recognition of changing obstetric practices such as increasing cesarean delivery rates and changing maternal characteristics, could reduce maternal near misses and promote healthy pregnancy outcomes. Continual surveillance and reassessment of the influence of maternal disease and obstetric outcomes on maternal near miss

Table 1.2. Case mix, outcome, and length of stay for currently and recently pregnant admissions to UK critical care units, 2008 to 2010

Pregnancy status on admission to the critical care unit	Currently pregnant	Recently pregnant[a]
Number of admissions (%[b])	775 (0.3)	3579 (1.3)
Age (mean years (SD))	28.0 (6.6)	30.6 (6.4)
Gestation (No. (%))		
First trimester	114 (14.9)	270 (7.9)
Second trimester	326 (42.6)	217 (6.4)
Third trimester	326 (42.6)	2926 (85.7)
ICNARC physiology score (mean (SD))	12.3 (6.8)	11.7 (6.5)
APACHE II score (mean (SD))	11.3 (5.2)	10.1 (4.7)
Surgical status (No. (%))		
Non-surgical	685 (88.4)	1675 (46.8)
Elective/scheduled	11 (1.4)	176 (4.9)
Emergency/urgent	79 (10.2)	1728 (48.3)
No. critical care unit deaths (% (95% CI))	16 (2.1) (1.3–3.3)	46 (1.3) (1.0–1.7)
No. acute hospital deaths[c] (% (95% CI))	24 (3.2) (2.2–4.8)	67 (1.9) (1.5–2.4)
Readmissions within the same acute hospital stay (No. (%))	21 (2.7)	78 (2.2)
Days stay in critical care unit (median (IQR))		
All	2.1 (1.0) (4.0)	1.1 (0.7) (2.1)
Unit survivors	2.0 (1.0) (4.0)	1.1 (0.7) (2.1)
Unit non-survivors	6.3 (2.2) (22.2)	3.3 (0.7) (6.5)
Total days stay in acute hospital[c] (median (IQR))		
All	8 (5) (14)	7 (5) (13)
Hospital survivors	8 (5) (14)	7 (5) (13)
Hospital non-survivors	12 (2) (29)	8 (2) (22)

APACHE, Acute Physiological and Chronic Health Evaluation; CI, confidence interval; ICNARC, Intensive Care National Audit & Research Centre; IQR, interquartile range; SD, standard deviation
[a] Within 42 days prior to admission to the critical care unit.
[b] Percentage of all admissions to the critical care unit.
[c] Excluding readmissions to the critical care unit within the same acute hospital stay.

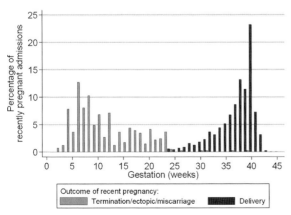

Figure 1.1. Gestation by outcome for recently pregnant admissions to UK critical care units, 2008 to 2010.

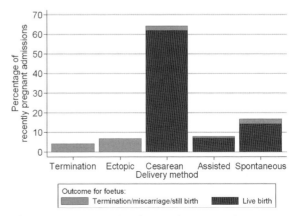

Figure 1.2. Delivery method for recently pregnant admissions to UK critical care units, 2008 to 2010.

5

prevalence should lead to the development or adoption of evidence-supported obstetric care interventions to effectively reduce maternal mortality and near miss. Effective prevention policies are necessary to influence the long-term outcomes associated with maternal near miss.

References

1. Pattinson R, Say L, Souza JP, van den Broek N, Rooney C. WHO maternal death and near-miss classifications. *Bull World Health Organ* 2009;**87**:733–804.

2. Say L, Souza JP, Pattison RC. WHO working group on maternal mortality and morbidity classifications. Maternal near miss: towards a standard tool for monitoring quality of maternal health care. *Best Pract Res Clin Obstet Gynaecol* 2009;**23**:287–296.

3. Lewis G (ed.) *Saving Mothers' Lives: Reviewing Maternal Deaths to Make Motherhood Safer, 2003–2005. The Seventh Report on Confidential Enquiries into Maternal Deaths in the United Kingdom.* London: CEMACH, 2007.

4. MacKay AP, Berg CJ, Liu X, Duran C, Hoyert DL. Changes in pregnancy mortality ascertainment: United States, 1999–2005. *Obstet Gynecol* 2011;**118**:104–110.

5. Maternal Health Study Group of the Canadian Perinatal Surveillance System. *Special report on maternal mortality and severe morbidity in Canada. Enhanced Surveillance: The Path to Prevention.* Ottawa: Health Canada; 2004.

6. Geller SE, Rosenberg D, Cox SM, *et al.* The continuum of maternal morbidity and mortality: factors associated with severity. *Am J Obstet Gynecol* 2004;**191**:939–944.

7. World Health Organization. *The International Statistical Classification of Diseases and Related Health Problems*, 9th revision. Geneva:World Health Organization, 2002.

8. Callaghan WM, MacKay AP, Berg CJ. Identification of severe maternal morbidity during delivery hospitalizations, United States, 1991–2003. *Am J Obstet Gynecol* 2008;**199**:e1–133e8.

9. Wen SW, Huang L, Liston RM, for the Maternal Health Study Group Canadian Perinatal Surveillance System. Severe maternal morbidity in Canada, 1991–2001. *CMAJ* 2005;**173**:759–763.

10. Goffman D, Madden RC, Harrison EA, Merkatz IR, Chazotte C. Predictors of maternal mortality and near miss maternal morbidity. *J Perinatol* 2007;**27**:597–601.

11. Brown HL, Small M, Taylor YJ, Chireau M, Howard D. Near miss maternal mortality in a multiethnic population. *Ann Epidemiol* 2011;**21**:73–7.

12. Lalonde AB, Butt C, Bucio A. Maternal health in Canadian Aboriginal communities: challenges and opportunities. *J Obstet Gynaecol Can* 2009;**31**:956–962.

13. Luo Z-C, Senécal S, Simonet F, *et al.* Birth outcomes in the Inuit-inhabited areas of Canada. *CMAJ* 2010;**182**:235–242.

14. Geller SE Adams MG, Kominiarek MA, Hibbard JU, Endres LK, Cox SM, Kilpatrick SJ. Reliability of a preventability model in maternal death and morbidity. *Am J Obstet Gynecol* 2007;**196**:57.e1–57.e4.

15. Pattinson RC, Hall M. Near misses: a useful adjunct to maternal death inquiries. *Br Med J* 2003;**67**:231–243.

16. Baskett TF. Epidemiology of obstetrical critical care. *Best Prac Clin Obstet Gynaecol* 2008;**22**:763–774.

17. Pollock W, Rose L, Dennis C-L. Pregnant and postpartum admissions to the intensive care unit: a systematic review. *Intensive Care Med* 2010;**36**:1465–1474.

18. Baskett TF, O'Connell CM. Maternal critical care in obstetrics. *J Obstet Gynecol Can* 2009;**31**:218–221.

19. Vincent JL, Moreno R, Takala J, Willatts S, De Mendonça A, Bruining H, *et al.* The SOFA (Sepsis-related Organ Failure Assessment) score to describe organ dysfunction/failure. On behalf of the Working Group on Sepsis-Related Problems of the European Society of Intensive Care Medicine. *Intensive Care Med* 1996;**22**:707–710.

20. Joseph KS, Young DC, Dodds L, *et al.* Changes in maternal characteristics and obstetric practice and recent increases in primary cesarean delivery. *Obstet Gynecol* 2003;**102**:791–800.

21. Kuklina E, Callaghan W. Chronic heart disease and severe obstetric morbidity among hospitalizations for pregnancy in the USA: 1995–2006. *BJOG* 2011;**118**:345–352.

22. Golombeck K, Ball RH, Lee H, *et al.* Maternal morbidity after maternal–fetal surgery. *Am J Obstet Gynecol* 2006;**194**:834–839.

23. Creanga AA, Kamimoto L, Newsome K, *et al.* Seasonal and 2009 pandemic influenza A (H1N1) virus infection during pregnancy: a population-based study of hospitalized cases. *Am J Obstet Gynecol* 2011;**204**; S38–S45.

24. Oluyomi-Obi T, Avery L, Schneider C, *et al.* Perinatal and maternal outcomes in critically ill obstetrics patients with pandemic H1N1 influenza A. *J Obstet Gynaecol Can* 2010; **32**:443–447, 448–452.

Service organization: hospital and departmental

Gerda G. Zeeman, Nadir Sharawi, and Geraldine O'Sullivan

Introduction

The evolution of critical care medicine started in the 1960s and guidelines for the design and staffing of critical care units were developed further during the following decades. The purpose of maternal high dependency or critical care is to provide specialized care to the sick parturient both antenatally and postpartum. The critically ill parturient is unique in that the needs of both the mother and fetus have to be considered.

Delivering high-quality care to this high-risk group can be challenging and involves a multidisciplinary approach. The needs of such patients can be quite complicated and may require input from obstetric, anesthetic, medical, and surgical teams. Although detailed guidelines for parturients in need of critical care are sparse, several national professional organizations have made recommendations pertaining to the role of critical care in the management of the obstetric patient [1].

Since the early 1990s, a multitude of reports, mainly retrospective with small sample sizes, has provided descriptive analyses of intensive care utilization by critically ill parturients. Such reports reflect significant variations in definitions of major morbidity, patient populations, unit design, admission criteria, usage rates, and outcomes [2–8]. Differences in access to healthcare, nursing policies, hospital settings, and management protocols add to the observed variations, which make comparisons of prognostic factors, standards of care, and recommendations for improvement difficult. Therefore, proposing maternal morbidity as an indicator for quality measures of maternal services is hampered.

Currently more research is needed to determine the optimal location in a hospital for the sick parturient. At present, such care is often provided in a dedicated critical care bay in or adjacent to the labor ward.

However the exact arrangement will depend upon the local hospital configuration and provisions within the regional area.

This chapter aims to provide an overview of hospital and departmental service delivery issues, which hospitals may use in formulating a service for the critically ill parturient. As levels of evidence vary, this overview is largely based on available consensus and expert opinion.

What is maternal critical care?

Critical care refers to patients who have life-threatening conditions and require continuous monitoring with the support of specialist staff, equipment, and medication. The term critical care encompasses the older terminology of "high dependency" and "intensive care." A very important goal of maternal critical care should be that of keeping mother and baby together unless precluded by the clinical situation.

Defining the level of critical care required by pregnant or puerperal women will generally depend on the type of support required as well as the number of organ systems involved. The levels of support are best based on clinical needs [9].

The UK Department of Health document *Comprehensive Critical Care* [10] has recommended a classification into four levels depending upon the level of care required:

level 0: patients whose needs can be met through normal ward care
level 1: patients at risk of their condition deteriorating and needing a higher level of observation or those recently relocated from higher levels of care
level 2: patients requiring invasive monitoring/ intervention that include support for a single

failing organ system (excluding advanced respiratory support)

level 3: patients requiring advanced respiratory support (mechanical ventilation) alone or basic respiratory support along with support of at least one additional organ.

The type of care provided to a patient should be independent of location. For example, level 2 care could be provided on the delivery suite (e.g. invasive blood pressure monitoring for massive hemorrhage or the management of severe pre-eclampsia).

The role of obstetric critical care

In general, critically ill parturients are cared for in the delivery unit or in an obstetric high dependency unit (HDU); alternatively they may be admitted or transferred to a medical or surgical intensive care unit (ICU). Use of HDU is a clinically appropriate and resource effective option when patients need more care than that provided on a general ward, such as frequent monitoring of vital signs and/or nursing interventions, but do not necessarily require ICU care. The need for critical care will largely be determined by the number of deliveries, the frequency and acuity of serious obstetric complications, and the institution's own critical care resources. Hospitals providing maternity services should have a clearly defined process for ensuring the early recognition of severely ill pregnant women and enabling prompt access to either HDU or ICU [11]. While tertiary care centers and hospitals providing maternity services of sufficient volume usually provide HDU care, smaller hospitals may not be able to fulfill the requirements for such a unit or they may not encounter enough critically ill women to maintain contemporaneous skills. In these situations, transfer to an institution with obstetric HDU services may be preferable to transfer to ICU.

The current evidence states that approximately 0.5–1% of pregnant or recently pregnant women would require treatment in a critical care unit [12,13]. The commonest reasons for admission are postpartum hemorrhage or hypertensive disorders of pregnancy. Furthermore, at least 50% of women who are admitted for ICU care can expect to be discharged back to the maternity unit within 24 hours.

The high dependency unit

The concept of care in HDU was proposed for patients who did not require advanced respiratory support but who needed more sophisticated care than could be provided on a general ward. Although HDU care has not been formally assessed nor adequately defined for obstetric patients, many referral centers in the USA and throughout Europe have incorporated this concept using guidelines that have been extrapolated from those describing intermediate care issues in the non-pregnant population [14]. Obstetric units providing HDU care are generally located in hospitals with adult and neonatal intensive care units. The advantages of an HDU within an obstetric setting are numerous:

- allows access to multidisciplinary expertise from midwives, obstetricians, anesthesiologists, obstetric medicine physicians, and so on
- has the ability to keep mother and infant together, thereby allowing early bonding
- allows appropriate monitoring of mother and fetus through access to specialized equipment (such as continuous fetal monitoring)
- provides a setting of familiarity with obstetric medicine and pathology, which often allows reduced use of invasive monitoring, without a negative impact on patient outcome
- should also reduce the need for maternal transfer to the general ICU [15].

The introduction of obstetric critical care facilities has been shown to be cost-effective, particularly as the most common reasons for obstetric admissions to ICUs are complications of pre-eclampsia and postpartum hemorrhage [16]. Obstetric HDUs should be able to manage the majority of these conditions and, therefore, potentially reduce admissions and length of stay to ICUs without increasing hospital length of stay.

Admission and discharge criteria

Identification of the high-risk parturient, whenever feasible, is key to the prevention of obstetric morbidity and mortality because it allows time to plan multidisciplinary management strategies. Generally, the HDU may be appropriate for pregnant or puerperal women who are conscious and who have single-organ dysfunction. Some examples of conditions that could qualify for HDU care and adopted in many tertiary referral centers throughout Europe and the USA are shown in Table 2.1. However clinical judgment remains paramount in any decision to admit a woman to HDU or ICU. Because of the often unexpected nature of obstetric complications, the operating

Table 2.1. Criteria for admission to an obstetric high dependency unit

System	Criteria
Cardiac	Low probability of, or excluded, myocardial infarction Hemodynamically stable myocardial infarction or arrhythmias Hemodynamically stable patient without myocardial infarction requiring temporary/permanent pacemaker Mild/moderate congestive heart failure without shock Severe hypertension without end-organ damage such as severe pre-eclampsia and/or HELLP syndrome Eclampsia
Pulmonary	Hemodynamically stable patients with evidence of compromised gas exchange with the potential for respiratory insufficiency/failure who require frequent observation (e.g. asthma or pneumonia) Patients who require frequent monitoring of vital signs (e.g. suspected/confirmed pulmonary embolism) or aggressive pulmonary physiotherapy
Neurological	Stable central nervous system, neuromuscular, or neurosurgical conditions that require close monitoring for signs of neurological deterioration or frequent nursing intervention
Drug overdose	A patient requiring frequent neurologic, pulmonary, or cardiac monitoring but who is hemodynamically stable
Gastrointestinal	Stable bleeding responsive to fluid therapy Liver failure with stable vital signs, such as acute fatty liver of pregnancy
Endocrine	Stabilization of a woman with diabetic ketoacidosis Thyrotoxicosis that requires frequent monitoring
Surgical	The postoperative patient who, following major surgery, severe hemorrhage or peripartum hysterectomy, is hemodynamically stable but may require close monitoring and/or fluid resuscitation Complicated cholecystitis, pancreatitis, or appendicitis
Miscellaneous	Appropriately treated and resolving early sepsis Patients whose condition requires closely titrated intravenous fluid management Any patient requiring frequent nursing observation such as in sickle cell crisis Hemofiltration/plasmapheresis

HELLP, hemolysis, elevated liver enzymes, and low platelets.

theater and HDU in the obstetric unit must always be prepared for emergencies such as massive hemorrhage, eclampsia, and maternal collapse.

Discharge of patients from the HDU to the general maternity ward is appropriate as soon as the woman has stabilized and the need for comprehensive monitoring is no longer compulsory. Alternatively, transfer to the ICU is appropriate for those women who need active life support or when this becomes highly likely.

Location, design, and utilities for maternity units

In general, maternity units consist of primary inpatient areas such as the birthing rooms, operating theaters and the HDU, with secondary areas consisting of the reception area, visitor's room, storage areas, and so on (Figures 2.1 and 2.2). Ideally, the HDU should be located in or in close proximity to the labor and delivery ward. Basic equipment required in a HDU setting is shown in Box 2.1 [17].

Personnel

The HDU physician director and nurse/midwife director can give clinical, administrative and educational direction through guidelines and education of the HDU nursing, medical, and other ancillary staff. There should be regular ward rounds, ideally multidisciplinary, and appropriate senior staff should always be available to provide ongoing daytime and out of hours supervision. Depending on local practice and staff availability, maternal–fetal medicine physicians, obstetric anesthesiologists, and/or critical care physicians are all well suited to provide specialized care for these patients and leadership in the HDU.

The ideal nurse to patient ratio is 1:1 or 1:2, depending on acute care needs. Ideally, obstetric nurses should rotate through the unit and they must have completed formal training in the care of the critically ill pregnant woman. Anesthetic personnel should be immediately available and intensivists should be on site. Medical and surgical specialties should also be available in the hospital and should be capable of providing 24 hour support when needed.

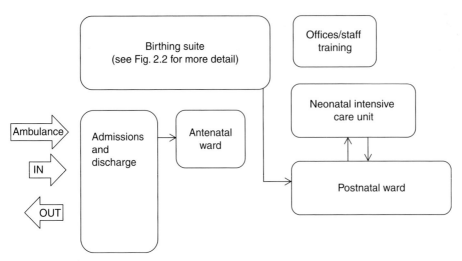

Figure 2.1. Plan of maternity services.

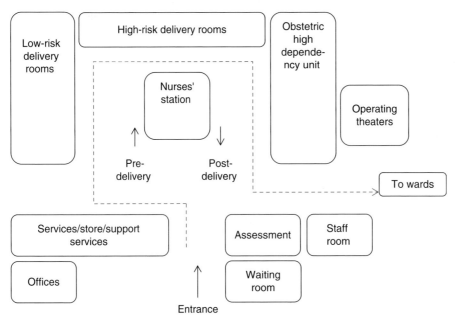

Figure 2.2. Relationships of the birthing suite.

Further discussion on personnel can be found in Chapter 3.

The intensive care unit

There is considerable variation in ICUs with respect to organizational characteristics, the services provided, and the level of expertise. Large medical centers frequently have multiple ICUs defined by (sub) specialty. Small hospitals may have only one ICU designed to care for a large variety of critically ill patients.

The major components of obstetric intensive care involve the monitoring and care of antepartum or postpartum women with severe physiological instability requiring technical and/or artificial life support [18]. Most obstetricians and specialized obstetric nurses do not see sufficient cases to acquire and maintain skills related to invasive monitoring and ICU support systems. The medical management of such

---

Box 2.1. Monitoring and equipment in the high dependency unit

Monitor for basic vital signs including electrocardiography and oxygen saturation; invasive pressure monitors (arterial, central) may be appropriate in some HDUs
Piped oxygen and suction
Intravenous fluid and forced air-warming device
Blood gas analyser
Infusion pumps
Massive hemorrhage trolley
Eclampsia box with standard medications
Transfer equipment, monitor and ventilator
Computer terminal to facilitate access to blood results, hospital system, guidelines
Resuscitation trolley with drugs, defibrillator, and airway management equipment

---

Box 2.2. Criteria for ICU admission and discharge

Patients requiring intense nursing care and titrated patient care for 12 to 24 hours a day
Patients with acute respiratory failure who are intubated or at imminent risk of requiring ventilatory support or who need airway maintenance
Patients requiring advanced invasive hemodynamic monitoring and/or cardiovascular organ support with vasoactive therapy such as inotropes, vasopressors, etc.
Patients requiring an intracranial pressure monitor
Patients with abnormal electrocardiography findings requiring intervention, including cardioversion or defibrillation
Patients in coma
Patients with multiorgan failure

---

women presents quite a challenge and often requires the input of several specialties such as the anesthesiologist/intensivist. The unique ethical and medical dilemmas and patient care decisions must be considered collaboratively between the intensivist, obstetrician, and neonatologist, and should involve the patient and her family.

Criteria for admission and discharge from intensive care units

Rather than using specific conditions or diseases to determine appropriateness of ICU admission, which can be found in various (inter)national guidelines, applying specific needs criteria may work best when considering the obstetric patient. Examples are women who require mechanical ventilation, usually as a result of massive hemorrhage and in anticipation of major fluid shifts or sepsis with pulmonary involvement. In addition, cardiovascular support using inotropic drugs or the need to support two or more organ

systems as well as those with chronic system insufficiency should be managed in an ICU setting (Box 2.2).

Alternatively, the objective parameters triage model applies specific criteria to trigger ICU admission, regardless of diagnosis [1]. Such criteria, although largely arbitrary, include parameters pertaining to vital signs, laboratory values, imaging, and physical findings. Research indicating improved outcome using such specific criteria levels are not available and when using such criteria it is paramount to realize that key laboratory and physical findings may be different in pregnancy (see Chapter 10).

When the need for ICU monitoring and care is no longer necessary, the patient can be discharged to the HDU or the maternity ward depending on the level of care required.

Labor and delivery in the intensive care unit

The optimal setting for the care of a critically ill woman in labor will depend on the viability of the fetus and, more importantly, on factors related to the safe support of the mother, such as availability of critical care interventions and staff expertise. The fetus is always secondary to optimal management of the maternal condition.

Delivery in the ICU comes with significant disadvantages, including limited availability of space for anesthetic, surgical, and neonatal resuscitation equipment. Frequently, assisted second stage of labor may be required, because of either an inability to push or contraindications such as underlying cardiac conditions. Adequate analgesia is often required as pain may result in hemodynamic derangements. Regional analgesia may be contraindicated secondary to patient positioning, coagulopathy, or hemodynamic instability.

The ICU staff are likely to be unfamiliar with obstetric procedures for labor and delivery. Nosocomial infections are also a hazard for mother and baby. Consequently, labor and delivery should not normally be conducted in an ICU setting. Cesarean delivery in the ICU should be restricted to absolute emergencies as transport to the operating theater or delivery room can usually be achieved safely or quickly.

Transfer of the critically ill obstetric patient

Smaller hospitals providing maternity care may not fulfill requirements for a HDU and may need to transfer a woman to another institution when she is in need of such care. Referring hospitals should have the ability to provide adequate stabilization and have resources and guidelines for the transfer of such patients to a center providing a higher level of care.

Standard guidelines for perinatal transfer that describe the responsibilities of the referring and receiving hospitals are available in many countries [19]. Antenatal rather than neonatal transfer is generally preferable. In the event that imminent delivery is expected or maternal transport is unsafe or impossible, alternative arrangements for neonatal transport should be available.

The appropriate arrangements, equipment, and documentation for inter- and intrahospital transfers for the obstetric patient are well described [1,9,19]:

- the patient should be meticulously resuscitated and stabilized prior to transfer
- the patient should be attended in transport by trained personnel

- venous access should be secured
- there should be regular assessment of vital signs, to include continuous pulse oximetry and electrocardiography
- if already *in situ*, arterial and central lines or other invasive monitoring devices should be monitored
- in the event of mechanical ventilation, the position of the endotracheal tube must be confirmed and secured before transport
- the adequacy of oxygenation and ventilation must also be assessed before transport
- aortocaval compression should be prevented by left uterine displacement
- supplemental oxygen should be available
- fetal monitoring, where technically feasible, may allow for advance preparation for intervention, including delivery by the receiving hospital.

Clinical governance and record keeping

The importance of clinical governance within modern obstetric care cannot be overemphasized. Clinical governance is the umbrella term that incorporates clinical audit, research, risk management, education, training, and information management. It is these mechanisms that allow the best outcomes in patient care within the available resources. The principal aim is that critically ill parturients should receive the same high-quality care whether they are cared for on the delivery suite, in maternal HDU, or a general ICU by staff with the appropriate competencies [20]. There are numerous auditable standards for maternal critical care and they encompass standards such as safety, effectiveness, and experience [21].

The results of local and national audits should reveal the main causes of major maternal morbidity and mortality. Units should have management guidelines and training schemes available for staff. For example, guidelines should be available for the management of massive hemorrhage, severe pre-eclampsia/eclampsia, and emergency hysterectomy. Application of audit recommendations need not be financially or resource expensive. There is much that can be achieved by appropriate use of resources and equipment.

Good record-keeping is an essential part of good obstetric practice. The use of computers has allowed the analysis of large quantities of data and the integration of the anesthetic, analgesia, and appropriate analysis of the maternal and fetal conditions. Accurate

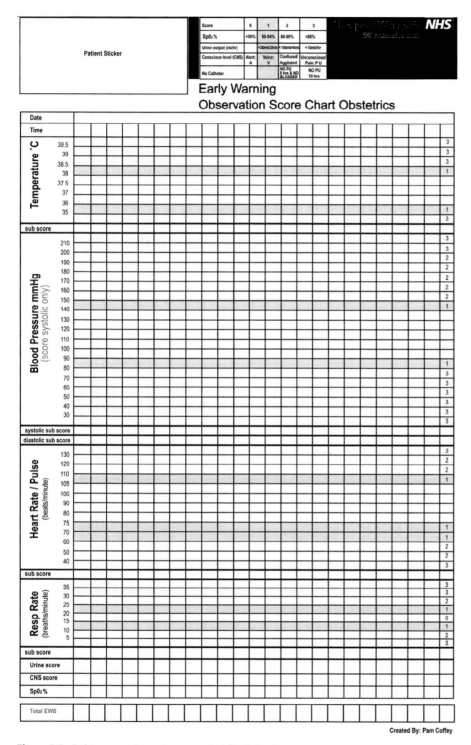

Figure 2.3. Early warning observation score chart for obstetrics.

records are essential in maintaining patient care to the highest standard and are a valuable source of information for medical coding and clinical audit. As management of the critically ill obstetric patient involves a multidisciplinary team, it is important that there is good communication between different members of the team and that records of every patient visit are documented. The nursing chart should clearly display all the maternal and fetal physiological parameters including [17]:

- conscious state/orientation
- temperature
- respiratory rate, oxygen saturation, inspired oxygen concentration
- blood pressure, central venous pressure, pulse rate, ongoing blood loss
- urine output
- daily blood results
- drains, wound, uterus, lochia
- motor/sensory function (if regional block present)
- fetal monitoring (if applicable).

Figure 2.3 shows an example of an obstetric observation chart [18].

Simulation and training

Simulation can encompass a large range of activities ranging from basic skills and drills to more sophisticated multidisciplinary training in purpose-built simulation centers. Currently there is considerable evidence to suggest that the use of simulation is lacking. However, obstetric emergencies, although rare, are frequently life threatening and staff working in maternal critical care must be seen to maintain their skills in managing life-threatening obstetric emergencies. Good simulation training can help to achieve this goal.

References

1. American College of Obstetricians and Gynecologists. Practice bulletin 100: critical care in pregnancy. *Obstet Gynecol* 2009;**113**:443–450.

2. Pollock W, Rose L, Dennis CL. Pregnant and postpartum admissions to the intensive care unit: a systematic review. *Intensive Care Med* 2010;**36**:1465–1474.

3. Leung NYW, Lau ACW, Chan KKC, *et al.* Clinical characteristics and outcomes of obstetric patients admitted to the intensive care unit: a 10-year retrospective review. *Hong Kong Med J* 2010;**16**:18–25.

4. Zeeman GG. Obstetric critical care: a blueprint for improved outcomes. *Crit Care Med* 2006;**34**:S208–S214.

5. Lataifeh I, Amarin Z, Zayed F, *et al.* Indications and outcome for obstetric patient's admission to intensive care unit: A 7-year review. *J Obstet Gynaecol* 2010;**30**:378–382.

6. Lewinsohn G, Herman A, Leonov Y, *et al.* Critically ill obstetrical patients: outcome and predictability. *Crit Care Med* 1994;**22**:1412–1414.

7. Martin SR, MR Foley. Intensive care in obstetrics: an evidence-based review. *Am J Obstet Gynecol* 2006;**195**:673–689.

8. Saravanakumar K, Davies L, Lewis M. High dependency care in an obstetric setting in the UK. *Anaesthesia* 2008;**63**:1081–1086.

9. Intensive Care Society. *Levels of Critical Care for Adult Patients. Standards and Guidelines.* London: Intensive Care Society. 2009 (www.ics.ac.uk/intensive_care_professional/standards_and_guidelines/levels_of_critical_care_for_adult_patients, accessed 29 January 2013).

10. Department of Health. *Comprehensive Critical Care.* London: The Stationery Office, 2000.

11. NHS Litigation Authority. *Clinical Negligence Scheme for Trusts. Maternity Clinical Risk Management Standards.* London: NHS Litigation Authority, 2009.

12. Zeeman GG, Wendel GD Jr., Cunningham FG. A blueprint for obstetric critical care. *Am J ObstetGynecol* 2003;**188**:532–536.

13. Mabie WC, Sibai BM. Treatment in an obstetric intensive care unit. *Am J Obstet Gynecol* 1990;**162**:1–4.

14. Society of Critical Care Medicine. Guidelines for intensive care unit admission, discharge and triage. Task Force of the American College of Critical Care Medicine. *Crit Care Med* 1999;**27**:633–638.

15. Wheatley E, Farkas A, Watson D. Obstetric admissions to an intensive therapy unit. *Int J Obstet Anaesth* 1996;**5**:221–224.

16. Intensive Care National Audit & Research Centre. *Female Admissions (aged 16–50 years) to Adult, General Critical Care Units in England, Wales and Northern Ireland, Reported as "Currently Pregnant" or "Recently Pregnant."* London: Intensive Care National Audit & Research Centre, 2009.

17. Vaughan D, Robinson N, Lucas N, Arulkumaran S (eds.) *Handbook of Obstetric High Dependency Care.* Oxford: Blackwell, 2010.

18. Maternal Critical Care Working Group. *Providing Equity of Critical and Maternity Care for the Critically Ill Pregnant or Recently Pregnant Woman.* London: Royal College of Obstetricians and Gynaecologists, 2011 (www.rcog.org.uk/womens-health/clinical-

guidance/providing-equity-critical-and-maternity-care-critically-ill-pregnant, accessed 29 January 2013).

19. American Academy of Pediatrics. *Guidelines for Air and Ground Transport of Neonatal and Pediatric Patients*, 3rd edn. Elk Grove Village, IL: American Academy of Pediatrics, 2006.

20. National Institute for Health and Clinical Excellence. *Acutely Ill Patients in Hospital (CG 50)*. London: NICE, 2007 (http://guidance.nice.org.uk/CG50, accessed 29 January 2013).

21. Baskett TF. Epidemiology of obstetric critical care. *Best Pract Res Clin Obstet Gynaecol* 2008;**22**:763–774.

Chapter 3

Competency and personnel

Helen Scholefield and Lauren A. Plante

Introduction

Childbirth is a major life event for women and their families. The few women who become critically ill during this time should receive the same standard of care for both their pregnancy-related and their critical care needs, delivered by professionals with the same level of competences, irrespective of whether these are provided in a maternity or general critical care setting [1]. This chapter will summarize standards and recommendations relevant to the care of the pregnant or recently pregnant critically ill woman for maternity and critical care.

What is maternal critical care?

The terms maternal critical care, high dependency care, and high-risk maternity care are not interchangeable, the term critical care having a more precise definition. In the UK, the Department of Health document *Comprehensive Critical Care* recommends that the terms "high dependency" and "intensive care" be replaced by the term "critical care" [2]. The document also proposes that the care required by an individual be independent of location, coining the phrase "critical care without walls." In this schema, care is subdivided into four levels, dependent on organ support and the level of monitoring required independent of diagnosis.

In the UK, the level of critical care required by the mother will be dependent on the number of organs requiring support and the type of support required, as determined by the Intensive Care Society's *Level of Care* document [3]. This term was first defined in *Comprehensive Critical Care* and subsequently updated in 2009 (Table 3.1). There are four levels of support (0–3).

> *Level 0*: patients whose needs can be met through normal ward care.

> *Level 1*: patients at risk of their condition deteriorating and needing a higher level of observation, or those recently relocated from higher levels of care.

> *Level 2*: patients requiring invasive monitoring/intervention that includes support for a single failing organ system (excluding advanced respiratory support).

> *Level 3*: patients requiring advanced respiratory support (mechanical ventilation) alone or basic respiratory support along with support of at least one additional organ.

The USA distinguishes among several types of intensive care and uses the intermediate or stepdown designation for units caring for patients who need more nursing care or more monitoring without specifically needing life-support interventions. These would be "low-risk monitor admissions" if admitted to a full-service intensive care unit (ICU) or would be admitted to an intermediate care unit. The Society of Critical Care Medicine has guidelines for admission to ICU, by prioritization (too sick or too well to profit from ICU), by diagnosis (aortic dissection, hyperosmolar coma, etc.), or, more applicable to obstetric populations, by objective parameters (vital signs, laboratory, imaging, etc.) [4]. The American College of Obstetricians and Gynecologists recommends the use of an objective parameters model to determine which obstetric patients to admit to ICU. High-acuity maternity services can manage many of these issues (hemorrhage, hypertensive crisis, etc.) on their ICU. A few American institutions have the obstetric equivalent of a stepdown unit.

In the UK, the nature of organ support is captured using the Critical Care Minimum Dataset [6]. Any area which satisfies the UK Department of Health definition for critical care setting will qualify for

Maternal Critical Care: A Multidisciplinary Approach, ed. Marc Van de Velde, Helen Scholefield, and Lauren A. Plante.
Published by Cambridge University Press. © Cambridge University Press 2013.

Table 3.1. Examples of maternity critical care required at the differing levels of support outlined by the Intensive Care Society

Level	Issues	Care required
0: normal ward care	None	Normal care of low-risk mother
1: additional monitoring or intervention, or stepdown from higher level of care	Hemorrhage	Risk of hemorrhage Oxytocin infusion
	Hypertension	Mild pre-eclampsia, taking oral antihypertensives, with fluid restriction, etc.
	Specific medical condition	For example, congenital heart disease or diabetic and on insulin infusion
2: single organ support	Basic respiratory support	50% or more oxygen via face mask to maintain oxygen saturation Continuous positive airway pressure, bi-level positive airway pressure
	Basic cardiovascular support	Intravenous antihypertensives to control blood pressure in pre-eclampsia Arterial line used for pressure monitoring or sampling Central venous line used for fluid management and pressure monitoring to guide therapy
	Advanced cardiovascular support	Simultaneous use of at least two intravenous, antiarrythmic/antihypertensive/vasoactive drugs, one of which must be a vasoactive drug Need to measure and treat cardiac output
	Neurological support	Magnesium infusion to control seizures (not prophylaxis) Intracranial pressure monitoring
	Hepatic support	Management of acute fulminant hepatic failure (e.g. from HELLP syndrome) or acute fatty liver, such that transplantation is being considered
3: advanced respiratory support alone or support of two or more organ systems above	Advanced respiratory support	Invasive mechanical ventilation
	Support of two or more organ systems	Renal support and basic respiratory support Basic respiratory support/basic cardiovascular support *and* an additional organ supported[a]

[a]Basic respiratory support/basic cardiovascular support occurring simultaneously during the episode count as a single organ support.
Source: adapted from Wheatly, 2010 [5].

submission of data. The advantage of using this dataset to reflect organ support in maternity units is obvious. A standardized platform will provide accurate data and facilitate comparative audit, utilizing the Intensive Care National Audit and Research Centre Case Mix Programme. This approach has been beneficial as it has facilitated some aspects of critical illness management, particularly some aspects of level 2 care, to be delivered in alternative clinical locations with the proviso that the non-critical care location possesses competent staff with appropriate clinical expertise to manage the clinical situation, either with or independently of critical care consultant medical/nursing/midwifery staff. An example of such care would be women requiring invasive cardiovascular monitoring and intervention for pre-eclampsia or massive hemorrhage on the delivery suite. Thus, maternal critical care can be distinguished from "high-risk" obstetrics [1,5] because:

- fetal issues are excluded
- maternal risk factors or obstetric complications that require closer observations or intervention, but not support of an organ system, are also outside the term.

The case study described through this chapter illustrates the use of these levels of need and the Early Warning Score (EWS) in the care of a pregnant woman.

Jane Smith is in her third pregnancy. Her body mass index (BMI) is 38. She has essential hypertension that is not well controlled because of her poor compliance with her antihypertensive medication. A growth scan at 28 weeks shows her baby to be on the 5th centile for gestational age with umbilical artery Doppler measurements at the upper end of normal. The liquor volume is reduced. The placenta is covering the internal cervical os. Ongoing fetal surveillance is instituted.

A week later, she presents to the maternity unit triage and assessment area with 300 mL of fresh vaginal bleeding. Her blood pressure is 144/95 mmHg, pulse 92, and hemoglobin 10 g/dL. She has no proteinuria. An intravenous line is sited. She is admitted to the maternity ward in view of a significant bleed associated with placenta previa and hypertension. She is started on iron. The bleeding settles and she appears stable over the next day.

Competencies required
She has a high-risk pregnancy on both fetal and maternal grounds. Her EWS is 1

Staff competent to cannulate, take, chart, monitor, and act appropriately on fetal and maternal observations

Midwifery/obstetric nursing skills.

The recognition of the acutely ill parturient

Successive maternal mortality enquiries in the UK [7] have highlighted delayed recognition of the acutely ill woman as a significant contributor to death and have recommended that early warning scores should be used to identify deterioration. In view of this, services should implement the UK National Institute for Clinical Excellence (NICE) guideline on the care of the critically ill in hospital [8]. Admissions to maternity services should have physiological observations recorded at the time of their admission or an initial assessment together with a clear written monitoring plan that specifies which physiological observations should be recorded and how often. The plan should take into account:

- whether the woman has a high- or low-risk pregnancy
- the reason for the admission
- the presence of comorbidities
- an agreed treatment plan.

Physiological observations should be recorded and acted upon by staff who have been trained to undertake these procedures and who understand their clinical relevance.

Physiological track and trigger systems should be used to monitor all antenatal and postnatal admissions. There are a number of charts in use nationally that take into account physiological changes that occur in parameters measured, such as blood pressure and respiratory rate. An example is given in Figure 3.1. There is not currently, however, a validated chart for use in pregnancy. A longer-term goal is the production of a validated system and observation chart for use nationally in maternity services that is compatible with the proposed National Early Warning Score (NEWS); this, in its current iteration, unfortunately excludes pregnancy [9]. Following labor and delivery, physiological observations should be monitored at least every 12 hours, unless a decision has been made at a senior level to increase or decrease this frequency for an individual patient or group of patients. The frequency of monitoring should increase if abnormal physiology is detected, as outlined in the recommendation on graded response strategy.

Staff caring for patients in acute hospital settings should have competences in monitoring, measurement, interpretation, and prompt response to the acutely ill patient appropriate to the level of care they are providing. Education and training should be provided to ensure staff have these competencies, and they should be assessed to ensure they can demonstrate them [10–12].

On the third day of her admission, Jane spends much of the time socializing with her family off the ward. On return, her blood pressure is 152/95 mmHg and pulse 107. Her EWS is 3. She has not had her antihypertensive medication. She is given this, and observations are repeated in an hour. Her blood pressure is 146/92 mmHg and pulse 110. There is a small amount of vaginal bleeding and she has abdominal pain. She collapses suddenly. Her blood pressure is unrecordable and pulse 115 and thready.

Competencies required
Assessment of the critically ill patient [10]
Advanced airway management and resuscitation [11]
Obstetric skills to assess cause collapse [12].

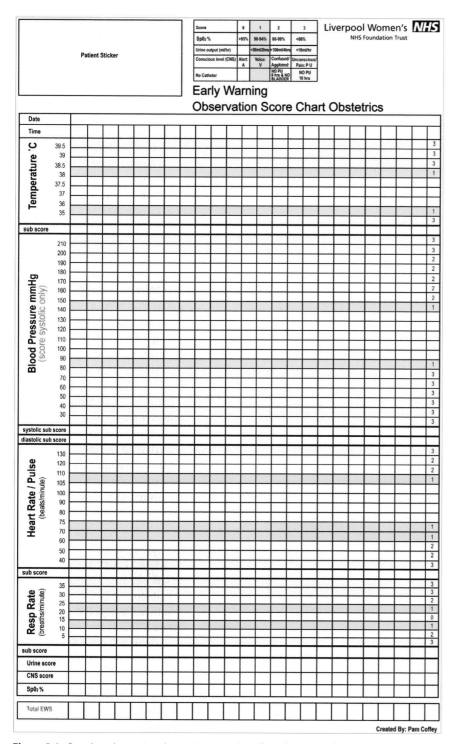

Figure 3.1. Sample early warning observation score chart (from the Liverpool Women's NHS Foundation Trust).

A graded response strategy for patients identified as being at risk of clinical deterioration should be agreed and delivered locally. It should consist of three levels [10] based on EWS score.

Level 1, low-score group (EWS, 3)

- low risk of deterioration
- increase frequency of observations and the midwife/nurse in charge alerted
- institute appropriate intervention
- rescore.

Level 2, medium-score group (EWS, 4 or 5)

- medium risk of deterioration
- urgent call to team with primary medical responsibility for the patient
- simultaneous call to personnel with core competences for acute illness
- these competences can be delivered by a variety of providers at local level, such as a critical care outreach team, a hospital-at-night team, or a specialist trainee in anesthesia, obstetrics, acute medical, or surgical specialty

- institute appropriate treatment
- hourly observations
- rescore.

Level 3, high-score group (EWS ≥6)

- high risk of deterioration
- emergency call to team with critical care competences and maternity team
- team should include a medical practitioner skilled in the assessment of the critically ill patient and who possesses advanced airway management and resuscitation skills
- an immediate response is required
- appropriate treatment instituted
- frequent observations
- rescore.

Figure 3.1 shows an example of an early warning observation chart and Figure 3.2 an associated escalation algorithm.

Obstetric early warning systems are not currently well developed in the USA. In general services, many places have a rapid response team that can be

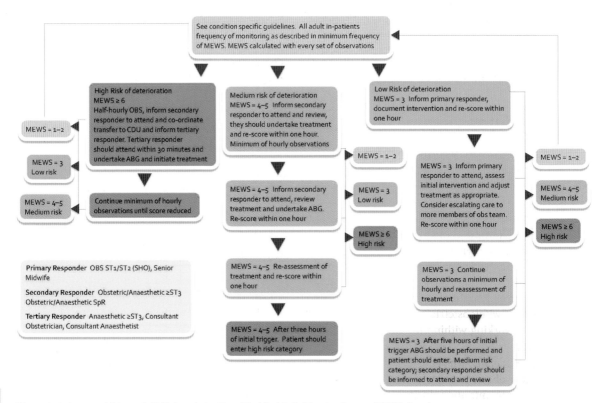

Figure 3.2. Liverpool Woman's NHS Foundation Trust Modified Early Warning System (MEWS) flowchart.

summoned for various physiological derangements in patients not in an ICU, with the idea that a rapid response and intervention can prevent a cardiac or respiratory arrest [13]. This has taken off in hospital medicine as a sort of critical care outreach, but it remains inadequately developed for obstetric patients. A few institutions are experimenting with an obstetric rapid response team [14], although it is early in the evolutionary phase.

Competences for recognition and care of the critically ill parturient: practical concerns

In the UK the acute care competences needed for staff are defined within the Department of Health document *Competencies for Recognising and Responding to Acutely Ill Patients in Hospital* [10]. The competences are targeted at staff who are involved in the care of acutely ill patients in hospital but they may be adapted for use in other settings, such as maternity, or across sectors. They define the knowledge, skills, and attitudes required for safe and effective treatment and care along the chain of response. It is likely that one staff group or banding will cover more than one role in the chain; for example, the recognizer may also fulfill the role as primary responder or on occasions may fulfill the recorder role. Units should define who fulfills the following roles in their own service:

non-clinical supporter, who may also be the "alerter" and may include the woman or visitor

recorder, who takes designated measurements, records observations and information; in maternity services this could be a maternity support worker, healthcare assistant, or midwife/nurse

recognizer, who monitors the patient's condition, interprets designated measurements, observations, and information, and adjusts the frequency of observations and level of monitoring; in the maternity setting, this could be a midwife/obstetric nurse, recovery or other nurse working within the unit or a junior doctor

primary responder, who goes beyond recording and further observation by interpreting the measurements and initiating a clinical management plan (e.g. commencing oxygen

therapy, insertion of airway adjuncts, selection and administration of a bolus of intravenous fluids); this would be a junior doctor

secondary responder, who is likely to be called to attend when the patient fails to respond to the primary intervention or continues to "trigger" or "re-trigger" a response; this individual (a more experienced obstetrician or anesthesiologist) will assess the clinical effect of the primary intervention, formulate a diagnosis, refine the management plan, initiate a secondary response, and will have the knowledge to recognize when referral to critical care is indicated

tertiary responder, this role encompasses the acute care competencies such as advanced airway management, resuscitation, clinical assessment, and interpretation of acutely ill obstetric patients; this would be a senior anesthesiologist or intensive care physician in most cases, but might be a senior obstetrician or maternal–fetal medicine physician with specialized training.

The acute care competencies required focus primarily on the clinical and technical aspects of care and the delivery of effective patient management. They assume the possession and application at every level of complementary generic competencies such as record-keeping, team working, interpersonal skills, and clinical decision making. Of particular note in this context is the ability to rapidly access hospital information systems and retrieve patient information, such as blood results and radiographs.

For units providing level 2 (intermediate/step-down) care, obstetricians and midwifery staff should have additional training in the care of the critically ill women to achieve the relevant competencies.

Case 3.1. A 39-year-old woman in her third pregnancy: Part 3

Her airway is intact and she is breathing. Oxygen is administered. Fluid resuscitation is begun. Blood is sent for urgent cross-matching, full blood count, and clotting screen. The amount of external bleeding is not consistent with the clinical condition. A systolic blood pressure is achieved, but Jane remains very unwell with tachycardia and tachypnea and a EWS of 7. She is transferred to the maternity high dependency unit with ongoing resuscitation.

After colloid, her blood pressure is 110/80 mmHg, pulse 120, respiratory rate 26 breaths/min, and her EWS 4.

The fundal height is much larger than dates and getting bigger.

Ultrasound scan finds no fetal heart pulsations. There is a large retroplacental clot.

Her clotting studies are extremely deranged, with no measurable fibrinogen, platelets 16×10^9/L and hemoglobin 7 g/dL.

Competencies required
Assessment of the critically ill patient [10]
Advanced airway management and resuscitation [11]
Hematology
Obstetric skills [12]
Midwifery/obstetric nursing
Team working/shared decision making.

Implementing competences in care

Maternity services should define which of their staff take on each one of the above acute care responder roles and ensure that they have suitable training and assessment of the competencies they require. The medical clinical competencies required to provide a critical care service irrespective of location in the UK are described in the Curriculum for Intensive Care Medicine. The provision of a level 2 service within a maternity unit requires consultant anesthetic staff to have the minimum of step 1 competencies in intensive care medicine [11]. Nursing competencies for critical care should be in place in any maternity unit undertaking level 2 (intermediate/stepdown) critical care. The point at which there is a need to bring professionals with the required competences into the maternity unit, or transfer the woman to a setting where they are available, should also be defined using this framework while the continuation of obstetric and midwifery care is ensured. Arrangements made locally should reflect the recognition that the holistic needs of the woman, including maintaining contact with her baby, are paramount. The quality of critical care she receives should not be compromised by providing for holistic needs where required competencies are not available within the maternity unit or through critical care outreach. Equally, the quality of her maternity care should not be compromised if circumstances require transfer to a general critical care setting [1]. It is essential to ensure a seamless pathway to provide for both her critical care and her maternity needs. Clinical areas of responsibility for both of these should be identified in local policies. Implementing the competences will require a system-wide approach with effective leadership and rigorous change management from board through to ward [1]. This may include the following:

- identifying a designated clinical and managerial lead and implementation team, who will also secure training provision
- monitoring outcomes at all levels with board reporting and intervention
- critical incident analysis and peer supervision with regular multidisciplinary meetings to review severe maternal morbidity cases
- the incorporation of recommendations for education/training and assessment of competence into induction and ongoing provision, as well as into formal performance review and development processes
- making sure that resources, such as equipment, are in place
- adapting local policies to support people meeting the competences and clarifying levels of authority and responsibility
- developing team working, assertiveness, and interprofessional working relationships; it is essential that staff have confidence in the competence of colleagues and are willing to challenge and to be challenged.

Case 3.1. A 39-year-old woman in her third pregnancy: Part 4

The working diagnosis is placental abruption causing severe coagulopathy associated with her hypertension and abnormally sited placenta. Jane's blood pressure improves with fluid and blood transfusion. She has platelets, fresh frozen plasma, and cryoprecipitate. Her coagulopathy is improving on bedside testing with thromboelastography. The uterus continues to enlarge and is now term sized and very tense.

The team decides to do a cesarean section while she is more stable, anticipating that, with continuing expansion of the retroplacental hemorrhage and likely uterine atony, she will decompensate again without delivery. A difficult procedure with high risk of bleeding is predicted. The consultant obstetrician and anesthesiologist are directly involved, with input from the consultant hematologist. Blood and blood products are available in the delivery suite. A consultant gynecological oncologist is on standby in case hysterectomy is required to control bleeding.

Dialogue with the intensivists takes place. She has an emergency cesarean section under general anesthesia with cell salvage. The uterus is Couvelaire and filled with about 3 L of clot. A stillborn infant weighing 800 g is delivered. The placenta has completely separated.

There is ongoing bleeding that does not respond to uterotonics. A brace suture is inserted, which controls the bleeding.

She has invasive arterial blood pressure monitoring. A central venous line is considered but not placed as she is much more stable and concerns about coagulopathy continue. Her total blood loss is about 5 L.

She is transferred from obstetric theater recovery to the ICU for ventilation [15].

Competencies required
Assessment of the critically ill patient [10]
Advanced airway management and resuscitation [11]
Hematology
Obstetric and obstetric anesthetic skills [12]
Theater skills: anesthetic assistant, scrub and supporting
Team working/shared decision making
Transfer [15]
Handover [8,16].

Workforce development

Lead professionals in maternity services have a responsibility to ensure staff are deemed competent in the early recognition of acutely ill and deteriorating patients and are able to perform the initial resuscitation and management. A suggested curriculum is included at the end of this chapter (Appendix 3.1). Training is essential to develop the competencies. This can be through internal training or external courses, such as Acute Illness Management (AIM) or Acute Life-threatening Events: Recognition and Treatment (ALERT) in the UK or, in the USA, the Advanced Cardiac Life Support (ACLS), the Advanced Trauma Life Support for Physicians, the Advanced Life Support in Obstetrics (ALSO), or Fundamentals of Critical Care Support (FCCM).

Whichever training program is selected, assessment of competences is essential. Scenario-based or simulation-based training has been found to be valuable, particularly when developing team drills for life-threatening clinical situations. In addition to these resources, a number of services have been developed; local teaching initiatives, acute care sessions at clinical

simulation centers, and some e-learning packages are also being developed. There are a number of national certified courses available to support workforce development.

Case 3.1. A 39-year-old woman in her third pregnancy: Part 5

Jane is ventilated in ICU. By the following afternoon, she is stable enough to be extubated. She returns to the maternal high dependency unit and is cared for by a midwife with both maternity and critical care competencies, together with the obstetric anesthesiologists and obstetricians. She has time with her baby and bereavement support. Mementos are prepared for her. She has suppression of lactation. Her family come in to see their brother.

She is well enough to go home on day 5. Initial debriefing is done before discharge and arrangements made for follow-up to discuss events and plan for future pregnancies.

Competencies required
Assessment of the critically ill patient [10]
Advanced airway management and resuscitation [11]
Obstetric and obstetric anesthetic skills [12]
Midwifery/obstetric nursing postnatal care [16]
Nutrition
Emotional and bereavement support
Other allied professionals as required
Team working/shared decision making.

Conclusions

The care of a critically ill pregnant or recently delivered woman poses challenges to health professionals because of the uniqueness of childbirth as a life event and alterations in physiology and pathology. The use of competencies for all of the woman's care needs, including both maternity and recognition and management of acute illness, is a means of ensuring her healthcare and holistic needs are met.

References

1. Maternal Critical Care Working Group. *Providing Equity of Critical and Maternity Care for the Critically Ill Pregnant or Recently Pregnant Woman*. London: Royal College of Obstetricians and Gynaecologists, 2011 (www.rcog.org.uk/womens-health/clinical-guidance/providing-equity-critical-and-maternity-care-critically-ill-pregnant, accessed 29 January 2013).

23

2. Department of Health. *Comprehensive Critical Care: A Review of Adult Critical Care Services*. London: The Stationery Office, 2000 (www.dh.gov.uk/en/ Publicationsandstatistics/Publications/ PublicationsPolicyAndGuidance/DH_4006585, accessed 29 January 2013).

3. Intensive Care Society. *Levels of Critical Care for Adult Patients. Standards and Guidelines*. London: Intensive Care Society, 2009 (www.ics.ac.uk/intensive_care_ professional/standards_and_guidelines/levels_of_ critical_care_for_adult_patients, accessed 7 January 2013).

4. Task Force of the American College of Critical Care Medicine, Society of Critical Care Medicine. Guidelines for intensive care unit admission, discharge and triage. *Crit Care Med* 1999;**27**:633–638.

5. Wheatly S. Maternal critical care: what's in a name? *J Obstet Anesth* 2010;**19**:353–355.

6. Information Standards Board for Health and Social Care. *Critical Care Minimum Dataset*. Leeds: Information Standards Board for Health and Social Care, 2010 (www.isb.nhs.uk/documents/isb-0153, accessed 29 January 2013).

7. Cantwell R, Clutton-Brock T, Cooper G, *et al.* Saving Mothers' Lives: Reviewing Maternal Deaths to make Motherhood Safer 2006–2008. The Eighth Report of the Confidential Enquiries into Maternal Deaths in the United Kingdom. *BJOG* 2011; **118**(Suppl 1):1–203.

8. National Institute for Health and Clinical Excellence. *Acutely Ill Patients in Hospital (CG 50)*. London: NICE, 2007 (http://guidance.nice.org.uk/CG50, accessed 29 January 2013).

9. Royal College of Physicians. *NHS Early Warning Score (NEWS)*. London: Royal College of Physicians, 2011 (http://www.rcplondon.ac.uk/resources/national- early-warning-score-news, accessed 29 January 2013).

10. Department of Health. *Competencies for Recognising and Responding to Acutely Ill Patients in Hospital*. London: The Stationery Office, 2008 (www.dh.gov.uk/ en/Publicationsandstatistics/Publications/ PublicationsPolicyAndGuidance/DH_096989, accessed 29 January 2013).

11. Faculty of Intensive Care Medicine. *The CCT in Intensive Care Medicine Part IV Core and Common Competencies*. London: Faculty of Intensive Care Medicine, 2011.

12. Royal College of Obstetricians and Gynaecologists. *Maternal Collapse in Pregnancy and the Puerperium*. London: Royal College of Obstetricians and Gynaecologists, 2011.

13. Jones DA, DeVita MA, Bellomo R. Rapid-response teams. *N Engl J Med* 2011;**365**:139–146.

14. Gosman GG, Baldisseri MR, Stein KL, *et al.* Introduction of an obstetric-specific medical emergency team for obstetric crises: implementation and support. *Am J Obstet Gynecol* 2008;**198** :367. e1–367.e7.

15. Intensive Care Society. *Guidelines for the Transport of the Critically Ill Adult*. London: Intensive Care Society, 2002.

16. Royal College of Obstetricians and Gynaecologists. *Improving Patient Handover (Good Practice No. 12)*. London: Royal College of Obstetricians and Gynaecologists, 2010 (www.rcog.org.uk/womens- health/clinical-guidance/improving-patient-handover- good-practice-no-12, accessed 29 January 2013).

APPENDIX 3.1. SUGGESTED CORE CURRICULUM, MATERNAL CRITICAL CARE

General

Normal physiology of pregnancy

Respiratory system

- Anatomy and physiology of airway and respiratory function
- Respiratory failure
- Optimizing airway and respiratory function
- Arterial blood gas and oxygen therapy
- High-flow oxygen therapy and continuous positive airway pressure
- Chest radiography interpretation

Cardiovascular system

- Anatomy and physiology of heart and conductive system
- 12-lead electrocardiography interpretation
- Cardiac disease in pregnancy

Other systems

- Hypertensive disease in pregnancy
- Hepatorenal disease in pregnancy
- Diabetes in pregnancy
- Obesity in pregnancy
- Neurological disease or altered conscious level in pregnancy
- Coagulation and blood products within the high dependency setting

General critical care topics

- Transfer of critically ill woman
- Shock and sepsis
- Midwifery Early Warning Score in obstetrics and the outreach team
- Infections in pregnancy: human immunodeficiency virus and swine flu
- Infection control

Others

- Sudden collapse in pregnancy
- Complications of anesthesia and pain relief in labor and pregnancy
- Fluid balance in critical care (including massive hemorrhage)
- Advanced resuscitation in pregnancy including the 5 minute CS rule
- Audit and documentation
- Competency-based training
- Psychological care after critical illness

Chapter 4

Planning for elective and emergency problems

Clemens M. Ortner, Ruth Landau, Clare Fitzpatrick, and Leanne Bricker

Introduction

Caring for the obstetric patient is particularly challenging as physiological changes during pregnancy may significantly affect the risk status of pregnant women and fetal well-being. In addition, the otherwise healthy woman may develop life-threatening peripartum complications; consequently, providers of obstetric services must at all times be prepared to deliver safe and effective care in the most timely manner to both planned and unexpected emergencies. Anesthesia and critical care providers have become invaluable partners involved more and more in obstetric care, and even more so in the context of the high-risk parturient. Despite significant efforts in maternity care in Europe and the USA, maternal mortality has become static over the last few decades [1,2]. Progress in medical and obstetric management has resulted in a steady reduction in the number of direct pregnancy-related deaths. However, indirect causes of maternal deaths, such as those from cardiac or psychiatric diseases, are rising and mirror the constantly increasing proportion of high-risk pregnancies, indicating that women with significant comorbidities are no longer discouraged from considering a pregnancy [2,3]. As a result, measures to prevent and diagnose early comorbidities and complications during pregnancy and at the time of delivery have become indispensable in this century and are constantly emerging.

The goal of the current chapter is to present an overview on the current recommendations and guidelines that may be implemented to improve the management of planned and unplanned urgent high-risk obstetric patients and prevent fatal outcomes for both mothers and their babies. The proposed measures include pre-pregnancy counseling, improvements in patient communication and multidisciplinary specialist care, development of high-risk pre-anesthesia clinics, novel strategies to improve medical training and preparedness for potentially rare cases, such as the use of simulation training and emergency drills, and the introduction of modified early warning scoring (MEOWS) systems and rapid response teams (RRTs).

Maternal morbidity and mortality

Despite a low prevalence for each specific comorbidity in the context of pregnancy in the developed world, overall morbidity remains high, with up to 50% of women suffering at least one complication during the course of pregnancy and the peripartum period [4]. According to the most recent report of the UK Confidential Enquiries into Maternal Deaths (CEMACH), published in 2011, maternal deaths occurred in more than 11 per 100 000 maternities in the UK during the 2006–2008 triennium (Figure 4.1) and pre-existing cardiac diseases are the leading cause nowadays for maternal death (Figure 4.2) [2]. In the USA, the absolute risk of pregnancy-related death was 15 per 100 000 births for 2005 (Figure 4.3) [5].

Since the early 1900s, many lives of mothers and babies have been saved through regularly renewed health authority recommendations and newly implemented guidelines that focus on improving policies, procedures, and medical practice. However, epidemiological reports analyzing each cause of death uniformly indicate that more than 50% of maternal deaths could have been prevented by better medical patient care, and human- and/or system-related factors [2,6,7]. Maternal death is the result of a continuum of adverse events, starting from normal/healthy pregnancy and moving through morbidity to severe morbidity, to near miss and to death [8,9]. In a high proportion of cases, the progression along this continuum was deemed preventable by an expert commission, through improvements in (1) patient and

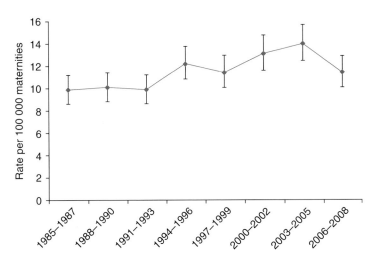

Figure 4.1. Maternal mortality rates per 100 000 maternities in the UK, 1985–2008 [2].

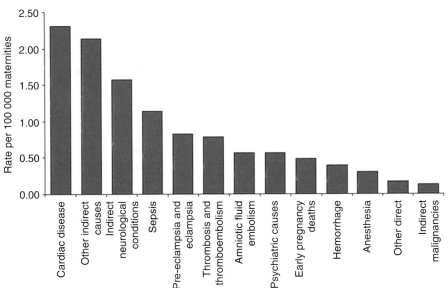

Figure 4.2. Leading causes of maternal deaths per 100 000 maternities in the UK, 2006–2008 [2].

medical staff communication, (2) identification of the high-risk status of the parturient, (3) specific staff training, and (4) healthcare processes [8].

Pre-pregnancy counseling

Pre-existing diseases or medical conditions can severely affect the outcome of pregnancy and often require specialized care and modified medical and obstetric management. Reviewing morbidity and mortality data over the 10 years from 2000 reveals an increase in the proportion of indirect causes of maternal deaths and demonstrates that many of the case-fatalities were

women who did not receive pre-pregnancy counseling or any specific medical management [2]. With a large proportion of pregnancies being unplanned, particularly in the sociodemographic groups that are more prone to suffer pre-existing diseases and insufficient antenatal care, women of childbearing age should be informed whenever possible about the impact of pregnancy on their pre-existing disease and should be enrolled in an antenatal program to have a management plan for any pregnancy-related problem by experienced high-risk obstetric providers.

The report by CEMACH recommends that women with the following pre-existing diagnoses are offered

27

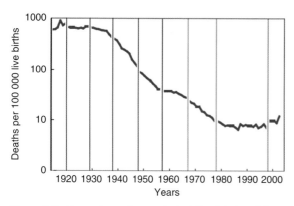

Figure 4.3. Maternal mortality rates in the USA 1915–2003 [4]. Note that prior to 1933, only birth registration data are available. Breaks in the lines show transition between successive revisions of the *International Classification of Diseases*.

counseling prior to considering and starting a pregnancy [2]:

- congenital or acquired cardiac disease
- asthma
- diabetes
- epilepsy
- autoimmune disorders
- renal disease
- liver disease
- obesity with body mass index >30
- human immunodeficiency virus (HIV) infection
- severe pre-existing or past mental illness.

Patient communication and multidisciplinary specialist care

Optimizing patient communication

According to the 2010 Report of the Joint Commission on Accreditation of Healthcare Organizations in the USA [10] and the 2011 CEMACH report in the UK [2], root causes for the majority of peripartum death and injury are related to problems in patient communication, team work, and organizational culture.

In order to provide optimal patient communication, the importance of professional interpreter services was emphasized in the 2011 CEMACH report [2] as a means to reduce maternal mortality. In many European countries, as well as in the USA, the proportion of childbearing women with immigrant background is increasing. The use of family members for translation, which often involve children of school age or close members from the social community, is

particularly not suitable as women may be uncomfortable addressing sensitive topics that are related to pregnancy. Providers of maternity services should, therefore, ensure that professional and independent interpretation services are available in the primary and secondary care settings. Indeed, the basis for effective two-way communication between the patient and the healthcare provider relies on core values such as understanding and trust.

Multidisciplinary care plans

Interdisciplinary care planning and communication among professionals is essential. In many cases of substandard care, major failures of communication between obstetricians and specialists have contributed to some extent to maternal morbidity and mortality. With the increasing proportion of women with comorbidities becoming pregnant, a woman's pregnancy status, risk status, and additional comorbidities need to be clearly communicated to all caregivers and appropriate referral to a tertiary care center needs to occur. However, lack of appropriate and timely referrals to specialists remains a problem, and reasons for this are multiple. To overcome the problem of missed or inappropriate referrals, as well as potentially incomplete or lacking information from some providers, organizing a streamlined pathway by one care provider is one way to reduce mishaps [2]. Based on the medical system and national guidelines, high-risk obstetric patients may be managed during pregnancy by their primary care physicians (e.g. the primary care physician or general practitioner) or by their obstetrician as long as there is a multidisciplinary approach and ongoing concerted management with medical (or surgical) specialists, obstetric anesthesiologists, critical care medicine specialists and the neonatologists.

Multidisciplinary care of the pregnant woman at risk of significant obstetric complications

Two examples of multidisciplinary care planning are given: for women who have placenta previa with acreta and have had a previous cesarean section and for women with a serious comorbidity.

Placenta previa with acreta in women with previous cesarean section

With increasing cesarean section rates and rising maternal age, the occurrence of placenta previa and complications of morbid adherence (acreta, increta, or percreta) is likely to present more commonly with significant risk to both mother and baby. One of the top recommendations from the CEMACH 2003–2005 report was that all woman with previous cesarean section have a scan to determine placental localization and, if there is previa, a detailed assessment (by ultrasound and possibly magnetic resonance imaging (MRI) if necessary) to determine whether there is accreta, increta, or percreta [11]. The management of the placenta accreta, increta, and percreta is challenging and requires involvement of senior clinicians with appropriate resources to hand and a multidisciplinary approach. Even if there is not thought to be morbid adherence in women with previous cesarean and low-lying placenta or major placenta previa, clinicians should err on the side of caution and assume there may be clinical difficulties at delivery. In view of this, the National Patient Safety Agency in the UK developed a care bundle entitled *Placenta Previa after Cesarean Section* [12] to enable optimizing management and reducing harm in these difficult cases. The bundle advocates that all women undergoing cesarean section at high risk of placenta accreta should be managed in line with this care bundle; this includes women with one or more previous cesarean section and placenta previa, and women with a previous scar where imaging of placental localization has found the placenta to be lying over the previous scar, even if it is well clear of the internal cervical os. The six elements of the *Placenta Praevia after Caesarean Section Care Bundle* are outlined in Box 4.1 [12]. The elements include multidisciplinary assessment and planning and provides a good example of optimizing care by planning effectively ahead of potential difficulties and involving the appropriate clinicians and ensuring the availability of appropriate resources. It also demonstrates how all eventualities and treatment options must be considered and discussed with the woman herself. With all the elements in place, the team would be well prepared in the event of massive hemorrhage at the time of cesarean section. It is also important for all services dealing with these high-risk cases to have an agreed approach to massive hemorrhage, and if this were in a general hospital setting this would need some adaptation for obstetric purposes. Appendix 4.1 shows the UK Mersey Regional Massive Hemorrhage Algorithm adapted for obstetric cases.

Pregnant women with serious comorbidity

Women who are planning pregnancy or are pregnant but have significant comorbidities require appropriate

---

Box 4.1. The Placenta Previa After Cesarean Section Care Bundle

1. Consultant obstetrician planned and directly supervising delivery
2. Consultant obstetric anesthesiologist planned and directly supervising anesthesia at delivery
3. Blood and blood products are available on-site
4. Multidisciplinary involvement in preoperative planning
5. Discussion and consent includes possible interventions (such as hysterectomy, leaving placenta *in situ*, cell salvage, and interventional radiology)
6. Local availablility of level 2 critical care bed

Source: National Patient Safety Agency, 2010 [12].

---

assessment and planning with involvement of all disciplines responsible for her care. This is aimed at optimizing all aspects of her and her baby's health. The planning should include considerations relating to current medication and treatment, disease status (active, quiescent, well controlled, etc.), effect of pregnancy on disease, effect of disease on pregnancy, and considerations for labor and delivery, including potential anesthetic issues.

Medication and treatment. It is important when considering whether to continue or modify medication to balance risks of stopping with benefits of continuing. A common problem faced by obstetric staff looking after women with comorbidities is that they stop medication themselves or are inappropriately advised to do so and their disease/condition flares, which may result in adverse effects on her health or that of her unborn child. At times getting treatment back on track can prove problematic too.

Effect of pregnancy on disease. Pregnancy may have lasting effects on the underlying medical condition and this needs to be considered when planning care, particularly with regard to postnatal follow-up. Furthermore, medications need to be reviewed in light of women wishing to breastfeed, again considering benefits and risks.

Effect of disease on pregnancy. The effects of the condition on pregnancy need to be considered, including the additional concerns related to the physiological adaptations in pregnancy.

Considerations for labor and delivery. A specific care plan for labor and/or delivery should be developed such that specific instructions are given with regard to monitoring, limitations, and special circumstances. The plan should include contingency instructions for common complications such as preterm labor, hemorrhage.

Ideally joint multidisciplinary consultations are most effective in planning care before and during pregnancy. For example, in the UK Northwest Region, cardiologists, anesthesiologists, and maternal medicine specialists have developed a regional guideline for the reproductive management of women with acquired or congenital heart disease and there are two regional clinics where women are seen in a joint consultation with an obstetrician, cardiologist, and anesthesiologist to plan care for the preconception, antepartum, intrapartum, and postpartum period, thus ensuring a seamless transition through these epochs of time. Appendix 4.2 is an example of the care plan used for women with cardiac disease. In most cases, the requirement for a joint consultation/communication is such that the plan can be developed once and women can then continue with normal care, being referred back only if clinical circumstances change.

Development of an obstetric high-risk pre-anesthesia clinic

Maternal morbidity and mortality reports demonstrate repeatedly the continuously rising proportion of expectant mothers who are at increased risk for severe complications during pregnancy as a result of pre-existing conditions [1–4,6,13–15]. The same reports identify poor recognition of pre-existing conditions and life-threatening illness as major risk factor for maternal mortality. In response to these observations, hospitals that care for a high-risk obstetric population have recognized the need and introduced obstetric high-risk pre-anesthesia assessment clinics [15]. Anesthestists have become invaluable partners in managing emergency obstetric cases, as emphasized by the fact that anesthesia services are called for in up to 50% of cases resulting in a maternal death [2]. Even though only a small number of catastrophic events

resulting in maternal death are directly related to anesthesia, a review of these fatal cases revealed that some were caused by delay in the call to the anesthesia team and fewer to provision of substandard of anesthesia care.

The primary goal of the pre-anesthesia assessment process is to create a delivery plan that integrates concerns of different specialties involved in the care of the patient and her baby. As medical conditions often undergo significant changes throughout pregnancy, patient assessments may require repeated visits, and various algorithms adapted to the delivery plan and specific care modalities will need to be proposed. Initial plans may change as the condition of the fetus or the mother can suddenly deteriorate and flexibility in care planning needs to occur. In a joint statement developed by the American Society of Anesthesiology and the American College of Obstetricians and Gynecologists, the availability of anesthesia and surgery personnel to enable the start of a cesarean delivery within 30 minutes has been defined as a standard for good obstetric care [16]. Despite this arbitrary timing being recently revisited, it does emphasize the need for obstetricians, nursing staff, anesthesiologists – and possibly hematologists, cardiologists, nephrologists, interventional radiologists, surgeons, urologists, and neonatologists – to be aware of high-risk cases and their individual formulated plan and potentially be available if and when needed A survey performed in the UK in 2005 showed that 30% of maternity clinics run a dedicated obstetric high-risk pre-anesthesia clinic for that purpose [15]. Not surprisingly, the higher the delivery rate of the maternity clinic was, the more likely it was that a pre-anesthesia clinic would exist. No clinic with fewer than 1000 deliveries offered this service, and in units with more than 4000 deliveries, 40% of obstetric clinics offered at least fortnightly a high-risk pre-anesthesia consultation.

In maternity clinics that do not run a dedicated pre-anesthesia clinic, anesthesiologists rely on ad-hoc referrals by their obstetric colleagues. As a consequence, some high-risk women will not be evaluated by any anesthesiologist at all or the delivery plan might be formulated too late. Even when a pre-anesthesia clinic is available, the referral process is crucial as women that should be seen may end up not been referred for other specialty consultation. Using an unstructured referral system may unduly burden a high-risk clinic with low-risk patients with mild

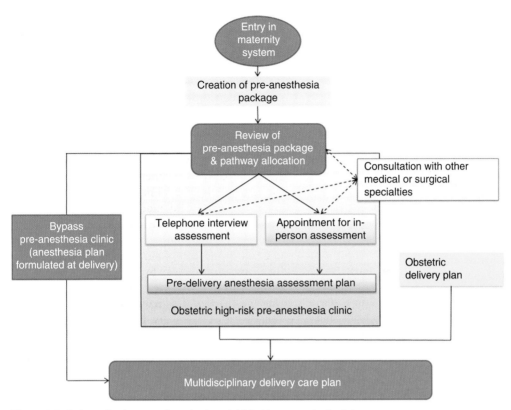

Figure 4.4. Patient referral process through obstetric high-risk pre-anesthesia clinic.

conditions unlikely to worsen during pregnancy or alter anesthetic management. Creating an "anesthesia review package" as a pre-screening system operated by the obstetric anesthesia team would ideally allow a referral plan for each pregnant woman admitted to the maternity clinic. This package would include (1) an entrance questionnaire filled by the parturient, (2) an obstetric summary with a formulated delivery plan (or plans), and (3), if available, medical records and notes from other specialty consultations. The package may be adapted to suit each institutions' requirements and case mix. Once reviewed, this initial pre-screening would allow the obstetric anesthesia team to define the appropriate pathway; for example the woman:

- may bypass the pre-anesthesia clinic
- will be contacted for a telephone interview to gather further details
- will have a scheduled anesthesia consultation for an in-person evaluation.

During or resulting from this process, the expectant mother may be referred for further specialized evaluations or consultations. The information gathered should then be reviewed, and the woman may be reassigned on the algorithm (Figure 4.4). At the end of this dynamic process, an anesthesia plan may be formulated and integrated into a final delivery plan based on the obstetric care plan and input from other providers involved with the clinical management. This plan should be made readily accessible to all providers in charge of the patient when admitted into the labor and delivery unit.

Anesthesia preoperative assessment

Medical conditions that require specific care during pregnancy and delivery include some of the diagnoses listed below; therefore, anesthesiologists planning for labor and delivery in the pre-anesthesia clinic should be aware that a detailed care plan will be necessary. More specific management may be found in dedicated chapters throughout this book.

- *Assessment and recognition of the difficult airway:*
  - airway complication is the leading cause of anesthesia-related death [13]

- failed intubation incidence is 1:300 (10× higher than normal population) [17]
- airway disasters are predictable in 90% of the cases [18]
- Mallampati score plus thyromental distance predicts difficult intubation with specificity 98% and sensitivity 80% [19]
- obesity is associated with a substantial increase in morbidity and mortality, in part through increased operative deliveries (either planned or unscheduled cesarean deliveries)
- all direct anesthesia-related deaths are associated with obesity [2]
- pre-anesthesia assessment is indicated for all who are morbidly obese to evaluate upper airway/intubation difficulties; bronchoaspiration has been shown to occur also at the time of extubation and during unattended transport to recovery room [20]
- neuraxial analgesia placed in laboring obese women will be useful to reduce the need for a general anesthetic in the event of an urgent unplanned cesarean delivery
- thromboembolic prophylaxis is indicated (stockings and low-molecular weight heparin)
- obstructive sleep apnea requires appropriate after-delivery monitoring, particularly after a cesarean delivery (and with concomitant opioids for postdelivery analgesia).

- *Pregnancy in an HIV-positive woman*:

  - the majority of women in developed countries are taking highly active antiretroviral therapy and are seemingly healthy
  - consider CD4 cell count and viral load within 3 months of delivery; if the CD4 cell count is 200×10^6 cells/L and viral load is high, patients are susceptible for opportunistic infections and malignancies
  - assess general status, drug side effects, and coagulation, liver, and kidney status
  - consider electrocardiography and chest radiography
  - neuraxial analgesia and anesthesia and general anesthesia can be provided as usual [21,22].

- *Allergies and the pregnant patient*:

  - 10% of patients allergic to penicillin are allergic to cephalosporins
  - 15% of asthmatics are allergic to non-steroidal anti-inflammatory drugs
  - latex allergy is associated with allergies to kiwi fruit, chestnuts, avocado, and banana and is more common in healthcare workers and patients with spina bifida.

Novel approaches to improve medical training and preparedness for obstetric emergencies

Comprehensive reviews of pregnancy-related mortality have shown that lack of training and clinical skills as well as the delayed identification and appropriate management of the very sick parturient were important root causes for preventable maternal deaths during the last decade [2,4,23]. As a consequence, hospital quality improvement initiatives in the USA [10,22–26] and the UK [11,27] have emphasized the importance of emergency drill training, MEOWS systems, and RRTs as training and medical management tools to further improve patient safety.

Simulation and emergency drills

Obstetrics is a medical specialty in which stable clinical conditions carry the potential to quickly deteriorate into a critical event. At any given time, quick decisions and actions are made and carried out in order to manage effectively and safely emergencies within the challenging realm of a multiprofessional environment. In smaller maternity clinics, such situations may occur so rarely that an appropriate and standardized medical response may create an extremely stressful challenge to the team. Simulation offers an opportunity of unlimited exposure to uncommon, complicated, and critical clinical events in a safe environment for patients and trainees, along with useful debriefing and continuous opportunities for improvements of individual performances as well as team achievements. During recent years, simulator options have tremendously increased and have been systemically embedded in medical training programs; nowadays, they form an integral part of numerous professional certification and credentialing programs [28].

Contextually, simulation-based training methods can be implemented at three levels: task, clinical, and environmental. Task-level simulation typically focuses on practicing skills that are required to complete a procedure. Examples of task-level skill simulation training include intubation and airway management, laparoscopic camera navigation, placing a central venous catheter or simply placing an intravenous line; for obstetricians, managing a shoulder dystocia is typically an example of a task that can be trained in a simulator. Task-level exercises can lead the learner through a sequence of more complicated skills until she/he reaches a certain point where proceeding to the procedure itself is the natural progression. Clinical-level simulation addresses the practice of defined clinical situations such as postpartum hemorrhage, eclampsia [29], or anesthesia induction for emergency cesarean section [30]. The goals of simulating clinical events are to develop improved clinical reasoning, decision making, diagnostic judgment, and resource management. However, as most preventable errors that occur in healthcare are associated with team behaviors and communication, effective training warrants simulation on a contextual or environmental level. In other words, clinical scenarios and emergencies have to be simulated in the clinical environment itself, including different medical professions interacting with each other as they would during the real event. Simulation on an environmental level should allow team members to learn and practice together and to develop interdisciplinary team competencies and optimize crisis resource management (Box 4.2). Based on multidisciplinary simulation on an environmental level, role responsibilities can be newly redefined and practiced. Concepts of communication, such as direct or closed-loop communication, can be exemplified and trained. Last, but not least, processes that lie beyond an obvious mistake, such as target fixation, can

be revealed; decision-making processes can be analyzed, and scenarios can be retrained until participants feel comfortable in handling the situation.

Reviewing literature from recent years indicates that simulation, team training, and emergency drills improve clinical outcome, knowledge, practical skills, communication, and team performance [29,31–36].

In a retrospective cohort study performed in the UK, after the introduction of a simulation-based training on the management of obstetric emergencies (shoulder dystocia, postpartum hemorrhage, eclampsia, twin/breech extraction, adult and neonatal resuscitation), the number of children with 5 minute Apgar scores <6, as well as the incidence of hypoxic–ischemic encephalopathy, was significantly reduced, with sustained improvements over time [31]. The observed improved outcomes were attributed to improved decision-making processes as a direct result of training. Task and clinical scenario trainings using mannequins have demonstrated improvements in clinical skills for management of shoulder dystocia, breech extraction, and treatment of postpartum hemorrhage or eclamptic seizure [29,32,33]. As an additional result, commonly occurring management errors such as delayed transfer of the bleeding patient to the operating room, lack of familiarity with prostaglandin administration to reverse uterine atony, or poor cardiopulmonary resuscitation techniques, were identified and this information was then incorporated when new checklists were created [29].

Simulation-based training focusing on interpersonal skills demonstrated better team performances from midwives and physicians after practicing emergencies (adult/neonatal resuscitation, eclampsia, shoulder dystocia, postpartum hemorrhage, electronic fetal monitoring, fetal cord prolapse, twin and breech extraction) compared with lecture-based teaching [34,35]. Another interesting approach during critical event simulation involves the use of patient-actors in lieu of mannequins; this more plausible approach to provide simulation seems to enhance perception of good communication and safety [36].

Therefore, even though a clear association between simulation-based programs and tangibly improved clinical outcomes in rare urgent events is complicated to establish, there is some evidence suggesting that simulation training promotes patient safety and better clinical outcome through improvements of clinical skills, knowledge, communication, and team performance.

Box 4.2 Crisis resource management

1. Role responsibility
   - role clarity
   - performance as a leader/helper
2. Communication strategies
   - direct communication
   - closed-loop communication
   - transparent thinking
   - orient self/other members
3. Situational awareness
   - resource allocation
   - target fixation
4. Decision making
   - prioritization

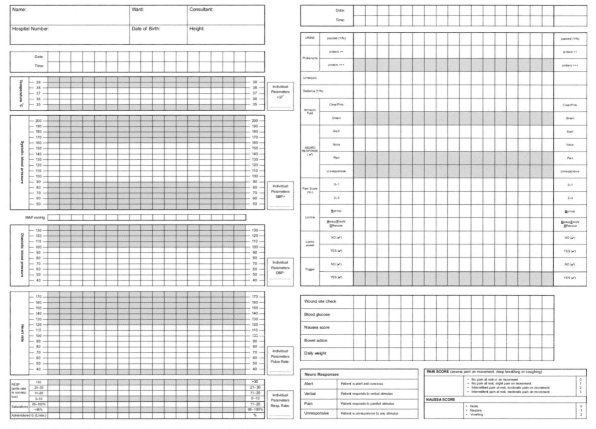

Figure 4.5. Modified early warning scoring system chart [40].

Early warning scoring systems

Analyzing clinical antecedents of in-hospital cardiac arrests and deaths reveals that 66–84% of patients experiencing a medical crisis show signs of clinical deterioration within the 6–8 hours preceding the critical event [37–39]. According to the 2007 and 2011 CEMACH Reports [2,11], the same could be demonstrated for the obstetric patient, where early warning signs of impending maternal collapse went unrecognized too often. In a significant number of maternal deaths, healthcare professionals either failed to identify that a woman was becoming seriously ill or failed to manage the critical situation outside their area of expertise. The relative rarity of such critical events, combined with the normal changes in physiology with pregnancy and childbirth, can make early detection of severe illness in the parturient especially challenging. Health service authorities in the UK have, therefore, urgently recommended the introduction of MEOWS systems to be applied for all pregnant or postpartum woman entering the acute hospital setting [11]. This measure includes the regular recording of clinical parameters on defined charts that allow early recognition of critical changes and prompt fast referral to an appropriate practitioner (Figure 4.5) [40]. A full set of observations includes the physiological parameters:

- respiratory rate
- pulse rate
- blood pressure
- temperature
- mental status.

It is assessed at regular intervals defined by the cause of admission, with a minimum interval of 12 hours. These physiological parameters include a minimum set. Additional clinical parameters, such as oxygen saturation, urine output and fluid balance, symphysis fundal height, abdominal girth, peripheral temperature, and laboratory investigations are included to the scoring chart defined by the clinical condition.

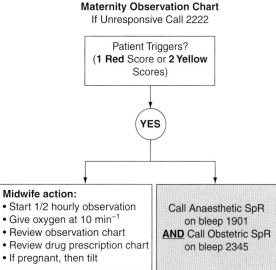

Action:
- Attend within 10 min or send deputy
- Confirm observations
- Take history & examination
- Decide on differential diagnosis

Options:
- Reset trigger levels
- Make intervention (fluid, oxygen, etc.)
- Decide on relocation (CLOMA, theater, ITU)
- Consider involvement of PART team on bleep 2525
- Make referral and consider appropriate escalation

Must:
- Decide when to review
- Write clear plan in notes

Maternity Observation Chart
If Unresponsive Call 2222

Patient Triggers?
(**1 Red** Score or **2 Yellow** Scores)

YES

Midwife action:
- Start 1/2 hourly observation
- Give oxygen at 10 min^{-1}
- Review observation chart
- Review drug prescription chart
- If pregnant, then tilt

Call Anaesthetic SpR on bleep 1901 **AND** Call Obstetric SpR on bleep 2345

Figure 4.6. Callout algorithm for triggers of early warning scoring system [40].

One or several measurements reaching a certain threshold trigger immediate following of steps in the defined algorithms (Figure 4.6) including:

- referral to the appropriate medical level
- increased monitoring
- review of the clinical condition and situation
- additional investigations
- adapted plan of care.

Triggering a response does not necessarily imply a new diagnosis but definitely indicates that a worsening clinical condition was recognized and acknowledged, warranting further monitoring and investigations on an appropriate level. A number of hospitals in the UK have implemented the use of the MEOWS chart in daily routine as a valuable clinical predictor for morbidity [40,41]. Ideally, each maternity clinic will audit all critical events and determine which observations or clinical events require which level of bedside personnel. The most critical conditions will require a defined medical emergency response team (RRT) bringing critical care expertise and equipment within shortest time to the bedside.

Rapid response teams

In 2005, the Institute for Healthcare Improvement's 100 000 Lives Campaign recommended the implementation of RRTs as one of six strategies to reduce preventable in-hospital deaths in the USA [24]. Since then, numerous hospitals in the USA have implemented these as part of their improvements strategies. Despite the challenge of defining the impact of such strategies on patient outcome, several studies have demonstrated a decrease in unplanned intensive care unit admissions and cardiac arrests in and outside of the units [42,43]. Based on these observations, the American College of Obstetricians and Gynecologists has included the recommendation for implementing RRTs in obstetrics in their latest consensus on planning for clinical emergencies [23].

The goal of such RRTs is to bring critical expertise and equipment to the patient without delay, in a timely manner, and to provide a solution to the problem in a standardized manner. Establishing a rapid response system involves a multistep approach [44] and includes the definition of:

- who is authorized to activate the RRT
- criteria for activation of the RRT
- identified roles and tasks within the RRT
- means of evaluation and process improvement.

In general, an RRT can be structured into four components (Figure 4.7):

- activator
- responder
- quality improvement
- administration.

The activators are those individuals who are eligible to call the RRT and may include non-medical personnel on the unit, the patient, or a family member. Most

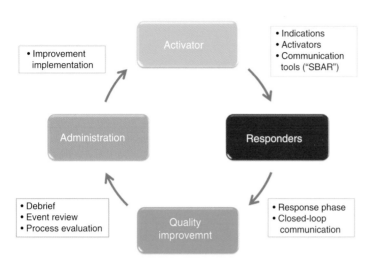

Figure 4.7. Structure of rapid response system: if the patient meets predefined clinical thresholds, the activator at the patient's bedside calls for the emergency response team. Responders rushing to the bedside attempt to treat the medical emergency. An integral part of the response system is the event review and process evaluation in order to plan process improvements in the future.

importantly is the creation of an atmosphere where activators feel free to start the process without fear of being blamed if they have wrongly estimated the gravity of a clinical condition.

Further, indicators that serve as triggers have to be determined; in obstetrics, this may be defined as any condition possibly causing harm to fetus or mother, such as acute vaginal bleeding, difficulty documenting fetal heart rate, severe abdominal pain, fetal distress, severe intrapartum bleeding, or eclampsia. Indicators and activators vary from one setting to the other, and their definition should be based on hospital chart review on past critical events or near misses. An example of successful RRT implementation comes from Shands Jacksonville Medical Center, in Jacksonville, Florida, USA [45], where criteria for staff to activate the RRT include the following:

- heart rate <40 or >120 beats/min, or significant change from baseline
- systolic blood pressure <90 mmHg or significant change from baseline
- respiratory rate <8 or >24 breaths/min
- oxygen saturation <92% or a fall of 4 points from baseline
- unexplained temperature fall <35.5°C or rise >38.8°C
- acute mental status change, decrease in consciousness and/or new agitation or delirium
- acute significant bleeding
- urinary output <50 mL in 4 hours
- seizures
- uncontrolled pain
- arrhythmias.

Experiences from Shands Jacksonville Medical Center emphasize the usefulness of the patient or the family member as an activator. Reasons for activation were more general and may vary, but the most frequent reason why the patient or family member activated the RRT was "something just does not feel right." In contrast to some people's concern, this did not lead to an overload of false positive calls. On the contrary, the introduction of a RRT system including the patient/family member as an activator seemed to have reduced non-intensive care codes, hospital mortality, and rescue failures at codes in the hospital [45].

Once the RRT is activated, responders arrive and act at the bedside. Different approaches can be taken in how to compose and define team size. In a so-called "ramp down" approach, a large team is called immediately at the bedside; following the first evaluation of the clinical condition, those team members not needed are dismissed. This approach has the disadvantage of consuming larger resources and taking hospital providers away from routine clinical duties. A less resource-consuming approach is the "ramp-up" approach: nurses, with an intermediate capability to assess the patient needs, start basic care to stabilize the patient and quickly triage the patient to the appropriate level of care, such as an intensive care unit [46]. However, a ramp-up approach bears the risk of slower response and delay in availability of needed workforce and equipment.

In order to reduce the risk of a huddle at the patient bed when responders arrive, activators must be prepared to exchange information, and the use of communication protocols, such as SBAR (situation, background, assessment, and recommendation) are recommended [47]. Such protocols should allow clear and concise information exchange between activator and responder. During the response phase, other communication tools may be implemented to enable organized management of the critical situation. For example, before getting into action, a "brief" should be used to assign essential roles, define expectations or goals, and to speak out. During the response phase, "check backs," "time outs," and "call outs" can keep the action organized and ensure closed-loop communication.

After the patient's condition is stabilized and the emergency is deemed under control, activators and responders review the events and evaluate the process. Optimally, the team is supported by a quality improvement team leading through this process with the aim to identify system factors that lead or had impact on the critical event. The loop is finally closed when the administration team provides organizational resources and accordingly implements changes in the care process.

Conclusions

The reduction of maternal mortality over the turn of the century has been impressive, with 99% fewer deaths since 2000 than in the early 1900s. However, epidemiological inquiries analyzing maternal deaths in the developed world still report that a significant number of mothers' lives could have been saved through improvements in health systems and processes in the mother's clinical pathway during and after pregnancy. Criteria for patients' transfer to tertiary care centers are critical in order to avoid high-risk deliveries in centers that cannot provide adequate care. Enhanced interdisciplinary strategies include high-risk clinics with targeted pre-anesthesia assessments by dedicated obstetric anesthesia experts leading to a streamlined plan of care, as well as drills and simulation to improve education and management of rare critical events. Recently developed tools such as MEOWS charts or RRTs in obstetrics are recommendations to further reduce maternal morbidity and mortality in the coming years.

References

1. Clark SL, Belfort MA, Dildy GA, et al. Maternal death in the 21st century: causes, prevention, and relationship to cesarean delivery. Am J Obstet Gynecol 2008;199:36. e31–36.e35; discussion 91–32.

2. Cantwell R, Clutton-Brock T, Cooper G, et al. Saving Mothers' Lives: Reviewing Maternal Deaths to make Motherhood Safer 2006–2008. The Eighth Report of the Confidential Enquiries into Maternal Deaths in the United Kingdom. BJOG 2011;118(Suppl 1):1–203.

3. Benhamou D, Chassard D, Mercier FJ, Bouvier-Colle MH. [The Seventh Report of the Confidential Enquiries into Maternal Deaths in the United Kingdom: comparison with French data.] Ann Fr Anesth Reanim 2009;28:38–43.

4. Berg CJ, Mackay AP, Qin C, Callaghan WM. Overview of maternal morbidity during hospitalization for labor and delivery in the United States: 1993–1997 and 2001–2005. Obstet Gynecol 2009;113:1075–1081.

5. Kung HC, Hoyert DL, Xu J, Murphy SL. Deaths: final data for 2005. Natl Vital Stat Rep 2008;56:1–120.

6. Hoyert DL, Danel I, Tully P. Maternal mortality, United States and Canada, 1982–1997. Birth 2000;27:4–11.

7. Nannini A, Weiss J, Goldstein R, Fogerty S. Pregnancy-associated mortality at the end of the twentieth century: Massachusetts, 1990–1999. J Am Med Womens Assoc 2002;57:140–143.

8. Geller SE, Rosenberg D, Cox SM, et al. The continuum of maternal morbidity and mortality: factors associated with severity. Am J Obstet Gynecol 2004;191:939–944.

9. Geller SE, Rosenberg D, Cox S, et al. A scoring system identified near-miss maternal morbidity during pregnancy. J Clin Epidemiol 2004;57:716–720.

10. Joint Commission on Accreditation of Healthcare Organizations. Root Cause of Sentinel Events, All Categories: 1995–2004. Oakbrook Terrace, IL: Joint Commission on Accreditation of Healthcare Organizations, 2010.

11. Lewis G (ed.) Saving Mothers' Lives: Reviewing Maternal Deaths to Make Motherhood Safer, 2003–2005. The Seventh Report on Confidential Enquiries into Maternal Deaths in the United Kingdom. London: Confidential Enquiries into Maternal Deaths, 2007.

12. National Patient Safety Agency. Placenta Praevia after Caesarean Section Care Bundle. NPSA Intrapartum Toolkit. London: National Patient Safety Agency, 2010 (http://www.nrls.npsa.nhs.uk/resources/? EntryId45=66359, accessed 7 January 2013).

13. Cooper GM, McClure JH. Maternal deaths from anaesthesia. An extract from Why Mothers Die 2000–2002, the Confidential Enquiries into Maternal Deaths in the United Kingdom: Chapter 9: Anaesthesia. Br J Anaesth 2005;94:417–423.

14. Lang CT, King JC. Maternal mortality in the United States. Best Pract Res Clin Obstet Gynaecol 2008;22:517–531.

15. Rai MR, Lua SH, Popat M, Russell R. Antenatal anaesthetic assessment of high-risk pregnancy: a survey of UK practice. Int J Obstet Anesth 2005;14:219–222.

16. American College of Obstetricians and Gynecologists. Committee Opinion 433: Optimal Goals for Anesthesia Care in Obstetrics. Washington, DC: American College of Obstetricians and Gynecologists, 2009.

17. Hawthorne L, Wilson R, Lyons G, Dresner M. Failed intubation revisited: 17-yr experience in a teaching maternity unit. *Br J Anaesth* 1996;**76**:680–684.

18. Sia RL, Edens ET. How to avoid problems when using the fibre-optic bronchoscope for difficult intubation. *Anaesthesia* 1981;**36**:74–75.

19. Frerk CM. Predicting difficult intubation. *Anaesthesia* 1991;**46**:1005–1008.

20. Mhyre JM. Anesthetic management for the morbidly obese pregnant woman. *Int Anesthesiol Clin* 2007;**45**:51–70.

21. Hughes SC, Dailey PA, Landers D, *et al.* Parturients infected with human immunodeficiency virus and regional anesthesia. Clinical and immunologic response. *Anesthesiology* 1995;**82**:32–37.

22. Gershon RY, Manning-Williams D. Anesthesia and the HIV infected parturient: a retrospective study. *Int J Obstet Anesth* 1997;**6**:76–81.

23. American College of Obstetricians and Gynecologists. Preparing for clinical emergencies in obstetrics and gynecology. *Obstet Gynecol* 2011;**117**:487.

24. Berwick DM, Calkins DR, McCannon CJ, Hackbarth AD. The 100 000 lives campaign: setting a goal and a deadline for improving health care quality. *JAMA* 2006;**295**:324–327.

25. Institute of Medicine. *Health Professions Education: A Bridge to Quality*. Washington, DC: National Academies Press, 2003: 19–63.

26. American College of Obstetricians and Gynecologists Committee on Quality Improvement and Patient Safety. Patient safety in obstetrics and gynecology. *Int J Gynaecol Obstet* 2004;**86**:121–123.

27. Lewis G (ed.). *Why Mothers Die 2000–2002. The Sixth Report of the Confidential Enquiries into Maternal. Deaths in the United Kingdom*. London: RCOG Press, 2004.

28. Andreatta PB, Bullough AS, Marzano D. Simulation and team training. *Clin Obstet Gynecol* 2010;**53**:532–544.

29. Maslovitz S, Barkai G, Lessing JB, Ziv A, Many A. Recurrent obstetric management mistakes identified by simulation. *Obstet Gynecol* 2007;**109**:1295–1300.

30. Scavone BM, Sproviero MT, McCarthy RJ, *et al.* Development of an objective scoring system for measurement of resident performance on the human patient simulator. *Anesthesiology* 2006;**105**:260–266.

31. Draycott T, Sibanda T, Owen L, *et al.* Does training in obstetric emergencies improve neonatal outcome? *BJOG* 2006;**113**:177–182.

32. Crofts JF, Bartlett C, Ellis D, *et al.* Training for shoulder dystocia: a trial of simulation using low-fidelity and high-fidelity mannequins. *Obstet Gynecol* 2006;**108**:1477–1485.

33. Ellis D, Crofts JF, Hunt LP, *et al.* Hospital, simulation center, and teamwork training for eclampsia management: a randomized controlled trial. *Obstet Gynecol* 2008;**111**:723–731.

34. Crofts JF, Ellis D, Draycott TJ, *et al.* Change in knowledge of midwives and obstetricians following obstetric emergency training: a randomised controlled trial of local hospital, simulation centre and teamwork training. *BJOG* 2007;**114**:1534–1541.

35. Birch L, Jones N, Doyle PM, *et al.* Obstetric skills drills: evaluation of teaching methods. *Nurse Educ Today* 2007;**27**:915–922.

36. Crofts JF, Bartlett C, Ellis D, *et al.* Patient-actor perception of care: a comparison of obstetric emergency training using manikins and patient-actors. *Qual Saf Health Care* 2008;**17**:20–24.

37. Franklin C, Mathew J. Developing strategies to prevent inhospital cardiac arrest: analyzing responses of physicians and nurses in the hours before the event. *Crit Care Med* 1994;**22**:244–247.

38. Hillman KM, Bristow PJ, Chey T, *et al.* Antecedents to hospital deaths. *Intern Med J* 2001;**31**:343–348.

39. Schein RM, Hazday N, Pena M, Ruben BH, Sprung CL. Clinical antecedents to in-hospital cardiopulmonary arrest. *Chest* 1990;**98**:1388–1392.

40. Singh S, McGlennan A, England A, Simons R. A validation study of the CEMACH recommended modified early obstetric warning system (MEOWS). *Anaesthesia* 2012;**67**:12–18.

41. Swanton RD, Al-Rawi S, Wee MY. A national survey of obstetric early warning systems in the United Kingdom. *Int J Obstet Anesth* 2009;**18**:253–257.

42. Chan PS, Jain R, Nallmothu BK, Berg RA, Sasson C. Rapid response teams: a systematic review and meta-analysis. *Arch Intern Med* 2010;**170**:18–26.

43. Dacey MJ, Mirza ER, Wilcox V, *et al.* The effect of a rapid response team on major clinical outcome measures in a community hospital. *Crit Care Med* 2007;**35**:2076–2082.

44. Gosman GG, Baldisseri MR, Stein KL, *et al.* Introduction of an obstetric-specific medical emergency team for obstetric crises: implementation and experience. *Am J Obstet Gynecol* 2008;**198**:367 e361–367.

45. Gerdik C, Vallish RO, Miles K, *et al.* Successful implementation of a family and patient activated rapid response team in an adult level 1 trauma center. *Resuscitation* 2010;**81**:1676–1681.

46. Devita MA, Bellomo R, Hillman K, *et al.* Findings of the first consensus conference on medical emergency teams. *Crit Care Med* 2006;**34**:2463–2478.

47. Haig KM, Sutton S, Whittington J. SBAR: a shared mental model for improving communication between clinicians. *J Qual Patient Safety* 2006;**32**:167–175.

APPENDIX 4.1. UK MERSEY REGIONAL MASSIVE HAEMORRHAGE ALGORITHM, ADAPTED FOR OBSTETRICS

Transfusion Management of Massive Haemorrhage in Obstetrics

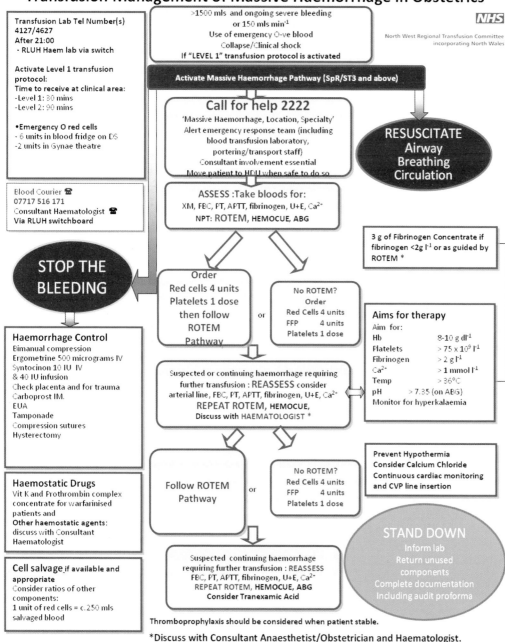

Transfusion Lab Tel Number(s)
4127/4627
After 21:00
- RLUH Haem lab via switch

Activate Level 1 transfusion protocol:
Time to receive at clinical area:
-Level 1: 30 mins
-Level 2: 90 mins

•Emergency O red cells
- 6 units in blood fridge on DS
-2 units in Gynae theatre

Blood Courier ☎
07717 516 171
Consultant Haematologist ☎
Via RLUH switchboard

>1500 mls and ongoing severe bleeding
or 150 mls min⁻¹
Use of emergency O-ve blood
Collapse/Clinical shock
If "LEVEL 1" transfusion protocol is activated

NHS
North West Regional Transfusion Committee
incorporating North Wales

Activate Massive Haemorrhage Pathway (SpR/ST3 and above)

Call for help 2222
'Massive Haemorrhage, Location, Specialty'
Alert emergency response team (including blood transfusion laboratory,
portering/transport staff)
Consultant involvement essential
Move patient to HDU when safe to do so

RESUSCITATE
Airway
Breathing
Circulation

ASSESS :Take bloods for:
XM, FBC, PT, APTT, fibrinogen, U+E, Ca²⁺
NPT: ROTEM, HEMOCUE, ABG

3 g of Fibrinogen Concentrate if fibrinogen <2g l⁻¹ or as guided by ROTEM *

STOP THE BLEEDING

Order
Red cells 4 units
Platelets 1 dose
then follow
ROTEM
Pathway

or

No ROTEM?
Order
Red Cells 4 units
FFP   4 units
Platelets 1 dose

Aims for therapy
Aim for:
Hb   8-10 g dl⁻¹
Platelets   > 75 x 10⁹ l⁻¹
Fibrinogen > 2 g l⁻¹
Ca²⁺   > 1 mmol l⁻¹
Temp   > 36°C
pH   > 7.35 (on ABG)
Monitor for hyperkalaemia

Haemorrhage Control
Bimanual compression
Ergometrine 500 micrograms IV
Syntocinon 10 IU IV
& 40 IU infusion
Check placenta and for trauma
Carboprost IM.
EUA
Tamponade
Compression sutures
Hysterectomy

Suspected or continuing haemorrhage requiring further transfusion : REASSESS consider
arterial line, FBC, PT, APTT, fibrinogen, U+E, Ca²⁺
REPEAT ROTEM, HEMOCUE,
Discuss with HAEMATOLOGIST *

Prevent Hypothermia
Consider Calcium Chloride
Continuous cardiac monitoring
and CVP line insertion

Haemostatic Drugs
Vit K and Prothrombin complex
concentrate for warfarinised
patients and
Other haemostatic agents:
discuss with Consultant
Haematologist

Follow ROTEM
Pathway

or

No ROTEM?
Red Cells 4 units
FFP   4 units
Platelets 1 dose

STAND DOWN
Inform lab
Return unused
components
Complete documentation
Including audit proforma

Cell salvage if available and
appropriate
Consider ratios of other
components:
1 unit of red cells = c.250 mls
salvaged blood

Suspected continuing haemorrhage
requiring further transfusion : REASSESS
FBC, PT, APTT, fibrinogen, U+E, Ca²⁺
REPEAT ROTEM, HEMOCUE, ABG
Consider Tranexamic Acid

Thromboprophylaxis should be considered when patient stable.

*Discuss with Consultant Anaesthetist/Obstetrician and Haematologist.

ABG – Arterial Blood Gas	APTT – Activated partial thromboplastin time	ATD- Adult Therapeutic Dose
FFP- Fresh Frozen plasma	MHP – Massive Haemorrhage Pack	NPT – Near Patient Testing
PT- Prothrombin Time	TEG/ROTEM - Thromboelastography	XM – Crossmatch

July 2012

APPENDIX 4.2. OBSTETRIC CARDIOLOGY CARE PLAN

Cardiac diagnosis/interventions

NYHA classification (see reference table below)

Comorbidities

Level of care (see reference table below)

Medication:

Long-term thromboprophylaxis/anticoagulation   Yes/No
If Yes see haematology care plan

Parity   EDD

Past Obstetric Hx

Anaesthetic referral   Yes/No; if Yes see anaesthetic
care plan

Fetal echocardiography   Yes/No

IF PATIENT ADMITTED TO LABOUR WARD PLEASE INFORM THE FOLLOWING:

Consultant Obstetrician on call   Yes/No
Consultant Anaesthetist on call   Yes/No
SpR Obstetrician on call   Yes/No
SpR Anaesthetist on call   Yes/No
SpR Cardiology   Yes/No_____
Consultant Cardiologist   Yes/No_____
Other_____

Planned mode of delivery: Elective CS   Trial of Vaginal Delivery
Indication for Elective CS:

Elective CS. If patient admitted in spontaneous labor inform doctors identified previously

Preterm labor Atosiban should be first-line management

Vaginal delivery first stage management USE A WEDGE TO AVOID SUPINE HYPOTENSION

HDU Chart	Yes/No	Note: cardiac patients can use entonox
ECG in labour	Yes/No	
Prophylactic antibiotics	Yes/No	
Arterial BP monitoring	Yes/No	
Early epidural analgesia	Yes/No	
Central Venous Access	Yes/No	

Syntocinon [synthetic oxytocin] augmentation of labour guidance: _____

Vaginal delivery second stage management

Normal second stage	Yes/No
Active second stage	Yes/No
Duration _____ min/hours	
Elective forceps/delivery only	Yes/No

Vaginal delivery third stage management

Normal active management	Yes/No

Syntocinon: infuse 5 IU in 20 ml saline over 20 minutes

Postpartum haemorrhage

- Inform   Consultant Obstetrician/SpR Obstetrician
                   Consultant Anesthesiologist/SpR Anesthesiologist
- Mechanical compression methods preferable
- Close fluid balance: count all pads/hourly urometer/CVP/arterial line
- Caution using uterotonics: misoprostol in preference to hemabate

Post delivery
Minimum stay on labour ward   _____hours/days
Length of hospital stay   _____days

Postnatal medication plan

Breastfeeding advice

Postnatal follow up arrangements

Other considerations/instructions

New York Heart Association (NYHA) classification of cardiovascular disease

Class	Description
I	Patients who are not limited by cardiac disease in their physical activity Ordinary physical activity does not precipitate the occurrence of symptoms such as fatigue, palpitations, dyspnea and angina
II	Patients in whom the cardiac disease causes a slight limitation in physical activity
III	Patients in whom the cardiac disease results in a marked limitation of physical activity. They are comfortable at rest but less than ordinary physical activity will precipitate symptoms
IV	Patients in whom the cardiac disease results in the inability to carry on physical activity without discomfort. Symptoms may be present even at rest, and discomfort is increased by any physical activity

Level of care

Level 1   Highly complex lesions:
               repairs with conduits, Rastelli, Fontan, Marfan syndrome with dilated aortic root, Ebstein anomaly, pulmonary atresia, Eisenmenger syndrome, repaired transposition of great arteries (arterial switch or atrial switch), congenitally corrected transposition of great arteries, pulmonary hypertension, cynanotic congenital heart disease

Level 2   Lesions of moderate complexity:

coarctation of aorta (repaired/native), repaired atrioventricular septal defect, aortic stenosis, pulmonary stenosis/regurgitation, tetralogy of Fallot, ventricular septal defect and aortic regurgitation, mechanical valves, hypertrophic cardiomyopathy, dilated cardiomyopathy

Level 3   Simple lesions:

repaired patent ductus arteriosus/ventriculoseptal defect/total anomalous pulmonary drainage/atrial septal defect, mild pulmonary stenosis/pulmonary regurgitation, small ventricular septal defect

Level 1 = Exclusive care in specialized unit
Level 2 = May have shared care with regional adult cardiology unit
Level 3 = Care predominantly in a general adult cardiology unit

Chapter 5

Midwifery and nursing issues in the intensive care setting

Wendy Pollock and Kate Morse

Introduction

The admission of a critically ill pregnant or post-partum woman to an intensive care unit (ICU) provides unique challenges to nursing staff for a variety of reasons. The physiological adaptations of pregnancy underscore a different set of "what is normal." Obstetric conditions that ICU staff may be unfamiliar with, nursing needs unique to this population, such as checking the fundus and supporting the establishment of lactation, and the presence of the fetus, all contribute to making the pregnant and postpartum woman a challenge. Similarly, midwives and obstetric nurses may find caring for critically ill pregnant and postpartum women testing given the potential instability of each woman's condition and the additional monitoring and technological support she may require. It can present a challenge for two healthcare teams, critical care and maternal health, and requires clear communication, explicit patient goals, and sometimes negotiation to promote the health of the mother and fetus.

Little research has been done to provide an evidence base to guide the management of critically ill pregnant and postpartum women. Consequently, much that has been written is experiential observational work or extrapolated from the non-obstetric critical care literature [1]. The purpose of this chapter is to provide meaningful information for nurses and midwives caring for critically ill pregnant and postpartum women. This chapter discusses the various clinical settings in which critically ill parturients may be cared for, along with the common nursing and midwifery staffing arrangements. Modifications to routine ICU care for pregnant women are outlined as well as the routine maternity care for pregnant women in ICU. Maternity care for critically ill postpartum women is described in detail.

Background and context

Critical illness is characterized by the presence of actual or potential life-threatening health problems where there is a requirement for continuous observation and intervention to prevent complications and restore health where possible. Critically ill patients often require invasive monitoring, technological support, and intense nursing surveillance and intervention to maintain basic organ function. Critically ill pregnant and postpartum women may be cared for in a variety of clinical settings, such as a general adult ICU, a specialist obstetric ICU, a high dependency unit (HDU), or in a birth suite within the maternity hospital. Approximately two thirds of women with severe maternal morbidity remain in the care of maternity services with one third admitted to an ICU [2].

However, the term ICU may mean different things in different places and the admission criteria vary across institutions and countries. Generally speaking, an ICU is a defined geographical area within a hospital where the necessary professional skills and competencies, technical equipment, and resources are assembled for patients with life-threatening illnesses, injuries, or complications; usually admission requires advanced respiratory support or support of two or more failing organ systems. An HDU refers to a dedicated space (which may or may not be within an ICU) that provides comprehensive monitoring and intervention to patients with, or at risk of developing, single organ failure, with the exception of those needing advanced respiratory support. The HDU may also be referred to as a stepdown unit or intermediate care unit in the USA or a medium care unit in certain mainland European countries.

Various terminology and training requirements exist for nurses and midwives providing care to pregnant and postpartum women. For example, in

---

Maternal Critical Care: A Multidisciplinary Approach, ed. Marc Van de Velde, Helen Scholefield, and Lauren A. Plante.
Published by Cambridge University Press. © Cambridge University Press 2013.

Australia, Belgium, and the UK, an individual may complete a Bachelor of Midwifery and obtain registration to practice as a midwife with no nursing prerequisite, qualification, or experience. The midwife is the health professional prepared to care for and support the woman and her partner/family through the journey of pregnancy and childbirth. Midwifery is based within the wellness paradigm, with pregnancy and childbirth viewed as normal healthy life events. A registered nurse may complete a specialist postgraduate formal study program, such as a Graduate Diploma of Midwifery, to obtain registration to practice as a midwife. Normally, only staff with a midwifery qualification are employed to care for pregnant and postpartum women in a maternity setting (e.g. hospital, primary health clinic) or are able to establish an independent practice. The title midwife is protected by legislation, with only those who have completed the required education and registered as a midwife able to use the title. The term obstetric nurse is not used in Australia, New Zealand, the UK, or much of Europe.

The education and training of staff caring for pregnant and postpartum women in North America has evolved along a different path. According to the American College of Nurse Midwives, there are three possible designations for midwifery credentials in the USA: certified nurse–midwife, certified midwife, and certified professional midwife. The certified nurse–midwife requires a nursing degree whereas the certified midwife does not require an active nursing license. The certified nurse–midwife is awarded a master or doctoral degree and the certified midwife is awarded a master degree; both are eligible to sit for the American Midwifery Certification Board examinations. The certified nurse–midwife and certified midwife are eligible to be licensed in 50 states plus the District of Columbia and US territories, whereas the certified professional midwife is not board eligible and a degree is not required. The certified professional midwife is currently regulated in 26 states. Prescriptive authority varies from state to state and the focus is on the healthy, normal pregnancy. Care may be provided in a variety of settings, including the home, hospital, and birthing centers, which may or may not be freestanding or geographically associated with a hospital. Midwives work in collaboration with medical providers. In Canada, the Canadian Association of Midwives describes the midwife as a professional who provides primary care to women and their babies during pregnancy. There are six midwifery programs in Canada and the schools offer baccalaureate programs taking 4 years. However, in both the USA and Canada, most women give birth in hospital under the care of obstetricians and specially trained registered nurses. Nurses working with active labor patients are commonly referred to as labor and delivery nurses, while the before and after care is provided on the maternity floor by nurses commonly referred to as obstetric nurses. For the purposes of this chapter, both these specially trained registered nurse roles will be referred to as obstetric nurses.

The one constant that critically ill pregnant and postpartum women require the world over, regardless of training and employment models, is the receipt of both critical care nursing and midwifery care. Few nurses and midwives are specialist in maternal critical care and there is a potential knowledge and skill gap, with critical care nurses ill-equipped to cater for the woman's maternity needs and midwives not educated to care for critically ill women [3,4]. Ideally, nurses and midwives caring for critically ill pregnant and postpartum women should undergo a specialized education program to provide the necessary knowledge and competencies to meet the needs of women. Such a program may be modular and some topics may involve nurses and midwives learning together. Educational programs may be conducted by health service providers or academic institutions; preferably, any program should offer the opportunity for the study to articulate with an academic award for advanced standing/credit (recognition of prior learning). Suggested content for a maternal critical care education program includes the physiological adaptations of pregnancy and how they relate to critical illness; assessment, monitoring, and interventions to support the critically ill woman; specific conditions of pregnancy and their management; medical conditions in pregnancy; maternity care during pregnancy (including assessment of fetal well-being); maternity care postpartum; communication and psychosocial care of critically ill women; and emergency situations and their management. Content on clinical audit and evaluation of care specific to maternal critical care would also be of benefit [5].

Maintaining knowledge and competency in the care of critically ill parturients is also a challenge given that many staff care for women infrequently and there is limited opportunity to build consolidated experience in the set of skills. Dedicated resource manuals, special interest journal club meetings, regular emergency drills involving the whole maternal critical care team, and combined seminar events with critical care nurses and midwives would assist in maintaining the knowledge base. Other options to maintain competency include staff rotations between areas; for example midwives/obstetric nurses could rotate to a general ICU for supernumerary time to be reacquainted with skills in a concentrated block, such as zeroing arterial lines and taking blood samples from arterial lines. Additionally, care can be planned jointly – the ICU nurse addressing the critical care needs and the obstetric nurse or midwife addressing those pregnancy-specific needs, with daily case conference to plan care. In the USA, midwives rarely continue care in the ICU, but it may be a future practice model. Similarly, ICU nurses could spend supernumerary time on a postnatal ward checking fundal height and condition with a midwife and consolidating their understanding of how to support the establishment of lactation. A further notion would be to have dedicated "maternal critical care" personnel who are always drawn upon to care for critically ill pregnant and postnatal women. These staff would have completed a maternal critical care education program and have developed competencies in the care of critically ill pregnant and postpartum women.

The type of collaborative program will be partially driven by state or countrywide regulation, scope of practice, and hospital policies regarding practice. The ideal collaboration would be between the midwife, the obstetric team (which may include physicians and nurses), the critical care team (which may include nurse practitioners, physician assistants, nurses, physicians, respiratory therapists, pharmacists), and the broader healthcare team (social worker, case manager, allied health).

Midwifery and nursing care of pregnant women

Pregnant women admitted to ICU are more likely to be admitted with a non-obstetric diagnosis than as a result of a complication of pregnancy. The ICU length of stay will vary according to clinical need and, although many pregnant women have a relatively short ICU length of stay (i.e. 2 days), some women require a long period of ICU support (i.e. extending to weeks). Conditions that may require long ICU stays include Guillain–Barré syndrome, influenza/pneumonia, and trauma.

Regardless of the length of stay, pregnant women in ICU have maternity care needs as well as a need to modify routine ICU care because of the physiological changes of pregnancy and presence of the fetus. The

mnemonic "MUM'S FAST HUG" is one way to assist nurses and midwives to remember how to incorporate all of the pregnant woman's needs into the care provided (Table 5.1). The "MUM'S" element (or MOM's in the USA) contains all the additional care required related to the pregnancy and the "FAST HUG" is an adaption of the usual ICU mnemonic [6] to modify routine ICU care to accommodate for the pregnancy. These components are discussed below and listed in Table 5.1.

Monitoring fetal well-being

There are two components of fetal well-being to be considered in a pregnant woman in ICU. The first is assessment of the normal growth and development of the fetus. The second is assessment of the real-time well-being of the fetus needed to aid decision making around the optimal time for delivery. Fetal assessment is discussed fully in Chapter 13.

Normal growth and development is routinely monitored by measuring the symphysis pubis–fundal height and, more accurately, by serial ultrasound measurements. In the ICU setting, the fetus may be considered at risk for restricted growth, and serial ultrasound measurements should be undertaken. Women who may require serial fetal growth assessment are those with long ICU stays, for example pregnant women in ICU with Guillain–Barré syndrome. Standard tools to assess real-time well-being of the fetus include biophysical profile and cardiotocography. Early research on the measurement of hypoxia-induced mRNA in maternal blood to detect fetal hypoxia in utero is showing some promise [7]. The main challenge is in the interpretation of the standard tools used, as the interpretation may be impacted by the medication that the woman is receiving. A sedated woman may result in a sedated fetus, resulting in reduced movements, reduced cardiotocography variability, and reduced biophysical profile scores. Furthermore, current mRNA blood tests cannot distinguish between fetal and maternal hypoxemia. Theoretically, uterine artery and fetal middle cerebral artery Doppler flow studies may be of benefit, but they have not been investigated in the setting of maternal critical illness.

Undertake/observe routine antenatal care

Routine antenatal care consists of confirming the pregnancy and gestation, preventing rhesus isoimmunization, multidisciplinary planning for labor/delivery as

45

Table 5.1. "MUM'S FAST HUG" covers the incorporation of all of the pregnant woman's needs into the care provided

	Item	Features
M	Monitor fetal well-being	Growth & development Real-time well-being
U	Undertake routine antenatal care (UK) or Observe routine antenatal care (USA)	Confirmation of pregnancy and estimation of gestation Rhesus isoimmunization prevention Surveillance of maternal complications Multidisciplinary planning for labor/delivery
M	Maternal complications	Gestational diabetes Pre-eclampsia Preterm rupture of membranes Preterm labor
S	Special considerations	Effective communication between critical care and maternity teams Impact of normal physiology of pregnancy on: • patient assessment • ventilation and airway management • patient positioning • oral care • medications Preparation for delivery
F	Feeding	Additional nutrition needs in pregnancy Consider supplements (e.g. folic acid, vitamin D)
A	Analgesia	Woman should not experience pain but excessive analgesia should be avoided Consider impact of maternal analgesia on interpretation of fetal well-being tests and ability of neonate to establish respiration when born
S	Sedation	Woman should not experience discomfort; excessive sedation should be avoided Consider impact of maternal sedation on interpretation of fetal well-being tests and ability of neonate to establish respiration when born
T	Thromboembolic prophylaxis	Active thromboprophylaxis in the form of antiembolic stockings or sequential compression devices All critically ill pregnant women should be considered for medical thromboprophylaxis.
H	Head-of-bed elevation	Optimal is 45°, unless contraindicated – if intubated to prevent ventilator-acquired pneumonia Consider patient positioning and potential for aortocaval compression
U	Stress ulcer prevention	Consider histamine H_2 antagonists or proton pump inhibitors
G	Glucose control	Avoid hypoglycemia and hyperglycemia Mild hyperglycemia is associated with worse perinatal outcomes

appropriate, and surveillance of the common complications of pregnancy that may arise during an ICU admission.

Confirmation of pregnancy and estimation of gestation

The presence of pregnancy should be considered in all female patients of childbearing age, although whether all such women admitted to ICU should undergo a pregnancy test is not clear. Enquiries should be made for every woman of childbearing admitted to ICU, as to whether the woman is known to be pregnant. A pregnancy can be detected by the presence of human chorionic gonadotropin in serum or urine; gestation as early as 3 weeks can be detected in this way, with the level of human chorionic gonadotropin doubling to its peak level at 10–12 weeks of gestation before reducing and stabilizing at an elevated level for the remainder of the pregnancy [8]. Ultrasound can determine a relatively accurate gestation by measuring the crown–rump length of the fetus. For women who are obviously pregnant, a quick non-technical way to estimate gestation is to measure the length from the pubis to the top of the fundus – the number of centimeters equates roughly to the number of weeks of gestation (e.g. 24 cm indicates 24 weeks). Otherwise, the fundus at the level of the umbilicus is often representative of about 20 weeks of gestation. Factors such as multiple pregnancy and polyhydramnios will impact on these estimations.

Prevention of rhesus isoimmunization

Rhesus isoimmunization occurs when rhesus-positive fetal blood enters the rhesus-negative maternal circulation, resulting in the development of anti-D antibodies by the mother. These antibodies then cross the placenta and destroy the rhesus-positive fetal red blood cells in a subsequent pregnancy. Events that are likely to result in fetal blood entering the maternal circulation include miscarriage, abdominal trauma, and antepartum hemorrhage. Anti-D immunoglobulin should be administered proactively following any known potential sensitizing event. The dose of anti-D immunoglobulin required is dependent on the volume of fetomaternal hemorrhage. The Kleihauer–Betke test is a commonly used test on maternal blood to estimate the volume of fetomaternal hemorrhage. However, sensitization of the maternal blood can occur without any "event" as such, and it is standard maternity practice to administer anti-D to all rhesus-negative women, usually at around 28 weeks and 34 weeks of gestation, and again within 72 hours of delivery, in the absence of any notable "event" [9].

Maternal complications surveillance

Pregnant woman admitted to ICU have the potential to develop complications of pregnancy just as any pregnant woman, and the complication may not be related to the diagnosis that led to ICU admission. Notable pregnancy complications include gestational diabetes, pre-eclampsia, preterm prelabor rupture of the membranes, and preterm labor. As detailed below, gestational diabetes and pre-eclampsia are difficult to identify in the setting of critical illness. Identification of prelabor ruptured membranes and preterm labor both require an alert clinician and warrant early referral to maternity staff.

Gestational diabetes

Pregnant women are routinely screened for gestational diabetes in many developed countries, during the second half of the second trimester, as it is associated with adverse perinatal outcomes. Treatment usually commences with dietary and exercise changes, with insulin common as the first-line medical treatment. However, given that critical illness is associated with altered carbohydrate metabolism, screening for gestational diabetes while a pregnant woman is in ICU would not be indicated. Rather, assessing blood glucose levels as one normally would during critical illness is required, keeping in mind that maternal hyperglycemia should be actively avoided.

Pre-eclampsia

Pre-eclampsia is a systemic disorder of pregnancy characterized by hypertension and sometimes by multisystem involvement (see Chapter 36). The classic triad of symptoms – hypertension, proteinuria, and edema – is no longer required for diagnosis. The problem with identifying the onset of pre-eclampsia in a critically ill pregnant woman is that organ dysfunction/failure may occur because of the underlying cause of critical illness. For example, raised liver enzymes, renal impairment, and low platelet levels may result from the cause of the critical illness or may represent the development of pre-eclampsia. It is important to keep an open mind when considering the causes of organ dysfunction and to manage the woman based on multidisciplinary advice.

Preterm/prelabor rupture of the membranes

Preterm (<37 weeks of gestation) and/or prelabor (before the onset of labor) rupture of the membranes may occur and result in leakage of amniotic fluid from the vagina. This is of concern because of the risk of ascending infection, resulting in chorioamnionitis, and the loss of amniotic fluid, which could result in insufficient amniotic fluid for normal fetal lung growth and development. Preterm rupture of the membranes is usually diagnosed by the clinical presentation (leaking or sudden gush of fluid from vagina). It can be confirmed by a sterile speculum examination that demonstrates a pool of liquid in the vagina, a positive nitrazine test (shows the liquid has a ph >6.5) or positive "ferning" pattern of the liquid when viewed under the microscope. More recently, tests have been developed to identify a specific biochemical marker present in amniotic fluid, such as placental alpha-microglobulin-1 or alpha-fetoprotein, with mixed success. The test for placental alpha-microglobulin-1, the Amnisure product, has demonstrated the best sensitivity and specificity in the detection of ruptured amniotic membrane [10] and is achieved with a single vaginal swab (no speculum needed). It may be of benefit to nurse a pregnant woman in ICU with a sanitary napkin *in situ* to assist in the identification of any possible amniotic fluid leak. A major potential sequela of preterm rupture of the membranes is chorioamnionitis; characterized by maternal pyrexia and tachycardia, fetal tachycardia, uterine tenderness, and offensive vaginal discharge: it is a key cause of neonatal sepsis. The other chief consequence may be the onset of labor.

Preterm labor

Identification of the onset of labor may be challenging in a pregnant woman in ICU, particularly if she is sedated. Labor is normally recognized by the commencement of regular, painful contractions, the loss of the cervical mucus plug (a "show"), cervical dilatation and effacement, and fetal descent. However, the only sign that may initially be evident in a ventilated and sedated pregnant woman may be increasing agitation, with increasing sedation needs. Use of a sanitary napkin will help to identify the presence of a mucus plug. The uterus contracts during pregnancy, although these are usually painless. The frequency of such contractions is not a useful sign of the likelihood for preterm labor. Despite uterine contraction being normal during pregnancy, it remains worthwhile to assess the contractions to assess whether labor may have started. Contractions, felt by gently pressing fingertips into the fundus to assess the tone of the uterus – whether it is contracted and hard or relaxed and soft – can be assessed for regularity and pattern. Preterm labor may be experienced more as lower back or pelvic pain rather than the more classic uterine contraction pain. However, the back/pelvic pain is usually not constant but rather more rhythmic in pattern when indicative of labor. The maternity team should be informed and attend the woman if there are regular uterine contractions, or vaginal loss of clear fluid or a cervical mucus plug.

Transvaginal cervical ultrasound is very helpful in assessing the risk of preterm delivery; women with a long cervical length (>3.0 cm) are very unlikely to deliver in the following week [10]. Likewise, a negative fetal fibronectin test in cervical/vaginal fluids reduces the chance that the woman will go into preterm labor. However, none of the studies that has led to these findings have been conducted in a critically ill pregnant population.

Planning for labor/delivery

Multidisciplinary discussions should be held to plan for labor and delivery in a woman with a viable pregnancy who is in the ICU setting. The anesthesiologist, intensivist, home team consultant (e.g. cardiologist, respiratory specialist), and maternity team caring for the woman should develop a plan including what maternal condition would trigger elective delivery; preferred type of anesthesia, delivery, and third stage management; and the resources and staff required if delivery becomes necessary (e.g. neonatal team). If feasible, the woman should be involved in planning for labor/delivery.

In ICU settings that care for pregnant women, the possibility of unplanned delivery should be considered and a strategy in place to manage such a delivery. This strategy should include appropriate skill mix of clinical staff, equipment (e.g. cardiotocography machine, humidicrib), and medication (e.g. to treat third stage, neonatal naloxone) for support during labor, delivery, and potential resuscitation of the newborn. This is discussed further under the heading Preparing for delivery.

Special considerations for pregnancy in intensive care setting

Pregnant women have unique needs in the critical care setting and effective communication of the critical care and maternity teams is necessary. The physiology of pregnancy impacts particularly on what may be considered "normal" parameters when conducting a patient assessment, as well as on the provision of mechanical ventilation, patient positioning, and oral care. Medication use in pregnancy and preparation for delivery are also "special considerations" when caring for a pregnant woman in ICU.

Communication and coordination of the healthcare team

Non-ICU medical specialists consulting on the patient in ICU (e.g. obstetrician, neurologist) commonly do not communicate with each other, which leaves the ICU nurse/team as the central hub for communication. Consequently, the bedside nurse/midwife allocated to the patient in the ICU setting is often the coordinating health professional in the care of a critically ill woman. The nurse at the bedside is fully up to date with the patient's condition and is usually present when various medical specialties consult on the patient. It is important to ensure that any visiting medical staff document their visit and consultation in the medical notes; they may need assistance with this if the ICU is using a paperless clinical information system that visiting medical staff are unfamiliar with. Daily patient care conferences with specialists may improve team communication and planning.

Communication with the patient and family regarding plan of care is critical to the well-being of both.

Critical care staff should record a named midwife and obstetrician to maintain communication about the woman's well-being. The midwife and obstetrician should visit the woman as part of a daily round and they should have input into the care of the woman. The plan for transfer from ICU should be made in conjunction with the maternity team.

Also important is for the bedside nurse to communicate the scope of practice that she/he is competent in regarding the care of critically ill pregnant and postpartum women. General nurses (with no obstetric nursing or midwifery training) must communicate any limitations in their scope of practice to the nurse in charge. For example, it would be inappropriate for such a nurse to assist with induction of labor and to monitor the progress of labor in a pregnant woman in ICU. Similarly, midwives (without additional highly acute care education) should not care for women on continuous intravenous antihypertensive medication or with invasive monitoring. Nurses and midwives are accountable for the care they provide and they should not provide care that is outside of their scope of practice. On occasions, it may be necessary to have both a critical care nurse and a midwife (labor and delivery nurse) caring for a woman throughout a shift together. More often the midwife (labor and delivery nurse) provides intermittent care only (e.g. once a shift), and clear communication between the critical care nurse and midwife/labor and delivery nurse is necessary.

Patient assessment

The basis for any patient assessment is an understanding of what is "normal." Chapter 10 outlines the normal physiological adaptations of pregnancy that need to be considered when conducting a patient assessment. Additionally, other pertinent information should be obtained when a pregnant woman is admitted to an ICU environment, including relevant past medical history; mental health history, including social supports; routine medications prior to the onset of acute illness; past obstetric history; and targeted questioning on the clinical presentation of the current illness. Relevant details will inform the individualized care plan.

Any physical assessment must be interpreted in relation to normal physiology (see Chapter 10). For example, the hemodynamic profile in a pregnant woman may

be mistaken for a septic picture, given the high cardiac output and low systemic vascular resistance that are normal in pregnancy. Every system is affected by physiological adaptations during pregnancy and, as a consequence, assessment of a pregnant woman must take these changes into consideration. Table 5.2 outlines key changes to the assessment criteria to take into account when conducting an assessment of a pregnant woman in the ICU setting.

Although fever in critical illness may be left untreated if the patient's hemodynamic stability is not compromised by the fever, this is not the case when the patient is pregnant. Maternal fever has the potential to have a negative impact on the fetus at all stages of gestation and should be avoided [11], keeping in mind that fetal temperature is commonly 0.5°C higher than maternal temperature [12]. In particular, prolonged and/or high maternal fever (e.g. >38.5°C) may be problematic. Maternal fever is associated with fetal hypoxemia, acidosis, and tachycardia, and with an increase in uterine activity. An antipyretic, such as acetaminophen (paracetamol), may be used to treat fever in the first instance (as long as there are no contraindications such as liver failure), or other cooling mechanisms should be used to achieve normothermia. Non-steroidal anti-inflammatory medications are probably best avoided, particularly if the woman is near term or delivery is imminent, because of potential patent ductus and reduced fetal urine production. While managing fever is important in pregnancy, the underlying cause of the fever should be investigated and treated.

Ventilation and airway management

It is well acknowledged that the airway in pregnancy is considered "high risk," with the failure to intubate rate estimated to be eight times higher in pregnancy. There are a host of physiological adaptations that contribute to this increased risk [13] (see Chapter 17). Additionally, clinicians rarely need to intubate the airway of a pregnant woman in contemporary maternity care, with as many as 95% of cesarean sections conducted under regional anesthesia in developed countries. From a nursing perspective, it is important to ensure that any artificial airway is secured appropriately and that there is a plan prepared for accidental extubation or failure to intubate. Nurses working in ICU environments that cater for intubated pregnant women should be familiar with the hospital's "failure to intubate" policy or emergency airway procedures in their institution, and with the equipment

Table 5.2. Pregnancy-specific considerations related to physical assessment

System	Variance to "normal" assessment criteria[a] during pregnancy
Neurological system	Severe headache and/or visual disturbances (e.g. blurred vision, black spots in vision) may be associated with pre-eclampsia
Cardiovascular system	Heart rate up to 110 beats/min is normal High cardiac output and low systemic vascular resistance is normal during pregnancy and may not be indicative of sepsis Central venous pressure and pulmonary artery pressures are unchanged during pregnancy and can be interpreted using the same normal parameters as non-pregnant values Serum albumin levels are reduced during pregnancy With a reduced colloid osmotic pressure, dependent edema is common; non-dependent edema (e.g. facial) is abnormal Elevated D-dimer and fibrinogen levels during pregnancy; by 36 weeks of gestation, virtually all pregnant women have D-dimer values at or above the conventional cut-off point for thromboembolism With a larger circulating volume and hyperdynamic state, the cardiovascular system can accommodate significant blood loss before a sudden and deleterious deterioration occurs; this required awareness of subtle changes in vital signs
Respiratory system	Respiratory rate unchanged in pregnancy; respiratory rate >20 breaths/min at rest is abnormal Up to 75% of pregnant women experience a feeling of "breathlessness," associated with needing to accommodate a 40–50% higher minute volume; dyspnea at rest is an abnormal sign Pulse oximetry should remain ≥95% even with exertion Arterial blood gas analysis interpretation should be based on the normal values for pregnancy, e.g. partial pressure for CO_2 28–32 mmHg (see Chapters 10 and 17)
Renal system	Although the "normal pregnancy" urine output has been poorly examined, a minimum urine output of 0.5 mL/kg should be expected Serum urea and creatinine are lower during pregnancy: BUN in pregnancy 1.7–4.9 mmol/L (4.8–13.7 mg/dL; normal non-pregnant range is 2.1–8.2 mmol/L (6–23 mg/dL); creatinine 43–74 μmol/L (0.5–0.8 mg/dL) up to 35 weeks of gestation before increasing towards the end of pregnancy up to 87 μmol/L (normal non-pregnant range 53–88 μmol/L (0.6–1.0 mg/dL)) [29] Up to 300 mg proteinuria per day and some glycosuria are normal during pregnancy; this is because of an overloading of the renal tubule active transport systems Assess for and treat asymptomatic bacteriuria associated with pyelonephritis (and preterm labor); minimize use of an indwelling urinary catheter
Gastrointestinal system	Heartburn is not uncommon in pregnancy owing to a relaxed cardiac sphincter; however severe or unrelieved epigastric pain may be a sign of pre-eclampsia The liver enzymes aspartate aminotransferase and alanine aminotransferase maintain normal non-pregnant values during pregnancy, although they may rise slightly above normal non-pregnant values during the postpartum phase [29] Both obstetric and non-obstetric causes of abdominal pain (e.g. appendicitis, bowel obstruction) should be considered when examining an acute abdomen; abdominal organs shift and are compressed by the expanding uterus and signs of non-obstetric conditions may be missed Cholestasis is more common in pregnancy Constipation is more common in pregnancy

[a]Non-pregnant values and assessment.

that is available to address a failed intubation (e.g. emergency airway tray). Note that pregnancy is associated with a poor tolerance of short-term apnea, for example during induction of anesthesia and/or intubation, and preoxygenation is important. Also, pregnant women are more likely to aspirate because of delayed gastric emptying and relaxed cardiac sphincter. The application of cricoid pressure during cardiopulmonary resuscitation is no longer recommended; its role during airway instrumentation in the non-arrest situation is debatable, with questions around the safety and effectiveness recently raised [14]. If applied, cricoid pressure should be done by adequately trained staff only.

The provision of mechanical ventilation is covered in detail in Chapter 17, with little available evidence to guide the "best practice" for pregnant women. Principles to remember include:

- fetal arterial carbon dioxide partial pressure (Pa_{CO_2}) is is higher than maternal Pa_{CO_2} as carbon dioxide passively diffuses across the placenta
- normal maternal Pa_{CO_2} is in the range 28–32 mmHg

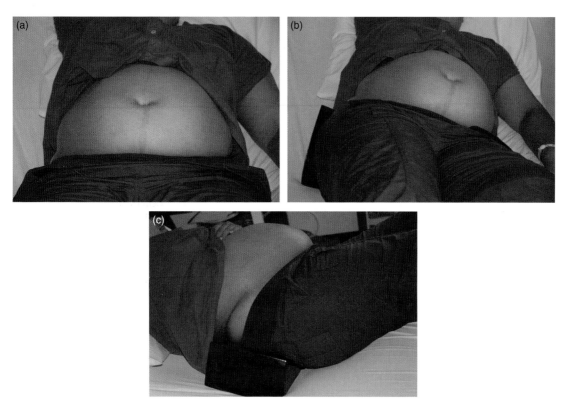

Figure 5.1. Different positions for pregnant patients admitted in order to optimize uteroplacental perfusion. (a) Patient is flat on her back. (b) Patient positioned supine with left lateral tilt from the wedge. (c) A wedge under the right hip tips the patient and relieves aortocaval compression.

- permissive hypercapnia, although a commonly adopted ventilation strategy, has not been evaluated in pregnant women
- fetal hemoglobin has a higher affinity for oxygen than adult hemoglobin
- increasing the ventilator rate to meet the required higher minute volume is more common than increasing the tidal volume ("normal" physiology is 40% increase in tidal volume) although no study has examined this area
- no mode of ventilation is recommended over any other in the setting of pregnancy.

Patient positioning

Once the pregnancy reaches 20 weeks of gestation and thereafter, it is advisable to nurse the woman on her side or with a left lateral tilt if she is lying on her back. At 20 weeks of gestation, the fundus is commonly at about the umbilicus. In the second half of pregnancy, the weight of the uterus compresses the main vessels (aorta and inferior vena cava) and impedes both cardiac output and venous return. While positioning the woman on her side is preferred, if the woman is nursed on her back then a wedge/pillow needs to be placed under one hip to shift the weight of the uterus off the main vessels, achieving a tilt of about 15° (Figure 5.1) [15]. However, taking into consideration the current recommendations for maximizing placental blood flow, minimizing the risk of ventilator-acquired pneumonia, and optimizing the tolerance of enteral nutrition, it is unclear what the best position is to routinely nurse the critically ill pregnant woman in the ICU setting. Monitoring of maternal breathing effort, oxygen saturation, arterial blood gas results, heart rate, blood pressure, cardiac output, and fetal heart rate may be useful to determine a suitable position.

Nevertheless, it is important to keep the weight of the uterus off the main vessels after 20 weeks of gestation. During cardiopulmonary resuscitation, it is possible to manually shift the uterus off the main vessels by the nurse standing on the left side of the bed, placing two hands on the right side of the uterus, and displacing the uterus by lifting the uterus towards the nurse [16].

As with any critically ill patient, care should be taken to minimize pressure sore development, including assessment of any pressure points, regular movement to relieve pressure points, and use of any appropriate pressure-relieving products.

Oral care

Pregnant women have a propensity for gingivitis and bleeding gums as a result of vasodilatation of the vasculature. The gums may also become more sensitive. Oral care is particularly important during pregnancy because of the association between poor oral health and preterm labor. A soft-bristled toothbrush is recommended and oral care should be attended to with gentle brushing twice a day, in addition to any other mouth care routinely provided in the ICU [17]. Furthermore, poor oral health is associated with the development of ventilator-acquired pneumonia owing to the colonization of the oral cavity with pathological organisms.

Medication considerations in pregnancy

Pregnancy is a time when medication use is particularly scrutinized and the benefit and risk of taking the medication is weighed up before the decision is made to prescribe/take a medication. Unfortunately, many of the medications used in the critical care setting have not been evaluated for use by pregnant women, and in those medications where safety has been established, the efficacy of the medication has often not been studied. Many of the physiological adaptations of pregnancy have the potential to influence the effect of medication [18] including:

- reduced serum protein levels (reduced protein-binding capacity)
- increased circulating volume (potential for dilution)
- delayed gut motility (potential for increased gut absorption)
- increased glomerular filtration rate (potential for increased excretion)
- changes to maternal drug-metabolizing enzymes (difficult to predict metabolism pattern of regular drugs).

Consequently, pregnant women may require different dosing regimens to those used for men or for non-pregnant women, and monitoring of the drug is required to ensure that it is having the desired effect and that toxicity is not evident.

From a nursing perspective, it is worth noting that the timing of drug administration is also highly relevant when considering the delivery of medication to pregnant women. The first trimester, in particular, is associated with the risk of teratogenicity and Chapter 14 goes into the pharmacological considerations in detail. The 24 hours prior to delivery is also an important time as the baby may be affected by maternal sedation given in the day prior to birth and require respiratory support following birth. All babies born to women who are critically ill should involve the attendance of a neonatologist/pediatrician at the birth. For women expected to deliver prior to 34 weeks of gestation, a course of antenatal steroids to enhance fetal lung maturity is recommended. A common regimen is two doses of 11.4 mg betamethasone (or 12 mg depending on manufacturer), administered intramuscularly, 24 hours apart. However, administration of betamethasone to enhance fetal lung maturity to a pregnant woman who has a systemic infection (e.g. varicella, tuberculosis) or who is septic, is contraindicated [19]. There is increasing evidence that magnesium sulfate administered antenatally prior to a very preterm birth is protective against the development of cerebral palsy and should be considered [20] if not contraindicated.

Finally, it is worth mentioning the importance for women with pre-existing disease to remain on any medication unless advised otherwise by their medical doctor. In most circumstances, the benefits of maintaining a stable medical condition, such as in asthma or mental illness, outweigh any potential risk of taking the medication during pregnancy.

Preparation for delivery

Any pregnant woman may deliver while in the critical care environment. Many women who deliver while a patient in ICU do so by cesarean section [21]. Vaginal birth does occur in the ICU setting sometimes, which may be a planned event or unexpected. As with any situation, planning ahead and being proactive is helpful should the unexpected occur. For example, even hospitals that do not offer a maternity service usually have a delivery pack somewhere – most often in the emergency department. When caring for a critically ill pregnant patient, the minimum planning for delivery requirements include:

- name and contact details of the obstetrician and maternity team

- the continuous presence of a midwife/labor and delivery nurse to monitor the progress of labor and fetal well-being if the woman is in labor
- details on how to contact the neonatologist or newborn transport service
- equipment that is likely to be needed available (e.g. cardiotocography machine, delivery pack)
- medication that is likely to be needed available – particularly uterotonics such as oxytocin (Syntocinon) or ergometrine/methylergonovine (normally stored in the refrigerator), neonatal naloxone.

Feeding

It is important to recognize that critical illness invokes a range of inflammatory, metabolic, and endocrine responses that independently of pregnancy require specific nutritional support strategies (see Chapter 20). Nutritional support in the critical care setting is an area of intense research; however, pregnant patients are often excluded from trials and the evidence for providing adequate and appropriate nutrition to a critically ill pregnant woman is lacking. Nevertheless, the principles of nutritional support should still apply to the critically ill pregnant woman including early (i.e. within 24–48 hours of admission to ICU) commencement of enteral nutrition. Given the additional nutritional requirements of pregnancy, early referral to a dietician is warranted and the use of supplemental combined vitamins and trace elements should be considered, including routine pregnancy nutritional supplements such as folic acid and vitamin D. Additionally, commencement of nutritional support should not be delayed on the assumption that the woman may have a short stay in ICU.

The physiological adaptations of pregnancy include a relaxed cardiac sphincter, delayed emptying of the stomach, and slowed peristalsis, which contribute to an increased likelihood of aspiration and constipation and an overall unknown effect on enteral feeding tolerance. Common strategies, such as keeping the head of the bed elevated 45°, the use of a gastroprokinetic agent (e.g. metoclompramide), and the placement of a postpyloric feeding tube, may be helpful to optimize feeding delivery [22].

Analgesia

Analgesia should not be withheld from a critically ill woman because she is pregnant. Most analgesics are safe in pregnancy although, as mentioned above, non-steroidal anti-inflammatory drugs should be avoided. Opioids are safe, although it must be remembered that they may potentiate the constipation that is more common in pregnancy. Importantly, consider the impact of maternal analgesia on interpretation of fetal well-being tests and ability to establish respiration when born, if administered within a couple of days prior to delivery. A shorter acting opioid, such as fentanyl, may be preferred over longer-acting drugs. The aim is to provide adequate pain relief without giving excessive amounts of analgesia. Consideration should also be given to long-term use of opioids and the potential to generate neonatal withdrawal symptoms. Much of the literature on neonatal abstinence syndrome relates to maternal drug dependence and polypharmacy illicit drug use, and the impact of short-term opioid use in the management of a critically ill pregnant woman has not been examined.

Sedation

Likewise, sedation should not be withheld from a critically ill pregnant woman because of concerns for effects on the fetus. The ICU environment and associated treatments can be uncomfortable, and an agitated, uncooperative patient poses risks (e.g. self-extubation). Many sedation agents are safe in pregnancy, and a calm, comfortable, and collaborative patient should be the aim [6]. Advice from the pharmacist may be of benefit to determine the best sedation agents to use at different stages of pregnancy. As with analgesia, consider the impact of maternal sedation on interpretation of fetal well-being tests and the ability to establish respiration when born, if administered within a couple of days prior to delivery. Note that long-term use of benzodiazepines can also lead to neonatal withdrawal symptoms. The aim is to achieve a therapeutic effect by using the fewest drugs at the lowest doses and for the shortest durations possible.

Thromboprophylaxis

Pregnancy is associated with an increased risk of thrombus formation, and the immobility associated with an ICU admission along with the impact of critical illness contribute to a high risk of thrombosis and pulmonary embolism in the critically ill pregnant woman. Consequently, all pregnant women in the ICU setting should have active thromboprophylaxis in the form of antiembolic stockings or sequential compression devices as soon as practicable, and all critically ill pregnant women should be considered for medical thromboprophylaxis. Low-molecular-weight heparins are the preferred agents for antenatal thromboprophylaxis [23]. Administration should be stopped if the woman goes into labor or delivery is planned. The Royal College of Obstetricians and Gynaecologists guideline provides a useful antenatal thromboprophylaxis framework [23].

Head-of-bed elevation

When there are no contraindications, it is advised to position ventilated patients 45° upright, to reduce gastric reflux and the incidence of ventilator-acquired pneumonia [6]. However, the impact of the heavily gravid uterus, on both the respiratory physiology and hemodynamic status, in this position has not been examined.

Stress ulcer prevention

Histamine H_2 blockers and proton pump inhibitors are both safe for use during pregnancy although it is not known how pregnancy affects the likelihood of a gastric stress ulcer during critical illness [24,25].

Glucose control

The appropriate glycemic target is not clear given the adverse obstetric and neonatal outcomes associated with relatively mild hyperglycemia [26]. The appropriate target for glycemic control in the general ICU population is inconclusive, with some ICU clinicians sitting in the "tight" glycemic control camp (4.4–6.1 mmol/L (80–110 mg/dL)) and others in the moderate glycemic control camp (8.0–10.0 mmol/L (140–180 mg/dL)). While it is agreed that both hyperglycemia and hypoglycemia should be avoided, no glycemic target has been investigated in the critically ill pregnant population.

Care for postpartum women

Most obstetric patients admitted to ICU are postpartum; the 6 weeks following birth during which the woman's body returns to the pre-pregnant state. In addition, most of these women are within the first 24 hours following birth. Despite the onset of critical illness at this time, women still require their routine postpartum needs attended to. Many critical care nurses are taught patient assessment using the "head to toe" approach and the 7Bs of postpartum care adopts this approach to assist critical care nurses to remember the specific needs of postpartum women [27]. Importantly, the 7Bs of postpartum care include consideration of the mother–infant bond and the partner/broader family in recognition of the need to provide holistic care to critically ill patients. The 7Bs of postpartum care are blues, breasts, belly, bottom, body, baby, and beloved (Table 5.3).

Table 5.3. The 7Bs of postpartum care

B	Features
Blues	"The baby blues" are a normal psychological physiology of the postpartum; short-term tearfulness, anxiety or feelings of inadequacy, occurring 3–4 days postpartum Abnormal psychological physiology of the postpartum: postnatal depression, puerperal psychosis
Breasts	Examine the breasts at least once per shift: look for signs of mastitis Establishing lactation: at least six expressions within 24 hours (including one overnight) is recommended Suppress lactation: if the baby has died or the woman's preference is not to breastfeed
Belly	Uterine involution
Bottom	Assessment of perineum Assessment of lochia Diuresis is normal in the first few postpartum days Prevent constipation
Body	Assess for deep vein thrombosis and consider thromboprophylaxis Lowest serum albumin levels occur 7–10 days postpartum
Baby	Ensure any legalities of birth registration (and death registration if required) are met Nurture a healthy mother–infant attachment Creation of a momento if the baby has died
Beloved	Remember to include the partner; consideration for other children Foster and support the development of the family unit

Blues

The delivery of the placenta heralds a substantial drop in circulating maternal hormones and the "baby blues" is a common response in the first few days postpartum. The "blues" are characterized by short-term tearfulness, anxiety or feelings of inadequacy, labile emotions; they occur 3 to 4 days postpartum and last for a couple of days at most. They are considered normal psychological physiology of the postpartum. The "blues" are normally self-limiting and if severe or prolonged may indicate an increased likelihood of postnatal depression.

Postnatal depression is a non-psychotic depressive illness that usually presents within 1–3 months of giving birth. It is more common in women with a pre-existing mental health condition, women with poor social supports, with relationship conflict, and women who have experienced recent major life events. Most obstetric patients admitted to ICU postpartum are admitted in the early postpartum phase (within 24 hours following birth) and postpartum depression is not usually a concern at this stage.

Postpartum psychosis, also known as puerperal psychosis, is a rare complication of pregnancy when the woman presents with hallucinations and is frequently delusional. It commonly presents within the first 2 weeks postpartum and is a very serious mental health condition with a risk of infanticide and suicide. The onset of this condition is more common in women with a pre-existing mental health condition, such as bipolar disorder, and requires hospitalization of the woman for acute psychiatric treatment. Rarely, an affected woman may require ICU admission for a self-harm event associated with the condition.

The onset of critical illness around the time of birth is commonly sudden and not predicted, and the "blues" part of the 7Bs is also a reminder to assess the psychological well-being of the woman.

Breasts

The process of lactation is a hormone-mediated one and even in the setting of maternal critical illness it is possible to establish lactation. Normally, a small amount of colostrum is produced in the first few days; this is rich in protein and antibodies and is a highly valuable fluid for the newborn baby. The milk "comes in" within a few days postpartum in response to the drop in progesterone and maintained levels of prolactin and cortisol. Although very few studies have examined the establishment of lactation in the setting of maternal critical illness, it is likely that women will experience a delayed response, with milk "coming in" at a later stage than the normal 3–4 days postpartum [28]. However, the "coming in" of milk will likely occur regardless of whether the woman intends to breastfeed. If the woman has indicated that she would like to breastfeed her infant, then lactation can be commenced while she is in ICU. If the woman does not want to breastfeed, or if her baby has died, then breast milk production can be suppressed.

Establishing lactation

If the woman has indicated a desire to breastfeed her infant, it seems reasonable to support her decision and support the establishment of lactation. Most women admitted to ICU postpartum are admitted within 24 hours of birth, have a short length of stay, and recover from their acute illness fairly quickly. Consequently, there is a real potential to establish breastfeeding with long-term successful breastfeeding feasible. The basic premise of breast milk production is that milk removal stimulates milk production. If the mother's and baby's conditions allow, and there are no contraindications, then the baby can suckle at the mother's breast in ICU. More commonly, the mother and baby are separated (often in different hospitals), or the condition of either the mother or baby precludes this option. Therefore, the most frequent practice to commence lactation in ICU is by breast expression. A summary of initiating lactation by expression is in Table 5.4.

Hand expressing is recommended in the first few days postpartum until the milk comes in. Even when breast milk production is established, hand expressing is recommended to start and finish each expressing episode, along with the use of a breast pump. Hand expression achieves a better stimulus and promotes the "let-down" reflex, which increases the flow of milk. Hand and machine expression should not be painful. In the first couple of days, small amounts of colostrum may be expressed, which may be as little as 1 or 2 mL to begin with at each expression. A 2 or 5 mL syringe may be used to collect the drops to facilitate easy storage and use. As the volumes increase, a small container, such as those used to collect urine samples, may be more appropriate until the milk production increases and bottles can be used. Colostrum/milk should be collected in a new container for each

Table 5.4. Summary of initiating lactation when mother and baby are separated

	Factors
Expression timing	Expression and milk removal stimulates milk production Minimum of six expressions in 24 hours is recommended, with at least one overnight Commence expression as soon as practicable, the earlier the better
Expressing process	Wash hands before starting Use a clean container to collect milk for each expressing episode; do not top-up a container that has milk from an earlier expressing episode Use hand expression only until the milk comes in Use hand expression to start and finish an expressing episode, in conjunction with a breast pump when the milk has come in Expression should not be painful or cause nipple damage
Expressed amount	First day or two, only small amounts of colostrum are produced, 1–2 mL per expression to begin with, building to 5mL; there may be more than this but these small volumes are common in women who are critically ill Small volumes does not mean that milk production cannot be established Milk usually "comes in" around day 3 or 4 postpartum but may be delayed in women who are critically ill Once milk "comes in," the breasts may become engorged or have a full feeling; the volume of milk produced is now increased Removing more milk will stimulate more milk production; by 1 week postpartum, each expression may produce anywhere between 50 and 200 mL of milk
Storage of milk	Label each collected expressed milk with: mother's name and hospital number plus date and time of expression Keep expressed milk in the refrigerator Transport expressed milk in a cooler bag to where the baby is Expressed milk may be frozen

expression with the woman's details and the date and time clearly labeled. Colostrum/milk must be stored in the refrigerator and may be frozen.

Having been informed of the woman's intent to breastfeed or obtaining approval to initiate lactation, the first step is to ensure that the woman is comfortable. A warm washer can be used, along with massage of any lumpy breast tissue, to facilitate the expressing episode. The thumb and forefinger are placed just outside the areola, where the collecting ducts are located. Gentle pinching together of the forefinger and thumb with a slightly inward motion will stimulate the breasts, release oxytocin, and produce small amounts of colostrum initially. Both breasts should be expressed, and shorter more frequent expressions are better than infrequent long expressions. Once the milk comes in, more volume will be produced with as much as 100 to 200 mL each expression possible, even in a woman who is critically ill. Care should be taken with the use of breast pumps, as nipple damage can occur if excessive suction is applied or if the pump is placed inappropriately.

Breast expression is recommended a minimum of six times in a 24 hour period, with at least one expression overnight, to establish milk production. More frequent expression and more milk removal will stimulate more milk production. Common ICU drugs may affect milk production, for example dopamine inhibits milk production while metoclopromide enhances it.

Suppressing lactation

If the baby has died or the woman has chosen to formula feed her infant, the process of lactation can be suppressed. In the past, medications such as bromocriptine were used to inhibit milk production, but there were a number of serious side effects observed, including puerperal psychosis and cardiovascular and cerebrovascular events; consequently, such drugs are prescribed less commonly now. The common method to suppress lactation consists of providing no stimulus to the breasts (i.e. no breast expression) and comfort measures to the woman to relieve any discomfort associated with the milk coming in (hard, hot, engorged breasts), including the use of cool compresses and mild analgesics (e.g. acetaminophen). In practice, major problems with engorged breasts are not likely when a woman has experienced critical illness around the time of birth. However, breast engorgement, even in the absence of mastitis, can produce fever.

Signs and symptoms of mastitis

Whether the woman is intending to breastfeed or not, the clinician should observe for any signs and symptoms of mastitis. Mastitis occurs when there is a blocked milk duct in the presence of infection. Milk engorgement or stasis, for example when the milk first "comes in" or if there is a sudden reduction in milk removal, can lead to blockage in the milk duct and milk is forced in to the surrounding breast tissue, causing inflammation. Infection is commonly caused by staphylococci and is more likely if there is nipple damage such as a cracked nipple (providing a portal of entry). Mastitis is characterized by both systemic and local signs and symptoms, including high temperature and general aches and pains; locally there may be a reddened, hot and painful spot or wedge of breast. Antibiotics are usually required to treat mastitis. Other important treatment is continuing the process of breast milk removal, whether by breast expression (hand and pump) or the baby suckling if the mother's and baby's conditions allow. Use of a warm compress and massage of the blocked duct prior to expression may be useful, along with a cool compress following expression to ease any local pain associated with the mastitis.

Medication considerations in the lactating woman

When the mother is receiving medication, there are a number of factors to consider regarding the safety of the breast milk for the infant. The amount of medication in the breast milk, the oral bioavailability of the medication, and the condition of the neonate to clear the medication (e.g. very premature infant, infant with liver failure) are each relevant. Consequently, the hospital pharmacist and the infant's medical team may collaborate in determining whether the breast milk is safe for the infant. Breast milk has many positive effects, for the premature infant in particular, and breast milk may be recommended to be given to the infant in the absence of any proven harm associated with the mother's medication. If the mother is taking medication that is harmful to the infant, if it is likely to be long-term medication usage, and there are no other safer options, then it is probable that the mother will need to suppress lactation and choose another infant feeding regimen. If the medication is short term only, then the milk can be discarded and the establishment of lactation continued to be supported in readiness for when the medication stops and the mother can commence breastfeeding.

Belly

The main focus of the "belly" is assessment of the uterine fundus (the upper edge of the uterus) to ensure that normal involution is occurring. Uterine involution is the normal process by which the uterus returns to the non-pregnant state. Assessment of the fundus includes the height of the fundus in relation to the umbilicus or symphysis pubis, the centrality of the fundus, and the "feel" of the fundus, to determine its state of contraction. Immediately following birth, the uterine fundus usually sits at about or just below the umbilicus. The fundus should be centrally located and well contracted (feels very hard when palpated – unable to push the fingertips in). If the fundus is not central (i.e. located to the side), then the most likely reason is a full bladder. A "boggy" uterus (one that feels "spongy" on palpation) indicates that the uterus is not contracting properly, which may be caused by uterine atony or retained products or clots. A "boggy" uterus can initially be treated by "rubbing up" the fundus, as the uterus is a tactile organ and will contract in response. A poorly contracted uterus may contribute to further postpartum blood loss, and a series of strategies may be required for effective treatment; for further details see Chapter 39. For the first 24 hours following delivery, the fundal height, position, and texture should be assessed initially hourly for the first 4 hours, and then every 2–4 hours depending on the findings and context (Figure 5.2). If there is ongoing blood loss and a poorly contracted uterus, assessment of the fundus may need to be done more frequently. After the first 24 hours, the fundal assessment can be done once a shift as long as the findings are normal. The date, time, and findings of fundal assessment should be documented. Fundal palpation and assessment should not be painful.

The rate of involution varies from woman to woman; however, it may be expected that the fundus reduces in height and recedes deeper each day; it should remain well contracted and central. Usually, the fundus is no longer palpable above the symphysis pubis by 7 to 10 days postpartum. Delayed involution or the reversal of fundal involution may indicate retained products or emerging infection. The final component of assessing normal involution is assessment of the lochia (the shedding of the uterine lining), which is outlined under "bottom" below.

The routine incision for a cesarean section is along the "bikini line" normally done for a "lower uterine segment cesarean section.". Sometimes a "classical" cesarean section is required when the uterus is incised medially through the uterine body. Sometimes this means that the skin incision looks like a laparotomy

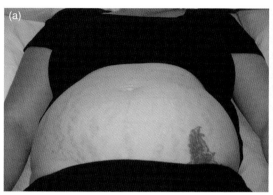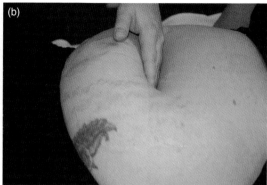

Figure 5.2. Assessing a fundus postpartum. (a) At day 1, the fundus is central and at the level of the umbilicus. (b) Manual evaluation of the height of the uterine fundus. This should not exceed the level of the umbilicus at postpartum day 1.

incision. Standard assessment of the wound is needed, regardless of the incision location. Obese women, in particular, are at risk of cesarean section wound infections, and care should be taken to keep all suture lines clean and dry. Obstetric advice should be obtained as to the management and removal of any sutures *in situ*.

Finally, in the early postpartum period, some women may have a diastasis rectus – separation of the abdominal muscles along the midline. For these women, a gap in the abdominal musculature of up to three or four fingerwidths is evident along the midline and may be particularly evident when she contracts the muscles to sit up. In the first few days postpartum, the woman should be assisted to roll on to her side to sit up and to avoid the "sit-up" action. As the connective tissue between the left and right sides of the muscle returns to the pre-pregnant state, the diastasis rectus should reduce in width. Women with a severe or persistent diastasis rectus should be referred for postnatal physiotherapy to optimize recovery.

Bottom

The focus of the "bottom" is essentially two-fold: assessment of the perineum and assessment of the lochia (vaginal loss occurring postpartum). Regardless of the mode of delivery, the woman's perineum should be inspected as part of an admission assessment following birth and then at the beginning of each shift. Even following an operative birth, vaginal varicosities or hematoma are possible, and visual inspection of the perineum to ensure that it is healthy is important.

If the woman has had an episiotomy or experienced a perineal tear, the wound needs to be assessed for alignment, signs of infection, and evidence of healthy healing. The common suturing material used to repair a perineal tear or episiotomy is self-absorbing and does not need to be removed. However, check the type of suturing material that has been used when assessing the area. If the woman is experiencing perineal pain in the first day or two following birth, an ice pack can be used to help to provide comfort, for 10–20 minute segments, in addition to any systemic analgesics. It is important to keep the area as clean and dry as possible to minimize the likelihood of a wound infection.

The color and volume of lochia changes as the involution of the uterus progresses. Immediately after birth, the lochia is a dark red color and may be quite heavy – requiring a sanitary napkin change every 3–4 hours. In the first 24 hours postpartum, regular assessment of per vagina loss is important, along with the fundus check, to assess for any postpartum hemorrhage. How frequently to check depends on the blood loss; if the loss is heavy (soaked pad within 1–2 hours) then the per vagina loss may need to be checked every hour. If the per vagina loss is minimal and the fundus is well contracted and central, the minimum check should be every 4 hours in the first 24 hours. The volume of loss should ease within the first few hours – it does not normally stay heavy for the first 24 hours (Figure 5.3). Any clots must be reported as they may be remnants of placental tissue. The per vagina loss is documented each time it is assessed and a record kept of when pads are changed.

Usually, by 3 or 4 days postpartum, the lochia changes to an old brownish color. The per vagina loss should now be far less and require less frequent

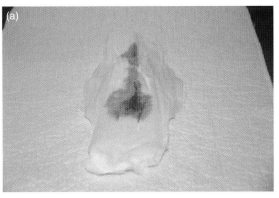

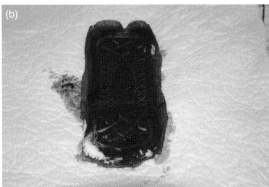

Figure 5.3. Normal (a) and abnormal (b) lochial loss.

pad changes. By 1 week postpartum, the lochia changes to a yellowy color. Lochia is not offensive to smell – any offensive per vagina loss or if the color of the lochia reverts back to red should be reported. Secondary postpartum hemorrhage occurs more than 24 hours postpartum and commonly occurs in the setting of a uterine infection – about 7 to 10 days postpartum. If the woman has had a hysterectomy, there will be no lochia and any per vagina loss will be coming from the surgical site.

Some women have trouble passing their first bowel motion postpartum because of constipation and fear of the potential pain that may result. All bowel actions should be documented on the observation chart and if the woman has not passed an action within 2 days postpartum, consideration should be given to the need for a laxative. It is normal in the first few days postpartum for a sustained diuresis to occur. This restores the cardiovascular volume to the pre-pregnant state.

Body

The "body" component of the 7Bs refers to the general return of the woman's body to the pre-pregnant state. Although the postpartum is defined as the 6 weeks following the birth/termination of pregnancy during which the woman's body returns to the pre-pregnant state, this time frame is rather arbitrary and parts of the body take shorter and longer than this time frame. For example, it is likely that the respiratory changes resolve fully by the end of the postpartum period, although some of the associated anatomical changes, such as flaring of the ribs, remain. In some women, cardiac output remains elevated for as long as 12 months postpartum. Notably, the lowest serum albumin levels are recorded in the first week or two postpartum before the levels start to climb back to pre-pregnant levels [29]. Overall, the major physiological adaptations of pregnancy pertinent to critical care practice resolve over the first couple of weeks postpartum, and with no fetus on board there is less motivation to match the normal physiology of the postpartum exactly.

The postpartum period is well recognized as a high-risk time for the development of deep vein thrombosis and pulmonary embolism. Women who experience critical illness around the time of birth have often undergone lengthy surgical procedures, had lengthy periods of relative immobility, and have experienced pre-eclampsia and/or obstetric hemorrhage. Each of these factors further increases the risk of deep vein thrombosis. Consequently, all postpartum critically ill women should have active thromboprophylaxis in the form of antiembolic stockings or sequential compression devices as soon as practicable and medical thromboprophylaxis, such as low-molecular-weight heparin, as soon as active bleeding is controlled.

Baby

Part of routine postpartum care is nurturing a healthy mother–infant attachment. The mother and infant should be kept together to facilitate that bond whenever possible. However, when the mother becomes critically ill around the time of birth, it is more common that the mother and baby are separated because of the organizational structures of adult ICU and neonatal care. If the mother has been sedated, it is important to orient her to the birth of her infant as she awakens. Obtain photographs of the infant to show the mother; some units use technological communications, such as Skype, to close the gap and to assist with the creation of a relationship. Another option is the use of diaries – one could be written for the woman's time in ICU and another for the infant's time away from the mother. Adult ICU diaries typically contain entries written by the nursing staff about the woman's condition and daily events, entries by visitors, and photographs of the ICU patient and key staff. Neonatal diaries contain photographs of key events, such as first weigh and first bath, and entries by staff about the infant's condition and daily events. However, the use of diaries to assist the mother–infant attachment has not been studied and is a theoretical option that may offer benefit. Furthermore, visiting of either the mother or the infant to each other, depending on which is able to be transported, should be facilitated.

If the baby has died, there are a number of options to consider which may support the mother. Many maternity units create a "memento" booklet that contains a handprint, footprint, lock of hair, and perhaps a photograph of the baby dressed. This is offered to the mother and her partner and if not taken remains in the medical history of the mother in case she changes her mind at a later date and wishes to retrieve it. The baby may be kept in the morgue until the mother is well enough to see and hold the baby if she wants to. Depending on the circumstances, it may be appropriate for an autopsy to be offered to identify a cause of death. At some point, the mother and/or the partner need to be informed about the practicalities of holding a funeral service if they wish to. The involvement of pastoral care staff or a social worker may assist with the early grieving process, with prayers or other support offered. Referral to a perinatal death community support group may also be warranted.

Finally, the registration requirements pertaining to "birth" and "death" need to be completed. What defines a "birth" varies from country to country. In Australia and New Zealand, any live or stillborn infant born after 20 weeks of gestation, or more than 400 g if the gestation is unknown, must be registered as a birth [30]. In the UK, a birth must be registered if it occurred after 24 weeks of gestation or showed signs of life [31]. Any liveborn infant that subsequently dies must have a death certificate filed and the death registered [32].

In the USA, the definition of live birth is based on the World Health Organization definition, with input from the American Academy of Pediatrics and the American College of Obstetricians and Gynecologists.

While there may be slight variations from state to state, a live birth is defined as the "expulsion or extraction from its mother of a product of human consumption" that demonstrates any signs of life. Duration of pregnancy does not define life and all states require the reporting of a live birth regardless of the weight or gestation. In the USA, fetal death is death prior to delivery and while reporting requirements vary from state to state, generally each fetal death of 350 g or more or, if the weight is unknown, of >20 weeks of gestation is required to be reported [32].

Beloved

The final B in the 7Bs is the woman's beloved – her partner – who must not be forgotten in the care of the woman. The critical illness of the woman can be very difficult for the partner when it is associated with pregnancy and birth, as some men feel partly responsible. There is further stress when the mother and infant are cared for separately, because the partner is unsure where to be – at the woman's bedside or their newborn child's. The partner should be kept informed about the condition of both mother and infant and encouraged to visit and talk with both. The partner can be involved in the care of the newborn (e.g. bathe the infant, change nappies) if the infant is well enough. Likewise, a partner may like to be involved in the woman's care (e.g. comb her hair, rub hand moisturizer in) if comfortable doing so. The partner may need referral to pastoral care or social work to assist them during the acute phase of the critical illness, even for essential practicalities like reduced hospital car parking fees and cafeteria vouchers. Partners may need to be encouraged to eat and drink and reminded of the need to look after themselves.

If there are other children, the partner may need assistance with organizing support at home or time off work. Also, depending on the age of the children, it may be appropriate for them to visit their mother and new sibling. If possible, nursing and midwifery staff should foster and support the development of the family unit by maintaining good communication, including family members, and welcoming them at the bedside.

Finally, many partners experience the acute phase of the maternal critical illness as though it were a dream or a blur. Both the woman and her partner may benefit from an ICU follow-up clinic visit, once the woman has recovered, where the events can be explained in detail and any questions answered.

Conclusions

Caring for pregnant and postpartum women in ICU provides challenges to all members of the healthcare team given the physiological adaptations and unique clinical needs. Nurses and midwives should undergo specialist additional education to ensure that they can cater for these women's complex needs. The woman and her family should be involved in care decisions whenever possible. Finally, effective communication and coordination of the health care team are important elements for the best outcomes to be achieved for the woman, her baby, and family.

Key learning points

1. Critically ill pregnant and postpartum women can present a challenge for two healthcare teams, critical care and maternal health, and require clear communication, explicit patient goals, and sometimes negotiation to promote the health of the mother and fetus.
2. Critical care staff should record a named midwife and obstetrician to maintain communication and contact details.
3. Critically ill pregnant and postpartum women may be cared for in a variety of clinical settings, such as a general adult ICU, a specialist obstetric ICU, a high dependency unit, or in a birth suite within the maternity hospital.
4. The one constant that critically ill pregnant and postpartum women require, regardless of training and employment models, is the receipt of both critical care nursing and midwifery care.
5. Ideally, nurses and midwives caring for critically ill pregnant and postpartum women should undergo a specialized education program to provide the necessary knowledge and competencies to meet the needs of critically ill parturient women.
6. Every system is affected by physiological adaptations during pregnancy; consequently, assessment and care of a pregnant woman must take these normal changes into consideration.
7. After 20 weeks of gestation, a woman should be nursed on her side or with a left lateral tilt of at least 15°.
8. The airway in pregnancy is considered "high risk;" nurses working in ICU environments that cater for intubated pregnant women should be familiar with the hospital's "failure to intubate" policy or emergency airway procedures in their institution.

9. While evidence for providing adequate and appropriate nutrition to a critically ill pregnant woman is lacking, the principles of nutritional support in critical illness should still apply – commencement of nutritional support should not be delayed on the assumption that the woman may have a short stay in ICU.
10. Both hyperglycemia and hypoglycemia should be avoided; the ideal target for glycemic control in critically ill pregnant and postpartum women is not known.
11. Pregnancy is associated with an increased risk of thrombus formation; consequently, all pregnant women in the ICU setting should be considered for active thromboprophylaxis.
12. It may be of benefit to nurse a pregnant woman in ICU with a sanitary napkin *in situ* to assist in the identification of any possible amniotic fluid leak or loss of mucus plug.
13. Rhesus isoimmunization prevention should not be overlooked in the pregnant ICU patient.
14. The timing of drug administration is relevant when considering the delivery of medication to pregnant women; the first trimester in particular carries the risk of teratogenicity. Medication administered in the 24 hours prior to delivery (e.g. sedative agents) may impact on the newborn's ability to establish respiration.
15. Any pregnant woman may deliver while in the critical care environment; staff should be proactive and plan ahead for any planned or unplanned delivery.
16. For women expected to deliver prior to 34 weeks of gestation, a course of antenatal steroids to enhance fetal lung maturity is recommended in the week prior to delivery. A course of magnesium sulfate should also be considered to reduce the risk of cerebral palsy developing in the neonate.
17. All babies born to women who are critically ill should involve the attendance of a neonatologist/pediatrician at birth.
18. Women who become critically ill postpartum still require their routine postpartum needs attended to – the 7Bs of postpartum care – blues, breasts, belly, bottom, body, baby, and beloved.
19. Hand expressing is recommended to start and finish each expressing episode, along with the use of a breast pump only once the milk has "come in;" more frequent expression and more milk removal will stimulate milk production.

20. Whether the woman is intending to breastfeed or not, the clinician should observe for any signs and symptoms of mastitis.
21. Postpartum assessment of the fundus includes the height of the fundus in relation to the umbilicus or symphysis pubis, the centrality of the fundus, and the "feel" of the fundus, to determine its state of contraction; it should remain well contracted and central.
22. Any cesarean wound or episiotomy/perineal tear should be assessed for alignment, signs of infection, and evidence of healthy healing.
23. All postpartum critically ill women should have active thromboprophylaxis in the form of antiembolic stockings or sequential compression devices as soon as practicable and medical thromboprophylaxis, such as low-molecular-weight heparin, as soon as active bleeding is controlled.
24. Nurses and midwives can actively nurture mother–infant attachment by communicating about the baby, providing pictures, and keeping a diary of events.
25. The partner should be included in the care of the woman and the practical and support needs of the partner and family must be considered.
26. The woman and her family should be involved in planning her care.

References

1. Pollock W. Caring for pregnant and postnatal women in intensive care: what do we know? *Aust Crit Care* 2006;**19**:54–65.

2. Zwart J, Dupuis J, Richters A, Öry F, van Roosmalen J. Obstetric intensive care unit admission: a 2-year nationwide population-based cohort study. *Intensive Care Med* 2010;**36**:256–263.

3. Kynoch K, Paxton J, Chang A. ICU nurses' experiences and perspectives of caring for obstetric patients in intensive care: a qualitative study. *J Clin Nurs* 2010;**20**:1768–1775.

4. Bench S. Recognition and management of critical illness by midwives: implications for service provision. *J Nurs Manag* 2007;**15**:348–356.

5. Maternal Critical Care Working Group. *Providing Equity of Critical and Maternity Care for the Critically Ill Pregnant or Recently Pregnant Woman*. London: Royal College of Obstetricians and Gynaecologists, 2011 (www.rcog.org.uk/womens-health/clinical-guidance/providing-equity-critical-and-maternity-care-critically-ill-pregnant, accessed 29 January 2013).

6. Vincent J-L. Give your patient a fast hug (at least) once a day. *Crit Care Med* 2005;**33**:1225–1229.

7. Whitehead CL, Walker SP, Mendis S, Tong S. Measuring hypoxia-induced mRNA in maternal blood to detect fetal hypoxia in-utero. *Aust N Z J Obstet Gynaecol* 2011;**51**:473.

8. Cole L. Human chorionic gonadotropin tests. *Expert Rev Mol Diagn* 2009;**9**:721–747.

9. Pilgrim H, Lloyd-Jones M, Rees A. Routine antenatal anti-D prophylaxis for RhD-negative women: a systematic review and economic evaluation. *Health Technol Assess* 2009;**13**: iii, ix–xi, 1–103.

10. Di Renzo GC, Roura LC, Facchinetti F, *et al*. Guidelines for the management of spontaneous preterm labor: identification of spontaneous preterm labor, diagnosis of preterm premature rupture of membranes, and preventive tools for preterm birth. *J Matern Fetal Neonatal Med* 2011;**24**:659–667.

11. Edwards MJ. Review: hyperthermia and fever during pregnancy. *Birth Defects Res A Clin Mol Teratol* 2006;**76**:507–516.

12. Miller M, Church C, Miller R, ME Fetal Thermal Dose Considerations During the Obstetrician's Watch: Implications for the Pediatrician's Observations. *Birth Defects Res C Embryo Today* 2007;**81**:135–143.

13. Munnur UMD, de Boisblanc BMD, Suresh MSMD. Airway problems in pregnancy. *Crit Care Med* 2005;**33**: S259–S68.

14. Fenton PM, Reynolds F. Life-saving or ineffective? An observational study of the use of cricoid pressure and maternal outcome in an African setting. *Int J Obstet Anesth* 2009;**18**:106–110.

15. Kinsella SM. Lateral tilt for pregnant women: why 15 degrees? *Anaesthesia* 2003;**58**:835–836.

16. Vanden Hoek TL, Morrison LJ, Shuster M, *et al*. American Heart Association guidelines for cardiopulmonary resuscitation and emergency cardiovascular care 2010. Part 12: cardiac arrest in special situations. *Circulation* 2010;**122**(Suppl 3): S829–S861.

17. Berry AM, Davidson PM, Masters J, Rolls K. Systematic literature review of oral hygiene practices for intensive care patients receiving mechanical ventilation. *Am J Crit Care* 2007;**16**:552–562.

18. Hodge LS, Tracy TS. Alterations in drug disposition during pregnancy. *Exp Opin Drug Metab Toxicol* 2007;**3**:557–571.

19. Miracle X, Di Renzo G, Stark A, for the WAPM Prematurity Working Group. Guideline for the use of antenatal corticosteroids for fetal maturation. *J Perinat Med* 2008;**36**:191–196.

20. Wolf HT, Hegaard HK, Greisen G, Huusom L, Hedegaard M. Treatment with magnesium sulphate in pre-term birth: a systematic review and meta-analysis of observational studies. *J Obstet Gynaecol* 2012;**32**:135–140.

21. Pollock W, Rose L, Dennis C-L. Pregnant and postpartum admissions to the intensive care unit: a systematic review. *Intensive Care Med* 2010;**36**:1465–74.

22. Canadian Clinical Trials Group. *Summary of Recommendations: Critical Care Nutrition*. Kingston, Canada: Canadian Clinical Trials Group, 2009 (http://www.criticalcarenutrition.com/docs/cpg/srrev.pdf, accessed 29 January 2013).

23. Royal College of Obstetricians and Gynaecologists. *Reducing the Risk of Thrombosis and Embolism during Pregnancy and the Puerperium (Green-top Guideline 37)* London: Royal College of Obstetricians and Gynaecologists, 2009.

24. Gill SK, O'Brien L, Einarson TR, Koren G. The safety of proton pump inhibitors (PPIs) in pregnancy: a meta-analysis. *Am J Gastroenterol* 2009;**104**:1541–1545; quiz 1540, 1546.

25. Gill SK, O'Brien L, Koren G. The safety of histamine 2 (H_2) blockers in pregnancy: a meta-analysis. *Digest Dis Sci* 2009;**54**:1835–1838.

26. HAPO Study Cooperative Research Group. Hyperglycemia and adverse pregnancy outcomes. *N Engl J Med* 2008;**358**:1991–2002.

27. Pollock W, Stanford J. The seven Bs of postpartum care for critical care nurses. *Aust Crit Care* 2013;**25**: in press.

28. Thompson J, Heal L, Roberts C, Ellwood D. Women's breastfeeding experiences following a significant primary postpartum haemorrhage: A multicentre cohort study. *Int Breastfeeding J* 2010;**5**:5.

29. Klajnbard A, Szecsi PB, Colov NP, *et al.* Laboratory reference intervals during pregnancy, delivery and the early postpartum period. *Clin Chem Lab Med* 2010;**48**:237–248.

30. Li Z, McNally L, Hilder L, Sullivan EA. *Australia's Mothers and Babies 2009 (Perinatal Statistics Series 25)*. Sydney: Australian Institute of Health and Welfare National Perinatal Epidemiology and Statistics Unit, 2011.

31. Centre for Maternal and Child Enquiries. *Perinatal Mortality 2009: United Kingdom*. London: CMACE, 2011.

32. Kowaleski J. *State Definitions and Reporting Requirements for Live Births, Fetal Deaths, and Induced Terminations of Pregnancy (1997 revision)*. Hyattsville, MD: National Center for Health Statistics (http://www.cdc.gov/nchs/data/misc/itop97.pdf, accessed 29 January 2013).

Chapter

6

Decisions related to the beginning and end of life

Frank A. Chervenak and Laurence B. McCullough

Introduction

Ethics is an essential dimension of maternal critical care [1]. This is an area of clinical practice with a high potential for ethical conflict in all cultural and national settings around the world. Rather than wait for such conflict to occur, it is far better for patients, their families, and healthcare professionals to anticipate and seek to prevent ethical conflicts. This chapter, therefore, emphasizes a transcultural, transnational, and transreligious preventive ethics approach that appreciates the potential for ethical conflicts and adopts ethically justified strategies to prevent those conflicts from occurring. Preventive ethics helps to build and sustain a strong physician–patient relationship. The chapter commences with a definition of ethics, medical ethics, and the fundamental ethical principles of medical ethics: beneficence and respect for autonomy. The ethical concept of the fetus as a patient is then considered before continuing to define critical care as a trial of management, with short- and long-term goals. Finally, an ethical framework for a preventive ethics approach to maternal critical care is provided.

Ethics, medical ethics, and ethical principles

Ethics has been understood in the global histories of philosophy and theology to be the disciplined study of morality. Medical ethics should, therefore, be understood to be the disciplined study of morality in medicine and to concern the obligations of physicians and healthcare organizations to patients as well as the obligations of patients. Medical ethics should not be confused with the many sources of morality that exist in particular societies. These can include, but are not limited to, law, the world's religions, ethnic

and cultural traditions, families, the traditions and practices of medicine (including medical education and training), and personal experience. Medical ethics since the eighteenth century European and American Enlightenments has been secular [2]. It makes no reference to God or revealed tradition, but to what rational discourse requires and produces. At the same time, secular medical ethics is not intrinsically hostile to religious beliefs. Therefore, ethical principles and virtues should be understood to apply to all physicians in all countries, regardless of their personal religious and spiritual beliefs [3]. The resulting professional responsibility model of obstetric ethics [4] is transnational and transcultural.

The traditions and practices of medicine provide an important reference point for medical ethics because they are based on the obligation to protect and promote the health-related interests of the patient. This obligation tells physicians what morality in medicine ought to be, but in very general abstract terms. Providing a more concrete, clinically applicable account of that obligation is the central task of medical ethics, using ethical principles [1–3].

The ethical principle of beneficence in its general meaning and application requires one to act in a way that is expected reliably to produce the greater balance of benefits over harms in the lives of others. To put this principle into clinical practice requires a reliable account of the *clinical* benefits and harms relevant to the care of the patient, and of how those *clinical* goods and harms should be reasonably balanced against each other when not all of them can be achieved in a particular clinical situation, such as a request for an elective cesarean delivery. In medicine, the principle of beneficence requires the physician to act in a way that is reliably expected to produce the greater balance of clinical benefits over harms for the patient [1–3].

Maternal Critical Care: A Multidisciplinary Approach, ed. Marc Van de Velde, Helen Scholefield, and Lauren A. Plante.
Published by Cambridge University Press. © Cambridge University Press 2013.

Beneficence-based clinical judgment has an ancient pedigree, with its first expression found in the Hippocratic oath and accompanying texts [5]. Beneficence-based clinical judgment makes an important claim: to interpret reliably the health-related interests of the patient from medicine's perspective. This perspective is provided by accumulated scientific research, clinical experience, and reasoned responses to uncertainty. As rigorously evidence-based, beneficence-based judgment is, therefore, not the function of the individual clinical perspective of any particular physician, it should not be based merely on the clinical impression or intuition of an individual physician. On the basis of this rigorous clinical perspective, focused on the best available evidence, beneficence-based clinical judgment identifies the benefits that can be achieved for the patient in clinical practice based on the competencies of medicine. The benefits that medicine is competent to seek for patients are the prevention and management of disease, injury, disability, and unnecessary pain and suffering, and the prevention of premature or unnecessary death. Pain and suffering become unnecessary when they do not result in achieving the other goods of medical care, for example allowing a woman to labor without effective analgesia [1–3].

Non-maleficence is an ethical principle that obligates the physician to prevent causing harm. Non-maleficence should be best understood as expressing the limits of beneficence. Non-maleficence is better known to physicians as *primum non nocere*, or "first do no harm." This commonly invoked dogma is really a Latinized misinterpretation of the Hippocratic texts, which emphasized beneficence while avoiding harm when approaching the limits of medicine. Non-maleficence should be incorporated into beneficence-based clinical judgment: when the physician approaches the limits of beneficence-based clinical judgment (i.e. when the evidence for expected benefit diminishes and the risks of clinical harm increase), then the physician should proceed with great caution. The physician should be particularly concerned to prevent serious, far-reaching, and irreversible clinical harm to the patient [1–3].

There is an inherent risk of paternalism in beneficence-based clinical judgment that must be responsibly managed. Beneficence-based clinical judgment, when it is *mistakenly* considered to be the sole source of moral responsibility and therefore moral authority in medical care, invites the unwary physician to conclude that beneficence-based judgments can be imposed on the patient in violation of his/her autonomy. Paternalism is a dehumanizing response to the patient and, therefore, should be avoided in the practice of maternal critical care.

The ethical principle of respect for autonomy stands in contrast with the principle of beneficence. Respect for autonomy obligates the physician to empower the patient to make informed decisions about his/her medical care and to implement his/her value-based preferences, unless there is compelling ethical justification for not doing so. The pregnant patient increasingly brings to her medical care her own perspective on what is in her interest. The principle of respect for autonomy translates this fact into autonomy-based clinical judgment. Because each patient's perspective on his/her interests is a function of his/her values and beliefs, it is impossible to specify the benefits and harms of autonomy-based clinical judgment in advance. Indeed, it would be inappropriate for the physician to do so, because the definition of benefits and harms and their balancing are the prerogative of the patient. Not surprisingly, autonomy-based clinical judgment is strongly anti-paternalistic in nature [1–3].

Beneficence and respect for autonomy both shape the informed consent process. The physician has the beneficence-based obligation to identify and present to the patient all of the medically reasonable forms of clinical management for the management of the condition, disease, or injury. "Medically reasonable" means that a form of clinical management is physically available, technically possible, and supported in evidence-based reasoning as having an outcome that, on balance, will be clinically beneficial. There is no ethical obligation to offer clinical management that meets only the first two criteria. Failure to recognize this creates preventable ethical conflict in critical care. The physician should describe the nature and expected outcomes of medically reasonable alternatives, along with their expected risks and how these will be managed should they occur.

The pregnant patient's role has iterative steps. She should (a) pay attention; (b) absorb, retain, and recall information about her condition and the medically reasonable alternatives for managing it; (c) understand these matters; (d) understand that these matters apply to her; (e) evaluate the outcomes of the medically reasonable alternatives based on her own values (i.e. what is important to her); and (f) express a value-based preference. The physician has a role to play in supporting each of these steps. The physician should recognize the capacity of each patient to deal with medical information (and not to underestimate that capacity), provide information (i.e. disclose and explain all medically reasonable alternatives), and recognize the validity of the values and beliefs of the patient. The physician should try not to interfere with but, when necessary, to assist the patient in her evaluation and ranking of diagnostic and therapeutic alternatives for managing her condition and then elicit and implement the patient's value-based preference [1].

In the USA, the legal obligations of the physician regarding informed consent were established in a series of cases during the twentieth century. In 1914, *Schloendorff v. The Society of The New York Hospital* established the concept of simple consent, that is, whether the patient says yes or no to medical intervention [6,7]. To this day in the medical and bioethics literature, this decision is quoted: "Every human being of adult years and sound mind has the right to determine what shall be done with his body, and a surgeon who performs an operation without his patient's consent commits an assault for which he is liable in damages" [6]. The legal requirement of consent further evolved to include disclosure of information sufficient to enable patients to make informed decisions about whether to say yes or no to medical intervention [7].

The ethical concept of the fetus as a patient

The ethical concept of the fetus as a patient is essential to maternal critical care in all cultural and national settings. Developments in fetal diagnosis and management strategies to optimize fetal outcome have become widely accepted, encouraging the development of this concept. This concept has considerable clinical significance because, when the fetus is a patient, directive counseling (i.e. recommending a form of management) for fetal benefit is appropriate, and when the fetus is not a patient, non-directive counseling (i.e. offering but not recommending a form of management for fetal benefit) is appropriate. However, there can be uncertainty about when the fetus is a patient. One approach to resolving this uncertainty would be to argue that the fetus is or is not a patient in virtue of personhood, or some other form of independent moral status. The following discussion shows that

this approach fails to resolve the uncertainty and, therefore, supports an alternative approach that does resolve the uncertainty.

One prominent approach for establishing whether or not the fetus is a patient has involved attempts to show whether or not the fetus has independent moral status. Independent moral status for the fetus means that one or more characteristic that the fetus possesses in and of itself and, therefore, independently of the pregnant woman or any other factor, generates and grounds obligations to the fetus on the part of the pregnant woman and her physician. Despite an ever-expanding theological and philosophical literature on this subject, there has been no closure on a single authoritative account of the independent moral status of the fetus. This is an unsurprising outcome because, given the absence of a single method that would be authoritative for all of the markedly diverse theological and philosophical schools of thought involved in this endless debate, closure is impossible. For closure ever to be possible, debates about such a final authority within and between theological and philosophical traditions would have to be resolved in a way satisfactory to all, an inconceivable intellectual and cultural event. In terms of the independent moral status of the fetus, the concept of the fetus as a patient has no stable or clinically applicable meaning. Maternal–fetal medicine, therefore, should abandon these futile attempts to understand the ethical concept of the fetus as a patient in terms of independent moral status of the fetus and turn to an alternative approach that makes it possible to identify ethically distinct senses of the fetus as a patient and their clinical implications for directive and non-directive counseling [1].

This alternative approach is based on the concept of the dependent moral status of the fetus and the recognition that being a patient does not require that one possesses independent moral status. Rather, being a patient means that one can benefit from the applications of the clinical skills of the physician. Put more precisely, a human being becomes a patient when two conditions are met: that a human being is presented to the physician, and that clinical interventions exist that are medically reasonable in that they are reliably expected to result in a greater balance of clinical benefits over harms for the human being in question. These two criteria are obviously transcultural, transnational, and transreligious. This is the sense in which the ethical concept of the fetus as a patient should be understood in all cultural and national settings.

The authors have argued elsewhere that beneficence-based obligations to the fetus exist when the fetus is reliably expected later to achieve independent moral status as a child and person [1]. That is, the fetus is a patient when the fetus is presented for medical interventions, whether diagnostic or therapeutic, that reasonably can be expected to result in a greater balance of goods over harms for the child and person the fetus can later become during early childhood. The ethical significance of the concept of the fetus as a patient, therefore, depends on links that can be established between the fetus and its later achieving independent moral status.

The viable fetal patient

One such link between the fetus and its later achieving independent moral status is viability. Viability, however, must be understood in terms of *both* biological and technological factors. It is only by virtue of both factors that a viable fetus can exist ex utero and thus achieve independent moral status. When a fetus is viable – that is, when it is of sufficient maturity so that it can survive into the neonatal period and achieve independent moral status given the availability of the requisite technological support – and when it is presented to the physician, the fetus is a patient.

Viability exists as a function of biomedical and technological capacities, which vary in different parts of the world. As a consequence, there is, at the present time, no worldwide, uniform gestational age to define viability. In developed countries, we believe, viability presently occurs at approximately 24 weeks of gestational age [8]. Clearly, in less developed countries viability can occur later because of variation in the technological ability to support premature infants. This variability may affect decision making about intrapartum management and resuscitation of the neonate.

The previable fetal patient

The only possible link between the previable fetus and the child it can become is the pregnant woman's autonomy. This is because technological factors cannot result in the previable fetus becoming a child. The link between a fetus and the child it can become when the fetus is previable can be established only by the pregnant woman's decision to confer the status of being a patient on her previable fetus. The previable fetus, therefore, has no claim to the status of being a patient independently of the pregnant woman's autonomy. The pregnant woman is free to withhold, confer, or, having once conferred, withdraw the status of being a patient on or from her previable fetus according to her own values and beliefs. The previable fetus is presented to the physician as a function of the pregnant woman's autonomy [1]. Some countries outlaw abortion of all previable fetuses, the result of which is ethically impermissible restriction of the pregnant woman's autonomy by state power. Physicians in these countries should work for change in such public policies.

When the fetus is a patient, directive counseling for fetal benefit is ethically justified. "Directive counseling" means that the physician should make recommendations that would benefit the fetus. It is emphasized that directive counseling for fetal benefit must occur in the context of balancing beneficence-based obligations to the fetus against beneficence-based and autonomy-based obligations to the pregnant woman. Any such balancing must recognize that a pregnant woman is obligated only to take reasonable risks of medical interventions that are reliably expected to benefit the viable fetus or child later.

Obviously, any strategy for directive counseling for fetal benefit that takes account of obligations to the pregnant woman must be open to the possibility of conflict between the physician's recommendation and a pregnant woman's autonomous decision to the contrary. Such conflict is best managed preventively through the informed consent process as an ongoing dialogue throughout a woman's pregnancy, augmented as necessary by negotiation and respectful persuasion [9].

Critical care as a trial of management

Critical care should be understood not as an all-or-nothing intervention but as a trial of management that can justifiably be discontinued when its goals are unlikely to be met. This may seem a jarring concept when a younger, previously healthy population of patients, such as pregnant women, is concerned. However, conditions, diseases, or injuries that warrant admission of a pregnant woman to a critical care unit are by definition very serious, which means that the limits of medicine to alter the course of disease or injury may be reached in the course of a critical care admission. Losing sight of this clinical reality sets up ethical conflict for the physician, the critical care team, the patient, and her family. Critical care may reach such limits with respect to either its short-term or its long-term goals.

Critical care has a short-term goal, the prevention of imminent death. Critical care is usually very effective at achieving this goal. When it is no longer reasonable in evidence-based consideration to expect that imminent death can be prevented, there is no beneficence-based obligation to continue.

Critical care also has a long-term goal, survival with an acceptable outcome. "Acceptable outcome" should be understood from either a clinical or a patient's perspective. The clinical perspective is beneficence based. When critical care is no longer expected to achieve survival with at least some interactive capacity, there is no beneficence-based obligation to continue. The patient's perspective is autonomy based. When critical care is expected to achieve survival with at least some interactive capacity but with a quality of life not acceptable to the patient, there is no autonomy-based obligation to continue. "Quality of life" means engaging in life tasks such as family life and pursuing meaningful activities and deriving satisfaction from doing so. There is no philosophical theory to support any claim about what life tasks are worth pursuing and how much satisfaction from doing so is enough. These are matters for each patient to determine for herself.

The stopping rules for critical care as a trial of intervention should be based on whether the short-term goal can be achieved. When it is no longer reasonable to expect this goal to be achieved, the beneficence-based obligation to continue critical care as a trial of intervention no longer exists. The stopping rules should also be based on the whether the long-term goals can be achieved. When it is no longer reasonable to expect that the long-term goals, from either a clinical or patient's perspective, can be achieved, then, respectively, the beneficence-based obligation or the autonomy-based obligation to continue critical care as a trial of intervention no longer exists.

Maternal critical care is ethically more complex when the fetus is a patient. After viability, discontinuation of critical care management should include delivery of the fetal patient. This is because there is beneficence-based obligation to protect the fetal patient's life and health, and delivery, including immediate postmortem delivery, does not violate

beneficence-based obligations to the pregnant woman. For the previable fetus, continuation of critical management for fetal benefit, including continuation after the pregnant woman is determined to be dead by accepted brain-function criteria, should be undertaken only when she has explicitly authorized this or when a valid surrogate authorizes it on the basis of the patient's wishes and there is a plan for the delivery of the viable fetal patient if continued critical care becomes ineffective in maintaining the pregnant woman in a stable condition.

A preventive ethics approach to decisions about maternal critical care

Preventive ethics uses the informed consent process to anticipate and prevent ethical conflict between patients and their physicians [9]. Preventive ethics should play a very prominent role in maternal critical care. There are distinctive, but complementary, roles for the physician and patient.

The physician's role is to explain to the pregnant patient before critical care is initiated its nature as a trial of management. The physician should explain both the short-term and the long-term goals and the possibility that they might not be achieved. The physician should explain that, if this becomes the case, discontinuing critical care management and discharging the patient to hospice care is the ethical standard of care. The patient's wishes should be elicited. The physician should make every effort to help patients who request that everything be done to understand that not every reduction in the risk of mortality is worth the disease-related and iatrogenic morbidity that result, because these can greatly reduce or even eliminate the ability of the patient to experience a quality of life that she would want for herself. Seriously ill patients who "want everything done" often do not appreciate what this means in clinical reality, setting up preventable ethical conflict.

It is now possible for patients to formally express their wishes about maternal critical care in the form of what in the USA are called "advance directives," a concept and practice pioneered in the USA. The practice of medicine in the American federal system of self-government is regulated by the individual states. Spurred by the famous case of Karen Quinlan in New Jersey in 1976 [10], the first end-of-life case to be adjudicated, all states have enacted advance directive legislation [11]. Some states do not allow an advance directive to be applied to limit life-sustaining treatment of a terminally or irreversibly ill pregnant patient. This restriction has not been challenged in the courts.

The basic ethical idea of an advance directive is independent of how it is implemented in law and public policy in the USA. The ethical idea is that a patient, when autonomous, can make decisions regarding her medical management in advance of a time during which she becomes incapable of making her own healthcare decisions. The ethical dimensions of autonomy that are relevant here are the following. A patient may exercise her autonomy now in the form of a request for or refusal of life-prolonging interventions. Autonomy-based request or refusal, expressed in the past and left unchanged, remains in effect for any future time during which the patient becomes non-autonomous (i.e. in the clinical judgment of her attending physician, she no longer has decision-making capacity). That past autonomy-based request or refusal, therefore, creates the physician's obligations at the time the patient becomes unable to participate in the informed consent process. In particular, refusal of life-prolonging medical intervention should translate into the withholding or withdrawal of such interventions, including discontinuation of maternal critical care as a trial of intervention. This ethical reasoning can be applied clinically in countries without advance directive legislation, guided by competent legal advice.

The living will or directive to physicians is an instrument that permits the patient to make a direct decision, usually to refuse life-prolonging medical intervention in the future. The living will becomes effective when the patient is a "qualified patient," usually terminally or irreversibly ill, and is also not able to participate in the informed consent process as judged by her physician. Court review is not required. Obviously, terminally or irreversibly ill patients who are able to participate in the informed consent process retain their autonomy to make their own decisions. Some states prescribe the wording of the living will, and others do not. A living will, to be useful and effective, should be as explicit as possible. Readers in jurisdictions that sanction such advance directives should become familiar with them and with organizational policies for their preparation, documentation in the record, and implementation.

The concept of a durable power of attorney or medical power of attorney is that any autonomous adult, in the event that that person later becomes unable to participate in the informed consent process, can assign decision-making authority to another person. The advantage of the durable power of attorney for healthcare is that it applies only when the patient has lost decision-making capacity, as judged by his or her physician. Court review is not required. It does not, as does the living will, also require that the patient also be terminally or irreversibly ill. However, unlike the living will, the durable power of attorney does not necessarily provide explicit direction, only the explicit assignment of decision-making authority to an identified individual or "agent." Obviously, any patient who assigns durable power of attorney for healthcare to someone else has an interest in communicating his or her values, beliefs, and preferences to that person. The physician can play a facilitating role in this process. Indeed, in order to protect the patient's autonomy, the physician should play an active role in encouraging this communication process so that there will be minimal doubt about whether the person holding durable power of attorney is faithfully representing the wishes of the patient. The pregnant patient is free to name anyone of her choosing to act as her agent.

The main clinical advantages of these two forms of advance directives are that they encourage patients to think carefully in advance about their request for or refusal of medical intervention, and that these directives, therefore, help to prevent ethical conflicts and crises in the management, particularly, of terminally or irreversibly ill patients who no longer have decision-making capacity and for whom the stopping rules of critical care as a trial of intervention apply. The reader is encouraged to think of advance directives as powerful, practical strategies for preventive ethics for end-of-life care, and to encourage patients who are candidates for maternal critical care to consider them seriously. The use of advance directives prevents the experience of increased burden of decision making in the absence of reliable information about the patient's values and beliefs [12].

For patients without advance directives, medical ethics accepts surrogate decision making. Many legal jurisdictions do as well. Two standards, in priority, guide surrogate decision making. The first is the "substituted judgment" standard. This standard is autonomy based. This calls for the surrogate, as best as he or she can, to make decisions based on the values and beliefs of the patient. The physician can help surrogates to implement this standard by asking the surrogate to describe what was important to the patient, particularly life tasks that she valued. The physician can then provide his or her best judgment about the projected functional status of the patient and its implications for undertaking those life tasks. Doing so helps the surrogate to make a reliable decision about whether the long-term goal of critical care from the patient's perspective can be achieved. When a surrogate cannot meet the substituted judgment standard, which is probably unlikely for a married pregnant patient, the best interests standard applies. This standard is beneficence based. The physician, therefore, plays a leading role in implementing this standard. When the short-term goal of critical care cannot be achieved, the physician should explain that this is the case and that it is consistent with good medical care to discontinue critical care and transfer the patient to a hospice program. The physician's role is the same when the long-term goal from a clinical perspective cannot be achieved.

Conclusions

Maternal critical care is an essential component of comprehensive obstetric care. Maternal critical care is ethically challenging because it involves recognizing the limits of medicine to alter the course of serious injury or disease in the context of pregnancy. Physicians should respond to these ethical challenges with a preventive ethics approach. Like all critical care, maternal critical care should be understood by physicians and presented to pregnant patients or their surrogates as a trial of management with both short-term and long-term goals. Beneficence-based and autonomy-based stopping rules for the trial of intervention should shape the physician's role in the informed consent process for continuation of maternal critical care. Patients in jurisdictions that provide for them should be encouraged to formalize their decisions with advance directives and to have open and honest discussions in advance with those who could become surrogate decision makers.

References

1. McCullough LB, Chervenak FA. *Ethics in Obstetrics and Gynecology*. New York: Oxford University Press, 1994.

2. Engelhardt HT Jr. *The Foundations of Bioethics*, 2nd edn. New York: Oxford University Press, 1995.

3. Beauchamp TL, Childress JF. *Principles of Biomedical Ethics*. 5th edn. New York: Oxford University Press, 2001.

4. Chervenak FA, McCullough LB, Brent RL. The professional responsibility model of obstetric ethics: avoiding the perils of clashing rights. *Am J Obstet Gynecol* 2011**315**:e1–e5.

5. Hippocrates. Oath of Hippocrates. In Temkin O, Temkin CL (eds.) *Ancient Medicine: Selected Papers of Ludwig Edelstein*. Baltimore, MD: Johns Hopkins University Press, 1976, p. 6.

6. *Schloendorff v. The Society of The New York Hospital*, 211 N.Y. 125, 126, 105 N.E. 92, 93 (1914).

7. Faden RR, Beauchamp TL. *A History and Theory of Informed Consent*. New York: Oxford University Press, 1986.

8. Chervenak FA, McCullough LB, Levene MI. An ethically justified clinically comprehensive approach to peri-viability: gynaecological, obstetric, perinatal, and neonatal dimensions. *J Obstet Gynaecol* 2007;**27**:3–7.

9. Chervenak FA, McCullough LB. Clinical guides to preventing ethical conflicts between pregnant women and their physicians. *Am J Obstet Gynecol* 1990;**162**:303–307.

10. In re *Quinlan*355 A.2d 647 (1976), *cert. denied sub nom.*

11. Meisel L. *The Right to Die*, 2nd edn. New York: John Wiley, 1995.

12. Braun UK, Beyth RJ, Ford ME, McCullough LB. The burdens of end-of-life decision making: voices of female African-American, Caucasian, and Hispanic surrogates. *J Gen Intern Med* 2008;**23**:267–274.

Support of the family and staff

Renee D. Boss and Carl Waldman

Introduction

A critical illness in a pregnant woman is often a crisis for her entire family – the woman herself, her fetus, her partner, other children, and extended family and loved ones. The family burden becomes even greater if the infant is delivered and requires intensive care while the mother remains critically ill. In addition to stabilizing and treating the patient's acute medical problems, interdisciplinary clinicians must also anticipate and address the family's needs; this optimizes their ability to be fully engaged in supporting the patient, supporting each other, and acting as surrogate decision makers. While individual families have unique challenges and needs, a number of resources from clinicians and the healthcare system can benefit most families.

Critical care staff caring for the patient and her fetus or newborn also benefit from systematic supports, as they are repeatedly exposed to patient trauma, family crisis, and loss. Failure to routinely address staff moral and emotional distress can result in compassion fatigue and burnout.

This chapter will review the supports that can be provided to both families and staff in these scenarios.

Case 7.1. A 32-year-old woman at 23 weeks of gestation with a male fetus: Part 1

Ana Martinez is a 32-year-old woman currently pregnant at 23 weeks of gestation with a male fetus. Today, her husband has just dropped off their healthy 5- and 7-year-old daughters at school when his phone rings. Ana tells him that the headache she has had since yesterday is getting much worse. Can he take her to the doctor? When Raul arrives at home, Ana is lying on the kitchen floor, unresponsive and pale. Raul calls an ambulance, and Ana is taken to the emergency department of the local community hospital.

After 3 hours, doctors tell Raul that his wife is being transferred to the university hospital in the nearest city. He calls a neighbor to arrange for her to pick up his children after school, then drives 100 miles to see his wife in the intensive care unit. There he is told that Ana has suffered a large stroke and is on a breathing machine. The doctors are performing tests to better understand why this happened. The fetal heart rate is good now, but they worry that Ana's condition could harm the fetus. When Raul asks, "But my wife and baby are going to be okay, right?" he is told the doctors are doing everything they can.

Practical concerns

For family members and loved ones faced with the critical illness of a pregnant woman, multiple practical concerns can impair their ability to assimilate complicated medical information and remain engaged with the medical team. Families who perceive a lack of clear and timely information about their loved one's condition in the intensive care unit (ICU) are more likely to display symptoms of acute stress disorder [1]. Therefore, it is vital both to deliver this information to families and, equally, to minimize practical stressors so that they can be ready to understand that information. Cost-effective interdisciplinary supports can be instituted upon ICU admission with a goal of keeping families from becoming so overwhelmed that they cannot adequately support the patient or each other [2–4].

Regionalization of hospitals equipped to manage both critically ill pregnant women and critically ill neonates means that many families will have to travel significant distances between home and hospital. Occasionally, it is possible that the mother may remain in a critical care unit in one hospital while the baby is transferred to a regional neonatal critical care facility

---

Maternal Critical Care: A Multidisciplinary Approach, ed. Marc Van de Velde, Helen Scholefield, and Lauren A. Plante.
Published by Cambridge University Press. © Cambridge University Press 2013.

some distance away; this puts relatives under added stress as they will have to be present in two hospitals. This can continue for weeks or months, even after the mother recovers if the infant remains in the neonatal ICU, resulting in both a logistical and a financial burden for many families [5]. Families place great importance on being able to remain physically close to the ICU patient [4,6]. Hospitals can assist families with vouchers for petrol, parking, taxis, and buses. Families can also benefit from opportunities to stay in hospital-sponsored housing, where families may stay from days to weeks during the hospitalization. It is important to be aware of which housing options are unavailable to young families, either because small children or parents younger than 18 years of age are not permitted.

Financial concerns are often very immediate and distressing to families, who may rely on the mother's income to meet living expenses. Not only is this income suddenly gone, but her ability to return to work may also be uncertain. In many settings, the woman's health insurance, and that for her infant, may also be threatened by the loss of her job or her partner's job. In addition, family members may also have inflexible leave policies and may have to choose between being present in the ICU and continuing to work to support the family. Helping families to negotiate these concerns, such as providing letters to explain work absences and flexible visiting hours, is beneficial. In situations where the mother's illness either leads to or occurs at the time of delivery, families must also manage the stressor of a newborn, and possibly a sick newborn. Developing strategies to support families that bridge the adult and neonatal ICUs can help families to divide their time between these locations.

Many families struggle to secure safe, flexible, and reliable child care for the patient's children while she is hospitalized. Small children require full-time care; older children need help maintaining routines of school and activities. Hospital and ICU policies may limit the visitation by children, which, in turn, limits visits by other family members. When children are allowed to visit their mother or new sibling in the ICU, it is important to help the family prepare children for what they will see, in order to minimize additional stress [7,8]. While staff may have concerns that children will be unduly upset by seeing their parent or sibling in the ICU, data suggest that properly supporting children through these visits can be beneficial, particularly when it is possible that the patient could die [8].

Benefits afforded to new mothers in the form of maternity leave and/or paid support differ widely and impact patients recovering from complicated pregnancies and deliveries. In the USA, a woman can take up to 12 weeks of leave by law but her employer is under no obligation to pay her for that time. Women in the UK have extensive statutory rights to maternity benefits. Patients may need help accessing the benefits that are due to them.

An important step toward making interventions for families both relevant and cost-effective is ongoing evaluation of family satisfaction. Examples of such instruments are the Critical Care Family Needs Inventory [9], the Critical Care Family Satisfaction Survey [10], and the Needs Met Inventory [11].

Case 7.1. A 32-year-old woman at 23 weeks of gestation with a male fetus: Part 2

Ana Martinez remains intubated and responsive to pain only. The first evening of her ICU stay, a social worker helps Raul Martinez to arrange for his sister to care for his children for at least a few days, and also arranges for local housing for him during that time. A letter is faxed to his employee explaining his absence. Raul receives vouchers for the hospital cafeteria. A nurse practitioner sends a prescription for his asthma medication to the hospital pharmacy as he forgot to bring his medicines with him. The ICU doctors tell him they will plan to meet again at 8 a.m. to discuss Ana's progress; Ana's nurse confirms that she will accompany Raul during the conversation. Although Raul speaks English very well, he is offered, and accepts, the presence of a Spanish medical interpreter for all conversations with the clinical team.

Informational needs

With systems in place to address the practical needs of families in ICU, clinicians can begin the ongoing process of helping the family to understand the patient's medical condition. Studies of families whose loved one is being transported to [5] and hospitalized in [4] the ICU suggest that families consistently want clinicians to provide them with timely information about their loved one's condition. This information can be broadly divided into three types: information about the current medical condition, information about management plans and options, and prognostic information about potential short- and long-term outcomes for mother and fetus. Depending on the individual family's composition, details of legal surrogacy, or concerns regarding protected patient information, not all family members will want or receive all types of information.

Before initiating conversations with family about the patient's condition, management, and prognosis, it is important to ask those individuals how detailed they would like this information to be. Some families will want to know about every aspect of the patient's care, from overall condition to names of medications. Other families can tolerate no more than a general understanding of what is happening. Clinicians should respect family preferences for information as much as possible. Recognizing that some situations are so urgent that only a brief conversation is possible prior to a change in patient status or need for management decision, whenever possible it is preferable to deliver smaller amounts of information over several conversations with the family. This allows them time to digest information and formulate questions more effectively.

For most families, the threats to the health of the mother and fetus will be sudden and unexpected. Families commonly have no preparation for understanding the medical complications or the realities of ICU care. In some situations, a woman's critical illness will be a known complication of a chronic medical condition, such as for women with pre-existing severe renal disease. In these scenarios, the family may be fairly well informed and ready to understand fairly complex information from early on in the hospitalization. Clinicians can tailor information to the family's understanding by first asking what they know about the current medical problems; the family's responses will offer clinicians insight into how detailed and sophisticated the initial conversations can be. It should always be remembered that intense emotion interferes with families' abilities to hear and process cognitive information; families should be given opportunities to have information repeated and ask questions as often as possible.

Intensive care units should develop routine times, locations, and triggers for meeting with families to deliver information. Particularly early on in the hospitalization, families appreciate clear explanations about the ICU routines, the types of personnel caring for the patient, and the technologies and equipment being used. Many ICUs invite families to be present for daily rounds. Families benefit from this opportunity not only to receive an update on the patient's condition but also to be engaged in the deliberation of management decisions [12]. Communicating with families regularly during rounds can also increase efficiency for clinicians, who are able to regularly anticipate when a family will be available for conversation.

Clinicians should strive to provide consistent information to families, as families are stressed by conflicting information about their loved one's care. This task is made challenging by the rapid rate of clinical change within an ICU environment and the number of different clinicians interacting with families. Communication strategies such as weekly interdisciplinary rounds to coordinate patient care can be very effective [13]. Developing regular expectations for communication among the medical team can also reduce distress among staff.

Families' needs for information may continue after ICU discharge. Families, including the patient herself, may have ongoing questions about the medical problems and implications for future health and pregnancies. Designating a team member to regularly contact the patient and/or family in the days or weeks following ICU discharge can identify these concerns; families with significant concerns should be offered an opportunity to meet face to face with clinicians.

In the UK, there is an increasing trend for patients managed in a critical care environment to be "followed-up" with their relatives in an ICU follow-up clinic. This should be a multidisciplinary service to ensure the physical, psychological, and cognitive aftermath of a stay in a critical care unit is addressed. In the UK, care of patients after critical care has been very limited and very variable. One large three-center study, PRaCTICAL, showed no difference in outcome after a nurse-led follow-up service was implemented for patients after critical illness [14]. It would be interesting in the future to do a similar study where follow-up was performed by a multidisciplinary team.

Shared decision making

When a pregnant woman becomes critically ill, the threats to her health and that of her fetus may necessitate multiple decisions about medical management. When the patient is not able to participate in these decisions, conversations about preferred management and informed consent may occur with surrogate decision makers from the family. These discussions may be fairly routine, such as obtaining informed consent for a transfusion, or they may require complex decision making that weighs risk and benefit to both mother and fetus.

The degree to which family members are involved in medical decision making certainly varies among cultures and countries. In some settings, clinicians make all management decisions with no expectation that the patient or family will be asked to participate or will even be made aware of management options. In many settings, patients and families are afforded significant autonomy, as when choosing among various treatment strategies for a disease or weighing the risks and benefits of non-standard therapies. Whether families have full or limited autonomy in medical decision making, feeling supported by clinicians throughout the process may be just as important to them as the decisions themselves [15].

Even in cultures where patients and families are expected to participate in decision making, clinicians should begin this process by assessing the individual patient's and family's desire for decision-making responsibility. Most patients and families want to make decisions with clinicians; a minority want to make decisions completely independently, and some prefer not to participate in decisions at all. Clinicians should be ready to respect a patient's or family's preferences. If a patient is not competent, identifying the legal surrogate decision maker is of paramount importance. The legal surrogate for the mother may not be the legal surrogate for the newborn. For example, the legal surrogate for a 16-year-old mother may be her parents, while the legal surrogate for the neonate may be mother's 17-year-old boyfriend and the father of the infant.

Unique conflicts may arise when the mother's health problems, or the medical treatments indicated for those problems, threaten the health of the fetus [16,17]. Deliberating decisions about the mother's care can be accompanied by significant conflict – among family members, between family members and clinicians, or among clinicians. Clinicians are not traditionally well trained to manage conflict, and they should incorporate institutional resources into the decision-making process. In some situations, it may be difficult to establish an approach to care that balances the competing interests of mother and fetus; in such settings, consultation with local ethicists or hospital ethics committees is indicated.

> **Case 7.1.** A 32-year-old woman at 23 weeks of gestation with a male fetus: Part 3
>
> Raul Martinez attends rounds in the ICU daily, nearly always with the Spanish medical interpreter. Ana has suffered a ruptured cerebral aneurism, and by day 4 of her ICU hospitalization it appears that her intracranial pressure is beginning to normalize and she is intermittently more responsive. Raul is the legal surrogate and has been asked to sign consent forms for transfusions and central lines. He often discusses these decisions with his brother and his sister-in-law; sometimes clinicians talk with the extended family by phone at Raul's request. The Martinez children plan to visit on the weekend with a child life consultant.
>
> On day 5 of the ICU admission, Ana begins to have contractions. Because premature delivery is possible, a neonatologist counsels the family about predicted outcomes and complications of prematurity. The family is very worried that the baby could be born early, and even more worried that childbirth could make Ana sicker. They are confused by discussions about steroids and fetal monitoring, and possible cesarean section. Raul wishes someone would tell him what is the right thing to do. Some staff members are also upset, particularly that a cesarean section might be performed for a baby who would be so likely to die even with neonatal intensive care.
>
> On hospital day 6, Ana's contractions continue and cervical dilation ensues. She remains intubated, with no increasing awareness. Her husband is sad and overwhelmed and becomes angry when the new ICU physician seems unaware of the conversations had the day before. The patient's nurse suggests a family meeting that afternoon, to be attended by Raul and his brother and sister-in-law, the interpreter, the social worker, a chaplain, two nurses, the neonatologist, three physicians regularly involved in the patient's care, and a member of the hospital ethics committee.

Emotional support for family members

Pregnant patients in the ICU who are conscious require the emotional and psychological support needed by any adult with a critical illness. This includes opportunities to articulate goals and values, to ask questions, and to express worries and fears. The pregnant patient often has unique stressors that, left unaddressed, can further complicate her recovery. The pregnant patient may feel tremendous responsibility and guilt that she has done something to harm her fetus, or that she could have premature labor [18]. Regardless of the outcome of the mother's critical illness, she may need support as she grieves the loss of a "normal" pregnancy. Clinicians should guide patients through discussions about how to hope for the best while preparing for the worst [19].

Staff should also anticipate that the patient's family will also need emotional support, as family members who feel emotionally abandoned by clinicians in the ICU are more likely to have acute stress disorder [1]. The patient's husband or next of kin must suddenly assume new responsibilities and roles that can be very overwhelming, and is likely to be afraid of losing both the patient and their baby. In situations where the patient delivers the infant, it can be very difficult to manage the care of the new baby with the mother's medical condition. Extended family members can also be devastated by the hospitalization. Practical and emotional support from ICU staff can help to maintain the integrity of the family.

For patients who have other children, staff should be prepared to help them to understand their mother's illness and the disruption of their family. In some scenarios, they will also need help in understanding their newborn sibling's illness. This support should be delivered in a developmentally appropriate way. Child life specialists can be wonderful resources for the ICU team.

Many families find solace in their religious or spiritual beliefs, and involving a chaplain early in the hospitalization can be helpful. Because a family's religious beliefs may impact their approach to health, disease, pregnancy, and decision making, it is important to explore these beliefs. While clinicians are not trained to engage in these discussions alone, a willingness to initiate these conversations and to involve members of the pastoral care team is necessary.

End-of-life issues

While maternal, fetal, and neonatal mortality rates continue to fall worldwide, there will still be situations where clinicians are unable to save the life of the mother and/or infant. Given that pregnant women are often young, without serious pre-existing medical problems, and with other small children, this loss can be completely unexpected and devastating for family and staff alike.

As opposed to other areas of critical care, very rarely does a pregnant woman, or a neonate, have an advance directive. Should the ICU patient at any point be able to participate in discussions regarding advance directives for herself or her infant, she should be asked to name a surrogate for herself and the infant should that become necessary. Decisions about life-sustaining therapies should be discussed and documented. Clinicians need to also be aware of legal exceptions related to advance directives during pregnancy. For example, several states in the USA invalidate advance directives during pregnancy, or require a dated and signed directive for each of a woman's pregnancies.

Where available, consultation from a palliative care team should be sought to assist with goals of care, end-of-life planning, promoting patient comfort and quality of life, and supporting staff. Prenatal palliative care is increasingly available for patients who anticipate or experience a fetal or neonatal death [20]. These supports will be particularly important for families who also anticipate the possibility of maternal death. For the pregnant patient with a life-limiting condition who does not need intensive care, the potential for labor requires specialized hospice arrangements, which includes guidelines for neonatal interventions.

Families require support in the ICU of their anticipatory grief surrounding the loss of the woman and/or her fetus. Bereavement support should be readily available to families both during the hospitalization and, whenever possible, for months to years following the death. Because bereaved families may most benefit from the support of family and friends, clinicians have an important role in making sure that these supports are engaged.

Supporting staff

The interdisciplinary team may struggle with the stress and emotions of caring for critically ill pregnant women. The patient's obstetrician or midwife may worry that he or she failed to prevent the pregnancy complications and may feel excluded from the ICU. Where a pregnant women is hospitalized in a medical ICU, the ICU nurses and doctors may be unfamiliar with the complexities of managing both mother and fetus. Staff may confront fears about their own pregnancies or children. Conflict may exist within the clinical team. Individual team members may experience moral distress if asked to provide care for the mother that could harm the fetus. Concerns about malpractice may add to the stress.

In 2009, the first influenza pandemic for 40 years developed through the novel 2009/H1N1 virus and became a worldwide challenge to modern intensive care medicine. In the *Journal of the Intensive Care Society*, a case was presented illustrating how a pregnant woman was managed. It was already well known that pregnancy increased susceptibility to influenza and the risk of complications was greater, but at the time of the pandemic, experience in the management of this group of patients in the critical care environment was limited.

The case of a young pregnant patient with 2009/H1N1 pneumonitis illustrates these issues by exploring the difficult decision to perform a potentially life-threatening procedure in the absence of consent and without knowledge of unequivocal benefit. While this case occurred during the "swine flu" pandemic, the issues raised equally well apply to the care of any pregnant, obtunded patients within the ICU [21].

In English law, the fetus has no rights until it is born. This may be morally difficult, but the legal position is clear [22].

If the mother lacked capacity to consent, then the fetus would still not accrue any rights, and treatment should be determined by the best interests of the mother (although this *might* include consideration for her unborn child).

Supporting staff members and enabling them to continue their important work requires a culture which permits expression of emotion, confusion, and conflict. Organizational supports such as regular debriefing opportunities with mental health professionals, rituals of patient remembrance, and educational offerings around coping with stress and grief can all be beneficial.

Case 7.1. A 32-year-old woman at 23 weeks of gestation with a male fetus: Part 4

One hour before the interdisciplinary team could meet with the Martinez family, fetal heart tones were lost. Because of ongoing worry about the patient's health and the periviable gestational age, a cesarean section was not performed. The chaplain and palliative care team were called to support the family and to help Raul prepare to tell his wife about the loss of their baby once she was more awake. Plans were made with the child life specialist for the children to visit their mother and to be told about fetal death.

References

1. Auerbach SM, Kiesler DJ, Wartella J, *et al.* Optimism, satisfaction with needs met, interpersonal perceptions of the healthcare team, and emotional distress in patients' family members during critical care hospitalization. *Am J Crit Care* 2005;**14**:202–210.

2. Maxwell KE, Stuenkel D, Saylor C. Needs of family members of critically ill patients: a comparison of nurse and family perceptions. *Heart Lung* 2007;**36**:367–376.

3. Kosco M, Warren NA. Critical care nurses' perceptions of family needs as met. *Crit Care Nurs Q* 2000;**23**:60–72.

4. Verhaeghe S, Defloor T, Van Zuuren F, Duijnstee M, Grypdonck M. The needs and experiences of family members of adult patients in an intensive care unit: a review of the literature. *J Clin Nurs* 2005;**14**:501–509.

5. Perez L, Alexander D, Wise L. Interfacility transport of patients admitted to the ICU: perceived needs of family members. *Air Med J* 2003;**22**:44–48.

6. Bijttebier P, Vanoost S, Delva D, Ferdinande P, Frans E. Needs of relatives of critical care patients: perceptions of relatives, physicians and nurses. *Intensive Care Med* 2001;**27**:160–165.

7. Knutsson SE, Bergbom IL. Custodians' viewpoints and experiences from their child's visit to an ill or injured nearest being cared for at an adult intensive care unit. *J Clin Nurs* 2007;**16**:362–371.

8. Clarke C, Harrison D. The needs of children visiting on adult intensive care units: a review of the literature and recommendations for practice. *J Adv Nurs* 2001;**34**:61–68.

9. Leske JS. Internal psychometric properties of the Critical Care Family Needs Inventory. *Heart Lung* 1991;**20**:236–244.

10. Wasser T, Matchett S. Final version of the Critical Care Family Satisfaction Survey questionnaire. *Crit Care Med* 2001;**29**:1654–1655.

11. Warren NA. Perceived needs of the family members in the critical care waiting room. *Crit Care Nurs Q* 1993;**16**:56–63.

12. Schiller WR, Anderson BF. Family as a member of the trauma rounds: a strategy for maximized communication. *J Trauma Nurs* 2003;**10**:93–101.

13. Halm MA, Gagner S, Goering M, *et al.* Interdisciplinary rounds: impact on patients, families, and staff. *Clin Nurse Spec* 2003;**17**:133–142.

14. Cuthbertson BH, Rattray J, Campbell MK, *et al.* The PRaCTICaL study of nurse led, intensive care follow-up programmes for improving long term outcomes from critical illness: a pragmatic randomised controlled trial. *BMJ* 2009;**339**:b3723.

15. Orfali K, Gordon EJ. Autonomy gone awry: a cross-cultural study of parents' experiences in neonatal intensive care units. *Theor Med Bioethics* 2004;**25**:329–365.

16. Digiovanni LM. Ethical issues in obstetrics. *Obstet Gynecol Clin North Am* 2010;**37**:345–357.

17. Powner DJ, Bernstein IM. Extended somatic support for pregnant women after brain death. *Crit Care Med* 2003;**31**:1241–1249.

18. MacKinnon K. Living with the threat of preterm labor: women's work of keeping the baby in. *J Obstet Gynecol Neonatal Nurs* 2006;**35**:700–708.

19. Back A, Arnold R, Tulsky J. *Mastering Communication with Seriously Ill Patients: Balancing Honesty with Empathy and Hope.* Cambridge, UK: Cambridge University Press, 2009.

20. Leuthner S, Jones EL. Fetal Concerns Program: a model for perinatal palliative care. *Am J Matern Child Nurs* 2007;**32**:272–278.

21. O'Leary RTJ, Nadella V, Bodenham A, Bell D. Termination of pregnancy without maternal consent during H1N1 critical illness. *J Intens Care Soc* 2011;**12**:320–323.

22. *S v St George's Hospital NHS Trust* [1998] 3All ER 673.

Chapter 8

Recovery from intensive care and the next pregnancy

Hennie Lombaard and Neil S. Seligman

Introduction

Severely ill obstetric patients are admitted to intensive care units for various reasons. These include the following [1–3]:

- pregnancy related, for example:
  - hypertensive emergencies
  - obstetric hemorrhage
  - amniotic fluid embolism
- medical conditions aggravated by pregnancy, for example:
  - congenital/acquired heart disease
  - renal failure
- conditions not related to pregnancy, such as trauma.

The process of recovery continues past the discharge from the intensive care unit (ICU). It is important that the healthcare provider understands that there are different types of morbidity that can occur in these patients. These morbidities can be grouped into two major groups [1,4,5]:

- physical morbidity
- non-physical morbidity

Following discharge from ICU, it is important to focus on the management of the condition that resulted in the admission to ICU, as well as the physical and psychological morbidities.

Physical morbidity

Physical morbidity can result from the complications of the primary condition, prolonged ventilation, sedation, and immobility in ICU. Admission to ICU often results in a prolonged period of immobility, which has the effects outlined in Table 8.1 [4,6].

Intensive care unit-acquired weakness

Weakness is caused by either critical illness polyneuropathy or critical illness myopathy. The diagnosis can be made using electrophysiological testing or muscle biopsies. Management of both conditions is the same and so it is more important to diagnose functional weakness and treat it than spending time on making an exact diagnosis [7].

The incidence of ICU-acquired weakness depends on the diagnostic tools used. It varies between 25 and 58% after 7 days of ventilation. In patients with sepsis, the incidence is as high as 50% to 100% [7]. Surveying patients' activity of daily living and instrumental activities of daily living and evaluating their walk distance in 6 minutes are commonly used tools to evaluate the ICU survivors' physical functioning [8].

The risk factors for developing ICU-acquired weakness are immobility, presence of systemic inflammatory response syndrome, multiple organ failure, mechanical ventilation, sepsis, length of ICU admission, malnutrition, hypercapnia, hypoxia, treatment with corticosteroids and neuromuscular-blocking agents, initial heavy sedation, and glycemic control [4,7,9]. Studies have found that tighter glucose control was associated with less muscle weakness.

Rehabilitation should be aimed at obtaining early mobilization. The process starts at the time of admission to ICU, with maintenance of the correct posture and passive mobilization of the limbs. As the patient improves, measures such as sitting up in bed, and thereafter sitting in a chair, are used. The aim of rehabilitation is the return of muscle strength so that the patient can perform basic activities of everyday life [4,6].

Early mobility helps with the recovery from ICU and decreases the time spent in hospital. Several studies have shown improved outcomes after early mobility [9]. In a study that used the following four level

Maternal Critical Care: A Multidisciplinary Approach, ed. Marc Van de Velde, Helen Scholefield, and Lauren A. Plante.
Published by Cambridge University Press. © Cambridge University Press 2013.

Table 8.1. A summary of the physical and non-physical effects associated with admission to intensive care

Morbidity	Changes
Physical	
Skeletal muscles	2% muscle protein loss per day 3–4% reduction in muscle fibers [6] Transformation of muscle fibers from type IIa to IIb Decrease in the number and density of mitochondria
Cardiovascular function and blood composition	Decreased cardiac output and stroke volume Increased heart rate during exercise Increased risk of thrombosis
Respiratory function changes	Decrease in the functional capacity Decreased lung compliance Retained secretions Atelectasis
Body composition	Bone demineralization Protein wastage Decrease in total body water and sodium Loss of body weight Increase in percentage of body fat
Central nervous system	Problems with proprioception Decrease in intellectual function
Non-physical effects	Depression Anxiety Post-traumatic stress disorder

early mobility program, the authors showed an improved outcome:

- level 1: unconscious patients received passive limb mobilization three times per day
- level 2: active limb mobilization in cooperative patients
- level 3: sitting on the edge of the bed
- level 4: active transfer to a chair or walking under strict supervision.

These levels of early mobilization should be adjusted as per the patient's condition. Obstetric patients who have been admitted to ICU because of an underlying medical condition will be able to mobilize earlier than those patients admitted following extensive surgery. It is important to initiate these steps as early as possible so that the patient can take care of herself and her newborn baby.

Other preventative measures for ICU-acquired weakness include aggressive management to prevent sepsis and multiorgan failure, judicious use of sedatives (i.e. avoid deep sedation, or if sedation is necessary, a process of daily interruption or downward titration of sedation), tighter glucose control, and the cautious use of corticosteroids [9,10].

The long-term outcome of ICU-acquired weakness has far-reaching consequences for the patient. In many cases, the physicians are satisfied when the patient is discharged from ICU and subsequently from hospital. Because of a lack of resources, patients are sometimes discharged prematurely from the ICU. The lack of complete recovery may have far-reaching implications for the patient. Studies in a general population have found that patients recovering from ICU have reported poor function as a result of muscle bulk loss, fatigue, and proximal muscle weakness. This had significant implications on their employment status [10]. If this is extrapolated to the obstetric patient, the surviving mother will have difficulties in caring for her baby and the rest of her family.

The basis for treatment of ICU-acquired weakness is early mobilization and prevention. The mobilization can start as early as 36 to 72 hours after intubation [8,10,11]. Advanced technology can also be included in the rehabilitation. This includes neuromuscular electrical stimulation and a dynamic tilt table. Cycling exercises that are started in ICU, even in ventilated patients, also improves their recovery time [8]. A randomized study found that a rehabilitation program of 6 weeks improved the physical outcome of the patients measured at the 8 weeks and 6 months post-ICU follow-up [11]. The UK National Institute for Health and Clinical Excellence guideline on rehabilitation after critical care recommends that an individualized, structured rehabilitation program should be initiated as early as possible during ICU care. This program should continue following transfer to the general ward from ICU. The patient should be discharged from hospital with a self-guided rehabilitation program [1,8]. Figure 8.1 summarizes causes and interventions for ICU-acquired weakness.

Non-physical morbidity

Healthy postpartum women are at increased risk of postpartum depression. Reported incidences of postpartum depression differ between studies. It ranges between 7 and 15% in the first 3 months after delivery [12], up to an overall incidence of 13–21% [13]. When postpartum women are assessed for major depressive disorder, the incidence is 5 to 7% [12].

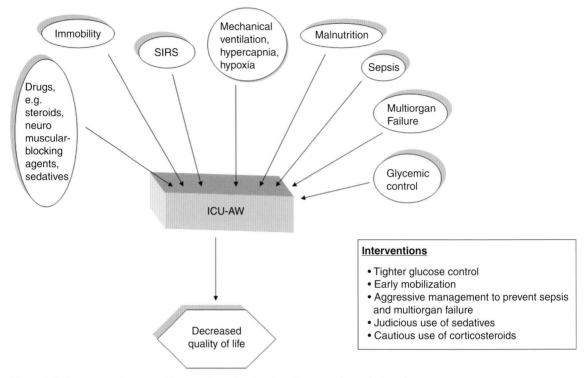

Figure 8.1. A summary of causes and interventions related to intensive care unit-acquired weakness.

Non-physical morbidity includes:

- depression in 25 to 50% of patients [11]
- anxiety, dependent on the oxygen partial pressure ratio and length of mechanical ventilation
- post-traumatic stress disorder (PTSD) in 5–63% [5]
- cognitive dysfunction
- decreased quality of life.

Depression

The risk factors for the development of depression in ICU survivors are [5,8,14,15]:

- young age
- significant alcohol dependence
- length of ICU admission
- duration of mechanical ventilation
- surgical trauma
- maximum organ failure score
- higher body mass index
- history of depression or anxiety
- mean benzodiazepine dose
- poor recollection of ICU stay

- memories of nightmares or fearfulness while in ICU that persist more than 5 days following discharge
- psychotic episodes
- depressive symptoms at the time of discharge
- cognitive impairment
- problems in physical function that persist for 2 to 6 months after discharge from ICU.

In addition, some women would have suffered a perinatal loss, while others may have babies who are also admitted to ICU. Suicide accounts for 20% of maternal deaths in the developed world [16].

The following are potential pathways for the development of psychiatric problems [14]:

- organ dysfunction
- medications
- pain
- sleep deprivation
- ICU treatment
- elevated cytokines
- stress-related activation of the hypothalamic–pituitary axis

- hypoxemia
- neurotransmitter dysfunction.

Depression is a significant risk factor in the obstetric ICU survivor. Screening for depression should form an integral part of the follow-up and rehabilitation of these patients. One of the tools that can be used in the screening of the postpartum ICU survivor is the Edinburgh Postnatal Depression Scale [17] (Table 8.2).

The screening should start at the time of discharge from the hospital and a depression scale assessment should continue at each visit following discharge from hospital. The patient should also be informed of the risk of developing depression and the danger signs to be aware of.

The treatment of postpartum depression has a biopsychosocial basis. Figure 8.2 illustrates the treatment.

Studies have shown that interpersonal psychotherapy and cognitive-behavioral therapy are effective interventions for the treatment of women with postpartum depression [18,19]. Group therapy benefits the woman who feels socially isolated.

In lactating women, group therapy and interpersonal psychotherapy can be the first line of therapy, but in ICU survivors it should form part of the treatment plan and not be the only option.

The antidepressant of choice in lactating women is the selective serotonin reuptake inhibitor (SSRI) [18]. Sertraline is regarded as the drug of choice because it has fewer side effects for the mother and neonate. Second-line options include paroxetine and nortriptyline. Since there is a risk of neonatal effects with antidepressants, the woman should be instructed to take the drug so that it does not have peak plasma concentrations at the time of breastfeeding [18].

Sleep disturbances should be minimized. Such disturbance may result from the inhibition of melatonin production through light exposure during the night while caring for the neonate. This can be reduced by wearing glasses, using blue-blocking light bulbs, or working in settings with very dim light [18].

Light therapy is commonly used for the treatment of postpartum depression. It has a favorable side effect profile, but there is limited research to support its efficacy. Aerobic exercise and walking outside with a pram can also be of value. The added benefit of weight loss and improved muscle tone seems to contribute to the feeling of well-being [18]. Studies have shown that

Table 8.2. Edinburgh Postnatal Depression Scale[a]

In the past seven days:

1. I have been unable to laugh and see the funny side of things	a. As much as I always could b. Not quite as much now c. Definitely not as much now d. Not at all
2. I have looked forward with enjoyment to things	a. As much as I ever did b. Rather less than I used to c. Definitely less than I used to d. Hardly at all
3. I have blamed myself unnecessarily when things went wrong	a. Yes, most of the time b. Yes, some of the time c. Not very often d. No, never
4. I have been anxious or worried for no good reason	a. No, not at all b. Hardly ever c. Yes, sometimes d. Yes, very often
5. I have felt scared or panicky for no very good reason	a. Yes, quite a lot b. Yes, sometimes c. No, not much d. No, not at all
6. Things have been getting on top of me	a. Yes, most of the time I have been unable to cope at all b. Yes, sometimes I haven't been coping as well as usual c. No, most of the time I coped quite well d. No, I have been coping as well as ever
7. I have been so unhappy that I had difficulty in sleeping	a. Yes, most of the time b. Yes, sometimes c. Not very often d. No, not at all
8. I have felt sad or miserable	a. Yes, most of the time b. Yes, sometimes c. Not very often d. No, not at all
9. I have been so unhappy that I have been crying:	a. Yes, most of the time b. Yes, quite often c. Only occasionally d. No, never
10. The thought of harming myself has occurred to me	a. Yes, quite often b. Sometimes c. Hardly ever d. Never

[a]Scores are 0, 1, 2, 3 for answers a–d, respectively. Questions 3, 5, 6, 7, 8, 9, and 10 are scored in reverse. A total score above 12/13 indicates the presence of depression.
Source: Cox JL, Holden JM, Sagovsky R. Detection of postnatal depression. Development of the 10-item Edinburgh Postnatal Depression Scale. *Br J Psychiatry* 1987; **150**: 782–786. [17]. © 1987 Royal College of Psychiatrists.

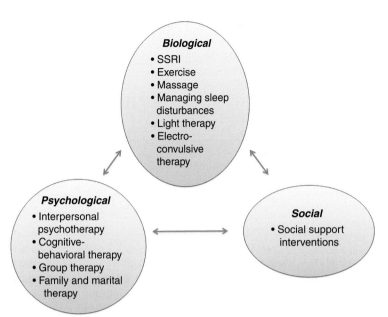

Figure 8.2. Treatment of postpartum depression.

massage by a partner for 20 minutes twice per week for 16 weeks significantly improved depression and anxiety symptoms [18].

In conclusion women recovering from ICU should be screened for depression regularly. Early detection and aggressive management with a multidisciplinary team and family involvement is important.

Post-traumatic stress disorder

The incidence of PTSD differs in the literature between 5% and 63% [6]. Improvement in PTSD may not be seen over the first 12 months after discharge and it can last up to 8 years. Risk factors for PTSD include the following [6,8]:

- recall of delusional memories
- prolonged sedation
- history of pre-existing psychological problems
- physical restraint without sedation
- agitation
- benzodiazepine use.

It is important to recognize women at risk for the development of PTSD and certain measures can be taken to reduce the risk of developing it. These include lighter sedation or daily interruption of sedation, preventing hypoglycemia, and using hydrocortisone, which may be protective [8].

The treatment of PTSD starts in ICU. During follow-up, it is important to ask patients about the symptoms of PTSD and refer appropriately.

Cognitive impairment and delirium

The incidence of cognitive impairment in ICU survivors is between 30 and 73% [8,14]. It appears that this is a long-term complication of critical illness, with 45% of patients still affected at 1 year and 25% at 6 years after discharge [8,14]. Risk factors include delirium, hypoxemia, inflammation, hypotension, hypoglycemia, and sedative and analgesic use. The areas of cognitive function that are affected are tasks requiring memory, executive functioning, and mental processing ability [8,14]. The level of affectation is in many cases severe, with patients falling below the 6th centile of the normal distribution [14], which results in a 41% disability in the patients [5].

Delirium can be present in up to 80% of ICU survivors [5,14]. Delirium results in altered perfusion of the brain, including the frontal, temporal, and subcortical areas. Decreased blood flow in the subcortical area is associated with impaired executive functioning [14]. Magnetic resonance imaging studies have shown brain atrophy and ventricular enlargement in patients with delirium [8,14].

Delirium is linked to the following adverse outcomes [14]:

- prolonged hospitalization
- poor surgical recovery
- increased morbidity
- increased mortality.

In order to help the obstetric patient to recover fully from ICU and enable her to have a good quality of life, measures must be taken to prevent cognitive impairment and delirium. A good understanding of the potential risk factors will help the attending physician to manage the patient in such a way that these risks are limited.

Pregnancy after critical illness

Fertility and pregnancy after recovery from critical illness presents a challenge because of the limited data on which to base counseling. Interest in long-term outcomes is growing because of improvements in survival [20], yet there is a paucity of information and particularly information that would be generalizable to women of reproductive age. Most patients report their health status to be as good as or better than their baseline [21]. However, patients with certain illnesses fare worse than others. For example, survivors of acute respiratory distress syndrome suffer significant decrement in quality of life [20]. Severe illness may have a wide range of adverse consequences on reproductive function through psychosocial maladjustment (see non-physical morbidity above) and/or sexual dysfunction, infertility, and changes in maternal medical condition that predispose to adverse obstetric and neonatal outcomes [22]. This is particularly true following traumatic brain injury. The female reproductive system is sensitive to stress and injury to the central nervous system [22]. Alterations in follicle-stimulating hormone and luteinizing hormone have been documented in women following traumatic brain injury, leading to menstrual irregularities such as skipped periods or amenorrhea [22,23]. In telephone interviews, significantly more women reported skipped periods following traumatic brain injury (23.3% before injury versus 90% after injury; $p < 0.001$) [22]. In this study, the duration of amenorrhea ranged from 20 to 344 days and correlated with the severity of brain injury; amenorrhea resolved after approximately 2 months in 50% of women regardless of the severity of injury. Additionally, there were no reported differences in items measuring fertility; however, only a small number of women ($n = 4$) reported ever becoming pregnant.

In our review of the literature, only a few studies assessed fertility and pregnancy following critical illness. Colantonio *et al.* [24] evaluated 29 women who attempted to conceive or became pregnant after traumatic brain injury compared with matched controls They found no differences in fertility but the number of live births was lower in the brain injury group (62% versus 91%; $p = 0.0045$). Additionally, significantly more women in the brain injury group reported postpartum difficulties, most common of which were fatigue, pain, depression, and mobility problems. The reproductive sequelae of severe maternal morbidity during pregnancy is unclear. Murphy and Charlett [25] reported a high percentage of fertility loss in women admitted to the ICU during pregnancy, labor, or postpartum. Camargo *et al.* [26] suggested that the effect on fertility was at least in part "surgical consequences of childbirth complications." Excluding women who had a hysterectomy or tubal ligation in the index pregnancy, they reported no difference in the rate of subsequent pregnancy compared with healthy healthy controls (92% versus 90.7%).

A novel finding of the study by Camargo *et al.* [26] was that the survivors of a maternal near miss events were more likely to experience complications in the subsequent pregnancy (odds ratio, 5.15; 95% confidence interval, 1.12–23.64). The effects of critical illness on subsequent pregnancy outcomes, if any, are at least partially dependent on the type of illness or injury and treatment. For example, pregnancy following spinal cord injury is associated with an increase in urinary tract infections and pyelonephritis, worsening respiratory impairment, unattended preterm or term birth, autonomic dysreflexia, and other complications [27,28]. Another example is hemorrhage during delivery, which may require admission to ICU. Uterine artery embolization, an alternative to surgical therapy, has been used to control life-threatening bleeding while preserving fertility [29,30]. Pregnancies conceived following uterine artery embolization are generally successful but may be at risk for growth restriction and recurrent hemorrhage [31]. Likewise, gestational hypertensive disorders such as pre-eclampsia also occasionally require admission to the ICU. Fertility is typically unaffected but recurrence rates of 25–65% have been reported, depending on severity (mild pre-eclampsia versus HELLP syndrome), gestational age at onset, and underlying medical conditions, particularly chronic hypertension [32].

It is difficult to generalize recommendations for women who wish to conceive or are currently pregnant after recovery from admission to the ICU because of the significant heterogeneity in the reasons for ICU admission, course of illness and recovery, prior state of health, and sequelae. Ideally, women who wish to conceive after recovery from critical illness should be seen for preconception consultation by a specialist in maternal–fetal medicine. Since approximately half of all pregnancies in the USA are unplanned [33], adequate contraception and a daily prenatal vitamin with at least 400 µg folic acid should be routinely recommended prior to discharge from the hospital. Reproductive-age women in the ICU for conditions unrelated to pregnancy are probably not routinely counseled about prenatal vitamins and contraception as it falls outside the purview of most intensivists/specialists.

A comprehensive preconception consultation should include discussion about pregnancy timing, and a review of the medical history, reason for hospitalization and course, and changes in medical condition resulting from the illness or injury. The World Health Organization (WHO) [34] recommends an interpregnancy interval (the number of months between the date of outcome the preceding pregnancy and conception of the subsequent pregnancy) of at least 24 months following a live birth. A meta-analysis of 26 observational studies concluded that both short and long interpregnancy intervals are associated with an increased risk of adverse perinatal outcomes [35]. Conde-Agudelo *et al.* [35] demonstrated that pregnancies conceived within 18 months of the preceding pregnancy were at increased risk of preterm birth, low birth weight (<2500 g), small for gestational age (birth weight <10th percentile), and stillbirth. Our counseling is consistent with the WHO recommendations regardless of whether the pregnancy was complicated by admission to the ICU. The optimal timing of pregnancy following admission to the ICU for non-obstetric reasons is unclear. Nonetheless, we suggest delaying conception when there are modifiable risk factors. For example, a woman with diabetes who was recently admitted to the ICU for diabetic ketoacidosis and whose hemoglobin A1c is still elevated should be counseled to improve her blood sugar control before conceiving.

Equally, if not more, important is a thorough review of the medical history, reason for hospitalization and course, and changes in medical condition resulting from the illness or injury. Most maternal–fetal medicine specialists are well versed in counseling about medical conditions ranging from asthma to solid organ transplant; however, counseling for women who have recovered from critical illness is much more complex. As discussed above, the risks of pregnancy following recovery from critical illness are not generalizable; myocardial infarction, for example, cannot be compared with pregnancy after a motor vehicle accident. Counseling should address any risks to the pregnancy that might result from the inciting event or condition as well as any new risks resulting from sequelae (e.g. progression of a pre-existing illness such as worsening glomerular filtration rate in a woman with chronic renal disease).

For most conditions, counseling can be divided into two parts: the risk of pregnancy on the condition (e.g. the risk of maternal mortality with dilated cardiomyopathy) and the risk of the condition on pregnancy (e.g. chronic hypertension and pre-eclampsia). In some circumstances, pregnancy may not be advisable (e.g. pulmonary hypertension, Eisenmenger syndrome). It is our practice to attempt to obtain and review all of the records pertaining to the illness and follow-up care. Often the reason for ICU admission needs to be interpreted within the context of the resources of the treating hospital. In other words, an illness or injury requiring ICU management in one hospital may be equally well managed on a regular unit in another hospital. Medications may be added or changed. The decision to continue any medication during pregnancy should be based on a careful assessment of the risks and benefits. Useful resources for assessing medication risks during pregnancy and lactation include Reprotox [36], TERIS [37], Drugs in Pregnancy and Lactation [38], Drugs During Pregnancy and Lactation [39], and Lactmed [40].

Depression is a common problem in ICU survivors (see above), which exemplifies several of the issues in counseling women who are pregnant or are contemplating pregnancy after recovery from critical illness. Depression during pregnancy increases the risk of poor prenatal care, poor weight gain, comorbid psychiatric conditions, self-medication, worsening depression, and postpartum depression. Other adverse outcomes such as low birth weight and preterm birth have been reported, but a causal link has not been clearly established [41]. Neonates of depressed parents are at increased risk of psychiatric problems and non-psychiatric medical disorders compared with infants of non-depressed parents [41]. Selective SSRIs are commonly used as the first-line agent for medical treatment of depression. There are no confirmed birth defects associated with their use and most fall into US Food and Drug Administration category C (risks cannot be ruled out in humans) [38]; however, SSRI use during pregnancy has been associated with transient neonatal withdrawal issues and an unconfirmed increase in primary pulmonary hypertension (6–12 per 1000 women) [42]. Relapse of depression is much more common among women who discontinue medication during pregnancy (68% versus 25%) [43]; therefore, we recommend that women continue antidepressant medications during pregnancy.

The ususal preconception recommendations about lifestyle should be offered. Women who become pregnant should be referred for counseling as soon as possible after conception. While preconception counseling is ideal, the principles of counseling women who are already pregnant are essentially the same, including a review of the history, condition that led to ICU admission, hospital course, and sequelae. Since critical illness and severe maternal morbidity can be so emotionally intense that it leads to psychological sequelae, the need for added and frequent patient and family support should be anticipated. Intimate partner, family, and other social support should be carefully evaluated. Care should be structured in such a way that the woman feels that she is in control, and situations which could potentially trigger anxiety, depression, or PTSD symptoms should be avoided. Quality interactions with office/hospital staff at all levels from the reception desk to the obstetrician is important in maintaining a positive experience for these women.

Case 8.1. A 37-year-old woman at 36 weeks of gestation with vaginal bleeding and severe abdominal pain

A 37-year-old gravida 1 para 0 presented to the hospital at 36 weeks with vaginal bleeding and severe abdominal pain. With the exception of maternal age over 35 years, her antenatal course was uncomplicated. In the spirit of non-intervention, she had declined aneuploidy screening and antenatal surveillance. Her birth plan was for labor without induction or augmentation, no analgesia, intermittent fetal monitoring, skin-to-skin after birth, and rooming in with her infant. In the hospital, she was diagnosed with abruption and intrauterine fetal demise. The patient rapidly developed a consumptive coagulopathy and became hemodynamically unstable. She

was transferred to the ICU and transfused blood and blood products. The patient survived the event and was discharged home.

After several months of physical and psychological recovery, the patient conceived her second pregnancy. When she presented for prenatal care, she was highly anxious and sought frequent medical surveillance and intervention including serial ultrasound, fetal non-stress tests, and requesting cesarean section at 36 weeks. Ultimately the patient settled for cesarean section on maternal request after demonstrating fetal lung maturity by amniocentesis. She delivered a healthy baby girl and had an unremarkable postpartum course.

Conclusions

An area of future research of value would develop a self-help manual that focused on PSTD for the women discussed in this chapter.

A careful follow-up plan should be made upon discharge of the woman from hospital. This should include follow-up appointments at which the physical and mental health of the patient can be evaluated. Care should be taken to identify women at risk of developing delirium, depression, and PTSD after a period in ICU.

References

1. National Institue for Health and Clinical Excellence. *Rehabilitation after Critical Illness Pathway (CG83).* London: National Institue for Haealth and Clinical Excellence, 2009 (www.nice.org.uk/CG83, accessed 29 January 2013).

2. Pollock W, Rose L, Dennis CL. Pregnant and postpartum admission to the intensive care unit: a systematic review. *Intensive Care Med* 2010;**36**:1465–1475.

3. Trikha A, Singh PM. The critically ill obstetric patient: recent concepts. *Ind J Anaesth* 2010;**54**:421–427.

4. Nava S, Piaggi G, De Mattia E, Carlucci A. Muscle retraining in the ICU patients. *Minerva Anestesiol* 2001;**68**:341–345.

5. Flaatten H. Mental and physical disorders. *Curr Opin Crit Care* 2010;**16**:510–515.

6. Griffiths RD, Jones C. Seven lessons from 20 years of follow-up of intensive care unit survivors. *Curr Opin Crit Care* 2007;**13**:508–513.

7. Griffiths RD, Hall JB. Intensive care unit-acquired weakness. *Crit Care Med* 2010;**38**:779–787.

8. Desai SV, Law TJ, Needham DM. Long-term complications of critical care. *Crit Care Med* 2011;**39**:371–379.

9. De Jonghe B, Lacherade JC, Sharshar T, Outin H. Intensive care unit-acquired weakness: risk factors and prevention. *Crit Care Med* 2009;**37**(Suppl):S309–S319.

10. Kress P. Clinical trials of early mobilization if critical ill patients. *Crit Care Med* 2009;**37**(Suppl):S442–S447.

11. Jones C, Skirrow P, Griffiths RD, *et al*. Rehabilitation after critica illness: a randomized, controlled trail. *Crit Care Med* 2003;**31**:2456–2461.

12. Hirst KP, Moutier CY. Postpartum major depression. *Am Fam Phys* 2010;**82**:926–933.

13. Wylie L, Hollins Martin CJ, *et al*. The enigma of post-natal depression: an update. *J Psychiatry Mental Health Nurs* 2011;**18**:48–58.

14. Jackson JC, Mitchell N, Hopkins RO. Cognitive functioning, mental health, and quality of life in ICU survivors. An overview. *Anesth Clin* 2011;**29**:751–764.

15. Davydow DS, Gifford DS, Desai SV, Bienvenu OJ, Needham DM. Depression in general intensive care unit survivors: a systemic review. *Intensive Care Med* 2009;**35**:769–809.

16. Meltzer-Brody S. New insights into perinatal depression: pathogenesis and treatment during pregnancy and postpartum. *Dial Clin Neurosci* 2011;**13**:89–100.

17. Cox JL, Holden JM, Sagovsky R. Detection of postnatal depression. Development of the 10-item Edinburgh Postnatal Depression Scale. *Br J Psychiatry* 1987;**150**:782–786.

18. Breese McCoy SJ. Postpartum depression: an essential overview for the practioner. *South Med J* 2011;**104**:128–132.

19. Lusskin SI, Misri S. Post-partum blues and depression. *UpToDate*, Feb 2011 (http://www.uptodate.com/contents/postpartum-blues-and-depression, accessed 29 January 2013).

20. Dowdy DW, Eid MP, Dennison CR, *et al*. Quality of life after acute respiratory distress syndrome: a meta-analysis. *Intensive Care Med* 2006;**32**:1115–1124.

21. Capuzzo M, Moreno RP, Jordan B, *et al*. Predictors of early recovery of health status after intensive care. *Intensive Care Med* 2006;**32**:1832–1838.

22. Ripley DL, Harrison-Felix C, Sendroy-Terrill M, *et al*. The impact of female reproductive function on outcomes after traumatic brain injury. *Arch Phys Med Rehabil* 2008;**89**:1090–1096.

23. Bazarian JJ, Blyth B, Mookerjee S, He H, McDermott MP. Sex differences in outcome after mild traumatic brain injury. *J Neurotrauma* 2010;**27**:527–539.

24. Colantonio A, Reg OT, Mar W, *et al*. Women's health outcomes after traumatic brain injury. *J Womens Health* 2010;**19**:1109–1116.

25. Murphy DJ, Charlett P. Cohort study of near-miss maternal mortality and subsequent reproductive outcome. *Eur J Obstet Gynecol Reprod Biol* 2002;**102**:173–178.

26. Camargo RS, Pacagnella RC, Cecatti JG, *et al*. Subsequent reproductive outcome in women who have experienced a potentially life-threatening condition or a maternal near-miss during pregnancy. *Clinics (Sao Paulo)* 2011;**66**:1367–1372.

27. American College of Obstetrics and Gynecology. Committee opinion 275: obstetric management of patients with spinal cord injuries. *Int J Gynaecol Obstet* 2002;**79**:189–191.

28. Signore C. Pregnancy in women with spinal cord injuries. *Contemp Obstet Gynecol* 2012;**57**:23–26.

29. Soncini E, Pelicelli A, Larini P, *et al*. Uterine artery embolization in the treatment and prevention of postpartum hemorrhage. *Int J Gynaecol Obstet* 2007;**96**:181–185.

30. Chauleur C, Fagnet C, Tourne G, *et al*. Serious primary post-partum hemorrhage, arterial embolization and future fertility: a retrospective study of 46 cases. *Hum Reprod* 2008;**23**:1553–1559.

31. Oyelese Y, Scorza WE, Mastrolia R, Smulia JC. Postpartum hemorrhage. *Obstet Gynecol Clin North Am* 2007;**34**:421–441.

32. August P, Sibai B. Preeclampsia: clinical features and diagnosis. *UpToDate*, Jan 2013 (http://www.uptodate.com/contents/preeclampsia-clinical-features-and-diagnosis, accessed 29 January 2013).

33. Henshaw SK. Unintended pregnancy in the United States. *Fam Plann Perspect* 1998;**30**:24–29.

34. Marston C. *Report of a WHO Technical Consultation on Birth Spacing*. Geneva: World Health Organization, 2006.

35. Conde-Agudelo, Rosas-Bermúdez A, Kafury-Goeta AC. Birth spacing and risk of adverse perinatal outcomes. *JAMA*. 2006;**295**:1809–1823.

36. Reproductive Toxicology Center. *Reprotox* [website]. Washington, DC: Reproductive Toxicology Center, 2012 (http://www.reprotox.org, accessed 5 December 2012).

37. Teratogen Information System (TERIS). *Clinical Teratology Web* [website]. Seattle, WA: University of Washington (http://depts.washington.edu/terisweb, accessed 5 December 2012).

38. Briggs G, Freeman RK, Yaffe SJ. *Drugs in Pregnancy and Lactation: A Reference Guide to Fetal and Neonatal Risk*. Philadelphia, PA: Lippincott Williams & Wilkins, 2011.

39. Schaefer C, Peters P, Miller RK. *Drugs During Pregnancy and Lactation: Treatment Options and Risk Assessment*. London: Elsevier, 2007.

40. US National Library of Medicine. *Drugs and Lactation Database (LactMed)*. Bethesda, MD: Specialized Information Services (http://toxnet.nlm.nih.gov/cgi-bin/sis/htmlgen?LACT, accessed 5 December 2012).

41. American College of Obstetrics and Gynecology. Practice bulletin 92: clinical management guidelines for obstetrician-gynecologists number 92, April 2008: Use of psychiatrics medications during pregnancy and lactation. *Obstet Gynecol* 2008;**111**:1001–1020.

42. Chambers CD, Hernandez-Diaz S, Van Marter LJ, *et al*. Selective serotonin-reuptake inhibitors and risk of persistent pulmonary hypertension. *N Engl J Med* 2006;**354**:579–587.

43. Cohen LS, Altshuler LL, Harlow BL, *et al*. Relapse of major depression during pregnancy in women who maintain or discontinue antidepressant treatment. *JAMA* 2006;**295**:499–507.

Chapter 9

Maternal critical care in the developing world

Fathima Paruk, Jack Moodley, Paul Westhead, and Josaphat K. Byamugisha

Introduction

Global maternal mortality exceeds 287 000 each year, and almost all of these deaths occur in the developing world. For every maternal death, there are many more women who have severe morbidity. Recent appraisal at the half-way stage of the United Nations' Millennium Development Goal 5 (to improve maternal care and specifically to reduce the maternal mortality ratio by 75% by 2015) suggests that progress has been disappointingly slow and particularly poor in South Asia and sub-Saharan Africa [1]. There are 49 countries classified as least developed, 32 in Africa, 8 in Asia and 9 Island nations. The burden of disease in these countries necessitates the need for critical care, yet there is a paucity of infrastructure, transport, skilled human resources, and basic resuscitative and life-saving equipment in many regions.

Riviello *et al.* [2] noted that critical care faces the same challenges as other aspects of healthcare in the developing world. However, critical care faces an additional challenge in that it has often been deemed too costly or complicated for resource-poor settings. This lack of prioritization is not justified. Hospital care for the sickest patients affects overall mortality, and public health interventions depend on community confidence in healthcare to ensure participation and adherence. Some of the most effective critical care interventions, including rapid fluid resuscitation, early antibiotics, and patient monitoring, are relatively inexpensive. Although cost-effectiveness studies on critical care in resource-poor settings have not been done, evidence from the surgical literature suggests that even resource-intensive interventions can be cost-effective in comparison with immunizations and care of those with HIV infection. In the developing world, where many critically ill patients are younger and have fewer comorbidities, strategies for early recognition of the deteriorating woman, triage, and critical care management present a remarkable opportunity to provide significant incremental benefit, arguably much more so than in the developed world (Table 9.1).

Obstacles to overcome for access to maternal critical care in low to middle income countries

Global and regional issues

The marked disparities of health expenditure in developed and what the World Bank describes as low to middle income countries parallels the "10/90 gap," where 10% of the global expenditure on health research and development is disproportionately directed towards 90% of the global disease burden [3]. Over half of governments in Africa spend less than $10 per person per year on health, and health financing is often dominated by inequitable, catastrophic, and impoverishing direct out-of-pocket payments [4]. Even if aid funds are given, there are problems with disbursement and accounting from multiple donors. With extremely limited material and human resources, and low government spending on health, they must also cope with the weak absorptive capacity in terms of administrative and managerial support and a huge burden of disease [2].

Inter- and intraregional socioeconomic differences have, however, resulted in the emergence of modern critical care facilities in select areas. The provision of resources to manage critically ill patients (including obstetric patients) varies enormously between countries in the middle and low income group, from the sophisticated intensive care units (ICUs) of urban centers in South Africa to the very limited facilities of much of sub-Saharan Africa. In these units, where the supply of oxygen, electricity, drugs, and disposables

Maternal Critical Care: A Multidisciplinary Approach, ed. Marc Van de Velde, Helen Scholefield, and Lauren A. Plante.
Published by Cambridge University Press. © Cambridge University Press 2013.

Table 9.1. Key areas of consideration in developing maternal critical care in resource-poor settings

Area	Features
Personnel and training	
The value of human resources	Some effective critical care interventions, are more labor intensive than technology intensive
Skill development and staff retention	Strategies for training *and* retaining skilled labor including: tying education to service commitment, incentives to stay, training modules that require less personal teaching time
Essential skills training	Early recognition of the sick woman, emergency obstetric care skills, resuscitation
Training in protocols and checklists	Surgical safety checklist, surviving sepsis, intensive care unit bundles (see text)
Equipment and support services	
Cardiopulmonary monitoring	Non-invasive monitoring can be adequate; manual devices at each bedside in case of equipment malfunction or power loss
Oxygen and pulse oximetry	Oxygen cylinder tanks are bulky and expensive but do not require electricity; concentrators are cheaper but require electricity and may be difficult to maintain over several years; piped oxygen could be ideal but requires underlying infrastructure and capital funds (see Lifebox provision of oximeters in text)
Ventilators	Focus on one model to maximize availability, cost of parts, and availability of skilled biotechnicians
Laboratory, radiology, reliable electricity, and administrative capacity.	Increasing support services for critical care can raise the level of care for all patients in the hospital
Relevant technology	This should not be an excuse for poorly made devices but rather an opportunity to develop devices particularly suited to the context; concomitant uses for military and humanitarian emergencies can increase incentives for development of relevant technology
Ethics	
Global disparity in healthcare	Efforts to increase resources for poor patients must be an ongoing endeavor; the United Nations' Millenium Development Goal 5 is to improve maternal health; sustainable aid programs
Prioritizing limited resources	Daily decisions must be made in the reality of constrained resources; factors that can help include data on prognosis and cost, transparent discussions and policies on how to make difficult decisions with critically ill patients
Research and audit	
Research performed in the developing world	This should include critical care illness epidemiology, current available services, and perceived needs across regions and for individual hospitals; needs assessments; prognostic scores; cost-effectiveness, including relative value of different interventions and difficult-to-measure benefits

Source: adapted from Riviello *et al.*, 2011 [2]

may be erratic, the ICU may provide little more than better monitoring and care from a superior quality of nursing staff, and dependence on oxygen concentrators and generators rather than piped gas supplies may be the norm.

Inequity in resource, facilities, and knowledge

Internationally, many countries, including well-resourced ones, are often characterized by superior devices for the more financially privileged everyone else, with a dichotomy between the public and private healthcare sectors. In the public sector, the vast majority of the ICUs are located in developed areas, or attached to centers of academic excellence/universities.

For example, in Indonesia, Adisasmita *et al.* [5] reported that close to a fifth of admissions in public hospitals were associated with maternal mortality near miss, and the critical state in which the women arrived suggest important delays in reaching the hospitals.

Even though the private sector takes an increasingly larger share of facility-based births in Indonesia, managing obstetric emergencies remains the domain of the public sector. The prevalence of near miss was much greater in public than in private hospitals. Hemorrhage and hypertensive diseases were the most common diagnoses associated with near miss, and vascular dysfunction was the most common criterion of organ dysfunction. The majority (70.7%) of woman with near miss in public hospitals were in a critical state at admission, but this proportion was much lower in private hospitals (31.9%).

Maternal critical care is not a formalized discipline and, as such, access to this scarce resource constitutes a major concern. The quality of maternal critical care may vary from the provision of state-of-the-art medicine to a complete absence of the basic requirements of critical or emergency obstetric care.

In South Africa, the socioeconomically advantaged population (about 10% of the population) is serviced by a very well-resourced private medical sector with outcomes comparable to that in highly developed countries. The majority of the population in South Africa, however, relies on an overburdened public health service, and in other countries there may be no universal public sector health system at all. While academic and central hospitals are reasonably resourced, the majority of the South African population is often disadvantaged through lack of healthcare facilities, accessibility issues, or a lack of essential services. This is particularly true in the rural regions. The annual South African Government health expenditure per person of US $114 is a far cry from the annual expenditure in the USA of $2548 per person [6]. This is reflected in the unacceptably high maternal mortality rate. The plan by the South African Government to implement a national health insurance in the near future has involved discussions between the government and key opinion leaders in the health sector.

The per capita budget for healthcare in Uganda is £10 per year [7]. As with most developing countries, costs for inpatient treatment easily exceed the government provision. Some form of formal or informal cost-sharing process or direct subsidy is necessary for standard hospital care, and when the cost of intensive care is added to this burden, then the clinician must consider the overall sustainability of the unit [8]. The limited data comparing ICU care in Africa and Europe show that the overall age of the African patient is younger and the prior health status better. Good outcomes from ICU in Africa are, therefore, more likely to result in a healthier patient who will also have good economic potential [9,10].

While the lack of antenatal care and the delay in seeking medical assistance are patient-related factors, it is not known if this reflects lack of patient knowledge or accessibility issues. The identification of administrative factors such as accessibility issues, transport issues, the lack of healthcare facilities, the absence of blood products, and the paucity of adequately trained staff is helpful as a national health strategic plan can address these issues. Healthcare worker issues such as inappropriate assessment and substandard care need to be addressed nationally as they will be present at all levels of healthcare. The higher prevalence of healthcare worker issues at level I institutions (clinics and district hospitals) compared with level III institutions (academic and central hospitals) is probably related to the lack of adequately trained staff at the former; consequently, an effective and sustainable educational strategy needs to be identified and implemented. The occurrence of a greater number of deaths at district and regional hospitals compared with tertiary health facilities may be attributed to administrative problems or inappropriate care –or it may be attributed to a shortage of tertiary health facilities and poor referral mechanisms and systems.

> **Case 9.1.** A 35-year-old woman at term in her fifth pregnancy: Part 1
>
> Carol is a 35-year-old woman at term in her fifth pregnancy. She had developed quite strong contractions while at home but was only able to attend the local birth center once a family member arrived to help with her other children.
>
> On arrival at the center, she expressed concern that this labor seemed more painful than her others, but the staff at the clinic reassured her that this was normal and although the midwife was not sure of the position of the head, she and Carol felt that the clinic could deliver her again particularly in view of her previous deliveries.

The burden of morbidity

In South Africa, the estimates of maternal mortality ratio vary between 150 and 625 per 100 000 live births [11,12]. The National Committee for the Confidential

Enquiries into Maternal Deaths (NCCEMD) has set in place a mechanism to improve the reporting of maternal deaths. The major causes of maternal mortality are non-pregnancy-related infections (mainly HIV related), hemorrhage, hypertensive disorders of pregnancy, pregnancy-related infections, and pre-existing medical disease (largely cardiac disease). The main causes of maternal mortality are once again infections, hemorrhage, and hypertensive disorders. Maternal mortality statistics for 2010 reveal rates for South Africa of 300 per 100 000 live births, compared with the sub-Saharan Africa as a whole in the region of 500 per 100 000 live births.

There is a dearth of information pertaining to maternal morbidity in South Africa [13–18]. A report pertaining to ICU utilization by obstetric patients in South Africa indicates an ICU utilization rate of 9/1000 deliveries [19]. Mortality rates are difficult to compare because of the disparate patient populations and the different periods in time that the studies were conducted [19–21]. In Africa, the majority of ICU admissions are attributed to infections, hemorrhage, and hypertension. Other important indications include severe malaria, viral hepatitis, tuberculosis, tetanus, rheumatic valve disease, and anemia; this can be compared with admissions to ICU in the UK reported by the Intensive Care National Audit & Research Centre (see Chapter 1). It is evident from these figures that there is a substantial need for obstetric critical care services in Africa.

Elsewhere in the world, differences in admissions to obstetric critical care services have also been noted between different populations. Munnur *et al.* [22] compared admissions in an American and an Indian public hospital. The most common diagnosis in patients from both hospitals was pre-eclampsia/eclampsia, which was seen in 417 (44.9%) patients. The HELLP syndrome (puerperal sepsis, placental anomalies, and peripartum cardiomyopathy) were more common in US women admitted to ICU, whereas intrauterine fetal death was more common in Indian patients. Other abnormalities were equally common in both hospitals. There were also differences in medical disorders responsible for ICU admission. Malaria, viral hepatitis, cerebral venous thrombosis (confirmed angiographically), central nervous system infections, leptospirosis, tetanus, and typhoid were seen exclusively in Indian patients whereas drug abuse, trauma, and anaphylaxis were seen only in the US patients. Of the other disorders which occurred in both groups of patients, complicated urinary tract infection, acute abdomen, peripartum cardiomyopathy, primary bacteremia, malignancy, and bronchial asthma were more frequent in American patients, whereas cardiac arrest prior to ICU admission was more common in Indian ICU patients.

The HIV status of a patient does not impact on material outcomes for unrelated ICU admission indications [23,24]. There are many ethical problems in treating ICU patients in a developing country, which include the potential for financially impoverishing the patient's entire extended family, particularly if in the end the result is death or a poor outcome. However, for carefully selected patients, the prospects for survival in ICU are much greater than with care in the general ward, where one trained nurse cares for 70 patients or more, many of whom are seriously ill [7].

While South Africa is much more developed than the majority of Africa, it does have better data collection and provides useful information that is transferable to less developed regions. It is believed that maternal deaths are still under-reported in South Africa. Although the *Saving Mothers Report* [25] describes an improvement in institution-based maternal death notification with each progressive triennium, it is still believed that only 20–66% of rural deaths occur in health institutions, with the remainder being unreported. The report by the NCCEMD for the triennium 2005–2007 illustrates that women younger than 20 years of age are at greatest risk of hypertension-associated mortality and that women older than 35 years of age are at particular risk of mortality associated with hemorrhage, embolism, ectopic pregnancy, acute collapse, and pre-existing medical disease [25]. Of the maternal deaths, 38% were classified as avoidable from a health system perspective (administrative- and healthcare worker-related issues). Patient-related factors, administrative issues, healthcare worker issues, or inappropriate resuscitative measures were identified in many cases and are summarized in Table 9.2.

Thaddeus and Maine [26] identified many issues that contribute to maternal mortality. As pregnancy is considered a normal event, death during labor and delivery may sometimes be considered expected. Such fatalistic views can lead to the perception that the condition is not amenable to treatment and can, thus, act as effective barriers to a timely decision to seek care.

Table 9.2. The *Confidential Enquiries into Maternal Deaths* in South Africa for the triennium 2005–2007: avoidable factors

Avoidable factors	Major areas	Percentage
Patient orientated	No antenatal care, infrequent antenatal care, delay in seeking medical help, unsafe abortion	45.9
Administrative	Transport from home to institution or between institutions, barriers to entry, lack of accessibility, lack of specific healthcare facilities or intensive care facilities, lack of blood for transfusion, lack of personnel or appropriately trained staff, communication problems	29.9
Health worker related	Initial assessment, problem with recognition/diagnosis, delay in referring patient, managed at inappropriate level, incorrect management (incorrect diagnosis), substandard management (correct diagnosis) but not monitored/infrequently monitored, prolonged abnormal monitoring without action	
Health worker related at district (level 1)		58
Health worker related at regional (level 2)		49
Health worker related at tertiary (level 3)		30.1
Resuscitation		22.7

Source: National Committee on Confidential Enquiries into Maternal Deaths [25].

Culture

The status of women in many parts of the world means that women do not decide on their own to seek care; the decision belongs to a spouse or to senior members of the family. Obtaining medical care for women with obstetric complications begins with the recognition of danger signs. Access to such information and understanding of the gravity of symptoms, such as bleeding or prolonged labor, help a woman and her family to seek timely treatment. Beliefs as they relate to the etiology of illness and maternal complications also play some part in the decision whether to seek modern obstetric care. These beliefs play a lesser role as societies change through urbanization and increasing recognition of the effectiveness of modern medicine [26].

Distance

Long distances can be an actual obstacle to reaching a health facility, and they can be a disincentive to even trying to seek care. In addition, the effect of distance becomes stronger when combined with lack of transportation and poor roads. The need to travel long distances also often results in delaying the decision to seek healthcare. This delay further exacerbates the patient's physiological derangement at the time of presentation for healthcare services. Presumably they waited longer because distance was acting as a disincentive to seek care earlier, thus delaying their decision [26].

Cost

The financial cost of receiving care include transportation costs, physician and facility fees (when they exist), the cost of medications and other supplies, and opportunity costs. Cost and distance often go hand in hand as considerations in the decision-making process as longer distances entail higher transportation costs. The other important component is the opportunity cost of the time used to seek health services. Time spent getting to, waiting for, and receiving health services is time lost from other more productive activities, such as farming, fetching water and wood for fuel, herding, trading, and cooking [26].

> **Case 9.1.** A 35-year-old woman at term in her fifth pregnancy: Part 2
>
> Because the center was busy, Carol was not examined until several hours later. The midwife was concerned that there was the possibility of a brow presentation. The midwife explained that the patient would need delivery at a center that had access to a theater. Carol expressed her fears that from her tribe's experience women only went there to die. The midwife also changed her mind and felt that in view of her previous deliveries there was a chance that this position may resolve and she remained at the birth center. After 2 hours, her pain became intense and she decided to seek help from the larger obstetric unit.

Unfortunately, the clinic had no access to an ambulance; therefore, a local taxi was used to transport Carol to the hospital. Although the distance was relatively short, the overcrowded and poorly maintained roads led to a travel time of a further 2 hours. During this time, the patient's birth attendant noticed she was no longer complaining of pain and that the bumps in the road no longer seemed to be bothering her. By the time they arrived at the hospital, Carol was completely unresponsive.

Key areas of consideration in developing maternal critical care in resource-poor settings

Human resources

There is a disparity in the distribution of the health workforce, with Africa having a workforce density of only 2.3 per 1000 population, much lower than the global average of 9.3 per 1000 population [27].

This difference is mirrored at a national/ regional level where the distribution of the health workforce is skewed in favor of towns and cities. This has enormous implications for the delivery of healthcare in rural settings, particularly in countries like India where 60% of the population is predominantly rural. Some of the major issues facing the workforce in developing countries are migration, illnesses, and absenteeism.

Skilled personnel (nurses and medical specialists) form the backbone of emergency obstetric services. Attracting and retaining such staff constitutes a major obstacle in the delivery of these services. The most skilled staff are lured by the better working conditions, higher salaries, or attractive opportunities associated with working in the urban private sector setting or emigrating. This often results in an understaffed and overworked scenario. Staff members are often tasked with responsibilities beyond their capabilities. The lack of appreciation and poor patient outcomes is demoralizing and creates work apathy or movement to greener pastures.

To overcome these issues, it is important to recognize the value of human resources. Many effective critical care interventions and monitoring of the sick woman are more labor than technology intensive [2].

Novel and creative methods are required to attract and retain skilled staff. Strategies may include the provision of improved working conditions, better living quarters, higher salaries, and contractual obligations for sponsored trainees. The build up of frustration and negativity should be anticipated. Strategies to address this include the use of motivational speakers, identification of burnout, debriefing, conveying appreciation of effort when necessary, and organizing group activities to permit "de-stressing." The introduction of mandatory community service as well as the rural and scarce skill allowance in South Africa for healthcare appointments attempts to address the issue of providing staffing. While the former provides health personnel in existing facilities, it does not address the issue of providing skilled personnel.

Training

Training needs to be delivered in innovative ways to reduce time away from delivering care. It should be targeted to provide essential skills, particularly effective triage and early recognition of the sick woman to reduce avoidable delay in providing appropriate care. The use of protocols and check lists has resulted in huge improvements in care, the Surviving Sepsis Campaign Bundle for the management of severe sepsis and septic shock [28] and the World Health Organization (WHO) surgical safety checklist [29] being good examples to consider. Examples of triage, modified early warning score, and escalation protocols used at Mulago Hospital in Kampala are included in Appendices 9.1–9.3. In most situations, timely appropriate monitoring and care will avoid the need for intensive care (level 3). Training needs to provide sufficient numbers of staff with the competencies to provide high dependency (level 2) care. A smaller number of staff will need training to provide intensive care competencies (see Chapter 3).

Towey and Ojara [7] have noted that trained nurses are vital for an effective ICU, but clinicians are rarely full time in the unit [30]. The nurse's role often encompasses duties that may be regarded as medical duties in some countries, although they rarely have any financial reward for increased responsibility and workload. Specific training for ICU nurses in sub-Saharan Africa is very rare. Nurses who remain in these posts may be attracted by the challenge and remain particularly motivated. Identification of such nurses and encouragement for them to remain in post can enhance the general quality of care offered. Often the hospital administration fails to appreciate the specialist nature of ICU nursing and rotates nurses throughout all wards as a routine. This practice can be detrimental to establishing a core of locally trained and experienced ICU nursing staff. In the larger units in sub-Saharan Africa, physician anesthesiologists provide the major medical input to ICUs. In rural areas, where physicians of any speciality are very few, this responsibility often falls on non physicians such as the anesthetic clinical officers, who may also be committed to a busy workload in the operating theater [7]. Emphasis on intensive care in the training of anesthetic clinical officers would be appropriate to prepare them for future developments in ICU for the rural areas.

Cost-effective and practical training solutions may include the following.

The implementation of check lists and protocol-driven care. The use of protocols and care bundles in the critical care setting has been shown to yield benefits in terms of patient outcomes. Their use in the scenario of limited skilled resources may lead to fewer errors of care.

Guidelines. Readily available guidelines are needed for cardiopulmonary resuscitation (for pregnant women and after delivery), medical emergencies, infection control, and the major causes of maternal deaths.

Language. Protocols, guidelines, and emergency algorithms should be available in all national languages as well as the languages of foreign employees.

Outreach. Scheduled on-site ward rounds, morbidity and mortality meetings, workshops, or educational meetings chaired by experienced nurses and physicians would not only impact on staff mortality but also improve knowledge and clinical practices.

Competency certification. Attendance at accredited practical courses that provide a competency certificate need to be supported. The spin-off may be that the more skilled attendees may be identified and encouraged to become course instructors and possibly in-house course directors for their region.

Communication technology. The availabilty of a toll-free call, telemedicine, Skype, or email could provide immediate guidance from a more experienced individual. A regional or national roster can be devised so that there is always someone "on-call" to advise. These strategies can be negotiated with and be sponsored by businesses in the private sector, including mobile network providers.

Skilled birth attendants. These provide important delivery services and should be educated on issues related to recognition of the need to refer patients as well as in basic resuscitation skills. This would be useful as many women die at home or present late with such advanced physiological derangement that the institution of medical care would be futile. The use of traditional birth attendants is more controversial.

Midwifery skill training courses and ongoing certification. This should be offered to staff at healthcare facilities as well as to midwives who serve the community in a private capacity. However, it should be remembered that attendance at courses or workshops, or even completion of a "test" following a course, is not synonymous with the ability to practically apply that knowledge.

Facilities

The situation in South Africa is illustrative of the issues elsewhere. Critical care provision is not considered to be a major priority as the focus is instead on primary healthcare provision. The ratio of ICU beds to hospital beds is 1.7% in the public sector and the ICU beds are largely confined to urban and academic centers; this is much lower than the US allocation of 13.4% [31]. A national problem in the public sector is the immense shortage of ICU beds in relation to the demand. This necessitates the practice of patient triage (Appendices 9.1 and 9.2). Ethical challenges are further compounded in the scenario of the pregnant patient with a living fetus. Design of ICUs often does not conform to acceptable standards as they are often created as "add-on" areas. The lack of critical care facilities in periurban and rural areas is further compounded by the inaccessibility of referral centers through transport and communications issues. In rural areas, home deliveries are not uncommon and they are often managed by traditional birth attendants. If such deliveries develop complications, the time to presentation at a healthcare facility is largely dependent on the obstacles discussed above.

The WHO recognize that one way of reducing maternal mortality is by improving the availability, accessibility, quality, and use of services for the treatment of complications that arise during pregnancy and childbirth. These services are collectively known

Table 9.3. Emergency obstetric care facilities

Facility	Provision
Basic	Administer parenteral antibiotics
	Administer parenteral oxytocin
	Administer parenteral magnesium sulfate
	Manually remove placenta
	Remove retained products of conception
	Perform assisted vaginal delivery
	Perform basic neonatal resuscitation
Comprehensive	As basic facility plus perform surgery and blood transfusion

as emergency obstetric care. The WHO minimum recommendation is there are at least five emergency obstetric care facilities (Table 9.3), including one comprehensive facility, per 500,000 population. They have developed indicators [32] to help countries assess if:

- there are enough facilities providing emergency obstetric care
- the facilities are well distributed
- enough women are using the facilities
- the appropriate patients (i.e. women with obstetric complications) are using the facilities
- enough critical services are being provided
- the quality of the services are adequate.

The scarcity of ICUs (level 3) makes it extremely important that basic emergency obstetric facilities function effectively to minimize the number of women becoming critically ill and that comprehensive emergency obstetric facilities can provide at least basic facilities for high dependency (level 2) care. Key decision makers in government need to be engaged with regarding the need for the equitable provision of emergency obstetric care and critical care facilities. There needs to be a plan to ensure that the facilities have adequate equipment, communication technology, essential drugs, and an adequate staff complement with appropriate skills. The inability to communicate (uncharged mobile, malfunctioning telephone/fax/internet, or no air time) is not uncommon and needs to be addressed.

Equipment and drugs

There is evidence that mortality in ICU is related to the availability of appropriate technical equipment [33]. Any planning for an ICU facility must relate to

the economic background of the community the hospital intends to serve. A clinical area where there is a rational use of oxygen, good basic nursing, and monitoring may be the entry point and an inexpensive first step. An appropriate ventilator independent of compressed gases and disposable circuits is ideal [34]. Invasive arterial monitoring and hemodialysis require a significant cost in disposables that make them beyond the scope of all except private hospitals in the major cities of sub-Saharan Africa, or university hospitals, where there is also a substantial patient cost-sharing input and is unlikely to be an option in the rural areas of Africa for many decades. Although donated equipment is usually sent with genuine desire to help, it is important that this equipment will be useful to the recipient. Sending broken or partially working equipment is not helpful as maintenance or spare parts can be difficult to obtain. Airport taxes may be needed to be paid by the recipient in some cases, which may nullify the benefit of the donation. It is usually best to ask the recipient exactly what they want and see if this can be matched rather than waste time and money on sending something unsuitable.

The lack of basic equipment and drugs and the purchase and use of exorbitantly expensive unfamiliar, complex and unnecessary equipment or drugs are equally important causes of ineffective care. There are a number of schemes, such as the Programme for Appropriate Technology in Health (PATH) [35] that are working to improve these issues. In rural regions, oxygen cylinders and oxygen concentrators may need to be relied upon rather than piped gases. Monitors, ventilators, defibrillators, manual sphygmomanometers, Ambu bags, and laryngoscopes are in short supply and may need to be shared by several patients and even a few wards. Blood and blood products are often unavailable. There needs to be a paradigm shift in terms of the requisites of critical care. The notion that expensive technology and drugs are essential needs reconsideration. The focus should be in individualizing and defining the essentials for emergency obstetric services and critical care for specific sites. The WHO publishes a model list of essential medicines [36]. In addition to this, a basic requisite equipment list needs to be determined.

Simple solutions can be very helpful; for example, basic equipment for observations that will allow early recognition of the deteriorating woman often goes missing. The Liverpool–Mulago Partnership have developed an equipment kit in a bag for midwives to wear during working hours (Figure 9.1). This is given to her as her own personal kit to be kept with her at all times so that she has an incentive to take care of it and have immediate access to the necessary basic equipment for taking physiological observations. The equipment kit shown includes a fob-watch, thermometer, fingertip pulse oximeter, an aneroid sphygmomanometer, and stethoscope in a bag. The total cost for each midwife is about £50. Other examples are the use of a condom and foley catheter for uterine tamponade in massive obstetric hemorrhage (Figure 9.2), rather than expensive bespoke catheters as described in Chapter 39. Sepsis bundles can be adapted for use in low resource settings by using the basic physiological observation parameters and developing systems for early access to antibiotics (see Chapter 31). Intramuscular magnesium sulfate regimens for eclampsia and severe pre-eclampsia avoid the need for expensive infusion devices (see Chapter 36).

Lifebox [37], in consultation with an international panel of experts, have developed a pulse oximeter that exceeds the highest World Federation of Societies of Anaesthesiologists/WHO specifications and is intended for targeted sale in low-resource countries. At $250 including delivery, the price is unmatched and within reach. It comes with an educational CD-Rom that contains an award-winning video and materials about oximetry for use in self-learning or classroom teaching; the project will make surgery safer for millions of patients around the world.

The equipment list for units should include cardiorespiratory monitoring tools, oxygen supply, airway management, back-up generator capacity, and electricity surge-protecting mechanisms and, in tertiary units, mechanical ventilators. The nature of the equipment (simple or sophisticated, new or previously used) would largely depend on purchasing capacity as well as the robustness, simplicity, and technical support/after-service for a particular brand of equipment. To minimize cost, items such as monitors and ventilators are best secured from a single supplier. Apart from obtaining a better price per unit, only one service contract will be required. Additionally, staff will require less in-house training and patient safety will be enhanced. Manual tools such as powerful torches, blood pressure manometers, Ambu bags, and oxygen cylinders need to be available to address the issue of malfunctioning of equipment or power outages. There is an increasing awareness for the "specialized needs" of under-resourced countries. This has resulted in investment in the development of equipment that addresses these issues. This includes equipment with longer battery lives and solar-powered equipment. Depending on the level of service, a drug list in addition to the South African Essential Drug List needs to be formulated. A mechanism needs to be created such that there is an adequate supply of these drugs at all times. Blood should be readily available to all institutions that provide obstetric services.

Water and electricity

A regular supply of water and electricity cannot be guaranteed even in the capital cities of many developing countries and the situation is often worse in the rural areas, where up to 80% of the population live [8]. An irregular supply of water is not in itself a limitation to the ICU as hospital staff become adept at managing with a system of rationing and storing water on the wards. Cross-infection is, no doubt, more of a risk, but an acceptable standard of care can be given. An

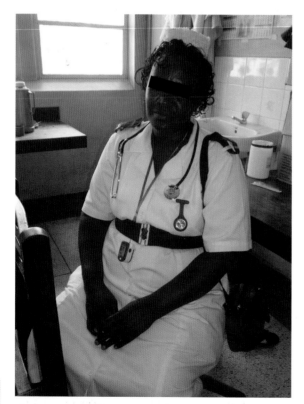

Figure 9.1. Midwife with basic equipment kit.

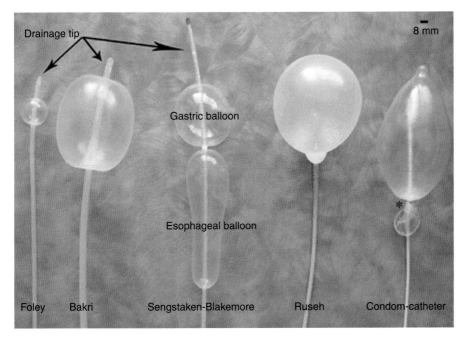

Figure 9.2. Ballon tamponade catheters.

irregular electricity supply is a more serious problem, particularly when oxygen concentrators are in use. Back-up generators in many hospitals provide an important source of power when main supplies fail, but this back-up may take a significant time to connect. Nursing staff must remain alert to this possibility if subsequent mortality and morbidity is to be avoided, particularly for the ventilated patient. Monitoring equipment and ventilators are at risk of damage from voltage surges, which should be prevented. An irregular supply of water and electricity to a hospital is, therefore, not a complete bar to developing some ICU facility, but staff need to be trained to deal with the local conditions [6].

Oxygen

Providing a regular supply of oxygen cylinders to any hospital in rural Africa is both expensive and logistically difficult [7]. The most important development in the last 15 years in oxygen supply is the oxygen concentrator [38]. Although the concentrator requires an initial capital outlay, the cost of oxygen production is then very low. A regular safe electricity supply is essential, although it may be obtained by varying methods over time, as well as technical support for maintenance. Rational oxygen therapy is most practically guided by pulse oximetry.

Supporting services

Basic laboratory services for emergency obstetric services should include the determination of hemoglobin, white cell count, platelet count, urea, and electrolytes, and microscopy. The quality of ICU care depends upon supporting laboratory and radiology departments. Hemoglobin, white cell counts, HIV testing, and blood transfusion capabilities are usually available in even remote areas of Africa, but even in major cities of sub-Saharan Africa, blood gas, creatinine, and serum electrolyte estimations are usually unavailable. This affects clinical care as well as the ability to estimate international severity sickness scores [7].

Blood transfusion services are usually under great strain and fewer than 70 of the 191 WHO Member States meet the WHO recommendations for a national blood program. Microbiological services are very rare and often unreliable. While many remote hospitals may have a basic radiology service, few have the ability to offer a portable service to the wards and the same is true of ultrasound imaging [7].

Case 9.1. A 35-year-old woman at term in her fifth pregnancy: Part 3

On arrival, Carol was assessed by the triage midwife who noted that the patient was peripherally shut down, tachycardic and her blood pressure was unrecordable. The midwife immediately contacted the senior house officer, who gave intravenous fluids. Fetal parts were easily palpable and the patient was taken straight to theater, where a laparotomy was performed. A ruptured uterus was confirmed and a fresh stillbirth was found. A large amount of blood was seen abdominally and an estimated blood loss of 3 L was made. The surgeon was unable to achieve hemostasis and a hysterectomy was performed. A blood transfusion was requested but was unavailable until later in the afternoon because of shortages in supply. Carol was transferred to the maternal high dependency unit and was followed using the African Midwifery Early Warning Score chart. She was given regular intravenous fluids to maintain her blood pressure while awaiting transfusion.

Organizational issues and policies

The head of the emergency obstetric services or critical care facility needs to have the support of the medical and financial administrator. Policies or protocols pertaining to standard operating procedures, admission criteria, triage (Appendices 9.1 and 9.2), patient referral patterns, emergency contacts, treatment withdrawal, sourcing of equipment, servicing of equipment, and disaster management need to be agreed upon and be available in a written format.

Box 9.1 illustrates the working of an intensive care unit in Uganda.

Community

Engaging with influential community leaders and even the formation of community advisory boards may be valuable as the communication may facilitate the involvement of the community. Initiatives to improve antenatal attendance, early presentation for medical assistance, or even training of traditional birth attendants may be viewed more positively.

Research/audits

The research agenda in the developing world should include [2]:

- epidemiology
- current available services
- perceived needs across regions and for individuals
- prognostic scores
- cost-effectiveness
- ascertaining reasons for poor antenatal attendance
- ascertaining if existing health facilities (clinic, hospitals, ICUs) are sufficient and appropriately distributed
- factors that influence staff retention in periurban areas
- cost-effective educational strategies

Box 9.1. St Mary's Hospital Lacor intensive care unit

St Mary's Hospital Lacor, Gulu, in Uganda is a church-supported general hospital of 476 beds where 87% of patient costs are subsidized. It is in a remote rural area where for the last 20 years there has been a significant security problem. For 10 years it has had a small four-bed ICU near the operating theater, which was recently upgraded to an eight-bed unit.

It is predominantly a general postoperative ICU but also accommodates women with eclampsia, which forms a major part of the workload, and recently delivered women after surgery.

The nurses and clinical officer anesthesiologists are trained in central line placement and its interpretation. The central lines are donated. One Glostavent and one Puritan Bennet ventilator with an internal compressor are available. There are no infusion pumps and inotropes are rarely used. Laboratory results are slow to reach the ward and there is a limited quantity of bedside Glucostix strips. There is no capacity for peritoneal dialysis or hemodialysis as, despite significant overseas assistance, this specialist area has not been sustainable. There is no fresh frozen plasma, platelets, parenteral nutrition, or activated protein C and no facility for invasive arterial monitoring. The nurse-to-patient ratio is approximately one trained nurse to four patients, but assistant nurses who have no formal training are present on each shift. The surgical and medical teams share care with one physician anesthesiologist and one non-physician medical clinical officer, both attached to the ICU full-time. One non-physician anesthetic clinical officer shares duties on the ICU with theater duties.

Source: adapted from Towey and Ojara, 2007 [7].

- cost-containment strategies in under-resourced countries
- audit and revision of existing practices at individual centers.

Early identification of the critically ill woman

Early identification of the critically ill woman in developing regions is equally important as focusing, for critically ill obstetric patients, on basic infrastructure (facilities, transport, and electricity), accessibility, basic equipment, essential drugs for advanced life support, blood, human resources, and quality of care. Strategies to reduce the demand for this scarce resource include:

- primary prevention: prevent pregnancy
- secondary prevention: strategies to reduce the occurrence of obstetric complications
- tertiary prevention: strategies to recognize life-threatening complications early.

The last is particularly important as delays in treatment initiation impact negatively on outcomes. Further, obstetric patients admitted to ICU have been demonstrated to have better outcomes than medical patients. The importance of early recognition of the severely ill pregnant patient is emphasized in the *Confidential Enquiry into Maternal and Child Health* report for the triennium 2003–2005 in the UK [39]. In the UK, these scoring systems to identify the severely ill pregnant patient include multiple physiological parameters, including oxygen saturation. Singh *et al.* [40] have published a validation study showing that pulse, blood pressure, and respiratory rate are the most significant parameters. This allows a simplified score to be used in a low resource setting where minimal equipment is available. Mulago Hospital Uganda has developed the African Midwifery Early Warning Score (AMEWS). This helps to identify deteriorating patients quickly and with minimal equipment (sphygmomometer and clock). Like many early warning systems, it applies a score to each physiological parameter and a cumulative score can be calculated (Appendix 9.3). The escalation algorithm used is also shown in Appendix 9.3. If the score is >6 then an immediate review is required, and if >4 a review within 30 minutes is expected. If this is not achieved, there is an escalation policy to mandate contact with more senior grades.

The parameters measured are pulse rate, blood pressure, respiratory rate, and consciousness level On review by the doctor, a thorough examination is performed and other parameters such as temperature are checked as indicated and management instituted as required.

Management of the critically ill obstetric patient in poorly resourced settings

The challenge in the management of the critically ill antenatal or peripartum patient in these settings is the need to tailor treatment around the significant cardiorespiratory, immunological, hematological, and metabolic alterations that accompany the gravid state.

These and other aspects of critical care are discussed in the relevant chapters. Patients with need for rigorous monitoring, single organ dysfunction or de-escalation from ICU can often be managed in a high dependency or high care unit (HDU; level 2) rather than an ICU (level 3). This can be provided at relatively low cost within the maternity unit. An example is the obstetric HDU at Mulago Hospital (Box 9.2).

Case 9.1. A 35-year-old woman at term in her fifth pregnancy: Part 4

Three hours later...

The midwife in the HDU found an increase from 4 to 6 on Carol's AMEWS chart and requested a review from the senior house officer. Along with the raised AMEWS score, the patient's hourly urine output was also noted to be low. The senior house officer initially increased the intravenous fluids but after 30 minutes the patient became increasingly tachycardic and hypotensive. The senior house officer requested a senior review. The specialist decided to take the patient to theater where a bleeding pedicle was found. The blood was availed during the operation and the patient was transfused. The patient was then taken back to the HDU for close monitoring. She remained stable and was discharged back to the postnatal ward after 2 days.

Acknowledgements

The authors would like to acknowledge the contributions of the team at Mulago Hospital. They would also like to thank Dr Helen Scholefield and Dr Paul Howell,

---

Box 9.2. The obstetric high dependency unit (level 2) at Mulago Hospital

Mulago Hospital is a free tertiary referral center in Kampala, Uganda. The maternity unit has 31 000 deliveries per annum. Patient load and referrals of moribund patients, combined with understaffing (midwifery ratio1:25) and general poor health of the patients, leads to a high maternal mortality rate, which varies between 300 and 550 per 100 000 live births. Many of these deaths occur in the postnatal period.

The Liverpool–Mulago Partnership with funding from the Tropical Health Education Trust has developed a postnatal HDU. An exchange program is in place for staff to move between Mulago and the Liverpool Women's Hospital. Ugandan visitors to Liverpool identified systems that could be implemented in Mulago to improve the situation. Support was given to the Mulago team to help them to develop guidelines and new roles, and in selecting and training staff and procuring equipment. Careful staff selection was crucial to ensure that those appointed had appropriate skills as well as the motivation to make the project succeed, particularly as there were no financial benefits. As the staff at Mulago deal with emergencies such as eclampsia, ruptured uteri, and massive obstetric hemorrhage on nearly a daily basis, they are highly competent in their management. Therefore the main focus of the training was on recognition of sick women, immediate resuscitation, and the longer-term management of these conditions. High-risk postnatal patients fitting strict admission criteria are admitted into a six-bedded monitored area with a minimum nurse to patient ratio of 1:6. Regular observations are performed every 30 minutes. There are close links with the hospital's ICU department and joint training programes are being developed. The caseload has been mixed but the most frequent reason for admission was ruptured uterus. To provide ongoing support and help in developing sustainable capacity, senior UK members of the Liverpool–Mulago Partnership, including obstetricians, midwives, and health systems experts, visit to provide clinical and administrative support and training several times a year. A junior doctor from the UK spends 12 months in placements as an Eleanor Bradley Fellow in the unit, working alongside their Ugandan colleagues and this helps to continue the link between the Liverpool Women's Hospital and Mulago teams throughout the year

The HDU opened in October 2010 and resulted in an initial 75% reduction in deaths. This increased expectations that the partnership can significantly affect the maternal mortality rate. This mortality rate has fluctuated because of difficulties in availability of blood and supplies at times, but there has been a sustained significant reduction in mortality. The difficulties with immediate availability of supplies such as antibiotics has been addressed by giving local ownership to the unit for its own ordering. The unit is now self-sustaining and continuing evaluation of the project is in place.

Consultant Anaesthetist at St Bartholomew's and Homerton Hospitals, London, UK; and the Chairman of the Obstetric Committee of the World Federation of Societies of Anesthesiologists for their contribution to the chapter.

References

1. Countdown Coverage Writing Group. Countdown to 2015 for maternal, newborn, and child survival: the 2008 report on tracking coverage of interventions. *Lancet* 2008;**371**:1247–1258.

2. Riviello ED, Letchford S, Achieng L, *et al.* Critical care in resource-poor settings: lessons learned and future directions. *Crit Care Med* 2011;**39**:860–867.

3. Global Forum for Health Research. *10/90 Report on Health Research 2003–2004.* Geneva: Global Forum for Health Research (http://announcementsfiles.cohred.org/gfhr_pub/assoc/s14789e/s14789e.pdf, accessed 29 January 2013).

4. Organisation for Economic Co-operation and Development. *Health Data 2011.* Paris: Organisation for Economic Co-operation and Development, 2011.

5. Adisasmita A, Deviany PE, Nandiaty F, Stanton C, Ronsmans C. Obstetric near miss and deaths in public and private hospitals in Indonesia. *BMC Pregnancy Childbirth* 2008;**8**:10 1471.

6. Kissoon N. Out of Africa: a mother's journey. *Crit Care Med* 2011;**12**:73–79.

7. Towey R, Ojara S. Intensive care in the developing world. *Anaesthesia* 2007;**62**(Suppl 1): 32–37.

8. Dare L, Buch E. The future of health care in Africa. *BMJ* 2005;**331**:1–24.

9. Nourira S, Roupie E, Atrouss ES, *et al.* Intensive care use in a developing country: a comparison between a Tunisian and a French unit. *Intensive Care Med* 1998;**24**:1144–1451.

10. Armaganidis A. Intensive care in developed and developing counties:are comparisons of ICU

performance meaningful? *Intensive Care Med* 1998;**24**:1126–1128.

11. Government of South Africa. *Maternal Deaths in South Africa*. Pretoria: Government Press, 2006.

12. Moszynski P. South Africa's rising maternal mortality is due to health system failures, says report. *BMJ* 2011;**343**:d5089.

13. Prual A, Bouvier-Colle MH, de Bernis L, *et al.* Severe maternal morbidity from direct obstetric causes in West Africa: incidence and case fatality rates. *Bulletin WHO* 2000;**78**:593–600.

14. World Health Organization, UNICEF, UNFPA and World Bank. *Trends in Maternal Mortality: 1990 to 2010*. Geneva: World Health Organization, 2012 (http://whqlibdoc.who.int/publications/2012/9789241503631_eng.pdf, accessed 29 January 2013).

15. Oladapo OT, Ariba AJ, Odusoga OL. Changing patterns of emergency obstetric care at a Nigerian University Hospital. *Int J Gynecol Obstet* 2007;**98**:278–284.

16. Filippi V, Ronsmans C, Gohou V, *et al.* Maternity wards or emergency obstetric rooms? Incidence of near miss events in African hospitals. *Acta Obstet Gynecol Scand* 2005;**84**:11–16.

17. Vandecruys HB, Pattinson RC, Macdonald AB, *et al.* Severe acute maternal morbidity and mortality in the Pretoria Academic Complex: changing patterns over 4 years. *Eur J Obstet Gynecol Reprod Biol* 2002;**102**:6–10.

18. Pattinson RC, Buchmann E, Mantel G, *et al.* Can enquiries into severe acute maternal morbidity act as a surrogate for maternal death enquiries? *BJOG* 2003;**110**:889–893.

19. Johanson R, Anthony J, Domisse J. Obstetric intensive care at Groote Schuur Hospital, Cape Town. *J Obstet Gynecol* 1995;**15**:174–177.

20. Taylor R, Richards GA. Critically ill obstetric and gynaecology patients in the intensive care unit. *South Afr Med J* 2000;**90**:1140–1144.

21. Platteau P, Engelhardt T, Moodley J, Muckart DJJ. Obstetric and gynaecological patients in an intensive care unit: a 1 year review. *Trop Doctor* 1997;**27**:202 206.

22. Munnur U, Karnad D, Bandi V, *et al.* Critically ill obstetric patients in an American and an Indian public hospital: comparison of case-mix, organ dysfunction, intensive care requirements, and outcomes. *Intensive Care Med* 2005;**31**:1087–1094.

23. Bhagwanjee D, Muckart P, Jeena P, Moodley P. Does HIV status influence the outcome of patients admitted to a surgical intensive care unit? A prospective double blind study. *BMJ* 1997;**314**:1077–1084.

24. Watters DAK, Sinclair JR, Luo N, Verma R. HIV seroprevalence in critically ill patients in Zambia. *AIDS* 1988;**2**:142–143.

25. National Committee on Confidential Enquiries into Maternal Deaths. *Saving Mothers 2005–2007: Fourth Report on Confidential Enquiries into Maternal Deaths in South Africa, Expanded Executive Summary.* Cape Town: National Committee on Confidential Enquiries into Maternal Deaths, 2007 (www.doh.gov.za/docs/reports/2007/savingmothers.pdf, accessed 13 January 2013).

26. Thaddeus S, Maine D. Too far to walk: maternal mortality in context. *Soc Sci Med* 1994;**38**:1091–1110.

27. Fitzhugh M. Doctors and soccer players: Africa professionals on the move. *N Engl J Med* 2007: 356:440–443.

28. Surviving Sepsis Campaign. *Management of Severe Sepsis and Septic Shock Bundle* [website]. (http://www.survivingsepsis.org/Bundles/Pages/default.aspx, accessed 13 January 2013.).

29. World Health Organization. *Safe Surgery Saves Lives.* Geneva: World Health Organization, 2008 (http://www.who.int/patientsafety/safesurgery/knowledge_base/SSSL_Brochure_finalJun08.pdf, accessed 29 January 2013).

30. Dunser MW, Baelani I, Ganbold L. A review and analysis of intensive care medicine in the least developed countries. *Crit Care Med* 2006;**34**:1234–1242.

31. Baker T. Critical care in low income countries. *Trop Med Int Health* 2009;**14**:143–148.

32. World Health Organization, UNFPA, UNICEF and Mailman School of Public Health. *Monitoring Emergency Obstetric Care. A Handbook.* Geneva: World Health Organization, 2009 (http://whqlibdoc.who.int/publications/2009/9789241547734_eng.pdf, accessed 29 January 2013).

33. Bastos PG, Knaus WA, Zimmermann JE, *et al.* The importance of technology for achieving superior outcome from intensive care. Brazil APACHE 111 Study Group. *Intensive Care Med* 1996;**22**:664–669.

34. Eltringham RJ, Fan Qiu Wei. Experience with the Glostavent anaesthetic machine. *Update Anaesth* 2003;**16**:31–35.

35. Programme for Appropriate Technology in Health. *The Right Technologies Lead to Widespread Change* (website). Seattle, WA: Programme for Appropriate Technology in Health, 2012 (http://www.path.org/health-technologies.php, accessed 29 January 2013).

36. World Health Organization. *Model Lists of Essential Medicines*, 17th List. Geneva: World Health Organization, 2011 (http://www.who.int/medicines/

publications/essentialmedicines/en/index.html, accessed 29 January 2013).

37. Lifebox. *Saving Lives Through Safer Surgery* (website). London: Lifebox, 2012 (http://www.lifebox.org/project, accessed 29 January 2013).

38. Dobson M. Oxygen concentrators for district hospitals. *Update Anaesth* 1999;**10**:61–63.

39. Lewis G (ed.) *Saving Mothers' Lives: Reviewing Maternal Deaths to Make Motherhood Safer, 2003–2005. The Seventh Report on Confidential Enquiries into Maternal Deaths in the United Kingdom.* London: CEMACH, 2007.

40. Singh S, McGlennan A, England A, Simons R. A validation study of the CEMACH recommended modified early obstetric warning system (MEOWS]. *Anaesthesia* 2012;**67**, 12–18.

APPENDIX 9.1. THE MULAGO HOSPITAL GUIDE TO TRIAGE (PRIORITISATION OF PATIENTS) ON ADMISSION TO THE LABOUR WARD

The aim of triage is:

- To identify those patients who are sickest, at the point of admission to the labour ward so that prompt medical attention can be given to those who need it most, first.
- To ensure a more streamlined patient journey through the labour suite so that:
  i. those who do not require emergency care can be seen in a more appropriate environment such as the antenatal clinic or managed an outpatient and sent home
  ii. those who need immediate intervention, receive definitive care in as short a time as possible.
- This will hopefully reduce mortality and long-term morbidity for mothers and babies who are treated on the labour suite.

Note: Triage is aimed ONLY at categorising patients on admission, and is not a replacement for clinical judgement, nor does it dictate what happens to the patient for the rest of their stay on labour suite.

HOW TO USE THE TRIAGE ASSESSMENT FORM

- All patients are to have the primary survey (Appendix 9.3) completed in full as soon as possible on arrival on labour suite.
- **Triage patients in order of arrival by admission midwife or shift in charge or labour suite in charge or other designated person**. The doctors will initially participate in this process as it is being streamlined.
- If several patients arrive at the same time, triage those with any obvious life-threatening obstetric emergency and any that have been referred from Old Mulago or other clinics first.
- Once you have completed the primary survey (i.e. the first page) check the findings against the table. If the patient has any of the findings listed in the table, she fails the primary survey and is automatically categorised as triage code RED. She requires immediate medical review. The doctor should be requested to attend immediately – if not present on labour ward contact by telephone. The time of informing the doctor should be noted on the triage sheet. It is not necessary to proceed to secondary survey, as this will not change the patient's triage category. They still need to see a doctor urgently. **In case the intern sees them first, after initial resuscitation he or she ought to inform the SHO [senior house officer] and or specialist as soon as possible**.
- If the patient passes the primary survey, proceed to the secondary survey (focused triage). The secondary survey should complete in full.
- Once you have completed the secondary survey you should be able to reach a differential diagnosis. If you are unable to reach a diagnosis or are unsure as to the appropriate triage category, seek medical advice. The doctor will then see the patient fully and triage accordingly.
- Check your differential diagnosis against the triage category table on the wall [shown below], and assign a triage category.

CATEGORY	ACTION
Red	The patient requires immediate medical attention. Place the file in the red tray in time order, and inform the doctor on duty, either in person or by telephone. These patients should be prioritised over other categories, as they have potentially immediately life-threatening problems.
Yellow	The patient requires medical review soon, but not immediately, and does

CATEGORY	ACTION
	not take priority over red patients. If the doctor is not present on the labour ward they should be informed that there are patients waiting for review. Patients who are categorised as yellow have the potential to deteriorate if not reviewed in a timely manner.
Green	The patient does not require a medical review and can be assessed and examined by a midwife. If the midwife has any cause for concern after she has assessed her patient, she should seek medical review/advice.
Blue	The patient does not need to be reviewed on labour suite, and can be given an appointment for the next antenatal clinic and sent home.

REMEMBER THAT TRIAGE IS A SORTING PROCESS THAT SHOULD IDENTIFY THOSE THAT NEED TO BE SEEN SOONEST. PATIENT CONDITION CAN CHANGE. MEDICAL ADVICE SHOULD ALWAYS BE SOUGHT IF YOU ARE IN DOUBT OR HAVE ANY CONCERNS ABOUT YOUR PATIENT.

Once patient is triaged, she will be sent to the relevant healthcare professional for review

If a further problem is detected, the patient's triage category can be revised.

Midwives and doctors assessing patients should perform a routine physical examination, including a detailed obstetric examination.

Where a midwife assesses a patient, if she feels that

- there is a malpresentation
- there is a malposition
- there is clinical evidence of an obstructed labour
- there is an undiagnosed multiple pregnancy
- if she has any other specific concern

she should discuss the case with the doctor on duty at the earliest possible opportunity, and if appropriate the patient should be recategorised and reviewed.

APPENDIX 9.2. MULAGO HOSPITAL OBSTETRIC TRIAGE PROFORMA

Patient Name……………… Hospital ID………………………....

Date of admission………… Time of admission……………

Name of Midwife or other designated person

triaging……………………………………………………

Primary Survey – ALL PATIENTS (At admission table; triage patients in order of arrival by admission midwife or shift in charge or labour suite in charge or other designated person).

Airway	Patient able to talk	No ☐	Yes ☐
	Noisy breathing, i.e. stridor	Yes ☐	No ☐
Breathing	Respiratory Rate ………………… Breaths/min		
Circulation	Pulse Rate ………………………/min		
	BP ……………/………… mmHg		

Disability assessment: (*Tick best response*)

Alert ☐

Responds to Voice ☐

Responds to Painful Stimuli ☐

Unresponsive ☐

Restless/uncooperative ☐

Obvious Obstetric Emergency

- Massive Obstetric Haemorrhage   Yes ☐ No ☐
- Sudden Maternal Collapse   Yes ☐ No ☐
- Eclamptic Fit   Yes ☐ No ☐
- Cord Prolapse   Yes ☐ No ☐
- Direct Abdominal Trauma   Yes ☐ No ☐
- Severe Chest Pain   Yes ☐ No ☐

Findings and Action: Tick (√)Triage code RED or Other triage Code then proceed

Airway	Unable to talk/noisy breathing	Needs immediate medical review
Breathing	Respiratory rate more than 29 or less than 5	Triage code RED

Circulation	**Pulse** greater than 120 beats/min
	Blood Pressure
	Systolic more than 160 or less than 90 mmHg
	Diastolic more than 100 mmHg
		THESE PATIENTS HAVE FAILED THEIR PRIMARY
		  SURVEY
		DO NOT PROCEED TO SECONDARY SURVEY
		  THEY ARE CATEGORY RED

Disability	Unresponsive to voice or pain/restless	
Obvious obstetric emergency	Any of the above listed problems	
Patient does not have any of the above findings		Triage other Then secondary survey

Secondary Survey: (At admission table; by admission midwife or shift in-charge or labour suite in-charge or other designated person)

Booked/Unbooked (Cross out as applicable)

Gravidity ………………………………

Parity ………………………………..

Number of previous cesarean sections…………………………………

Gestational Age

                          EDD from LMP …………………………..

                          EDD from USS …………………………..

Contractions   Yes □ No □   Unsure □

      Frequency …………………………………………….

      Strength   Mild □   Moderate □   Strong □

      Duration ……………………………………………………..

Spontaneous Rupture of Membranes   Yes □ No □ Unsure □

      Clear   Yes □   No □

      Blood stained   Pink □   Red □

      Meconium   Thin □   Thick □

Bleeding   Yes □   No □

                   Light □   Moderate □ Heavy □

Headache   Yes □ No □

Visual Disturbance   Yes □ No □

Seizure/Blackout   Yes □ No □

Oedema   Face □   Hands □   Feet □ None □

Urinary problems   Yes □ No □

Fetal Movements   Yes □ No □

                   If no, when were fetal movements last felt?

Abdominal Pain (NOT contractions)

                   Yes □ No □

                   Mild □ Moderate □   Severe □

Fever   Yes □ No □   Temp…………

Other problem (specify) ………………………………………………

DIFFERENTIAL DIAGNOSIS …………………………………………

TRIAGE CATEGORY   **RED YELLOW   GREEN   BLUE**

(Circle as appropriate; use triage categories version 2 document if not sure)

Doctor informed? Yes □ Time………….. No □

APPENDIX 9.3. AFRICAN MIDWIFERY EARLY WARNING SCORE

The table below shows the data that give the early warning score.

Score	0	1	2	3
Systolic blood pressure	90–140 mmHg	140–150 or 80–90 mmHg	150–200 mmHg	> 200 mmHg or <80 mmHg
Pulse	75–105 bpm	105–110 or 60–70 bpm	110–130 or 40–60 bpm	> 130 bpm or < 40 bpm
Respiratory rate	15–20 resps/min	20–25 or 10–15 resps/min	25–30 or 5–10 resps/min	> 30 or < 5 resps/min
Conscious level (AVPU score)	Alert	Responds to voice	Confused or agitated	Unconscious or unresponsive to pain

The escalation algorithm shown below is used for patients with scores above or below 4 (SHO, senior house officer).

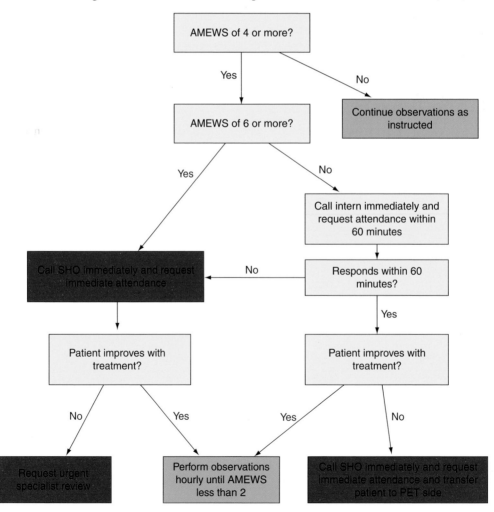

Chapter

10

Physiological changes of pregnancy

Lisa E. Moore and Nigel Pereira

Introduction

The physiological changes of pregnancy consist of adaptations designed to enable adequate oxygen and nutrient delivery to both the mother and developing fetus. Thorough understanding of these changes is essential to differentiate between normal physiological alterations of pregnancy and pathological abnormalities. Many physiological and biochemical changes of pregnancy can modify the reference ranges of common laboratory results during different trimesters. Using reference ranges derived from non-pregnant women to evaluate and interpret laboratory values in pregnant women may lead to erroneous clinical implications. This chapter, therefore, reviews the major physiological adaptations during pregnancy and also highlights changes in the reference ranges of common laboratory values encountered in pregnancy.

Body fluid homeostasis

The expansion in total body fluid volume is one of the most significant changes during pregnancy, and this increase is distributed throughout the maternal–fetal unit. At term, the overall increase in body fluid volume is estimated to be 6.5 to 8.5 L [1]. While the fluid volume of the fetus, placenta, and amniotic cavity account for about 3.5 L, maternal blood volume increases 1.5–1.6 L, of which 1.2–1.3 L is plasma volume and 0.3–0.4 L is red blood cell volume [1,2]. The rest is attributed to the expansion of maternal extracellular fluid volume, breast as well as adipose tissue [1].

Immediately following conception, expansion of the plasma volume begins; this, in turn, decreases serum osmolality [1,3]. At 12 weeks of gestational age, serum osmolality is 8 to 10 mOsm/kg lower than the non-pregnant state [3]. In addition, the osmotic threshold for thirst and antidiuretic hormone release is lowered by 10 mosmol, resulting in increased water intake and retention [3]. Over the course of an entire pregnancy, 500–900 mmol sodium and 350 mmol potassium are usually retained. However, despite retention, the mean sodium and potassium concentrations are lower (3–4 mEq/L (mmol/L) and 0.2 mEq/L (mmol/L), respectively) after 12 weeks of gestational age compared with the non-pregnant state [3]. This decrease in the serum sodium and potassium concentrations is attributed to water retention, which exceeds sodium and potassium retention [3]. Table 10.1 summarizes the effects of maternal plasma volume expansion on the reference values of common serum electrolytes during pregnancy.

Cardiovascular system

Pregnancy induces a myriad of changes in the cardiovascular system, which include changes in cardiac output, heart rate, blood pressure, vascular compliance, capacitance, vascular resistance, and ventricular dimensions [5]. Many of these changes are thought to be caused by the hormonal milieu of pregnancy, and they may occur as early as 4–5 weeks of gestational age [6].

Maternal heart rate increases 10 to 20 beats/min over the course of pregnancy, peaking in the early third trimester, which in combination with a 25% increase in stroke volume, produces a 50% increase in overall cardiac output (i.e. heart rate multiplied by stroke volume) (Figure 10.1). Most of this increased cardiac output is directed towards the gravid uterus, placenta, and breasts. At term, the uterus and breasts receive 17% and 2% of cardiac output, respectively [1].

Labor and the immediate puerperium are associated with additional increases in cardiac output, which increases 12% in the first stage of labor and is primarily mediated by an increase in stroke

Maternal Critical Care: A Multidisciplinary Approach, ed. Marc Van de Velde, Helen Scholefield, and Lauren A. Plante.
Published by Cambridge University Press. © Cambridge University Press 2013.

Table 10.1. Reference ranges of serum electrolytes in pregnancy

Serum electrolyte	Non-pregnant adult	First trimester	Second trimester	Third trimester
Bicarbonate (mEq/L or mmol/L)	21–30	20–24	20–24	20–24
Calcium, ionized (mmol/L [mg/dL])	1.1–1.4 (4.5–5.6)	1.1–1.3 (4.5–5.1)	1.1–1.2 (4.4–5.0)	1.1–1.3 (4.4–5.3)
Calcium, total (mmol/L [mg/dL])	2.2–2.6 (9.0–10.5)	2.2–2.6 (8.8–10.6)	2.0–2.2 (8.2–9.0)	2.0–2.4 (8.2–9.7)
Chloride (mEq/L or mmol/L)	98–106	101–105	97–109	97–109
Magnesium (mmol/L [mg/dL])	0.8–1.2 (1.8–3.0)	0.7–0.9 (1.6–2.2)	0.6–0.9 (1.5–2.2)	0.4–0.9 (1.1–2.2)
Osmolality (mOsm/kg or mmol/kg serum water)	285–295	275–280	276–289	278–280
Phosphate (mmol/L [mg/dL])	1.0–1.4 (3.0–4.5)	1.0–1.5 (3.1–4.6)	0.8–1.5 (2.5–4.6)	0.9–1.5 (2.8–4.6)
Potassium (mEq/L or mmol/L)	3.5–5.0	3.6–5.0	3.3–5.0	3.3–5.1
Sodium (mEq/L or mmol/L)	136–145	133–148	129–148	130–148

Sources: Kratz, *et al.*, 2004 [3]; Abbassi-Ghanavati, *et al.*, 2009 [4].

volume [1]. This increase is thought to occur as a result of increased preload from additional blood expressed from the uterus during each contraction, a phenomenon sometimes called "uterine autotransfusion" [6]. During the second stage of labor, cardiac output can increase by up to 34%, with an initial increase from an increase in stroke volume following which additional increase in cardiac output mainly reflects increased heart rate [1]. Immediately postpartum (i.e. 10 to 30 minutes following delivery), approximately 300–500 mL of blood, which had previously been shunted to the uterus, is transferred to the maternal circulation, [6,7]. This increase in preload and stroke volume leads to a further increase in cardiac output by 10–20% [6]. This represents a particularly delicate time for patients with underlying cardiovascular disease for the development of pulmonary edema or congestive heart failure. Cardiac output values then return to pre-pregnancy levels by 2 weeks postpartum and to non-pregnant levels by 6 weeks postpartum [6,7].

Cardiac output is also affected by maternal position, with greatest output noted in knee–chest or lateral recumbent positions [1]. The gravid uterus compresses the inferior vena cava in the supine position and may completely occlude venous return from the lower extremities. Of note, 5–10% of pregnant women may experience nausea, diaphoresis, light-headedness, or even syncope because of the supine position, which can be alleviated by gentle leftward tilt [1].

Progesterone-mediated smooth muscle relaxation causes vasodilatation and a fall in systemic vascular resistance by approximately 20% [1]. This effect begins at 5 weeks and will nadir between 20 and 32 weeks of gestation, after which systemic vascular resistance will gradually rise until term [1]. The decrease in systemic vascular resistance manifests as decreased blood pressure, even in light of increased cardiac output. Diastolic blood pressure decreases by 12 mmHg in mid-pregnancy, followed by a gradual increase of 10 mmHg by term [3]. Systolic blood pressure shows minimal change until a slight rise at 36 weeks of gestational age [3]. Therefore, the mean arterial blood pressure nadirs by mid-gestation, returning to pre-pregnancy levels by term [1,3].

Although all four chambers of the heart will increase in some size from the first trimester to the end of the third trimester, left ventricular hypertrophy and dilatation are particularly significant [1,3]. An increase in left ventricular end-diastolic volume can be seen by 10 weeks of gestation that peaks in the third trimester (Figure 10.1). The structural changes of the left ventricle are consistent with eccentric hypertrophy, which are similar to changes in exercise [1,9]. This is in contrast to concentric hypertrophy, which is usually seen as a long-term adaption to chronic hypertension. Eccentric hypertrophy enhances the efficiency and pumping capacity of the heart in the context of increased left end-diastolic volumes.

Central hemodynamic measurement may sometimes become necessary for critically ill pregnant

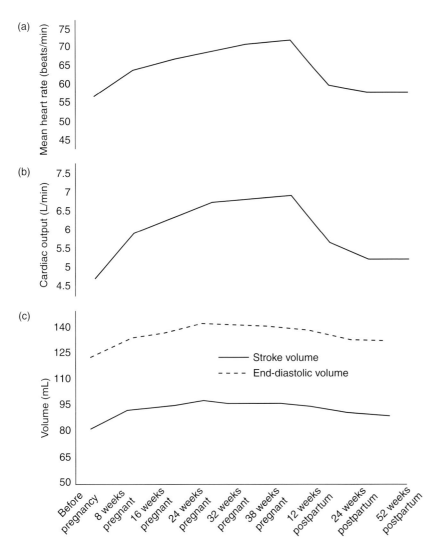

Figure 10.1. Variations in heart rate (a), cardiac output (b), stroke volume, and end-diastolic volume (c) before, during, and after pregnancy [6].

patients. Table 10.2 summarizes central hemodynamic measurements obtained via arterial lines and Swan–Ganz catheters in term pregnancies [8]. Pulmonary edema may develop when pulmonary capillary wedge pressure exceeds a threshold of 24 mmHg, and also when it exceeds the colloid oncotic pressure by more than 4 mmHg [1,8]. However, because colloid oncotic pressure decreases in pregnancy, pregnant patients may develop pulmonary edema at lower pulmonary capillary wedge pressures.

Respiratory system

Marked changes occur in the structure and function of the respiratory system during pregnancy. Apart from connective tissue changes in the upper airway and thorax, pregnancy affects static lung volumes, gas exchange, and ventilation [9].

The upper respiratory tract becomes edematous, hyperemic, congested, and friable at the beginning of the first trimester [9,10]. These changes, which are thought to be mediated by estrogen, persist throughout pregnancy, and peak in the third trimester [9,10]. The effects of estrogen on the nasal mucosa may explain why 30% of pregnant women experience rhinitis-like symptoms during pregnancy, as well as occasional nosebleeds [9].

The enlarging uterus constantly changes the configuration and dimensions of the thoracic cavity during pregnancy [1,9]. With progressive increases in uterine size, the circumference of the abdomen and lower chest wall increases, the costal angles widen, and

Table 10.2. Central hemodynamic measurements in normal term pregnancies

Hemodynamic measurement	Term pregnancy (36–38 weeks of gestation)	Change from non-pregnant state
Heart rate (beats/min)	83 ± 10	↑
Cardiac output (L/min)	6.2 ± 1	↑
Systemic vascular resistance (dyne.s/cm^5)	1210 ± 266	↓
Colloid oncotic pressure (mmHg)	18 ± 1.5	↓
Pulmonary capillary wedge pressure (mmHg)	3.6 ± 2.5	No change
Central venous pressure (mmHg)	3.6 ± 2.5	No change

Source: Clapp and Capeless, 1997 [5].

Table 10.3. Changes in static lung volumes observed during pregnancy

Lung volume	Definition	Change in pregnancy
Tidal volume	Volume of air inspired and expired in a normal breath	↑ (30 to 40%)
Inspiratory reserve volume	Maximum volume of air that can be inspired at the end of a normal inspiration	No change
Expiratory reserve volume	Maximum volume of air that can be expired at the end of a normal expiration	↓ (15–20%)
Inspiratory capacity	Maximum volume of air that can be inspired at the end of a normal expiration	↑ (5–10%)
Vital capacity	Maximum volume of air that can be forcibly expired after a maximal inspiration	No change
Functional residual capacity	Volume of air remaining in the lungs at the end of a normal expiration	↓ (17–20%)
Residual volume	Volume of air remaining in the lungs at the end of a maximal expiration	↓ (20–25%)
Total lung capacity	Total volume of air in the lungs at the end of a maximal expiration	No change to ↓ (5%)

Sources: Gabbe, *et al.*, 2012 [1]; Crapo, 1996 [8]; Bobrowski, 2010 [9].

the resting position of the diaphragm elevates [9]. During pregnancy, both the anterior–posterior and transverse diameters of the chest wall increase, leading to an overall increase of 5–7 cm of the circumference of the lower chest wall [9]. The costal angles also widen by 50%, from 68° to 103° [9,10]. Furthermore, the resting position of the diaphragm is elevated 4–5 cm [9,10]. Although most of these changes are primarily mechanical effects of the enlarging uterus, relaxation of the ligamentous attachments to the ribs may contribute to earlier changes in the shape of the thoracic cavity [9,10]. Changes in the configuration of the thoracic cavity appear to peak at about 37 weeks of gestation, returning to normal dimensions within 24 weeks following delivery [9].

Structural changes of the thoracic cavity can translate into functional changes of the respiratory system, particularly static lung volumes. The functional residual capacity (FRC) decreases 300 to 500 mL (i.e. 17–20%), and this decrease is a direct effect of the elevated resting position of the diaphragm. The FRC can be further subdivided into expiratory reserve volume and residual volume, which decrease 100–300 mL (15–20%) and 200–300 mL (20–25%), respectively. The reduction in FRC causes a concomitant increase in the inspiratory capacity volume by 100–300 mL (5–10%) [9,10]. This decrease in FRC is clinically important as it increases the uptake and clearance of inhaled anesthetic agents [10].

Although some lung volumes are affected by the pregnancy-related changes of the thoracic cavity, the total lung capacity and vital capacity remain relatively unchanged by pregnancy [10]. Similarly, spirometric measurements reveal unchanged bronchial flow, suggesting that airway function remains stable during pregnancy [1,10]. Table 10.3 summarizes the changes in static lung volumes observed during pregnancy.

Oxygen consumption increases in pregnancy by up to 20% to meet the increasing metabolic demands of the mother and developing fetus. Logically, multifetal gestation increases oxygen consumption even more [10]. Additionally, during labor, oxygen consumption may increase by up to 60% [10]. Increasing progesterone levels stimulate the respiratory center of the medulla, causing an increase in the respiratory drive [1,10]. By 8 weeks of gestation, the minute ventilation increases 30 to 50%, primarily owing to a 40% increase in tidal volume (minute ventilation = tidal volume × respiratory rate) (Table 10.3) [1,10].

Table 10.4. Variations in arterial blood gas values in a term pregnancy

Blood gas measurement	Non-pregnant adult	Third trimester
pH	7.38–7.44	7.39–7.45
Arterial partial pressure of oxygen (mmHg [kPa])	80–100 (11–13)	92–107 (12.3–14.3)
Arterial partial pressure of carbon dioxide (mmHg [kPa])	35–45 (4.7–5.9)	25–33 (3.3–4.4)
Bicarbonate (mmol/L or mEq/L)	21–30	16–22

Sources: Clark, *et al.*, 1989 [7]; Crapo, 1996 [8].

The increase in minute ventilation, combined with a physiological decrease in FRC, leads to a 50–70% increase in alveolar ventilation, thereby increasing alveolar oxygen partial pressure (P_{AO_2}), decreasing arterial carbon dioxide partial pressure (P_{ACO_2}), and mildly increasing blood pH [1,9,10]. Decreased P_{ACO_2} is critical in maintaining a carbon dioxide gradient that facilitates its transfer from the fetus to the mother. In addition, lower P_{ACO_2} leads to mild respiratory alkalosis, with renal compensation occurring by increased bicarbonate excretion [1,9,10]. Variations in arterial blood gas values in a term pregnancy are summarized in Table 10.4. Because of increased oxygen consumption and decreased FRC, the maternal oxygen reserve is reduced; therefore, pregnant women are more susceptible to effects of apnea, particularly during intubation [1]. Hence, preoxygenation prior to intubation becomes necessary to prevent acute hypoxia and respiratory acidosis.

Pregnancy is also associated with changes in sleep patterns and sleep disorders that may continue postpartum. Although a detailed discussion of pregnancy-associated sleep patterns and disorders is beyond the scope of this chapter, several key points are worth highlighting. First, pregnancy is associated with an overall decrease in rapid-eye movement (REM) sleep and stage 3 and 4 non-REM sleep [1,10]. Second, with increasing gestational age, sleep efficiency and continuity decrease, while daytime somnolence and night-time awakenings increase [1]. Third, women who complain of excessive daytime sleepiness, night-time awakening, loud snoring, or self-reported or witnessed apneic spells must be evaluated with polysomnography for obstructive sleep apnea [1,10].

As obstructive sleep apnea leads to chronic hypoxemia, women with this apnea are at an increased risk of developing intrauterine growth restriction and gestational hypertension [1,10]. Finally, pregnancy may cause restless leg syndrome, a neurological disorder that can prevent women from falling asleep [1]. Although the prevalence of restless leg syndrome in pregnancy is not known, up to 23% of pregnant women may develop some component of this disorder in the third trimester [1].

Gastrointestinal and hepatobiliary systems and nutrition

Pregnancy-related hormones substantially influence the motility and synthetic function of the gastrointestinal and hepatobiliary systems. Modifications of these functions may manifest as clinical symptoms during pregnancy or may cause variations in the results of common laboratory values.

Nausea and vomiting are perhaps the most common symptoms experienced, possibly complicating up to 70% of pregnancies [1]. These symptoms typically peak at 9 weeks of gestation, with 60% resolving by the end of the first trimester, and 90% by 20 weeks of gestation [11]. Although the precise physiological mechanisms underlying nausea and vomiting remain unclear, rising human chorionic gonadotropin levels causing estrogen production is thought to be the most likely mechanism [11]. In most women, these symptoms resolve with minimal support; however, a small minority may suffer from hyperemesis gravidarum, a condition associated with persistent vomiting, profound dehydration, electrolyte imbalance, and weight loss, necessitating hospitalization [1,11].

As pregnancy progresses, many women experience gastroesophageal reflux caused by a combination of progesterone-mediated reduction in gastroesophageal sphincter tone and gastric compression by the enlarging uterus [1,3]. Progesterone and estrogen also decrease gastrointestinal motility, tone, and gall bladder emptying, resulting in modification of bowel habits and propensity to develop biliary sludge and stones [1,3].

Despite minimal change in the absolute blood flow to the liver during pregnancy, its synthetic capacity and activity increases several fold [3]. In addition to increased production of serum albumin, prealbumin and total protein, hepatic synthesis of fibrinogen, transferrin, ceruloplasmin, and the binding proteins for sex steroids, corticosteroids, and thyroid hormones

Table 10.5. Variations in the measured concentrations of markers of hepatic synthetic activity

Serum analyte	Non-pregnant adult	First trimester	Second trimester	Third trimester
Alanine transaminase (U/L [μkat/L])	0–35 (0–0.58)	3–30 (0.05–0.5)	2–33 (0.03–0.55)	2–25 (0.03–0.42)
Albumin (g/L)	35–55	31–51	26–45	23–42
Alkaline phosphatase (U/L [nkat/L])	30–120 (0.5–2.0)	17–88 (0.28–1.47)	25–126 (0.42–2.1)	38–229 (0.63–3.82)
Alpha-1 antitrypsin (g/L)	0.8–2.1	2.2–3.2	2.7–3.9	3.3–4.9
Asparatate transaminase (U/L [μkat/L])	0–35 (0–0.58)	3–23 (0.05–0.38)	3–33 (0.03–0.55)	4–32 (0.07–0.53)
Bilirubin, total (mmol/L [mg/dL])	5.1–17.0 (0.3–1.0)	1.7–6.8 (0.1–0.4)	1.7–13.7 (0.1–0.8)	1.7–18.8 (0.1–1.1)
Bilirubin, unconjugated (mmol/L [mg/dL])	1.7–5.1 (0.1–0.3)	1.7–8.5 (0.1–0.5)	1.7–6.8 (0.1–0.4)	1.7–8.5 (0.1–0.5)
Bilirubin, conjugated (mmol/L [mg/dL])	3.4–12.0 (0.2–0.7)	0–1.7 (0–0.1)	0–1.7 (0–0.1)	(0–1.7 (0–0.1)
Ceruloplasmin (mg/L)	270–370	300–490	400–530	430–780
Gamma-glutamyl transpeptidase (U/L)	1–94	2–23	4–22	3–26
Lactate dehydrogenase (U/L [μkat/L])	100–190 (1.7–3.2)	78–433 (1.3–7.2)	80–447 (1.3–7.5)	82–524 (1.4–8.7)
Prealbumin (mg/L)	195–358	150–270	200–270	140–230
Protein, total (g/L)	55–80	62–76	57–69	56–67

Sources: Kratz, *et al.*, 2004 [3]; Abbassi-Ghanavati, *et al.*, 2009 [4].

increases during pregnancy [1,3]. It is estimated that albumin mass increases by 15% to 123 g at 28 weeks of gestation compared with 107 g in the non-pregnant state [3]. Alkaline phosphatase levels also increase dramatically after 24 weeks of gestation, although this is attributed to a heat-stable isoenzyme produced from the placenta [1,3]. The measured levels of other liver enzymes, however, remain unchanged during pregnancy. Circulating estrogen can influence bile acid production and secretion, leading to mild sub-clinical cholestasis, even though fasting levels of bile acids remain unaffected by pregnancy [1]. These variations in commonly reported laboratory results are highlighted in Table 10.5.

Some women may exhibit unique clinical and laboratory findings that, although are within the physiological norms of pregnancy, may otherwise be considered as signs of liver disease. These include estrogen-related spider angiomata and palmar erythema, which resolve soon after delivery, as well as lowered serum albumin and total protein concentrations [1,3]. Although the overall concentrations of serum albumin and total protein increase during pregnancy, dilutional effects of the expanded plasma volume will lower measured concentrations (Table 10.5) [1,3]. The decreased serum albumin concentration may be reflected in the measurement of albumin-bound substances such as unconjugated

bilirubin, calcium, and zinc, even though their total circulating levels may be higher (Table 10.5) [3].

In the absence of clinically significant nausea and vomiting, most women experience increased appetite, with caloric intake increasing by almost 300 kcal/day [1]. Pica, a peculiar craving for odd food such as iron, clay, detergent, or ice, may also occur [1]. In addition, many women may also complain of increased salivation. This condition, also known as ptyalism, may lead to losses of 1–2 L of saliva per day and actually represents the inability of nauseated women to swallow normal amounts of saliva rather than a true overproduction of saliva [1].

Cholesterol and triglyceride concentrations also change throughout pregnancy [3]. By 12 weeks of gestation, high density lipoprotein-cholesterol levels have increased by 20% compared with non-pregnant levels and continue to increase until term [3]. Similarly, low density lipoprotein-cholesterol levels begin to increase at 18 weeks of gestation, continuing to term [3]. Triglyceride levels increase by 40% at 18 weeks of gestational age, and are almost 250% higher than non-pregnant levels at term [3]. Table 10.6 summarizes the changes in lipid, cholesterol and triglycerides levels during pregnancy.

Adequate quantities of vitamins and certain trace minerals are necessary to ensure proper growth and

Table 10.6. Lipid, vitamin and mineral concentrations during pregnancy

Serum analyte	Non-pregnant adult	First trimester	Second trimester	Third trimester
Cholesterol, total (mmol/L [mg/dL])	<5.17 (<200)	3.65–5.44 (141–210)	4.56–7.74 (176–299)	5.67–9.04 (219–349)
High density lipoprotein-cholesterol (mmol/L [mg/dL])	1.03–1.55 (40–60)	1.03–2.02 (40–78)	1.35–2.25 (52–87)	1.24–2.25 (48–87)
Low density lipoprotein-cholesterol (mmol/L [mg/dL])	<2.59 (<100)	1.55–3.96 (60–153)	1.99–4.77 (77–184)	2.62–5.80 (101–224)
Very low density lipoprotein-cholesterol (mmol/L [mg/dL])	0.16–1.04 (6–40)	0.26–0.47 (10–18)	0.34–0.60 (13–23)	0.54–0.93 (21–36)
Triglyceride (mmol/L [mg/dL])	<1.8 (<160)	1.0–4.1 (40–159)	1.9–9.9 (75–382)	3.4–11.7 (131–453)
Apolipoprotein A1 (g/L)	1.2–2.4	1.1–1.5	1.4–2.5	1.4–2.6
Apolipoprotein B (g/L)	0.52–1.63	0.58–0.81	0.66–1.88	0.85–2.38
Retinol (vitamin A) (µmol/L [µg/dL])	0.7–3.5 (20–100)	1.1–1.6 (32–47)	1.2–1.5 (35–44)	1.0–1.5 (29–42)
Vitamin B_{12} (pmol/L [ng/dL])	205–712 (27.9–96.6)	87–323 (11.8–43.8)	96–484 (13.0–65.6)	73–388 (9.9–52.6)
Ascorbic acid (vitamin C) (µmol/L [mg/dL])	23–57 (0.4–1.0)	Not reported	Not reported	51–74 (0.9–1.3)
1,25-Dihydroxyvitamin D (pmol/L [ng/dL])	60–108 (2.5–4.5)	52–169 (2.0–6.5)	187–416 (7.2–16.0)	156–309 (6.0–11.9)
25-Dihydroxyvitamin D (nmol/L [µg/dL])	25–169 (1.0–6.8)	45–67 (1.8–2.7)	25–55 (1.0–2.2)	25–45 (1.0–1.8)
Alpha-tocopherol (vitamin E) (µmol/L [mg/dL])	116–279 (0.5–1.8	162–302 (0.7–1.3)	232–371 (1.0–1.6)	302–534 (1.3–2.3
Copper (µmol/L [µg/dL])	11–22 (70–140)	18–31 (112–199)	26–35 (165–221)	20–38 (130–240)
Zinc (µmol/L [µg/dL])	11–18 (75–120)	9–13 (57–88)	8–12 (51–80)	8–12 (50–77)

Sources: Kratz, et al., 2004 [3]; Abbassi-Ghanavati, et al., 2009 [4].

development of the fetus. While retinol (vitamin A) is lower during pregnancy, α-tocopherol (vitamin E) levels parallel the increase in cholesterol [3]. Overall levels of 1,25-dihydroxyvitamin D increase in pregnancy, but 25-hydroxyvitamin D generally does not change [1,3]. Circulating concentrations of trace minerals are influenced by their respective carrier proteins and serum albumin levels. In this context, copper concentrations increase in pregnancy because of increased hepatic synthesis of ceruloplasmin [1,3]. By contrast, lowered zinc concentrations correlate with lowered serum albumin levels [1,3]. These trends in vitamin and mineral concentrations during pregnancy are also listed in Table 10.6.

Genitourinary system

Similar to the cardiovascular and respiratory systems, the genitourinary system undergoes several anatomical and functional changes during pregnancy. The size and weight of the kidney increases during pregnancy through an increase in interstitial volume, renal vasculature, and urinary dead space [1,12]. Substantial dilatation of the renal calyx, pelvis, and ureters occurs, which contributes to the urinary dead space [1,3,12]. Dilatation of the ureters and renal pelves begins by the 8 weeks of gestation and peaks during the second trimester, when the ureteric diameter may be up to 2 cm. Often, dilatation of the right ureter exceeds that of the left [1]. On occasion, the physiological findings of ureteral and pelvicaliceal dilatation may interfere with radiological evaluation of urinary tract obstruction [1]. Pregnancy is also marked by anatomical changes in the bladder, which include elevation of the trigone and increased vascular tortuosity throughout the bladder. These changes primarily cause an increased incidence of microscopic hematuria [1]. Furthermore, bladder capacity decreases because of the enlargement of the uterus, leading to increased urinary frequency, urgency, and possibly stress incontinence [1].

Renal plasma flow increases gradually during the first half of pregnancy, reaching values that are 60–80% greater by mid-pregnancy. At term, renal plasma flow is about 50% greater than non-pregnant levels [3,12]. Similarly, the glomerular filtration rate rises 40–50% by 9–11 weeks of gestation, and this value is generally sustained until 36 weeks of gestation [3,12]. The net effect of these changes is represented by a decrease in plasma concentrations of creatinine, uric acid, and blood urea nitrogen. With creatinine clearance increasing to 150–200 mL/min in pregnancy, compared with 120 mL/min in the non-pregnant state, serum creatinine and blood urea nitrogen concentrations decrease concurrently [1,3]. Serum uric acid concentrations decline in early pregnancy as a result of the increased glomerular filtration rate, reaching a nadir by 24 weeks of gestation [1,3]. Shortly after, uric acid concentrations begin to rise and reach preconceptional levels by the end of pregnancy [1,3]. These changes in renal physiology are listed in Table 10.7.

Increased renal plasma flow and glomerular filtration rate also increase urinary excretion of glucose, amino acids, and protein [3,12]. As a result, glycosuria is common in most pregnant women, although the mechanism does involve modified tubular reabsorptive capability [1]. Pregnant women may also lose up to 2 g of amino acids per day, compared with <0.5 g in the non-pregnant state [3]. Similarly, total urinary protein and microalbumin excretion almost doubles, with upper limits of 300 mg for proteinuria and 30 mg for albuminuria considered the norm during pregnancy [1,3]. Urinary calcium excretion also increases steadily until term, reaching 8.75–15.5 mmol/day, compared with 2.5–6.25 mmol/day in non-pregnant women [1,3]. The physiological changes in urinary excretion are also summarized in Table 10.7. Importantly, changes in urinary excretion in conjunction with increased volume of distribution alter drug distribution during pregnancy, necessitating higher drug doses to compensate for urinary excretion.

Hematology and coagulation

During pregnancy, several changes occur in the maternal hematological system to support the growing maternal–fetal unit [2]. Total maternal blood volume increases by 1500 to 1600 mL, of which 1200 to 1300 mL is plasma volume and 300 to 400 mL is red blood cell volume [1,2]. Maternal blood volume begins to increase by 6 weeks of gestation, reaching its peak between 30 and 34 weeks of gestation, after which it plateaus until delivery [1,2]. The overall magnitude of maternal blood volume expansion is greater in multifetal gestations and multiparous women [3,9]. In contrast, lower than normal plasma volume expansion is known to be associated with intrauterine growth restriction as well as pre-eclampsia [3,9].

The necessity for red blood cell mass increase is obvious considering the increased physiological requirements of the developing maternal–fetal unit [2]. The mechanism of red blood cell production is complex and involves hormonal mediators such as erythropoietin, human placental lactogen, estrogen, and progesterone. Although red blood cell volume increases during pregnancy, this rate of increase differs from the rate of

Table 10.7. Variations in measured concentrations of serum and urine analytes reflecting renal physiological adaptations

Serum/urine analyte	Non-pregnant adult	First trimester	Second trimester	Third trimester
Creatinine (mmol/L [mg/dL])	38–69 (0.5–0.9)	30–53 (0.4–0.7)	30–61 (0.4–0.8)	30–69 (0.4–0.9)
Urea nitrogen (mmol/L [mg/dL])	3.6–7.1 (10–20)	2.5–4.3 (7–12)	1.1–4.6 (3–13)	1.1–3.9 (3–11)
Uric acid (mmol/L [mg/dL])	90–360 (1.5–6.0)	119–250 (2.0–4.2)	143–291 (2.4–4.9)	184–375 (3.1–6.3)
Calcium excretion, 24 hour (mmol)	<7.5	1.6–5.2	0.3–6.9	0.8–4.2
Creatinine excretion, 24 hour (mmol)	8.8–1.4	10.6–11.6	10.3–11.5	10.2–11.4
Potassium excretion, 24 hour (mmol)	25–100	17–33	10–38	11–35
Protein excretion, 24 hour (mg)	<150	19–141	47–186	46–185
Sodium excretion, 24 hour (mmol)	100–260	53–215	34–213	37–149

Sources: Kratz, *et al*., 2004 [3]; Abbassi-Ghanavati, *et al*., 2009 [4].

increase in the maternal plasma volume. As a result of the rapid increase in maternal plasma volume in early pregnancy and the later rise in the volume of red blood cells, the hematocrit falls by as much as 10% in the first trimester; this trend continues through the second trimester, finally stabilizing near term [1,2]. This apparent decrease in hematocrit and hemoglobin concentrations during pregnancy is often called the "physiological anemia of pregnancy" [1,2].

Following delivery and blood loss, maternal blood volume does not re-expand or redistribute to predelivery levels. Instead, an overall diuresis of the expanded plasma volume occurs in the postpartum period [1]. This results in a gradual increase in hematocrit and normalization of maternal blood volume [2]. If hematocrit and hemoglobin concentrations at 5–7 days following delivery remain considerably lower than predelivery levels, then either the magnitude of blood loss was underestimated or the degree of pregnancy-induced blood volume expansion was low – or possibly both [1,2].

In a normal pregnancy, the peripheral white blood cell count starts to increase by mid-first trimester, reaching its peak by 30 weeks of gestation [1,2]. White blood cell count increases with the onset of labor, possibly reaching levels of up to 25×10^9/L to 30×10^9/L [2] (Table 10.8). This physiological increase in white blood cell count is primarily caused by an increase in circulating numbers of segmented neutrophils and granulocytes [1,2]. Care should be taken when interpreting the white blood cell count to determine the presence of an infection, particularly during labor. Counts return to non-pregnant levels within 1–2 weeks following delivery [1,2].

Prior to the introduction of automated analyzers, studies of platelet counts during pregnancy revealed conflicting results [1,12]. However, even after the introduction of automatic counting machines, studies remained non-confirmatory, primarily due to discrepancies in methodology and variations in study populations [1,2]. Despite these limitations, several experts

Table 10.8. Variations in red blood cells, white blood cells, platelets, and other hematological analytes during pregnancy

Hematological analyte	Non-pregnant adult	First trimester	Second trimester	Third trimester
Erythropoietin (IU/L)	4–27	12–25	8–67	14–222
Ferritin (µg/L)	10–200	6–130	2–230	0–116
Folate, red blood cell (nmol/L [µg/dL])	340–1020 (15.0–45.0)	310–1335 (13.7–58.9)	213–1876 (9.4–82.8)	247–1502 (10.9–66.3)
Folate, serum (nmol/L [µg/dL])	7.0–39.7 (0.31–1.75)	5.9–34.0 (0.26–1.50)	1.8–54.4 (0.08–2.40)	3.2–46.9 (0.14–2.07)
Hemoglobin (g/L)	120–160	116–139	97–148	95–150
Hematocrit (%)	36.0–46.0	31.0–41.0	30.0–39.0	28.0–40.0
Iron, serum (mmol/L [µg/dL])	5.4–28.7 (30–160)	12.9–25.6 (72–143)	7.9–31.9 (44–178)	5.4–34.6 (30–193)
Mean corpuscular hemoglobin (pg/cell)	26–34	30–32	30–33	29–32
Mean corpuscular volume (µm³ or fl)	80–100	81–96	82–97	81–99
Platelet count (× 10^9/L)	165–415	174–391	155–409	146–429
Red blood cell count (× 10^9/L)	4.00–5.20	3.42–4.55	2.81–4.	2.71–4.43
Red cell distribution width (%)	11.5–14.5	12.5–14.1	13.4–13.6	12.7–15.3
White blood cell count (× 10^9/L)	4.5–11.0	5.7–13.6	5.6–14.8	5.9–16.9
Neutrophils (× 10^9/L)	1.4–4.6	3.6–10.1	3.8–12.3	3.9–13.1
Lymphocytes (× 10^9/L)	0.7–4.6	1.1–3.6	0.9–3.9	1.0–3.6
Monocytes (× 10^9/L)	0.1–0.7	0.1–1.1	0.1–1.1	0.1–1.4
Eosinophils (× 10^9/L)	0–0.6	0–0.6	0–0.6	0–0.6
Basophils (× 10^9/L)	0–0.2	0–0.1	0–0.1	0–0.1

Sources: Kratz, et al., 2004 [3]; Abbassi-Ghanavati, et al., 2009 [4].

agree that the platelet count in pregnancy seldom falls below 150×10^9/L [1,2]. Although a mild decrease in platelet count (70×10^9/L to 150×10^9/L) may be seen in women with gestational thrombocytopenia, dramatic decreases in platelet counts may be seen in conditions such as pre-eclampsia, placental abruption, or HELLP syndrome [1,2]. Changes observed in RBC, WBC platelet count, and other hematological parameters during pregnancy are summarized in Table 10.8.

The anatomical and physiological changes that occur during pregnancy increase the risk of thromboembolic events by four- to five-fold compared with non-pregnant women; these changes are consistent with Virchow's triad: vessel wall injury, increased venous stasis, and hypercoagulability [1,13]. Increased venous status in the lower extremities primarily results from compression of the inferior vena cava and pelvic veins by the enlarging uterus [1,13]. Pregnancy also alters the delicate balance of procoagulant, anticoagulant, and fibrinolytic activity, leading to overall hypercoagulability; while factors I (plasma fibrinogen), VII, VIII, and X are markedly increased, factors II, V, and IX remain unchanged [1,13]. In addition, pregnancy causes a decrease in the fibrinolytic activity through an increase in plasminogen activator inhibitor 1 and 2 [1,13]. Similarly, a progressive

Table 10.9. Changes in coagulation factors during pregnancy

Coagulation factor	Change from non-pregnant state
Antithrombin III	No change
Plasma fibrinogen (factor I)	↑
Factor II	No change
Factor V	No change
Factor VII	↑
Factor VIII	↑
Factor IX	No change
Factor X	↑
Free protein S	↓
Plasminogen activator inhibitor 1	↑
Plasminogen activator inhibitor 2	↑
Protein C	No change
von Willebrand factor	↑

Source: American College of Obstetricians and Gynecologists, 2011 [13].

decrease in the levels of total and free protein S is noted in pregnancy without alteration of protein C and antithrombin III [1,13]. These changes in activity of the coagulation system are summarized in Tables 10.9 and 10.10.

Endocrine system

Several biochemical and metabolic changes are mediated by the interaction of different protein and steroid hormones during pregnancy. These changes are not only necessary for early embryonic and later fetal growth but are also important in mobilizing energy stores and transporting nutrients during pregnancy. Hence, endocrine disorders during pregnancy can adversely affect maternal and fetal outcome [1,3]. Table 10.11 summarizes physiological alterations of hormone levels during different trimesters of pregnancy.

Adrenal glands

Pregnancy is associated with an overall increase in the serum concentrations of total cortisol, free cortisol, aldosterone, deoxycorticosterone, corticosteroid-binding globulin, and adrenocorticotropic hormone [1,3]. Although the weight of the adrenal glands do not change significantly during pregnancy, expansion of the zona fasciculate is observed [1]. Corticosteroid-binding globulin concentrations begin to increase during the second trimester and rise to twice non-pregnant levels by term; total and free cortisol concentrations show a parallel increase beginning early second trimester (Table 10.11) [3]. Diurnal pattern of cortisol production is maintained during pregnancy, with significantly higher values found in the morning than in the afternoon [1,3]. The adrenal gland is more responsive to adrenocorticotropic hormone during pregnancy, causing a greater rise in cortisol concentration for a given dose of adrenocorticotropic hormone [3]. Despite these changes, the urinary excretion of catecholamines, vanillylmandelic acid, and metanephrines do not change during pregnancy (Table 10.11) [3].

Pancreas

Pregnancy results in fasting hypoglycemia, postprandial hyperglycemia, and hyperinsulinemia [1]. Early in pregnancy, estrogen and progesterone stimulate islet cell enlargement, hyperplasia of beta-cells, insulin secretion, and increased sensitivity of peripheral

Table 10.10. Changes in the levels of coagulation factors during pregnancy

Coagulation factor	Non-pregnant adult	First trimester	Second trimester	Third trimester
Antithrombin III, functional (% [U/L])	80–130 (0.8–1.3)	89–114 (0.89–1.14)	88–112 (0.88–1.12)	82–116 (0.82–1.16)
D-dimer (mg/L)	<0.5	0.05–0.95	0.32–1.29	0.13–1.7
Plasma fibrinogen (factor I) (g/L)	1.5–4.0	2.44–5.1	2.91–5.38	3.73–6.19
Factor VII (%)	60–140	100–146	95–153	149–211
Factor VIII (%)	50–200	90–210	97–312	143–253
International normalized ratio	0.9–1.04	0.89–1.05	0.85–0.97	0.80–0.94
Partial thromboplastin time, activated (s)	22.1–35.1	24.3–38.9	24.2–38.1	24.7–35.0
Prothrobin time (s)	11.1–13.1	9.7–13.5	9.5–13.4	9.6–12.9
Protein C, functional (%)	70–140	78–121	83–133	67–135
Protein S, total (%)	70–140	39–105	27–101	33–101
Protein S, free (%)	70–140	34–133	19–113	20–65
Tissue plasminogen activator (µg/L)	1.6–13	1.8–6.0	2.4–6.6	3.3–9.2
Tissue plasminogen activator inhibitor 1 (µg/L)	4–43	16–33	36–55	67–92
Von Willebrand factor (%)	75–125	Not reported	Not reported	121–260

Sources: Kratz, *et al.*, 2004 [3]; Abbassi-Ghanavati, *et al.*, 2009 [4].

Table 10.11. Physiological alterations in different hormone levels during pregnancy

Hematological parameter	Non-pregnant adult	First trimester	Second trimester	Third trimester
Aldosterone (pmol/L [ng/dL])	55–250 (2–9)	166–1885 (6–104)	250–1885 (9–104)	416–2802 (15–101)
Angiotensin-converting enzyme (U/L [nkat/L])	<670 (<40)	1–38 (16–633)	1–36 (16–600)	1–39 (16–650)
Cortisol (nmol/L [µg/dL])	0–690 (0–25)	193–524 (7–19)	276–1159 (10–42)	331–1379 (12–50)
Estradiol (nmol/L [ng/dL])	0.07–1.63 (2.0–44.3)	0.69–9.17 (18.8–249.7)	4.69–26.40 (127.8–719.2)	22.53–127.0 (613.7–346.0)
Hemoglobin A1c (%)	3.8–6.4	4–6	4–6	4–7
Parathyroid hormone (ng/L)	10–60	10–15	18–25	9–26
Parathyroid hormone-related protein (pmol/L)	<1.3	0.7–0.9	1.8–2.2	2.5–2.8
Progesterone (nmol/L [µg/dL])	0.64–64 (0.02–2.0)	25.4–153 (0.8–4.8)	Not reported	315–1088 (9.9–34.2)
Prolactin (µg/L)	0–20	36–213	110–330	137–372
Sex hormone-binding globulin (nmol/L)	18–114	39–131	214–717	216–724
Thyroid-stimulating hormone (mU/L)	0.5–4.7	0.60–3.4	0.37–3.6	0.38–4.04
Thyroxine, free (pmol/L [ng/dL])	10.3–35.0 (0.8–2.7)	10.3–15.5 (0.8–1.2)	7.7–12.9 (0.6–1.0)	6.4–10.3 (0.5–0.8)

Sources: Kratz, *et al.*, 2004 [3]; Abbassi-Ghanavati, *et al.*, 2009 [4].

tissues to insulin [3]. The overall result is an anabolic state associated with increased glucose utilization, decreased gluconeogenesis, and increased glycogen storage [3]. In the latter half of pregnancy, however, rising levels of progesterone, cortisol, glucagon, human placental lactogen, and prolactin, along with decreased insulin receptor binding, contribute to insulin resistance [3]. After feeding, insulin resistance maintains high blood glucose levels, thereby enhancing glucose transport to the fetus [3]. These diabetogenic changes in some pregnant women may result in gestational diabetes [1,3].

Pituitary gland

Pituitary enlargement occurs in pregnancy by estrogen-mediated proliferation of prolactin-producing cells. This enlargement may render the pituitary gland more susceptible to alterations in blood supply, specifically increasing the risk for infarction in the context of excessive postpartum hemorrhage [1,3]. Serum prolactin levels begin to increase early first trimester and are 10 times higher at term. In non-lactating women, prolactin levels return to baseline by 3 months after delivery. However, in lactating women, this return may take several months and is influenced by the length and frequency of nursing [1]. Oxytocin levels increase throughout pregnancy: 10 ng/L in the first trimester, 30 ng/L in the third trimester, and 75 ng/L at term. These levels dramatically increase and peak during labor [1].

Thyroid

Pregnancy is an overall euthyroid state, although alterations in thyroid morphology and histology occur [1,3]. With adequate iodine intake, the size of the thyroid gland remains unchanged or increases slightly [1]. In addition, thyroid vascularity increases and histological evidence of follicular hyperplasia is noted [1]. However, the development of a goiter anytime during pregnancy is considered abnormal and should be evaluated [1,3].

During the first trimester of pregnancy, total thyroxine and total triiodothyronine concentrations begin to increase and peak at mid-gestation, primarily as a result of increased production of thyroid-binding globulin [1,3]. Free thyroxine concentrations, however, remain unchanged during the first trimester, after which there is a 25% decrease in mean concentrations during the second and third trimester [1,3]. Thyroid-stimulating hormone decreases transiently in the first trimester.

Following this initial decrease, concentrations rise to non-pregnant levels by the end of the first trimester and then remain stable throughout the remainder of pregnancy [1,3]. The transient decrease in thyroid-stimulating hormone is thought be to mediated by the thyrotropic effects of human chorionic gonadotropin and coincides with the first trimester increase in free thyroxine [1,3].

Immunology

The immunological adaptations of pregnancy, particularly at the maternal–fetal interface, comprise complex mechanisms that enable the fetus to grow while preventing the mother from rejecting the fetus [1,14]. These mechanisms include fetal factors such as altered major histocompatibility complex class I expression as well as maternal factors such as uterine natural killer cells and a shifting of the T-helper cell cytokine profile from type 1 to type 2 [1,14]. This shift in T-helper type 1-mediated cellular immunity to type 2-mediated humoral immunity may explain why pregnant women are more susceptible to viral infections [1,14].

References

1. Gabbe SG, Niebyl JR, Simpson JL, *et al.* (eds.) *Obstetrics: Normal and Problem Pregnancies*, 6th edn. Philadelphia, PA: Saunders-Elsevier, 2012.

2. Lockitch G. Biochemistry of Pregnancy. *Crit Rev Clin Lab Sci* 1997;**34**:67–139.

3. Kratz A, Ferraro M, Sluss PM, *et al.* Case records of the Massachusetts General Hospital. Weekly clinicopathological exercises. Laboratory reference values. *N Engl J Med* 2004;**351**:1548–1563.

4. Abbassi-Ghanavati M, Greer LG, Cunningham FG. Pregnancy and laboratory studies: a reference table for clinicians. *Obstet Gynecol* 2009;**114**:1326–1331.

5. Clapp JF III, Capeless E. Cardiovascular function before, during, and after the first and subsequent pregnancies. *Am J Cardiol* 1997;**80**:1469–1473.

6. Hunter S, Robson SC. Adaptation of the maternal heart in pregnancy. *Br Heart J* 1992 **68**:540–543.

7. Clark SL, Cotton DB, Lee W, *et al.* Central hemodynamic assessment of normal term pregnancy. *Am J Obstet Gynecol* 1989;**161**:1439–1442.

8. Crapo RO. Normal cardiopulmonary physiology during pregnancy. *Clin Obstet Gynecol* 1996;**39**:3–16.

9. Bobrowski RA. Pulmonary physiology in pregnancy. *Clin Obstet Gynecol* 2010;**53**:285–300.

10. Niebyl JR. Clinical practice. Nausea and vomiting in pregnancy. *N Engl J Med* 2012;**363**:1544–1550.

11. Dafnis E, Sabatini S. The effect of pregnancy on renal function: physiology and pathophysiology. *Am J Med Sci* 1992;**303**:184–205.

12. Arias F, Peck TM. Hematologic changes associated with pregnancy. *Clin Obstet Gynecol* 1979;**22**:785–798.

13. American College of Obstetricians and Gynecologists. Practice bulletin 123: thromboembolism in pregnancy. *Obstet Gynecol* 2011;**118**:718–729.

14. Poole JA, Claman HN. Immunology of pregnancy. implications for the mother. *Clin Rev Allergy Immunol* 2004;**26**:161–170.

Management of coagulopathy

Lawrence C. Tsen and Dianne Plews

Introduction

The enhancement of the coagulation system, which begins as early as fetal conception and extends into the 4th postpartum week, is among the most complex alterations induced by pregnancy [1]. However, these alterations may not fully mitigate the spectrum of coagulopathies that have continued from the non-pregnant state or are witnessed during the intra- or postpartum periods. Inherited bleeding disorders can produce significant management difficulties during pregnancy, although the most severe disorders are frequently diagnosed earlier in life and respond to discrete therapeutic interventions (e.g. individual factor replacement). Adverse drug events, particularly relating to the presence, dose, and timing of antiplatelet and coagulation-related medications (e.g. aspirin, heparin, thrombin inhibitors, thrombolytics, etc.), may also result in serious, critically relevant outcomes, but these are usually amenable to specific (e.g. protamine) or generalized (e.g. fresh frozen plasma) therapies.

By contrast, the management of major maternal hemorrhage, particularly when accompanied by disseminated intravascular coagulation (DIC) or the microangiopathies of pregnancy, can be complicated and controversial; admission and care in a critical care unit is frequently required. Maternal hemorrhage is the second leading cause, following pre-eclampsia-related complications, for admission of an obstetric patient to a critical care unit in both developed and developing countries (0.7/1000 deliveries; range 0.1–2.3) [2]. Disseminated intravascular coagulation can be a unifying factor between these and other entities; pre-eclampsia may also be associated with microangiopathy resulting in hemolysis, elevated liver enzymes, and low platelets (the HELLP syndrome). A final, equally complex microangiopathy that can complicate pregnancy is thrombotic thrombocytopenic purpura

(TTP). These three entities, DIC, HELLP, and TTP, represent unique and critical threats to the well-being of mother and fetus during the peripartum period and will consequently be the focus of this chapter.

Normal hemostasis in pregnancy

Normal hemostasis is a multistep process leading to stable clot formation and subsequent degradation at the site of vessel injury. It involves a dynamic relationship between the blood vessel epithelium, platelets, the coagulation cascade, anticoagulation elements, and the fibrinolytic system (Figure 11.1).

Following vascular injury, platelets rapidly adhere to exposed subendothelial collagen and von Willebrand factor. Various agonists (collagen, thrombin, epinephrine, ADP, and thromboxane A_2) then stimulate the platelets to release their alpha and dense granule contents, which promote further platelet recruitment, activation, and aggregation (primary hemostasis). Simultaneously, the coagulation cascade is activated, resulting in the generation of cross-linked fibrin, which interlaces with the platelet plug to form a stable clot (secondary hemostasis). Clot formation is limited by antithrombin, protein C, and protein S.

The normal thrombus undergoes degradation after endothelial healing occurs. An activated fibrinolytic system produces plasmin, which alters the cross-linked fibrin into degradation products. The degraded products from the thrombus are removed by normal blood flow.

During pregnancy, the majority of coagulation factors undergo a progressive increase, reaching maximal levels at time of delivery (Table 11.1). By contrast, levels of the natural anticoagulants and the activity of the fibrinolytic system decrease. The platelet count also decreases during normal pregnancy, most likely as a result of hemodilution and increased platelet destruction [1].

Maternal Critical Care: A Multidisciplinary Approach, ed. Marc Van de Velde, Helen Scholefield, and Lauren A. Plante.
Published by Cambridge University Press. © Cambridge University Press 2013.

Table 11.1. Hemostatic changes in pregnancy

	Coagulation factors	Fibrinolytic activity
Increased	Factors VII (up to 1000% by term), VIII, X, XII; von Willebrand factor, ristoceitin cofactor, fibrinogen	Plasminogen activator inhibitor 1 and 2, thrombin-activatable fibrinolysis inhibitor, D-dimers
Reduced	Factor XIII, protein S	Tissue plasminogen activator

Source: Thornton and Douglas, 2010 [1].

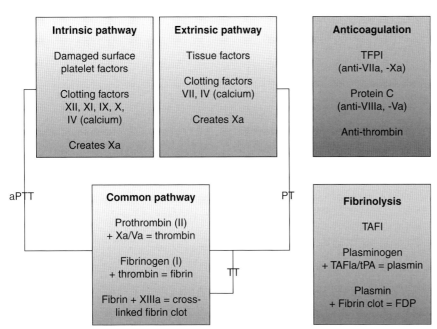

Figure 11.1. The process of normal hemostasis. aPTT, activated partial thromboplastin time; FDP, fibrinogen degradation products; PT, prothrombin time; TAFI, thrombin-activatable fibrinolysis inhibitor; TFPI, tissue factor pathway inhibitor (antithrombin); TT, thrombin time.

Tests of coagulation

Laboratory testing of coagulation is based on the time required to produce an in vitro clot. The tests are relatively insensitive, requiring a loss of up to 50% of coagulation factor activity before there is a significant prolongation of results. Interpretation is further complicated by pregnancy, when some of the expected physiological changes in coagulation factors produce a relative shortening of "normal" values.

The simple laboratory tests of coagulation are summarized in Table 11.2. As a screening test, the prothrombin time (PT) should be evaluated rather than the international normalized ratio, which is only validated for monitoring of patients on oral anticoagulants (e.g. warfarin). A platelet count is an additional useful screening tool, although it provides information limited to platelet numbers and not function. Fibrinogen levels may be derived using activated partial thromboplastin time/prothrombin time (aPTT/PT) assays or directly measured using the Clauss method; it must be remembered that fibrinogen levels are increased in pregnancy and apparently "normal" fibrinogen levels of 2 g/L can still be associated with maternal hemorrhage. The measurement of bleeding time, which requires making small, shallow incisions or puncture in the skin, is no longer recommended as it is invasive, unreliable, highly operator dependent, and unsuitable for repeated tests [1].

Thromboelastography provides useful real-time information about the various stages of coagulation and fibrinolysis and is now available in many centers, either as near-patient testing or within the laboratory. There are significant differences between pregnant and

Table 11.2. Tests of coagulation

Screening test	Abnormalities indicated by prolongation	Commonest causes of abnormality
Thrombin time	Deficiency or abnormality of fibrinogen or inhibition of thrombin by heparin or fibrinogen degradation products	DIC, heparin therapy
Prothrombin time	Deficiency or inhibition of one or more of the following coagulation factors: factors II, V, VII, and X, fibrinogen	Liver disease, vitamin K deficiency, warfarin therapy, DIC
Activated partial thromboplastin time	Deficiency or inhibition of one or more of the following coagulation factors: factors XII, XI, IX, VIII	Hemophilia A or B, von Willebrands disease DIC, heparin therapy, lupus anticoagulant

DIC, disseminated intravascular coagulation.

Table 11.3. Obstetric conditions associated with disseminated intravascular coagulation

Disease processes	Obstetric events
Acute fatty liver	Amniotic fluid embolism
Dilutional coagulopathy	Dilutional coagulopathy
Gestational trophoblastic disease	Intrauterine fetal demise
Hemolysis, elevated liver enzymes, low platelets	Placental abruption (most common cause)
Hemolytic transfusion reaction	Placental previa
Sepsis	Pre-eclampsia/eclampsia
Trauma	

non-pregnant women in all thromboelastography parameters and new reference limits have recently been recommended in pregnancy [2]. The absence of both standardized testing procedures and large clinical trials of its use during pregnancy have limited its routine application; however, as more experimental and clinical trial data become available, thromboelastography may provide accurate and needed interpretation of coagulopathies in pregnancy.

Platelet function assays measure the speed of formation of a platelet plug in vitro. Some studies in parturients suggest that such assays may be an effective bedside test of platelet function, but there is no evidence currently to support its routine use [1].

Disseminated intravascular coagulation

Disseminated intravascular coagulation is a syndrome characterized by systemic activation of pathways leading to and regulating coagulation (Figure 11.1), which can result in the generation of fibrin clots and consumption of coagulation factors and platelets; these clots may subsequently cause organ failure with concomitant consumption of platelets and coagulation factors that may result in clinical bleeding [3].

Etiology

Disseminated intravascular coagulation cannot originate spontaneously or in isolation [3] but rather arises in association with a spectrum of disorders or antecedent events, some of which are unique to pregnancy (Table 11.3).

The pathogenesis of DIC is believed to originate with the exposure of procoagulant surfaces or substances, or the enhanced generation of thrombin in vivo [3], which induces the formation and deposition of fibrin clot, the occlusion of small vessels, and subsequent tissue ischemia. Organ dysfunction, including cerebral infarction, acute respiratory distress syndrome, hepatic and renal failure, can result from DIC and may undergo further exacerbation with continued bleeding and hypoperfusion. Associated immunological or inflammatory mediators may further accentuate the coagulation distortion.

In obstetrics, thromboembolic phenomena, placental abruption, and pre-eclampsia are the most common precursors to DIC. A unifying factor associated with these entities appears to be the placental release of tissue immunological or inflammatory factors. The placenta contains fetal trophoblastic cells, which can alter hemostatic properties through the expression of tissue factor, suppression of anticoagulation and fibrinolysis, and presentation of anionic phospholipids [4]. Immune-mediated processes may assist in the biochemical signaling of the trophoblastic cell invasion of the uterine wall, or act as a potential cofactor in the production of coagulation abnormalities that result in DIC.

Placental abruption, separation, or partial retention interrupts the decidual–placental interface and allows the entry of tissue factor into the maternal systemic circulation; the degree of placental separation can correlate with the extent of fibrin formation and thrombocytopenia. Immunological and inflammatory factors have been associated with premature placental separation. Pre-eclampsia is also believed to originate from placental irregularities, with abnormal cytotrophoblast invasion of maternal spiral arteries in the endometrium causing placental hypoxia, intrauterine hypoxemia, and release of placental debris. Placental deterioration, as witnessed in multiple gestation, diabetes, prolonged pregnancy, sepsis, and intrauterine fetal demise, may invoke a similar sequence of events [5]. Mechanical disruption of placentation or pregnancy, as occurs with dilatation and evacuation or curettage, can provoke a similar cascade, particularly if the procedure is performed later in pregnancy and is associated with a fetal demise.

Clinical features

The clinical expression of DIC is variable. Acute DIC usually presents as difficulty in achieving hemostasis, which can be manifested by oozing from venipuncture sites, hematuria, pink-tinged pulmonary fluid, purpura, or petechiae. Chronic, compensated DIC is generally associated with thrombosis overbleeding and consequently more commonly presents as minor mucosal bleeding, hematuria, epistaxis, and easy bruising. Both hemorrhagic and thrombotic expressions of DIC are relevant to the management and final outcomes.

Investigations

There is no single diagnostic test for DIC. It is important to consider the clinical condition of the patient, the diagnosis, and all available laboratory results.

The dynamic nature of DIC is reflected in the need for serial measurements of coagulation factor consumption and activation (e.g. platelet count, PT, aPTT) as well as fibrin formation and lysis (e.g. fibrin D-dimers). An analysis of 900 patients in five independent reports indicated the most frequent laboratory abnormalities were, in decreasing order of frequency, thrombocytopenia, elevated fibrin degradation products (FDPs), prolonged PT, prolonged aPTT, and low fibrinogen [3]. Further studies are needed to examine whether the same order of prevalence is preserved in pregnant patients, given the many alterations observed in normal pregnancy, including thrombocytopenia, elevated FDPs, and enhanced fibrinogen.

Platelet count

A reduction or downward trend in platelet counts, even if within the "normal" range (150×10^9/L to 400×10^9/L), may reflect DIC caused by thrombin-induced platelet aggregation. Thrombocytopenia is a feature in up to 98% of those with DIC [3].

However, thrombocytopenia is not uncommon in pregnancy, with gestational thrombocytopenia being the most common (75%), followed by microangiopathic purpuras (21%; e.g. pre-eclampsia), auto- and alloimmune causes (3%), and other causes (<1%) [6]. These entities may often be distinguished from DIC by presentation earlier in pregnancy (first trimester: immune thrombocytopenic purpura; second trimester: gestational thrombocytopenia, pre-eclampsia); moreover, with gestational thrombocytopenia, it is exceptional for platelet counts to fall below 80×10^9/L [7].

Prothrombin time and activated partial thromboplastin time

Consumption of coagulation factors is the main reason for prolongation of PT or aPTT in 50–60% of those with DIC; however, impaired synthesis or loss of coagulation proteins may also be contributory [3]. Normal or shortened PT and aPTT values may exist during DIC because of activated clotting factors, which can accelerate the formation of thrombin.

Fibrin degradation products and D-dimers

Fibrin degradation products, which are measures of fibrinolytic activity, do not discriminate between degradation of cross-linked fibrin or fibrinogen. Levels may be increased in many conditions including normal pregnancy, recent surgery, trauma, and venous thromboembolic disease, as well as in DIC; FDP levels also may be altered by impairment of liver metabolism or kidney excretion. Raised FDPs and D-dimers are, therefore, not diagnostic of DIC as a stand-alone test and "significant" increases in FDPs have yet to be defined [3]. However, FDPs may be indicative of DIC when witnessed in the setting of a falling platelet count, prolonged coagulation times, and a consistent clinical evaluation.

The measurement of soluble fibrin monomers may more directly reflect thrombin's action on fibrinogen because such monomers are only generated intravascularly and, therefore, this avoids the potential contributions of extravascular inflammation or trauma. Although the presence of soluble fibrin monomers is associated with a 90–100% sensitivity for the diagnosis of DIC and an improvement in the specificity of the International Society on Thrombosis and Haemostasis DIC scoring system (noted below) when substituted for D-dimer, the very low specificity for DIC and wide discordance among assay systems limit its use [3].

Fibrinogen

The sensitivity of low fibrinogen levels for the diagnosis of DIC appears low (28%), with hypofibrinogenemia being detected only in very severe cases of DIC [3]. In addition, fibrinogen levels are significantly elevated during pregnancy, particularly during the third trimester. As a result, sequential measurements may be helpful in indicating a trend, although high FDPs may interfere with its measurement.

Other hemostatic markers

Fragmented red blood cells can be found in DIC but are rarely greater than 10% of the red cells and are neither sensitive nor specific for DIC. When seen in increased numbers, other causes (e.g. a thrombotic microangiopathy such as TTP) should be considered.

Antithrombin and protein C are frequently reduced in DIC but lack the sensitivity and specificity to diagnose the disorder.

Diagnosis

The diagnosis of DIC cannot rely on a single clinical sign, symptom or laboratory test; instead, a combination of clinical and laboratory information is necessary. The International Society of Thrombosis and Haemostasis has proposed a diagnostic algorithm to calculate a DIC score using the simple laboratory tests that are available at most hospitals (Tables 11.2 and 11.4) [3]. Overt DIC in either acute or chronic settings is indicated by cumulative score ≥5; this scoring threshold has 91% sensitivity, 97% specificity, 96% positive predictive value, and 97% negative predictive value for DIC diagnosed by blinded "expert" assessments [8]. Protein C, antithrombin, thrombin–antithrombin complexes, fibrinogen, and soluble fibrin varied significantly in patients with and without DIC, and did not increase the accuracy of the score [8].

Subsequent diagnostic scoring systems for DIC have been developed with different threshold values (Table 11.4); a prospective study of 413 mixed gender, older (mean age, 64 years) subjects with diseases associated with DIC evaluated the three most common

Table 11.4. Diagnostic algorithms for disseminated intravascular coagulation

Establish	Algorithm (points given for item)		
	JMHW	ISTH	JAAM
Underlying disease	Present (1)	Necessary (1)	Necessary (1)
Clinical symptoms	Bleeding (1[a]), organ failure (1)	NA	SIRS (1)
Platelet count (× 10^9/L)	>80 but <120 (1[a]), >50 but <80 (2[a]), <50 (3[a])	<100 (1), <50 (2)	>80 but <120 (1[b]), <80 (2[c])
Fibrin-related markers	FDP (mg/L): >10 but <20 (1), >20 but <40 (2), >40 (3)	FDP, SF, or D-dimer: moderate increase (2), severe increase (3)	FDP (mg/L): >10 but <25 (1), >25 (3)
Fibrinogen (g/L)	>1 but <1.5 (1)	<1 (1)	NA
Prothrombin time (s)	>1.25 but <1.5 (1), >1.67 (2)	>3 but <6 (1), >6 (2)	>1.2 (1)
Point accumulation to diagnose DIC	≥7	≥5	≥4

FDP, fibrinogen degradation products; ISTH, International Society on Thrombosis and Haemostasis, JAAM, Japanese Association for Acute Medicine; JMHW, Japanese Ministry of Health and Welfare; SF, soluble fibrin; SIRS, systemic inflammatory response syndrome; PT, prothrombin time; NA, non-applicable.
[a] In patients with hematopoietic malignancy, 0 points.
[b] Can also be a 30% reduction in platelet count.
[c] Can also be a 50% reduction in platelet count.

scoring systems [9]. The Japanese Association for Acute Medicine and the International Society on Thrombosis and Haemostasis criteria were found to have the highest sensitivity and specificity for DIC, respectively. Regardless of the criteria used, the early stages of DIC may be missed because of the limited ability of global coagulation tests (platelets, PT, aPTT, FDP) to identify such alterations. Ultimately, hemostatic molecular markers such as thrombin–antithrombin complexes and soluble fibrin may prove to be better indicators of early DIC stages [9].

Confounding issues

Major obstetric hemorrhage is frequently associated with coagulopathy, either from inadequate number or function of the coagulation components or from conditions unfavorable to the process.

Hemodilution has been associated with coagulation disorders, with increasing attention being placed on the type of intravenous solutions used for volume replacement and/or expansion. Colloid solutions (e.g. hydroxyethyl starch) have been observed to have both direct and indirect effects on hemostatic components, resulting in the inhibition of platelets, a reduction in coagulation factors and fibrinogen, and an augmentation of fibrinolysis [10]. The adverse hemostatic effects are more prevalent with colloids of greater molecular weight and degree of hydroxylation [10]. In an ex vivo model, dilution of blood with hydroxyethyl starch (130 kDa/0.4 and 200 kDa/0.5) at levels as low as 10% was associated with greater inhibition of platelet aggregation and fibrin formation when compared with saline [10]. Administration of crystalloid solutions, particularly when given in large volumes, can result in hemostatic alterations stemming from hypothermia, displacement of established clots, dilutional coagulopathy, acidosis, and tissue edema [11].

Acidosis and hypothermia have noted effects on coagulation. In (non-pregnant) adults without major brain injury or pre-existing coagulopathy and undergoing trauma resuscitation, the development of coagulopathy was associated with pH <7.1 (relative risk (RR), 12.3), core temperature <34°C, an injury severity score >25 (RR, 7.7) and a systolic blood pressure <70 mmHg (RR, 5.8) [12]. A pH of 7.0 reduces the activity of enzymatic enzymes, factor VIIa, factor VIIa/tissue factor complex, and factors Xa/Va (prothrombinase) complex by 55–90% [13]. Hydrogen ions interfere with ionic interactions between coagulation proteins as well as with the negatively charged phospholipids on activated platelets.

Each 1 °C decrease in temperature reduces the activity of coagulation factor enzymes by approximately 10%. Platelets have greater sensitivity to low temperatures, with the interaction between platelet glycoprotein Ib/IX and von Willebrand factor virtually non-existent at 30 °C [12]. Hypothermia can also result in decreased citrate metabolism, hepatic metabolism, drug clearance, and synthesis of acute phase proteins and clotting factors [13].

Resuscitation efforts with blood and fluids should always consider the potential for adverse reactions. Such reactions include transfusion-associated circulatory overload, transfusion-related acute lung injury, allergic reactions, hemolysis, and hypotension [14]. The incidence, etiology, prevention, and therapy for these complications have recently been reviewed [14]. Citrate, which is added to packed red blood cells to prevent clotting by complexing with calcium, may result in both hypocalcemia and hypomagnesemia when the packed red blood cells are transfused; these electrolyte disorders subsequently may impair coagulation and other cellular functions. Hyperkalemia from lysed red cells, particularly in older units of packed red blood cells, may also be observed with such transfusions and lead to electrical conduction and cellular function disorders. When replacing calcium, calcium chloride contains three times the amount of elemental calcium as calcium gluconate [13].

Management

The response to DIC must be directed primarily at treating the underlying conditions; however, supportive therapy is often required in the presence of bleeding or a high risk for bleeding (e.g. patients who are to undergo an invasive procedure or are recovering postoperatively). An understanding of the efficacy and safety of therapeutic measures is limited by the heterogeneity of DIC definitions and the paucity of evidence; in particular, there are very few studies evaluating a comparison with controlled groups using no-treatment or placebo.

Plasma and platelets

In non-bleeding patients with DIC, platelets and factor replacement should not be administered prophylactically or based on laboratory tests alone [3]. In the presence or perceived risk of bleeding, a platelet

Table 11.5. Considerations for transfusion of blood products

	Threshold for therapy		Therapy initial dose
	Bleeding patient	Non-bleeding patient	
Platelets ($\times 10^9$/L)	<50	10–20	240 (one pool of 5 units)
Plasma			10–15 mL/kg fresh frozen plasma
Fibrinogen (g/L)	<1	<1	Fresh frozen plasma 10–15 mL/kg, cryoprecipitate 5–10 mL/kg, fibrinogen concentrate 3 g

count of $<50 \times 10^9$/L or a prolonged PT/aPTT warrant consideration of platelet and fresh frozen plasma administration, respectively (Table 11.5) [3]. Severe hypofibrinogenemia (<1 g/L) that persists despite replacement with fresh frozen plasma may be treated with fibrinogen concentrate or cryoprecipitate. If the patient is currently fluid overloaded, factor concentrates (e.g. prothrombin complex concentrate) can be used, recognizing that only partial correction of the deficit will be observed because these complexes contain an incomplete panel of factors. There is a theoretical increased risk of thrombosis when factor concentrates are used in DIC, which must be considered prior to usage. Of interest, the use of high (versus low) ratios of plasma and platelets to red blood cells (≥1:2) may be of less benefit in women than in men, which may reflect gender-related differences in coagulation [15].

Anticoagulants

In the setting of DIC and thrombosis (e.g. arterial or venous thromboembolism, severe purpura fulminans associated with acral ischemia, or vascular skin infarction), anticoagulant therapy can be considered despite the absence of randomized, controlled clinical trials demonstrating improvement in clinical outcomes [3]. Heparin may partially inhibit the activation of coagulation in DIC and improve the associated laboratory anomalies. In patients at high risk of bleeding, unfractionated heparin may be administered by continuous infusion, as it has a short half-life and reversibility. Weight-adjusted doses (e.g. 10 mg/kg per hour) may be used without arbitrary therapy-directed goals (e.g. aPTT ratio of 1.5–2.5 times control), as these patients may be difficult to titrate [3]; clinical bleeding should serve as an important guide. Such therapies are standard care in patients with DIC, particularly in individuals at high risk of venous thromboembolic events

(e.g. advanced age, recent surgery, immobilization, in-dwelling vascular catheters, prior thromboembolic events) [3].

The replacement of low concentrations of anticoagulant agents, such as antithrombin III and protein C, in the setting of DIC is controversial; some guidelines advocate against their use, particularly in the absence of concomitant heparin use. Few studies have evaluated antithrombin III in this setting, particularly in the obstetric patient. In one randomized controlled trial of DIC secondary to placental abruption and postpartum bleeding, antithrombin III (3000 U/day) resulted in an improvement of coagulation parameters in 92% of patients; in the same study, gabexate mesilate (a serine protease inhibitor; 20–39 mg/kg per day) resulted in an improvement of coagulation paramaters in 53% of patients [16]. No adverse events were reported in either group. Pre- and postadministration levels of antithrombin III (goal >70%) can be predicted by the concentration of serum total protein and albumin (molecular weight 63 000) [17]; low levels of these proteins may indicate that capillary leak is present, particularly in DIC-related entities such as sepsis. Such capillary permeability would make it less likely for smaller molecules, such as antithrombin III (molecular weight 56 000), to stay intravascular.

Recombinant human activated protein C (24 mg/kg per hour continuous infusion for 96 hours) given in the setting of DIC and severe sepsis has been demonstrated to reduce the risk of 28-day mortality and thrombotic events when compared with placebo. In a cohort of 16 patients with DIC secondary to placental abruption, plasma-derived activated protein C (5000–10 000 IU for 48 hours) was noted to significantly modify all laboratory parameters except for platelet count; resolution of the DIC was observed at 24 hours [18]. Activated protein C is considered appropriate in the setting of severe sepsis but has not yet been recommended for other obstetric complications associated with DIC. Activated protein C should be discontinued prior to invasive procedures (elimination half-life is approximately 20 minutes) and resumed a few hours after, depending on the clinical situation. In patients at high risk of bleeding or with platelet counts $<30 \times 10^9$/L, protein C should not be given.

Additional therapies, including dermatan sulfate, recombinant factor VIIa, gabexate, plasma exchange, and thrombomodulin, appear to offer some promise in selected situations; however, they remain investigational and are not recommended at this time.

Antifibrinolytic agents

In the presence of DIC, the use of antifibrinolytic agents is generally not recommended; an exception would be in the setting of primary or secondary hyperfibrinolysis, which can be observed with some leukemias and malignancies.

The HELLP syndrome: hemolysis, elevated liver enzymes, and low platelet count

The HELLP triad represents a syndrome present in 0.5–0.9% of all pregnancies and 4–14% of those with severe pre-eclampsia/eclampsia [19]. Typically considered a variant or complication of severe pre-eclampsia, HELLP represents a serious condition with significant implications for mother and fetus.

Etiology

The pathogenesis of HELLP is believed to represent more than an epiphenomenon of hypertension or pre-eclampsia; plasma cellular fibronectin and markers of platelet activation and aggregation have been observed to precede the presence of severe pre-eclampsia [20]. Aberrant placental development and oxidative stress may play a role in releasing factors that injure the endothelium. The complement system (C1q and C5b–C9) may augment the thrombogenic properties of blood and induce an upregulation of platelet adhesion molecules on endothelial cells, resulting in coagulation and inhibition of endothelial-derived vasorelaxation [19].

Hemolysis represents red cell fragmentation from high-velocity passage through damaged endothelium; as such, HELLP is considered a form of microangiopathic hemolytic anemia.

Those with HELLP exhibit prominent endothelial damage in the liver, resulting in altered function,

congestion, ischemia, necrosis, and an elevation of liver enzymes. Recent investigations have evaluated the role of a ligand produced by the placenta, CD95 (APO01, Fas), which causes hepatocyte apoptosis; blocking this mediator has been observed to reduce cytotoxic and apoptotic activity in the hepatocytes of women with HELLP [19].

Renal dysfunction may occur from damaged microcirculation or intravascular volume depletion from plasma extravasation in the altered systemic microcirculation.

Clinical features

In 70% of cases, HELLP syndrome occurs before delivery with a frequency peak between the 27th and 37th gestational week [21]. When presenting in the postpartum period, HELLP usually develops within the first 48 hours (but can develop later as well), particularly in women who experienced proteinuria and hypertension prior to delivery. Postpartum onset is associated with a significantly greater risk of renal failure and pulmonary edema. In approximately 10–20% of cases, hypertension and proteinuria are absent, whereas excessive weight gain and generalized edema precede the syndrome in over 50%.

Typical clinical symptoms include right upper abdominal quadrant or epigastric pain, which may fluctuate in intensity and result in nausea and vomiting. Patients may present with a history of malaise or other non-specific flu-like symptoms several days prior to the presentation. Between 30 and 60% of HELLP patients may report a headache, with 20% also indicating visual symptoms; symptoms have been characterized by exacerbations during the night, with recovery during the day.

Hepatic Doppler blood flow examination in patients with HELLP indicates decreased flow and hypovolemia, with ischemia resulting in infarction, subcapsular hematomas, intraparenchymatous hemorrhage, and, although rarely, hepatic rupture [19]. Rupture usually occurs in the right liver lobe and is accompanied by sudden-onset, severe epigastric and right upper abdominal pain radiating to the back or right shoulder, anemia, and hypotension. Ultrasound, computed tomography (CT), or MRI examination can aid in the diagnosis.

Neurological complications associated with HELLP include cerebral and brainstem hemorrhage, thrombosis, infarction, and edema. Wound hematomas, placental abruption, and maternal hemorrhage are more common in the setting of HELLP, which may culminate in DIC; in women with HELLP, higher concentrations of fibronectin and D-dimer, and lower antithrombin levels, are observed when compared with women with normal pregnancies or preeclampsia only [21].

The HELLP syndrome can result in death of the mother, particularly when associated with cerebral hemorrhage or hepatic rupture. Fetal morbidity and mortality (range, 7–34%) in pregnancies associated with HELLP is greatly influenced by the gestational age of the fetus at birth. Prematurity, placental insufficiency, intrauterine growth restriction, placental abruption, and maternal hepatic rupture are associated with greater perinatal mortality. Neonatal thrombocytopenia occurs in 15–38% of cases of HELLP, which can augment the risk of intraventricular hemorrhage and other complications [21].

Investigations

The diagnosis of the HELLP syndrome relies on the demonstration of three elements (Table 11.6).

Hemolysis is demonstrated by an abnormal peripheral blood smear, the presence of unconjugated serum bilirubin, elevated lactate dehydrogenase (LDH), and low or undetectable haptoglobin. Red blood cells that are fragmented (schizocytes) or contracted with spicula (Burr cells) are representative of the hemolytic process, with increased reticulocyte counts reflecting a compensatory release of immature red cells into the peripheral blood. Destruction of red blood cells causes decreased hemoglobin concentrations and increased serum LDH. Hemoglobin is converted to unconjugated bilirubin in the spleen, or bound by haptoglobin and removed by the liver, resulting in very low or undetectable haptoglobin levels (<1 to <0.2 g/L).

Elevated liver enzymes

Liver biopsies demonstrate periportal hemorrhage, focal parenchymatous necrosis and macrovesicular steatosis in up to 33% of patients with HELLP; however, these histological findings are not specific for the disease process nor do they necessarily correlate with the clinical presentation [19]. Fibrin and hyaline deposits can be seen by immunofluorescence in the liver sinusoids. Elevation of liver enzymes reflects the hemolytic and liver processes. As noted above, hemolysis elevates levels of LDH; liver injury results in increased levels of aspartate aminotransferase, alanine aminotransferase, and gamma-glutamyltransferase). Elevation of plasma glutathione S-transferase-α_1 may represent a more sensitive earlier marker of liver damage, but its measuement is not widely available.

Thrombocytopenia is the result of increased consumption following greater platelet activation and adherence to endothelial cells.

Diagnosis

"True" or "complete" HELLP syndrome requires that the complete triad be present. The diagnosis has been complicated and obscured by different criteria, including the presence or absence of hypertension or preeclampsia, and the use of different biochemical levels [21]. Currently, two classifications of diagnostic criteria exist for HELLP syndrome (Table 11.7).

Partial or incomplete HELLP has been reported where only some of the elements (or thresholds) are present, including the complete absence of hemolysis (i.e. ELLP). The use of lower LDH and alanine aminotransferase thresholds has also been considered.

Differential diagnosis

The differential diagnosis of HELLP syndrome includes a number of disease entities (Table 11.8) [21,22].

Table 11.6. The HELLP triad

Entity	Characteristics	Severe maternal morbidity[a]
Hemolysis	Abnormal peripheral smear, total bilirubin ≥12 mg/L	Lactate dehydrogenase >1400 U/L
Elevated liver enzymes	AST >70 IU/L, GGT >70 IU/L	AST >150 U/L, ALT >100 U/L, uric acid (>460 mmol/L) (>7.8 mg/dL)
Low platelet count	<100 × 10^9/L	

ALT, alanine aminotransferase (also known as serum glutamic pyruvic transaminase); AST, aspartate aminotransferase; GGT, gamma-glutamyltransferase; HELLP, hemolysis, elevated liver enzymes, and low platelets.
[a] Criteria associated with >75% risk of serious maternal morbidity [21].

Table 11.7. Diagnostic criteria for the HELLP syndrome

HELLP class	Criteria	Tennessee classification	Mississippi classification
1	LDH (IU/L)	≥600	≥600
	AST (IU/L)	≥70	≥70 (or ALT)
	Platelets (× 10^9/L)	≤100	≤50
2	LDH (IU/L)		≥600
	AST (IU/L)		≥70 (or ALT)
	Platelets (× 10^9/L)		≤50 to 100
3	LDH (IU/L)		≥600
	AST (IU/L)		≥70 (or ALT)
	Platelets (× 10^9/L)		≤100 to 150

ALT, alanine aminotransferase; AST, aspartate aminotransferase; HELLP, hemolysis, elevated liver enzymes, and low platelets; LDH, lactate dehydrogenase.

Table 11.8. Differential diagnosis of the HELLP syndrome

Entity	Elements	Distinguishing differences
Acute fatty liver of pregnancy	30–38th gestational week; 1–2 weeks of malaise, anorexia, nausea, vomiting, epigastric or right upper abdominal pain, headache, jaundice; liver biopsy can confirm diagnosis	Hypertension and proteinuria usually absent; hypoglycemia and prolongation of prothrombin time often present; ultrasound and CT of liver may show increased echogenicity and decreased attenuation, respectively
Hemolytic uremic syndrome	Endothelial injury, platelet aggregation, microthrombi, thrombocytopenia, anemia; treated with plasma exchange and intensive care support	Microvascular injury affects primarily kidneys; usually develops postpartum Most cases in children and adolescents caused by enterotoxin (*Escherichia coli*) or rare genetic abnormality of complement system
Thrombotic thrombocytopenic purpura	Neurological dysfunction including headache, visual disturbances, confusion, aphasia, paresis, weakness, seizures; treated with plasma exchange and intensive care support	Rare during pregnancy; increased high-molecular-weight von Willebrand factor resulting from a virtually absence of the enzyme ADAMTS13
Systemic lupus erythematosus	Antigen–antibody deposits in capillaries affecting multiple organs (kidneys, lungs, heart, liver, and brain); can mimic severe pre-eclampsia; thrombocytopenia in 40–50% and hemolytic anemia in 14–23%	Anti-phospholipid antibodies (lupus anticoagulant and/or anti-cardiolipin) present in 30–40%; antibodies may result in recurrent thrombosis, and may be associated with HELLP

HELLP, hemolysis, elevated liver enzymes, and low platelets.

Thrombocytopenia can be observed with gestation (59%), immune thrombocytopenic purpura (11%), pre-eclampsia (10%), and HELLP (12%) [21]. Immune thrombocytopenic purpura has limited maternal or fetal morbidity or mortality. Folate deficiency may result in hemolytic anemia, thrombocytopenia, and coagulopathy.

Infectious and inflammatory diseases, not specifically related to pregnancy, may mimic HELLP, including viral hepatitis, cholangitis, cholecystitis, upper urinary tract infection, gastritis, gastric ulcer, or acute pancreatitis.

Management

Clinical management of HELLP is directed by maternal and fetal status, gestational age, presence of labor, cervical status, obstetric history, and laboratory or other associated findings. The treatment of HELLP involves monitoring and responding to maternal signs and symptoms, particularly when pre-eclampsia is present, and includes fluid management and the use of antihypertensive agents and magnesium sulfate for seizure prophylaxis

129

and fetal neuroprotection (to the 32nd week of gestation).

The use of corticosteroids for the promotion of fetal lung maturity has been advocated in the presence of a threatened preterm delivery, particularly between 24 and 33 weeks of gestation. Corticosteroids in this setting have been noted to reduce the risks of neonatal respiratory distress syndrome, as well as neonatal intraventricular hemorrhage and cerebral palsy. Betamethasone appears to have an improved therapeutic ratio when compared with dexamethasone for these neonatal effects.

The value of corticosteroid therapy in the treatment of HELLP has been questioned. A recent Cochrane analysis of women with HELLP concluded that maternal and perinatal/infant mortality or severe morbidity were not affected by corticosteroid therapy; however, significant increases in maternal platelet counts were observed, particularly with the use of dexamethasone compared with betamethasone [23]. Dexamethasone does not appear to be a useful treatment for postpartum HELLP.

Ongoing hemolysis, thrombocytopenia, and hypoproteinemia can require massive transfusion of red blood cells and platelets, and the administration of albumin. Severe biochemical derangements or progressive elevation of bilirubin or creatinine for more than 72 hours following delivery may benefit from plasma exchange with fresh frozen plasma or hemodialysis.

Rupture of subcapsular liver hematomas are often treated surgically by laparotomy (packing preferable to lobectomy), arterial ligation, and, in extreme cases, liver transplant; selective arterial embolization may also be performed. Recombinant factor VIIa has been used in the setting of preeclampsia with an expanding or ruptured subcapsular liver hematoma.

Antithrombin and glutathione offer some benefit in the treatment of severe pre-eclampsia but require further evaluation, particularly in the setting of HELLP [21]. Antithrombin supplementation has favorably altered levels of the plasmin–plasmin inhibitor complex, D-dimer, and platelets, and has improved fetal outcomes (gestosis index and biophysical profiles). S-Nitrosoglutathione in women with severe pre-eclampsia has been observed to lower mean arterial pressure, platelet activation, and uterine artery resistance without compromising fetal Doppler indices.

Thrombotic thrombocytopenic purpura

Thrombotic thrombocytopenic purpura is characterized by a pentad of thrombocytopenia, microangiopathic hemolytic anemia, renal impairment, fluctuating neurological signs, and fever, although all features do not have to be present to make the diagnosis (Table 11.9). It is a rare disorder with an incidence of 3.7 per million in the general population, although some reports indicate that as many as 20–25% of cases are associated with pregnancy, giving a pregnancy-related incidence up to 1 in 25 000 pregnancies [24].

Pathophysiology

Congenital and acquired deficiency of ADAMTS-13 (a disintegrin and metalloprotease, with thrombospondin-1-like domains) is now recognized as the key factor in the pathophysiology of TTP [24]. The gene for ADAMTS-13 maps to the long arm of chromosome 9. The enzyme is predominantly synthesized in the liver, with additional production in the endothelial cells. Several mutations of *ADAMTS13* have been described in familial forms of TTP, but inhibitory antibodies are detected in patients with acquired forms of the disease. The enzyme is a protease that cleaves von Willebrand factor; consequently, reduced or absent ADAMTS-13 allow the circulation of ultra-large von Willebrand factor fragments that mediate excessive platelet aggregation when the plasma is subjected to shear stress. Platelet microvascular thrombi develop, which primarily affect the renal and cerebral circulation.

Clinical features

Over 50% of pregnancy-associated TTP presents at or before 24 weeks of gestation [25]. Later presentation or postpartum TTP is harder to diagnose clinically because of the overlap of symptoms with other microangiopathic hemolytic anemias (Table 11.9), but correct diagnosis is essential to ensure appropriate management.

Renal function is normal in the majority of patients, however, the Canadian Apheresis Group have reported that 18% of their patients presented with renal impairment. Significant renal impairment can be evaluated by a biopsy, which indicates arteriolar and capillary thromboses largely composed of platelets and von Willebrand factor. Limited fibrin and

Table 11.9. Thrombotic microangiopathies in pregnancy [23]

Diagnosis	Classic TTP	Postpartum HUS	HELLP	Pre-eclampsia/eclampsia
Time of onset	<24 weeks	Postpartum	>34 weeks	>34 weeks
Histopathology of lesions	Widespread platelet thrombi	Thrombi in renal glomeruli only	Hepatocyte necrosis and fibrin deposition in peripheral sinusoids	Glomerular endothelial hypertrophy and occlusion of placental vessels
Hemolysis	+++	++	++	+
Thrombocytopenia	+++	++	++	++
Coagulopathy	–	–	+/–	+/–
Central nervous system symptoms	+++	+/–	+/–	+/–
Liver disease	+/–	+/–	+++	+/–
Renal disease	+/–	+++	+	+
Hypertension	Rare	+/–	+/–	+++
Effect on fetus	Placental infarct can lead to intrauterine growth retardation and death	None, if maternal disease is controlled	Associated with placental ischemia and increased neonatal mortality	Intrauterine growth retardation, occasional death
Effect of delivery on disease	None	None	Recovery, but may transiently worsen	Recovery, but may transiently worsen
Management	Early plasma exchange is imperative	Supportive ± plasma exchange	Supportive, consider plasma exchange if persists	Supportive ± plasma exchange

HELLP, hemolysis, elevated liver enzymes, and low platelets; HUS, hemolytic uremic syndrome; TTP, thrombotic thrombocytopenic purpura

fibrinogen contribution is observed, in contrast to the thrombi associated with DIC.

Multiple neurological manifestations may be seen, including headache, transient sensorimotor deficits, altered or bizarre behavior, seizures, and coma. Approximately 35% of patients have no neurological symptoms on presentation; the presence of coma is a poor prognostic indicator.

Hepatic ischemia is present in some patients, which can be reflected by increased biliribin and transaminase levels. Mesenteric ischemia may also be observed and presents with abdominal pain.

Investigations

Several different methods have recently been developed to measure ADAMTS-13 activity and detect the presence of inhibitors, but a rapid diagnostic test is still not widely available. Moreover, there is currently no international standard, quality control materials, or recognized units for measurement, further compounding the problems of accurate measurement and

interpretation [26]. Activity of ADAMTS-13 is reduced or absent in the acute phase of classical TTP, but levels may be normal in pregnancy-associated TTP. Baseline and repeated measurements in individuals with a prior history of TTP may be helpful during pregnancy, when decreasing levels may predict a relapse. Recommended diagnostic laboratory investigations at presentation of TTP are:

- full blood count and blood film
- reticulocyte count
- clotting screen including fibrinogen and D-dimers
- urea and electrolytes
- liver function tests
- LDH
- urinalysis
- direct antiglobulin test.

Abnormalities of von Willebrand factor multimers are observed in 86% of patients, including the presence of ultra-high-molecular-weight multimers or a relative decrease in the largest plasma forms [25]. The measurement of von Willebrand factor multimers is difficult and not widely available; therefore, they would be unlikely to provide rapid diagnostic information.

An association with thrombocytopenia is always seen in TTP and this is generally severe. A platelet count of $<20 \times 10^9/L$ at diagnosis is associated with a poor prognosis.

Microangiopathic hemolysis is generally present but may not be identifiable in the first 24–48 hours of diagnosis. The peripheral blood film demonstrates striking fragmentation of the red cells (schistocytes) and polychromasia. Other features of hemolysis are also present, including a raised LDH, raised bilirubin, and reduced, or absent, haptoglobins.

The coagulation profile is usually normal, although slight increases in D-dimers and FDPs may occur. Secondary DIC can result from ongoing tissue ischemia and is associated with a poor clinical outcome [25].

Renal function is abnormal in 18% of patients [3]. Liver function tests are generally normal, but transaminases may be raised if hepatic ischemia is present.

Management

Termination of pregnancy or early delivery of the fetus has not been shown to alter the clinical course in pregnancy-associated TTP and is, therefore, not recommended unless the mother fails to respond to standard treatment or there are fetal issues indicating a need for early delivery. The response to treatment is similar in pregnancy-associated TTP and classical TTP, with survival rates over 90% with optimal care. No cases of fetal thrombocytopenia have been reported in children born to mothers with TTP [25].

Plasma exchange is the treatment of choice for TTP and should be commenced as soon as practicable, and definitely within 24 hours of presentation. A delay in treatment may be associated with an increased risk of treatment failure. The response to plasma exchange does not appear to be reduced by pregnancy [25]. The optimal plasma exchange regimen has not been determined, but treatment is initiated with daily single volume exchanges. Exchanges should continue for a minimum of 2 days after complete remission is achieved, defined as normal neurological status, platelet count and LDH with an increasing hemoglobin level. Fresh frozen plasma is generally accepted as the standard exchange fluid, with current UK guidance advocating virally inactivated fresh frozen plasma. There is theoretical concern that methylene blue-treated plasma may not be as effective as solvent detergent-treated plasma in the management of TTP. Cryosupernatant (cryoprecipitate-poor plasma) lacks the largest von Willebrand factor multimers and appears to be as effective as fresh frozen plasma as an exchange fluid, particularly for resistant TTP.

Corticosteroids are frequently used in the management of TTP, although limited evidence exists to support their use, and there is no consensus on optimal dosing or route of administration [25].

Platelet transfusions are generally contraindicated in TTP and can worsen the immediate clinical state of the patient. Antiplatelet agents remain controversial in the management of TTP. No overall benefit has been demonstrated when low-dose aspirin and dipyridamole are added to plasma exchange in the initial treatment of TTP, but a trend towards reduced mortality is observed as platelet counts rise ($>50 \times 10^9/L$) [25].

The management of resistant TTP is complex and should be done in conjunction with specialists in this area. In general, an increased frequency of plasma exchanges is indicated and the use of other immunosuppressants (e.g. rituximab) should be considered.

Conclusions

Although pregnancy represents a state of heightened coagulation, disorders in this process, including DIC, HELLP, and TTP, are not uncommon and frequently require management within a critical care environment. The diagnosis, monitoring, and treatment of these disorders require knowledge of the relevant pathophysiology, diagnostic classifications, and specific laboratory tests and therapies. The optimal treatment regimen for obstetric coagulation disorders continues to evolve, given the frequently dynamic clinical situation, the presence and health of the fetus, and a growing interest in conducting investigations during the peripartum period.

References

1. Thornton P, Douglas J. Coagulation in pregnancy. *Best Pract Res Clin Obstet Gynaecol* 2010;**24**:339–352.

2. Polak F, Kolnikova I, Lips M, *et al.* New recommendations for thromboelastography reference ranges for pregnant women. *Thromb Res* 2011;**128**: e14–e17.

3. Levi M, Toh CH, Thachil J, Watson HG. Guidelines for the diagnosis and management of disseminated intravascular coagulation. British Committee for Standards in Haematology. *Br J Haematol* 2009;**145**:24–33.

4. Thachil J, Toh CH. Disseminated intravascular coagulation in obstetric disorders and its acute haematological management. *Blood Rev* 2009;**23**:167–176.

5. Ahn H, Park J, Gilman-Sachs A, Kwak-Kim J. Immunologic characteristics of preeclampsia, a comprehensive review. *Am J Reprod Immunol* 2011;**65**:377–394.

6. Hunt BJ, Missfelder-Lobos H, Parra-Cordero M, *et al.* Pregnancy outcome and fibrinolytic, endothelial and coagulation markers in women undergoing uterine artery Doppler screening at 23 weeks. *J Thromb Haemost* 2009;**7**:955–961.

7. Lefkou E, Hunt BJ. Bleeding disorders in pregnancy. *Obstet Gynaecol Reprod Med* 2008;**18**:217–223.

8. Bakhtiari K, Meijers JC, de Jonge E, Levi M. Prospective validation of the International Society of Thrombosis and Haemostasis scoring system for disseminated intravascular coagulation. *Crit Care Med* 2004;**32**:2416–2421.

9. Takemitsu T, Wada H, Hatada T, *et al.* Prospective evaluation of three different diagnostic criteria for disseminated intravascular coagulation. *Thromb Haemost* 2011;**105**:40–44.

10. Sossdorf M, Marx S, Schaarschmidt B, *et al.* HES 130/ 0.4 impairs haemostasis and stimulates pro-inflammatory blood platelet function. *Crit Care* 2009;**13**:R208.

11. Spoerke N, Michalek J, Schreiber M, *et al.* Crystalloid resuscitation improves survival in trauma patients receiving low ratios of fresh frozen plasma to packed red blood cells. *J Trauma* 2011;**71**:S380–383.

12. Hess JR, Lawson JH. The coagulopathy of trauma versus disseminated intravascular coagulation. *J Trauma* 2006;**60**:S12–S19.

13. Sihler KC, Napolitano LM. Complications of massive transfusion. *Chest* 2010;**137**:209–220.

14. Gilliss BM, Looney MR, Gropper MA. Reducing noninfectious risks of blood transfusion. *Anesthesiology* 2011;**115**:635–649.

15. Rowell SE, Barbosa RR, Allison CE, *et al.* Gender-based differences in mortality in response to high product ratio massive transfusion. *J Trauma* 2011;**71**:S375–379.

16. Maki M, Terao T, Ikenoue T, *et al.* Clinical evaluation of antithrombin III concentrate (BI 6.013) for disseminated intravascular coagulation in obstetrics. Well-controlled multicenter trial. *Gynecol Obstet Invest* 1987;**23**:230–240.

17. Kobayashi A, Matsuda Y, Mitani M, Makino Y, Ohta H. Assessment of the usefulness of antithrombin-III in the management of disseminated intravascular coagulation in obstetrically ill patients. *Clin Appl Thromb Hemost* 2010;**16**:688–693.

18. Kobayashi T, Terao T, Maki M, Ikenoue T. Activated protein C is effective for disseminated intravascular coagulation associated with placental abruption. *Thromb Haemost* 1999;**82**:1363.

19. Fang CJ, Richards A, Liszewski MK, Kavanagh D, Atkinson JP. Advances in understanding of pathogenesis of aHUS and HELLP. *Br J Haematol* 2008;**143**:336–348.

20. Hladunewich M, Karumanchi SA, Lafayette R. Pathophysiology of the clinical manifestations of preeclampsia. *Clin J Am Soc Nephrol* 2007;**2**:543–549.

21. Haram K, Svendsen E, Abildgaard U. The HELLP syndrome: clinical issues and management. *A Review.* *BMC Pregnancy Childbirth* 2009;**9**:8.

22. Mackillop L, Williamson C. Liver disease in pregnancy. *Postgrad Med J* 2010;**86**:160–164.

23. Woudstra DM, Chandra S, Hofmeyr GJ, Dowswell T. Corticosteroids for HELLP (hemolysis, elevated liver enzymes, low platelets) syndrome in pregnancy. *Cochrane Database Syst Rev* 2010: CD008148.

24. Gerth J, Schleussner E, Kentouche K, Busch M, Seifert M, Wolf G. Pregnancy-associated thrombotic thrombocytopenic purpura. *Thromb Haemost* 2009;**101**:248–251.

25. Allford SL, Hunt BJ, Rose P, Machin SJ. Guidelines on the diagnosis and management of the thrombotic microangiopathic haemolytic anaemias. *Br J Haematol* 2003;**120**:556–573.

26. Peyvandi F, Palla R, Lotta LA, Mackie I, Scully MA, Machin SJ. ADAMTS-13 assays in thrombotic thrombocytopenic purpura. *J Thromb Haemost* 2010;**8**:631–640.

Acute collapse and resuscitation

Larry Leeman and Alexandre Mignon

Introduction

Maternal collapse includes a variety of acute life-threatening events involving maternal cardiorespiratory or central nervous systems. Although these events have a variety of etiologies, the immediate consideration is rapid maternal resuscitation to prevent maternal mortality, long-term maternal morbidity, or adverse neonatal outcomes. Maternal resuscitation in pregnancy is based on standard Advanced Cardiac Life Support (ACLS) management guidelines [1]; however, resuscitative efforts must be informed by knowledge of pregnancy-related alterations in maternal anatomy and physiology (see Chapter 10), pregnancy-specific resuscitation recommendations, awareness of conditions unique to pregnancy, and consideration of perimortem cesarean delivery.

Causes of maternal collapse

Obstetrical hemorrhage is the most common cause of maternal mortality in the developing world, predominantly through uterine atony, and the most common cause of maternal collapse in developed nations (Table 12.1) [2]. In high-resource nations cesarean hemorrhage from invasive placental disease has become the leading cause of peripartum hysterectomy [3,4]. An increasing proportion of uterine atony in the USA is associated with primary or repeat cesarean delivery [5]. Pulmonary embolism from venous thromboembolic disease was the leading cause of maternal death in the UK Seventh Confidential Enquiries into Maternal and Child Health (CEMACH) 2003–2005 [2]. A review of pregnancy-related mortality in the USA from 1998 to 2005 demonstrated that six different etiologies were each responsible for 10–13% of maternal deaths: obstetric hemorrhage, hypertensive disorders of pregnancy,

pulmonary embolism, cardiomyopathy, cardiovascular disease, and infection [6]. If cardiomyopathy is combined with cardiovascular disease, then primary cardiac disease is the leading cause of maternal mortality [6]. Myocardial infarction and aortic dissection are the leading cardiovascular disease etiologies [7]. The growing population of reproductive-age women with congenital heart disease accompanied by pulmonary hypertension is another population at risk for cardiac arrest [8], which may occur in the setting of arrhythmias or heart failure.

Pregnancy-specific etiologies include amniotic fluid embolism, hypertensive disorders of pregnancy and peripartum cardiomyopathy. Amniotic fluid embolism may occur in the low-risk parturient, where sudden collapse may initially be confused with the more familiar entities of pulmonary embolism, myocardial infarction, and cerebrovascular accident until the other etiologies are ruled out or the often rapidly fulminant disseminated intravascular coagulation common to amniotic fluid embolism is recognized [9]. Maternal collapse can occur from iatrogenic drug toxicities, the most common being magnesium sulfate, which is commonly used either for seizure prophylaxis in preeclampsia or for tocolysis in preterm labor. Another very uncommon but potentially lethal drug reaction is the potential for local anesthetic agents to cause systemic toxicity resulting in neurological symptoms (including agitation, seizures, coma) and cardiovascular collapse (including cardiac arrhythmias, bradycardia, reduced cardiac output and cardiac arrest) [10]. Spinal or epidural anesthesia can cause an excessive anesthesia-related inhibition of sympathetic efferents, leading to massive vasodilatation and redistribution of blood to the splanchnic beds and lower extremities, in turn leading to decreased venous return and thereby decreasing preload and causing vagal stimulation. This

Table 12.1. Causes of maternal collapse

Obstetric	Non-obstetric
Postpartum hemorrhage	Myocardial infarction
Amniotic fluid embolism	Aortic dissection
Peripartum cardiomyopathy	Congenital heart disease
Hypertensive pregnancy disorders	Anaphylaxis
Magnesium toxicity	Sepsis
Local anesthetic toxicity	Status asthmaticus
	Status epileptiicus

may have an even more important role in those who have existing decreased preload (e.g. from hemorrhage). Careful attention to the level of anesthesia and blood pressure minute by minute in the first 15 minutes following spinal anesthesia and prophylactic treatment with vasopressors, such as phenylephrine, may decrease the incidence of this catastrophic accident. Finally, non-obstetric causes include anaphylaxis, sepsis, trauma, psychiatric disease, cerebrovascular disease, or status asthmaticus. Obesity, a condition which is increasing worldwide, increases the risk of both obstetric and non-obstetric causes of maternal mortality.

Prediction of maternal collapse or severe obstetric morbidity

Early warning systems (EWS) are used for hospitalized medical and surgical patients with abnormal physiological signs to identify patients at risk for death, intensive care unit admission, or severe morbidity. The audit of maternal morbidity in the UK CEMACH 2003–2005 identified several cases of maternal death that involved substandard care in which abnormal signs and symptoms were present but not identified during the time preceeding maternal collapse [2]. The Enquiry recommended the use of a modified obstetric EWS (MEOWS). Because of the low incidence of maternal mortality or need for intensive care, MEOWS was developed to predict serious obstetric morbidity, including obstetric hemorrhage, pre-eclampsia, infection, pulmonary embolism, central venous sinus thrombosis, intracranial bleed, acute asthma, status epileptic, diabetic ketoacidosis, myocardial infarction, pulmonary edema, and anesthesia complications [11]. The parameters are the usual vital signs, oxygen saturation, pain score, and ability

to respond to voice or pain. In a validation study, the MEOWS score when applied to 676 consecutive obstetric admissions had a 8% sensitivity with a 79% specificity and 39% positive predictive value [11]. A disease-specific morbidity predictor, the fullPIERS model, has been developed for patients with pre-eclampsia to identify women at risk for dying or serious obstetric complications. The model was found to have a high predictive ability in a prospective multi-center study [12].

Responding to maternal collapse

Initial response

The initial response to maternal collapse, regardless of etiology, is the rapid initiation of resuscitation directed to airway, breathing, and circulation, followed by consideration of fetal viability and well-being when collapse occurs prior to delivery. As the resuscitation progresses, it is important to consider etiologies requiring specific therapies, such as intravenous calcium gluconate for magnesium toxicity, decompression of tension pneumothorax, and initiation of antibiotics for sepsis. Specific etiologies are addressed in depth in other chapters.

When maternal collapse occurs in a labor and delivery setting, the nursing and maternity care provider staff should rapidly request assistance, which may include anesthesia personnel, a rapid response or code team based on hospital-specific protocols, and neonatal personnel if delivery of a viable infant is a possibility. When the collapse results from maternal hemorrhage or disseminated intravascular coagulation is occurring (e.g. amniotic fluid embolism), a massive transfusion protocol with involvement of blood bank or laboratory personnel will facilitate adequate supplies of blood products, including packed red blood cells, fresh frozen plasma, patient's blood, or cryoprecipitate, as well as consideration for factor VII replacement for life-threatening hemorrhage.

Intravenous access is critical and should include two large-bore catheters in peripheral veins and consideration of the need for central lines for rapid administration of crystalloid, colloid, or blood products, as well as monitoring of central venous process. A patient with hypotension or hypertension that does not respond to initial therapies may require an arterial line to accurately monitor pressures and facilitate management with vasopressor agents (norephinephrine, phenylephrine, dopamine) or antihypertensives (labetalol, calcium channel blockers, hydralazine). A Foley catheter should be placed to monitor urine output and as preparation for potential cesarean delivery if the gestational age warrants, and continuous cardiac and oxygen saturation monitoring should be initiated.

Cardiopulmonary resuscitation

Maternal resuscitation follows standard ACLS guidelines with a limited number of pregnancy-specific alterations. Little research has been done on cardiopulmonary resuscitation in pregnancy, as this is a rare event occurring in approximately one in 20 000 to 30 000 pregnancies [13]. Outcome is critically dependent both on the underlying cause of the arrest and on the speed of resuscitation efforts. All efforts including the most desperate must be performed, since cardiac arrest in pregnancy is a devastating event for the mother and fetus, as well as all involved in their care [13].

A systematic review was conducted in 2011 by Jeejeebhoy and colleagues pertaining to resuscitation of the pregnant patient with cardiac arrest [13]. They identified 1305 articles but only five were selected for further review, none of them being randomized trials. Chest compression, left lateral displacement, and the use of perimortem cesarean delivery were the only subjects studied.

The primary variation from non-pregnancy guidelines is the requirement to displace the gravid uterus laterally to increase cardiac output. Cardiac output during closed chest massage in cardiopulmonary resuscitation (CPR) is approximately 30% of normal. Since cardiac output in the normal supine pregnant woman is decreased 30–50% through aortocaval compression, the combined effect may be no cardiac output. Traditionally, displacement of the gravid uterus has been done by maternal tilt from 15 to 30° to facilitate increased venous return and cardiac output. The logistical difficulty is the maintenance of adequate chest compressions once tilt has been accomplished. The gravid uterus will adversely affect maternal resuscitation when it reaches the umbilicus at around 20 weeks of gestation. After this gestational age/uterine size, uterine displacement will be needed and perimortem cesarean considered if resuscitation is not successful within 4 minutes, even though fetal viability is not present until 23–24 weeks. Therefore, cesarean delivery may be undertaken as a component of maternal resuscitation even at a gestational age (20–23 weeks) at which perinatal survival is not expected.

As the degree of lateral maternal tilt increases toward 30°, cardiac output is improved; however, the ability to effectively compress the chest in CPR is decreased. A study by Rees and Willis [14] demonstrated that maximum force was 67% of body weight when supine compared with 36% of body weight when the patient was in the 30° left lateral tilt position. At more than 30°, the angle was sufficient to cause the body to roll on the incline. They recommended the 27° as optimal, and this is the maternal tilt provided by the Cardiff wedge through the use of a wooden frame. At this angle, 55% of body weight is transmitted through CPR, which is 80% of the force transmitted when the patient is supine [14]. The ACLS and European Resuscitation Council Guidelines in 2010 recommended 15–30° of tilt [1,7].

An alternative to maternal tilt is lateral manual uterine displacement, which allows for the maintenance of the supine position and maximizes the force of the chest compressions. A study randomizing women going for cesarean delivery to 15° table tilt or left lateral manual uterine displacement demonstrated an effect on blood pressure in the manual displacement group [15]. The American Heart Association's 2010 guidelines recommended initially performing manual displacement with a two- or one-handed technique (Figure 12.1) while performing chest compressions in the supine position. If this is unsuccessful, then using a firm wedge to support the pelvis and thorax and provide 27–30° of tilt is recommended (Figure 12.2) [1].

Special considerations for maintenance of the maternal airway and adequate breathing are based on the anatomic alteration of the airway, as well as the physiological need to maintain fetal oxygenation and the reduced functional capacity and increased carbon dioxide levels in pregnancy. The maternal airway in pregnancy is more edematous and hyperemic and has additional secretions; the upper airway appears to be narrowed in the third trimester [1]. These alterations to the maternal airway are responsible for the higher proportion of failed intubations in pregnancy (Box 12.1). Oxygen at 100% should be used throughout the resuscitation if available, and consideration given to obtaining a definitive airway sooner than might be the case in the non-gravid woman.

Chest compressions should be provided at a position that is slightly higher on the sternum to adjust for the elevation of the diaphragm and abdominal contents caused by the gravid uterus. Chest compressions

(a)

(b)

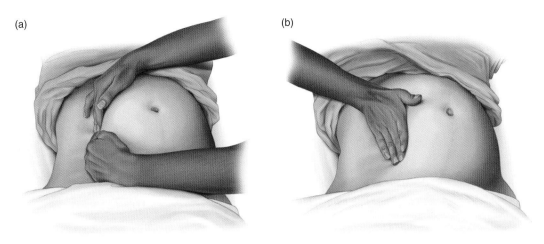

Figure 12.1. Manual displacement of the uterus during cardiopulmonary resuscitation using (a) a two-handed and (b) a one-handed technique. (With permission from Vanden Hoek TL, Morrison, LJ, Shuster M, *et al*. American Heart Association guidelines for cardiopulmonary resuscitation and emergency cardiovascular care. Part 12: Cardiac arrest in special situations. *Circulation* 2010; 122: S829–861 [1].)

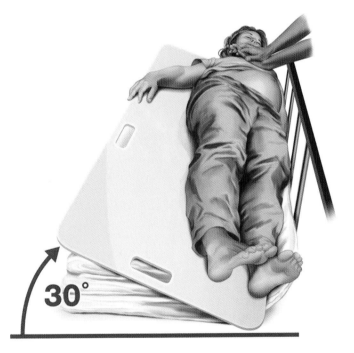

Figure 12.2. Left lateral tilt during cardiopulmonary resuscitation. (With permission from Vanden Hoek TL, Morrison, LJ, Shuster M, *et al*. American Heart Association guidelines for cardiopulmonary resuscitation and emergency cardiovascular care. Part 12: Cardiac arrest in special situations. *Circulation* 2010; 122: S829–861 [1].)

should be provided based on the American Heart Association's 2005 and 2010 guidelines to "push hard and fast," with the goal of 100 compressions per minute while allowing for full chest recoil between compressions. These guidelines also emphasize that compressions should be provided continually, while other resuscitative efforts are in place, with periods without compressions limited to less than 10 seconds other than for defibrillation.

Defibrillation is based on the standard ACLS algorithms and should not be delayed for obstetric or fetal concerns, as the earlier that defibrillation is provided in an arrest, the more likely it is to be effective. A study of transthoracic impedance in pregnant and postpartum women did not find a significant difference, supporting the use of standard energy requirements. Theoretical concerns for the potential arcing of electric current because of the presence of fetal monitors and

137

> **Box 12.1.** Alterations in cardiopulmonary resuscitation in pregnancy
>
> - Uterine displacement: manual displacement or 25–30° left tilt
> - Airway management: because of edema consider intubation sooner and the greater need for cricoid pressure
> - Chest compression site: hands midsternum (superior to non-pregnant) and deeper compressions
> - Advanced Cardiac Life Support medications: no change
> - Defibrillation: no change
> - Fetal assessment throughout if estimated to be >22 to 23 weeks of gestation
> - Five minute rule for initiating hysterotomy if estimated to be >20 weeks of gestation

amniotic fluid in the uterus have not occurred in practice and should not delay defibrillation, although it is acceptable to remove fetal monitors during cardiac arrest [1].

All ACLS medicines, including epinephrine, vasopressin, lidocaine, amiodarone, and pressor agents, should be administered as indicated by ACLS algorithms without delay based on any concerns regarding effect on uteroplacental perfusion. The restoration of maternal pulse and circulation will produce the best fetal outcomes. Perimortem cesarean section will be initiated at the 4–5 minute mark in the ALCS algorithms for asystole, ventricular fibrillation, pulseless ventricular tachycardia, and pulseless electrical activity.

If local anesthetic-induced systemic toxicity is suspected, it should be treated with the rapid infusion of a lipid emulsion (Intralipid 20% 1.5 mL/kg as a bolus followed by an infusion of 0.25 mL/kg per min; bolus can be repeated) [10]. Lipids are believed to bind local anesthetics and to improve myocardial energy production, hence reversing cardiac side effects of local anesthetics and significantly improving outcome. A whole series of isolated heart and intact animal experiments by Weinberg and coworkers [16] have conclusively demonstrated the benefit of administering lipid emulsions in this situation.

A study of videotaped resuscitation after a simulated cardiac arrest from amniotic fluid embolism demonstrated the difficulty obstetric personnel may have with effectively performing maternal resuscitation. Lateral displacement of the uterus and effective chest compression were only provided in 56% and effective ventilation in only 50% of simulated resuscitations done by provider groups containing obstetricians, labor and delivery nurses, and an anesthesiologist [17].

Diagnostic evaluation of maternal collapse

After initial resuscitative efforts have led to stabilization of the maternal airway, breathing, and circulatory functions, efforts are directed to determining or confirming the etiology of the collapse. The etiology may be readily apparent, such as the postpartum woman with severe vaginal bleeding from postpartum hemorrhage in uterine atony. Alternatively, sudden cardiac arrest may occur in the previously well parturient without apparent etiology, suggesting amniotic fluid embolism, pulmonary embolism, myocardial infarction, cardiac arrhythmias, or a cerebrovascular accident.

Initial laboratory studies will usually include a complete blood count, coagulation studies (prothrombin time, partial thromboplastin time international normalized ratio, fibrinogen), serum electrolytes, serum lactate, type and cross-match for blood products, and arterial blood gases. Magnesium sulfate should be obtained if a magnesium sulfate infusion is being administered. Diagnostic tests will include a chest radiograph if intubated to confirm tube position and exclude other pulmonary pathology, as well as a 12-lead electrocardiogram. Diagnosis of pulmonary embolism by a ventilation/perfusion scan or spiral CT may not be possible if maternal or fetal status precludes transfer from labor and delivery or an intensive care unit; however, lower extremity venous Doppler studies can often be carried out in these settings and, if positive, allow for presumptive diagnosis of pulmonary embolism if there are no other likely etiologies. The presence of severe disseminated intravascular coagulation in the setting of rapid maternal collapse in the previously healthy woman is supportive of amniotic fluid embolism.

Immediate mask ventilation and administration of supplemental 100% oxygen, followed by rapid control of the airway through endotracheal intubation early in the resuscitation effort, are particularly important in the pregnant cardiac arrest victim. In addition to the increased susceptibility of the mother to rapid development of hypoxia, because of her reduced functional residual capacity and increased oxygen consumption, pregnant patients are at increased risk of aspiration of gastric contents through their normally delayed gastric emptying and reduced lower esophageal sphincter tone. This risk of aspiration may be further exacerbated by gastric distention from air insufflation during prolonged bag-mask ventilation. It is, therefore, necessary to apply cricoid pressure as soon as possible, and early intubation is recommended. Airway access and intubation may be more difficult. Hyperemia and friability lead to increased risk of bleeding with introduction of gastric or tracheal tubes, which may limit visibility. This risk may be even higher in patients with complications such as thrombocytopenia occurring in association with pre-eclampsia or the HELLP (hemolysis, elevated liver enzymes, and low platelets) syndrome. Intubation is, therefore, often more difficult in the pregnant patient and a smaller endotracheal tube size may be necessary. Alternative airway devices, such as a laryngeal mask airways or video laryngoscopy, should also be immediately available.

Pharmacological interventions during ACLS are not modified during pregnancy, although alpha-adrenergic agents may theoretically reduce uteroplacental blood flow. There have been no studies evaluating medication dosing and pharmacokinetics during resuscitation in pregnancy. Therefore, recommendations are to follow the current adult ACLS medication guidelines. In case of refractory shock, extracorporeal life support may be considered, mainly when there is a reversible cause of cardiac arrest, by use of a femorofemoral bypass [18].

Finally, therapeutic hypothermia is now commonly used to improve neurological outcomes in eligible patients after cardiac arrest; however, no randomized study has included a pregnant woman. Rittenberger *et al.* [19] have reported a case of a patient with a cardiac arrest at 13 weeks of gestation who was resuscitated, underwent therapeutic hypothermia, and delivered a healthy baby at term. Despite the lack of evidence, the American Heart Association recommends consideration of hypothermia based on guidelines for non-pregnant patients, and to consider continuous fetal monitoring throughout the treatment [1].

Perimortem cesarean

Postmortem cesarean delivery dates back to the time of Roman law *Lex Regis de Inferendo Mortus* in 715 BC [20], which mandated that the abdomen be cut open as soon as possible to remove the baby if a mother died during a pregnancy. Neonatal survival was rare, and the primary motivation was religious to allow for proper burial. A study performed by the Berlin Obstetrical Society in 1864 demonstrated that only 3 of 147 postmortem cesareans resulted in the birth of live infants [20].

The modern introduction of perimortem cesarean delivery is attributed to a review by Katz *et al.* in 1986 [20]. Although historically advocated for fetal survival, the review described the potential for maternal benefits based on four case reports of intact maternal survival with cesarean delivery performed within 5 minutes of cardiac arrest [20]. Perimortem cesarean delivery is now performed for maternal benefit as well as fetal survival and should not be viewed as indicating that a maternal resuscitation will not be successful. The relief of aortocaval compression by the gravid uterus results in increased venous return and cardiac output, which can lead to a dramatic improvement in maternal resuscitative efforts and to a successful maternal outcome [21].

Perimortem cesarean delivery is indicated whenever maternal resuscitative efforts have not been successful for 4 minutes, and the estimated gestational age is 20 weeks or greater. The neonate should be delivered within 5 minutes of maternal arrest in order to maximize the chances of a successful neonatal outcome. The cut-off of 20 weeks of gestation is not for fetal viability, which does not occur until 22–24 weeks, but is based on the size of the uterus at which maternal uterine decompression through cesarean delivery has the potential for significant improvement in maternal venous return and cardiac output. A woman with an 18 week twin gestation resulting in a uterus closer in size to that at 24 weeks may benefit from perimortem cesarean even though her fetuses will not.

A perimortem cesarean delivery should be performed in the setting in which the resuscitative efforts have occurred, which may be a delivery room, operating room, or emergency room depending on the clinical scenario. The time required to transport the patient to a surgical facility will likely decrease the potential for a successful maternal or neonatal outcome and is not recommended. In these cases, in which time is of the essence, even physicians who are not fully trained or accredited in elective cesarean delivery may appropriately perform the cesarean delivery. Emergency room physicians, family medicine, or general practice physicians, or even a nurse–midwife with experience assisting cesarean delivery, all should be familiar enough with the anatomy and technique to successfully perform the procedure. Anesthesia is not required because of the time constraints and moribund maternal state. However, in some settings, the woman will have had endotracheal intubation and can be placed on ventilator support. A quick abdominal splash of an appropriate disinfectant material is indicated while the surgical team is preparing to initiate the procedure. A neonatal team, or at least a physician or nurse skilled in neonatal resuscitation, should be contacted as soon as it becomes apparent to the maternal resuscitation team that immediate delivery is being contemplated. Cardiopulmonary resuscitation including chest compressions and ventilation should continue through the cesarean delivery.

Few instruments are strictly required for a rapid perimortem cesarean delivery, which can be accomplished with a scalpel, manual retraction, and blunt dissection. If a cesarean delivery kit is available, this will be helpful in the event of adhesions needing lysis to accomplish delivery and for possible surgical closure after delivery. A vertical abdominal and uterine incision will be the most rapid route of delivery for most surgeons to accomplish delivery and minimize risk of injury to the urinary bladder and uterine arteries. Because of the deceased cardiac output despite chest compressions, the perimortem cesarean is usually a relatively bloodless delivery compared with typical cesarean deliveries.

After delivery has been accomplished, the uterus and peritoneal cavity do not need to be immediately closed if the team performing the emergency surgery is not skilled at closure. Pressure, packing, and surgical compression of bleeding vessels can temporize until appropriate surgical assistance is available. If after-delivery maternal resuscitative efforts are successful, then the uterus should be closed in the usual fashion after a careful examination for potential injury to bowel, bladder, and other organs. Antibiotic prophylaxis should be given as soon as possible in the scenario of successful resuscitation. If the resuscitation has not been successful, then the hysterotomy and abdominal incision do not need to be repaired and the decision regarding removal of intravenous lines, packing, or endotracheal tubes should be based on local forensic guidelines.

In 2005, Katz et al. [22] reviewed the case report literature that had evolved since the 1986 article recommending perimortem cesarean section and the adoption of the 4 minute rule by the American Heart Association. Only 12 of the 25 perimortem cesarean deliveries with a known time from cardiac arrest to delivery occurred in 5 minutes or less [22]. The authors did find that four of the seven infants delivered at over 15 minutes from arrest were apparently developmentally normal [22]. In 12 of the 22 cases with adequate information regarding the effect of the cesarean on maternal hemodynamics, there was a sudden and often impressive improvement in maternal status after cesarean [22]. Eight of the remaining 10 women were felt to have had lethal injuries that prevented any improvement in maternal status [22]. The authors acknowledged that the presence of reporting bias with regard to the collated case reports prevents an accurate determination of the likelihood of maternal and fetal benefits but found the results encouraging [22]. None of the women suffered a worsening of maternal status after her hysterotomy was performed [22]. A case series of 12 perimortem cesarean sections from the Netherlands demonstrated that none occurred within the 5 minute interval, and eight occurred in the range 15–45 minutes. Similar to the series of Katz et al. [22], the maternal response to perimortem cesarean section was good, with 8 of the 12 women regaining maternal cardiac output and 2 surviving to hospital discharge.

Perimortem delivery need not always require hysterotomy as operative vaginal delivery is an option in the rare situation when a patient has a cardiac arrest in the second stage of labor. There is one report in the literature of perimortem vacuum delivery [23]; however, obstetric forceps may be preferred as they are less dependent on maternal effort to effect a successful and rapid vaginal delivery.

Improving management of maternal collapse

The rarity of cardiac arrest in pregnancy fortunately prevents physicians, midwives, or nurses from learning through clinical experience. Alternatives include participation in simulations, inclusion of maternal collapse in standardized emergency care courses (ACLS, Advanced Trauma Life Support), and courses designed specifically for obstetric emergencies (Advanced Life Support in Obstetrics [24], Advances in Labour and Risk Management [25], and Managing Obstetric Emergencies and Trauma [26]). The use of perimortem cesarean is recommended in the standard ACLS and Advanced Trauma Life Support courses. The Advanced Life Support in Obstetrics course includes a workshop in maternal resuscitation, including a case requiring perimortem cesarean, as does the Managing Obstetric Emergencies and Trauma course [26].

Team training with obstetric simulation and drills is recommended by the Institute of Medicine and Joint Commission to prevent medical errors and improve patient safety [27,28]. The optimal approach to using simulations and drills remains controversial with regards to whether training is performed during standard clinical work hour times and settings or in distinct training course and simulation centers. Small studies of physicians in California and labor ward clinicians in Israel demonstrated a limited fund of knowledge of the basic concepts for maternal resuscitation [29,30]. A study of the utilization of perimortem cesarean delivery after implementation of the Managing Obstetric Emergencies and Trauma course in the Netherlands demonstrated increased utilization of the procedure from four in 11 years (12.5% of cardiac arrests) to eight in 5 years (35% of cardiac arrests), which was a statistically significant increase ($p = 0.01$) despite the small numbers [31].

Conclusions

Cardiac arrest is a rare event during pregnancy. The resuscitation protocol is the same as for non-pregnant victims of cardiac arrest, with a few important modifications, including early intubation, superior hand placement for chest compression, relief of aortocaval compression by the gravid uterus with left lateral displacement or if unsuccessful the use of a firm wedge to provide a 30° tilt, and rapid perimortem cesarean delivery when indicated. The use of these combined techniques may increase the ACLS success rate of the mother, as well as improve neonatal outcome. The immediate awareness of the need to perform perimortem cesarean delivery 4 minutes after persistent cardiopulmonary arrest and the availability of an emergency kit for surgery can result in faster delivery of the baby, faster return of the maternal circulation, and better clinical outcomes for both mother and child. Education and protocols should to be instituted in all maternity care units, while simulation exercises may maintain knowledge, performance, and skills of obstetric teams rarely confronted by maternal collapse.

References

1. Vanden Hoek TL, Morrison LJ, Shuster M, *et al.* American Heart Association guidelines for cardiopulmonary resuscitation and emergency cardiovascular care. Part 12: Cardiac arrest in special situations. *Circulation* 2010;**122**: S829–S861.

2. Lewis G (ed.) *Saving Mothers' Lives: Reviewing Maternal Deaths to Make Motherhood Safer, 2003–2005. The Seventh Report on Confidential Enquiries into Maternal Deaths in the United Kingdom.* London: CEMACH, 2007.

3. Tadesse W, Farah N, Hogan J, *et al.* Peripartum hysterectomy in the first decade of the 21st century. *J Obstet Gynaecol* 2011;**31**:320–321.

4. Wong TY. Emergency peripartum hysterectomy: a 10-year review in a tertiary obstetric hospital. *N Z Med J* 2011;**124**:34–39.

5. Bateman BT, Mhyre JM, Callaghan WM, Kuklina EV. Peripartum hysterectomy in the United States: nationwide 14 year experience. *Am J Obstet Gynecol* 2012;**206**:63.e1.

6. Berg CJ, Callaghan WM, Syverson C, Henderson Z. Pregnancy-related mortality in the United States, 1998 to 2005. *Obstet Gynecol* 2010;**116**:1302–1309.

7. Soar J, Perkins GD, Abbas G, *et al.* European Resuscitation Council Guidelines for Resuscitation 2010 Section 8. Cardiac arrest in special circumstances: electrolyte abnormalities, poisoning, drowning, accidental hypothermia, hyperthermia, asthma, anaphylaxis, cardiac surgery, trauma, pregnancy, electrocution. *Resuscitation* 2010;**81**:1400–1433.

8. Drenthen W, Pieper PG, Roos-Hesselink JW, *et al.* Outcome of pregnancy in women with congenital heart disease: a literature review. *J Am Coll Cardiol* 2007;**49**:2303–2311.

9. Conde-Agudelo A, Romero R. Amniotic fluid embolism: an evidence-based review. *Am J Obstet Gynecol* 2009;**201**:445 e1–e13.

10. Bern S, Weinberg G. Local anesthetic toxicity and lipid resuscitation in pregnancy. *Curr Opin Anaesthesiol* 2011;**24**:262–267.

11. Singh S, McGlennan A, England A, Simons R. A validation study of the CEMACH recommended modified early obstetric warning system (MEOWS)*. *Anaesthesia* 2012;**67**:12–18.

12. von Dadelszen P, Payne B, Li J, *et al.* Prediction of adverse maternal outcomes in pre-eclampsia: development and validation of the fullPIERS model. *Lancet* 2011;**377**:219–227.

13. Jeejeebhoy FM, Zelop CM, Windrim R, *et al.* Management of cardiac arrest in pregnancy: a systematic review. *Resuscitation* 2011;**82**:801–809.

14. Rees GA, Willis BA. Resuscitation in late pregnancy. *Anaesthesia* 1988;**43**:347–349.

15. Kundra P, Khanna S, Habeebullah S, Ravishankar M. Manual displacement of the uterus during Caesarean section. *Anaesthesia* 2007;**62**:460–465.

16. Weinberg G, Picard J, Meek T, Hertz P. *Lipid Rescue Resusucitation* [website] (www.lipidrescue.org, accessed 5 December 2012).

17. Lipman SS, Daniels KI, Carvalho B, *et al.* Deficits in the provision of cardiopulmonary resuscitation during simulated obstetric crises. *Am J Obstet Gynecol* 2010;**203**:179 e1–e5.

18. Hsieh YY, Chang CC, Li PC, Tsai HD, Tsai CH. Successful application of extracorporeal membrane oxygenation and intra-aortic balloon counterpulsation as lifesaving therapy for a patient with amniotic fluid embolism. *Am J Obstet Gynecol* 2000;**183**:496–497.

19. Rittenberger JC, Kelly E, Jang D, Greer K, Heffner A. Successful outcome utilizing hypothermia after cardiac arrest in pregnancy: a case report. *Critical Care Med* 2008;**36**:1354–1356.

20. Katz VL, Dotters DJ, Droegemueller W. Perimortem cesarean delivery. *Obstet Gynecol* 1986;**68**:571–576.

21. McDonnell NJ. Cardiopulmonary arrest in pregnancy: two case reports of successful outcomes in association with perimortem Caesarean delivery. *Br J Anaesth* 2009;**103**:406–409.

22. Katz V, Balderston K, De Freest M. Perimortem cesarean delivery: were our assumptions correct? *Am J Obstet Gynecol* 2005;**192**:1916–1920;discussion 1920–1921.

23. Solt I, Kim MJ, Rotmensch S. Perimortem instrumental vaginal delivery. *J Perinat Med* 2011;**39**:97–98.

24. Beasley JW, Damos JR, Roberts RG, Nesbitt TS. The advanced life support in obstetrics course.A national program to enhance obstetric emergency skills and to support maternity care practice. *Arch Fam Med* 1994;**3**:1037–1041.

25. Windrim R, Ehman W, Carson GD, Kollesh L, Milne K. The ALARM course: 10 years of continuing professional development in intrapartum care and risk management in Canada. *JOGC* 2006;**28**:600–602.

26. Johanson R, Cox C, O'Donnell E, *et al.* Managing obstetric emergencies and trauma (MOET): Structured skills training using models and reality-based scenarios. *The Obstetrician & Gynaecologist* 1999;**1**:46–52.

27. Kohn LT, Corrigan JM, Donaldson MS for the Committee on Quality of Health Care in America, Institute of Medicine. *To Err is Human: Building a Safer Health System.* Washington, DC: National Academies Press, 1999.

28. Joint Commission on Accreditation of Healthcare Organizations. *Sentinel Event Alert Issue 30: Preventing Infant Death and Injury During Delivery.* Oakbrook Terrace, IL: Joint Commission on Accreditation of Healthcare Organizations, 2004 (http://www.jointcommission.org/assets/1/18/SEA_30.PDF, accessed 29 January 2013).

29. Cohen SE, Andes LC, Carvalho B. Assessment of knowledge regarding cardiopulmonary resuscitation of pregnant women. *Int J Obstet Anesth* 2008;**17**:20–25.

30. Einav S, Matot I, Berkenstadt H, Bromiker R, Weiniger CF. A survey of labour ward clinicians' knowledge of maternal cardiac arrest and resuscitation. *Int J Obstet Anesth* 2008;**17**:238–242.

31. Dijkman A, Huisman CM, Smit M, *et al.* Cardiac arrest in pregnancy: increasing use of perimortem caesarean section due to emergency skills training? *BJOG* 2010;**117**:282–287.

Chapter 13

But what about the fetus?

Lauren A. Plante and Alex Sia

Introduction

The obstetrician with a patient in the intensive care unit (ICU) finds that "What about the fetus?" is very common question posed by colleagues in other specialties. Sometimes it is asked explicitly; sometimes it is only implied, as a background to a more specific question, for example "Is that safe for the baby?" This whole issue could probably be generally condensed into one sentence, maybe two: "Don't worry about the fetus. Keep the mother healthy and the rest will follow." Obstetricians are used to managing two patients at a time, one of whom (the fetus) is entirely dependent upon the other and not generally accessible to its own interventions. However, colleagues in other specialties may not be accustomed to this type of double perspective and may worry about the myth of maternal–fetal conflict. As a rule, however, the best way to maintain fetal stability is to maintain maternal stability.

While the principal goal of intensive care medicine remains unaltered, the presence of the fetus may affect management. For example, in women who are admitted to the ICU because of primary obstetric disorders, delivery may dramatically reverse the pathology. Similarly, cardiopulmonary resuscitation performed in a woman after mid-pregnancy is more effective when the uterus is empty. Aside from these situations, restoring maternal physiology is still key in ensuring the ultimate well-being of the fetus, and the interests of the fetus are not in conflict with those of the mother. In general, the fetus is relatively robust in spite of maternal illness, and any intervention or therapy that preserves or improves the physiological status of the mother is favorable to the fetus.

For the most part, obstetric patients who are admitted to the ICU have a better prognosis than their general medical non-obstetric counterparts, although both obstetric and non-obstetric critical illnesses may adversely affect fetal and neonatal outcomes.

The principles of pregnancy physiology are addressed in this textbook in Chapter 10, while the pharmacokinetics and pharmacodynamics are covered in Chapter 14. These important topics will not be discussed here except to note that normal pregnancy alters physiology and drug handling to a great extent and, therefore, must be kept in mind in intensive care management.

Fetal growth and development

Human pregnancy lasts an average of 266 days, counting from conception. More commonly, pregnancy is considered to last 280 days, counting from the first day of the last menstrual period: this equates to 40 weeks, even though – because conception usually occurs 2 weeks after the first day of the last menstrual period – the woman is not actually pregnant for the first 2 of those weeks. Implantation of the zygote into the uterus occurs 1 week after conception, at which time human beta-chorionic gonadotropin can first be detected and a sensitive pregnancy test shows as positive. By convention, gestational age (or weeks of pregnancy) is dated from the last menstrual period, since this is easier to fix than the conception date. These 40 weeks are divided into trimesters, which last roughly 13 weeks each. Organogenesis is complete by the end of the first trimester; growth, including brain growth, continues throughout. Because organogenesis is complete before 12 weeks, the only period in which teratogenesis is of concern is during that time. Exposures (drugs, radiation, etc.) after that time may affect fetal growth, neurodevelopment, or renal or cardiac function but cannot precipitate the development of congenital anomalies.

Maternal Critical Care: A Multidisciplinary Approach, ed. Marc Van de Velde, Helen Scholefield, and Lauren A. Plante. Published by Cambridge University Press. © Cambridge University Press 2013.

In 2012, the lower limit of gestational age at which extrauterine survival was feasible is about 24 weeks in high-resource settings. Preterm birth refers to delivery between 24 weeks (20 in some classification schemes) and 36 weeks, while term or full-term birth refers to 37–41 weeks. Pregnancies ending before 20 weeks are referred to as abortions, spontaneous abortions, or miscarriages.

Placental structure and function

The placenta is a temporary organ that serves multiple functions during mammalian pregnancy. These include gas exchange, excretory functions, water balance, elaboration of various hormones, immunological functions, nutrient transfer, and heat transfer. It substitutes in one way or another for lung, liver, endocrine system, gut, and kidney [1]. Remarkably, it develops from both embryofetal and maternal tissues, the former from chorion and the latter from endometrium.

The human placenta is a hemochorial barrier: that is, fetal and maternal blood never mix. The trophoblast is bathed in maternal blood once the trophoblast invades the uterine vessels supplying the myometrium and replaces the endothelium, a process which takes up to about 16 weeks of gestation. This leaves only fetal endothelium and the syncytiotrophoblast itself as interposing layers. Other mammalian placentae have as many as six layers.

The spiral arteries of the maternal endometrium discharge blood into the intervillous space of the placenta. Villi project into this space that contain fetal capillary units [2]. As maternal blood washes over placental villi, gas exchange and transfer of nutrients and waste products occur (Figures 13.1 and 13.2) [3,4].

Uteroplacental circulation and fetal well-being in the intensive care unit

Fetal well-being is intimately linked to, and critically dependent upon, the satisfactory perfusion of the uteroplacental unit. Up to 15% of the total maternal cardiac output supplies the uterus at term pregnancy. As invading trophoblast replaces vasoactive endothelium in the spiral arterioles of the uterus that supply the intervillous space in early pregnancy, uteroplacental perfusion becomes predominantly (if not entirely) dependent on arterial pressure; there is miminal capability for autoregulation. Consequently, the fetus does not tolerate maternal hypotension and great care must be exercised in preventing this condition, including avoiding supine aortocaval compression.

(a)

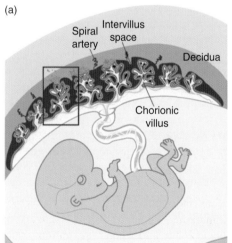

(b)

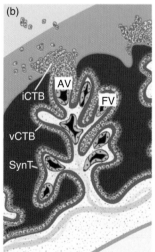

(c)

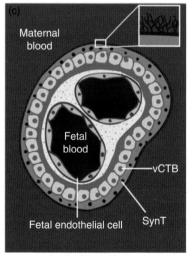

Figure 13.1. Maternal and fetal blood are separate in the placenta. (a,b) Maternal blood does not mix with fetal blood; the placental villi, containing fetal blood, project into the intervillous space, which contains maternal blood. The section in the square in (a) is expanded in (b) (c) Cross-section of a placental villus, bathed in maternal blood in the intervillous space. AV, anchoring villi; FV, floating villi; iCTB, invasive cytotrophoblast; vCTB, villous cytotrophoblast; SynT, syncytiotrophoblast. (With permission from Maltepe E, Bakardijev AI, Fisher SJ. The placenta: transcriptional, epigenetic physiological integration during development. *J Clin Invest* 2010; 120: 1016–1025 [4].)

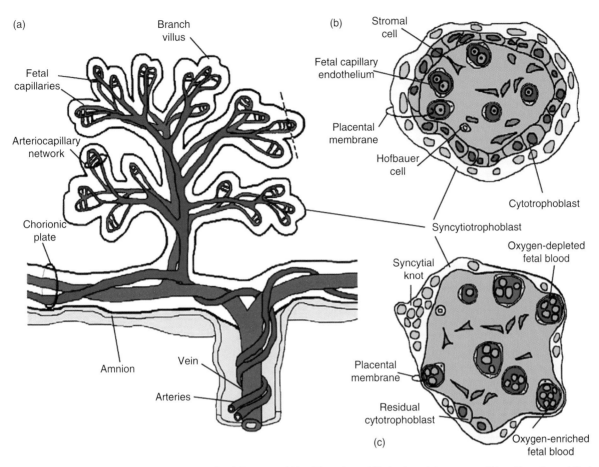

Figure 13.2. Fetal circulation within chorionic villi. (a) Oxygenated blood from the umbilical vein and deoxygenated blood from the umbilical arteries travel to the chorionic villi where gas and nutrient transfer occur. (b, c) Cross-section of villus at (b) 10 weeks and (c) full term. Note that as pregnancy progresses, the layer of cytotrophoblast atrophies, so the distance between fetal blood within the villus and maternal blood outside it decreases. (With permission from Gude NM, Roberts CT, Kalionis B, King RG. Growth and function of the normal human placenta. *Thromb Res* 2004; 114: 397–407 [3].)

As fetal blood is conducted to the placental villi by the two umbilical arteries (more highly oxygenated blood is returned from the placenta to the fetus by the single umbilical vein), exchange of oxygen and other substances happens in the intervillous space, which allows passive diffusion but distinctly separates maternal and fetal circulations. Transfer of oxygen and other molecules requires adequate perfusion and a concentration gradient; these factors can, to an extent, be altered in ICU. Other factors that may impede the transfer of substances between the maternal and fetal circulations, such as gross placental pathology or compression of the umbilical cord, are not amenable to supportive care in ICU. Fortunately, as these factors are unlikely to be primarily deranged in an otherwise normal pregnancy, and provided that the oxygen content of maternal blood is adequate, ensuring an uninterrupted uterine blood flow is the key issue in addressing the interest of the fetus in a critically ill mother.

Principles of placental gas exchange

Oxygen and carbon dioxide are transferred across the placenta by simple diffusion. Factors affecting oxygen transport to the fetus include maternal oxygen delivery to the placenta (blood flow multiplied by the oxygen content of maternal blood, which is a product of maternal hemoglobin and oxygen saturation), fetal umbilical arterial blood flow, oxygen capacity and oxygen affinity of fetal blood, efficacy of the exchange mechanism, oxygen-diffusing capacity of the placenta, and the metabolic requirements and oxygen consumption of the placenta itself [5].

Oxyhemoglobin saturation of maternal blood approximates 100% in most conditions. Because the oxygen affinity of fetal blood is much higher than that of maternal blood, transfer to the fetus is facilitated. The partial pressure of oxygen at which fetal hemoglobin is 50% saturated is about 20 torr (2.7 kPa) (NB under most conditions, 1 mmHg is approximately equal to 1 torr) compared with about 27 torr (3.6 kPa) in adult hemoglobin [6]. Fetal hemoglobin contains two α-chains that are identical to those in the adult, and two γ-chains, which differ from adult β-chains in their binding of 2,3-diphosphoglycerate. Although the fetus begins to produce some adult hemoglobin in the third trimester, conversion is not complete until after birth.

Normal fetal arterial oxygen partial pressure (Pao_2) ranges from 20 to 35 torr (2.7–4.7 kPa; i.e. 50–80% oxyhemoglobin saturation), and normal fetal pH is about 7.3. The carbon dioxide partial pressure (Pco_2) in the umbilical vein is 38–42 torr (5.1–5.6 kPa) (higher than the maternal arterial carbon dioxide partial pressure ($Paco_2$) because of the effect of pregnancy on maternal minute ventilation) and in the umbilical artery it is 49–55 torr (6.5–7.3 kPa). Oxygen delivery is maintained in the normal fetus by its higher hemoglobin concentration, its increased cardiac output relative to weight, and the higher oxygen affinity of fetal hemoglobin. Fetal Pco_2 is higher than maternal, being 42–50 torr (5.6–6.7 kPa) [7]. Both oxygen and carbon dioxide are transferred across the placenta down a maternal–fetal gradient. Diffusion across the villous interface is facilitated because the distance is short and the number of intervening layers minimal.

Although the placenta of some mammalian species is a counter-current exchanger, the human placenta appears to be a concurrent exchange model of placental gas transport [8]. The extreme example of concurrent exchange is a venous equilibrator [9]. Imagine two streams of blood flowing in the same direction, separated by a permeable membrane. Blood entering the arterial end of these streams differs in its Po_2: that in maternal blood is much higher than that in the fetal blood, which creates a gradient that drives oxygen into the lower-value fetal stream. However, as the streams continue toward the venous end, depending on the length of the path, the fetal stream becomes more highly oxygenated and the maternal less so. In a perfect venous equilibrator, of course, the two streams would have identical Po_2 at the venous end. This model assumes, however, that the dividing membrane has

no oxygen demands of its own, which would be a rash assumption given that it is known that the oxygen uptake of the placenta equals or exceeds that of the fetus. The placenta is highly metabolically active. The model, however, makes it clear that umbilical Po_2 venous relates more directly to uterine venous Po_2 than to maternal arterial Po_2 per se.

Changes in maternal Pao_2 can, certainly, affect umbilical venous Po_2, which is the most highly oxygenated blood in the fetus. As Meschia [9] makes clear, it would take a large decrement in maternal arterial oxygenation to effect enough of a difference in *uterine* venous saturation that the *umbilical* venous saturation would slide down the slope of the fetal oxyhemoglobin dissociation curve into territory associated with metabolic acidosis (less than 50% in the fetal lamb model). Table 13.1 shows a theoretical modeling of these differences, based on ovine data [10]. The "safe" lower level of maternal oxygenation is not known with any certainty in the human, despite repeated expert pronouncements that maternal oxygen saturation should be kept at or above 95%, or 90%. A small experimental trial of healthy volunteers in their third trimester breathing a hypoxic gas mixture with a fraction of inspired oxygen of approximately 0.1 for 10 minutes showed a fall in maternal oxygen saturation of 15% without an obvious change in non-invasive measures

Table 13.1. Theoretical exercise in acute hypoxemia (sheep model)

Vessel	Normoxemic	Hypoxemic
Uterine artery		
Po_2 (mmHg[a])	102	44
pH	7.45	7.50
Oxygen saturation (%)	96	85
Uterine vein		
Po_2 (mmHg[a])	35	27
pH	7.42	7.47
Oxygen saturation (%)	71	60
Umbilical vein		
Po_2 (mmHg[a])	28	20
pH	7.41	7.46
Oxygen saturation (%)	70	55

Po_2, oxygen partial pressure.
[a] 1 torr is approximately the same as 1 mmHg.
Source: Meschia 2011 [10].

of fetal oxygenation and acid–base balance. Fetal oxygenation was not sampled directly in this study, but the indices of fetal well-being reported (fetal heart rate tracing, Doppler velocimetry) are generally considered a proxy for fetal oxygenation and acid–base status. No adverse fetal outcomes were reported [11].

Fetoplacental oxygen delivery, of course, will also depend on uteroplacental blood flow, to a degree that is often underappreciated in the ICU. Factors that depress the maternal cardiac output will significantly affect fetal oxygen delivery: these may include maternal hypotension, positional compression of the inferior vena cava, or high levels of positive end-expiratory pressure, among others.

Understanding basic principles of placental gas exchange is important when caring for a pregnant patient in the ICU. Maintenance of uteroplacental perfusion is crucial. A lower limit of maternal oxygen saturation is not known, but analysis of the fetal heart rate tracing in many cases will help to determine whether the level of maternal oxygenation achieved is satisfactory for the fetus. There might be less concern about the maternal Pa_{O_2} than about the maternal Pa_{CO_2}, since fetal acid–base balance requires diffusion of fetally generated carbon dioxide across the placenta, following a fetomaternal gradient. The normally decreased maternal Pa_{CO_2} of 28–32 torr (3.7–4.3 kPa) during pregnancy allows this transfer to take place, but a policy of permissive hypercapnia, which is current standard of care in ventilation for acute respiratory distress syndrome, may preclude it. In a small trial of carbon dioxide rebreathing among healthy pregnant women, the Pa_{CO_2} was allowed to rise as high as 60 torr (8.0 kPa), and more than 50% of the fetuses demonstrated alterations in the fetal heart rate tracing that were suspicious for acidemia; most of these alterations reversed after maternal Pa_{CO_2} returned to normal [12].

Principles of management

Aside from the few cases in which delivery is the preferred therapy, managing a pregnant patient in ICU should focus primarily on maternal well-being and only secondarily on the effects of interventions on the fetus. These interventions may include pharmacotherapy, mechanical ventilation, surgery, and so on, which are covered elsewhere in this book. The physician, nurse, or other professional must be cognizant of uteroplacental physiology and transplacental pharmacokinetics. For example, maintaining adequate maternal blood pressure may require inotropes or vasopressors. The transplacental distribution of these agents may have repercussions for the fetus. For example, ephedrine, which formerly was the most widely used vasopressor in obstetric anesthesia, has been associated with an increased risk of fetal acidosis, possibly through a direct effect on fetal metabolism after its relatively uninhibited passage through the human placenta. This effect was not evident in previous studies on the sheep model because of the inherent difference: the ovine placenta does not allow free passage of ephedrine into the fetal circulation. A propensity for intrafetal accumulation of basic drugs of low molecular weight but high lipophilicity is also pertinent: fetal plasma has a lower pH and lower capacity for protein binding relative to maternal plasma. The interactions can be complex and ability to specifically assess the fetus is limited.

In the first trimester of pregnancy, the well-being of the fetus cannot separately be investigated at all. By the third trimester, however, electronic fetal monitoring is technically feasible and is believed to represent fetal acid–base status, level of oxygenation, and the integrity of the central nervous system. More subtle fetal effects such as interference with fetal growth or neurodevelopment cannot realistically be followed in ICU and, in fact, may not even be apparent at the time of birth.

While the practicioner would want, if possible to maintain normal maternal acid–base status, normal gas exchange, normal electrolytes, and normal hemodynamics when a pregnant patient is in ICU, it is not clear in all cases how to do so. Although the role of permissive hypercapnea is well established in nonpregnant patients for the acute respiratory distress syndrome, a high carbon dioxide tension (above 60 torr (8.0 kPa)) has been related to increased uterine vascular resistance and reduced uterine blood flow in the sheep model of pregnancy. Furthermore, hypercapnea may result in fetal acidosis through loss of the carbon dioxide gradient and a reduced oxygen-carrying capacity caused by the right shift of the hemoglobin oxygen dissociation curve. The institution of positive-pressure ventilation to ensure oxygenation may reduce perfusion to the uteroplacental unit either by decreasing venous return to the heart, and thereby decreasing cardiac output, or by increasing intra-abdominal pressure. Use of drugs to support maternal cardiorespiratory or other systems will result in exposure of the fetus to these agents, a risk which must be balanced against their benefit to the mother.

Enhancing fetal health: monitoring and interventions

External cardiotocography is technically feasible some time after 24 weeks, depending on maternal habitus, and can be employed on a continuous or intermittent basis. Although cardiotocography is not a consistently reliable predictor of fetal welfare, it is widely used. Normal fetal heart rate, normal baseline variability, and the presence of cardioaccelerations are all indicators that the fetal central nervous system has not been compromised by hypoxia or metabolic acidosis. Absence of these factors or the finding of heart rate decelerations would generally be a cause for concern and should prompt a search for remediable factors. Often, however, an alteration in the cardiotocograph tracing indicates that the maternal condition should be corrected, after which the fetal condition corrects itself. One should also be cautious not to overtreat. The classic example is in the treatment of severe maternal hypertension, when overaggressive lowering of blood pressure results in fetal heart rate decelerations. These are best treated by restoring maternal blood pressure to acceptable levels, since the placenta does not autoregulate. The presence of a non-reassuring fetal heart rate pattern, such as persistent fetal bradycardia or tachycardia, poor variability, and late decelerations, is used as an empirical surrogate for impending fetal decompensation, barring other causes such as cardiac anomalies and hypothermia. The suspicion of non-reassuring fetal status is often the trigger to provide intrauterine "resuscitation" such as maternal position changes or administration of an intravenous fluid bolus or supplemental oxygen.

Additional fetal assessment is possible with B-mode or Doppler ultrasound. Direct assessment of fetal acid–base status, while technically feasible by cordocentesis, would seldom if ever be indicated in ICU.

If preterm delivery is anticipated, administration of antenatal corticosteroids to the mother will decrease rates of common complications of prematurity for the newborn. Dexamethasone and betamethasone, which cross the placenta efficiently, have been shown to decrease rates of respiratory distress syndrome, intraventricular hemorrhage, and necrotizing enterocolitis among infants born at 24–33 weeks of gestation; the benefit is maximal for those infants delivered between 24 hours and 7 days after the mother receives a course of steroids [13]. There also seems to be a role for maternal magnesium sulfate in decreasing neurological morbidity (specifically, cerebral palsy) among infants born preterm; consequently, this too may be considered if a significantly preterm delivery is anticipated [14].

As discussed above, the usual rule is to optimize the maternal medical condition and allow the fetus and placenta to take care of themselves. Near term, however, delivery may be appropriate in order to simplify management or to allow interventions that would otherwise be logistically difficult (e.g. prone positioning). The major complications of prematurity are decreased after about 34 weeks of gestation, and delivery may be undertaken without the expectation of major neonatal morbidity to be added to the stresses on the family. Certain fetal conditions such as severe intrauterine growth restriction may also provide a reason to separate the fetus from the mother. There are a few conditions in which the presence of the fetus or placenta actually compromises maternal health and, therefore, delivery may be indicated for maternal reasons at any gestational age. Classic examples are eclampsia, severe pre-eclampsia, HELLP syndrome (hemolysis, elevated liver enzymes, and low platelets), acute fatty liver of pregnancy, and significant placental abruption.

Conclusions

The well-being of the fetus is strongly influenced by the status of the critically ill mother. It is imperative to ensure that homeostasis is maintained as close to the normal physiological state as possible. Under circumstances in which a preterm delivery is to be considered, administration of corticosteroids (betamethasone or dexamethasone, which cross placenta efficiently) to the mother will accelerate fetal lung maturity. In pregnancy-triggered critical illnesses such as severe or complicated pre-eclampsia, the separation of the fetus from the mother is the definitive treatment, hence the potential conflict of the mother's health (best served by delivery regardless of gestational age) with the infant's outcome (highly dependent upon gestational age). In most other critical maternal illness, this trade-off is not required.

A decision to effect delivery, whether for fetal or maternal indications, must be accompanied by a thoughtful analysis of the risks of labor or cesarean delivery. Both labor and major abdominal surgery impose risks upon a medically fragile mother, as well as imposing complicated logistics upon the resources and the staff providing care.

When making decisions about pregnant patients in ICU, we would urge a modification of the Hippocratic pronouncement to read *primum matrem non nocere*. Hasty modifications of standard care in an attempt to keep the fetus "safe" risk both the mother's health and, thereby, that of the fetus.

References

1. Bernirschke K, Kaufman P. *Pathology of the Human Placenta*, 4th edn. New York: Springer-Verlag, 2000.

2. Moore KL, Persaud TVN. *The Developing Human: Clinically Oriented Embryology*, 8th edn, Ch. 3: Placenta and fetal membranes. Philadelphia, PA: Saunders, 2008.

3. Gude NM, Roberts CT, Kalionis B, King RG. Growth and function of the normal human placenta. *Thromb Res* 2004;**114**:397–407.

4. Maltepe E, Bakardjiev AI, Fisher SJ. The placenta: transcriptional, epigenetic and physiological integration during development. *J Clin Invest* 2010;**120**:1016–1025.

5. Carter AM. Evolution of factors affecting placental oxygen transfer. *Placenta* 2009;**23**: S19–S25.

6. Ross MG, Ervin MG, Novak D. Fetal physiology. In Gabbe SG, Niebyl JR, Simpson JL (eds.) *Obstetrics: Normal and Problem Pregnancies*, 5th edn.

7. Philadelphia, PA: Churchill Livingstone, 2007, pp. 26–54.

7. Nageotte MP, Gilstrap LC, Intrapartum fetal surveillance. In Creasy RK, Resnik R, Iams JD, *et al.* (eds.) *Creasy & Resnik's Maternal Fetal Medicine: Principles and Practice*, 6th edn. Philadelphia, PA: Saunders-Elsevier, 2009, pp. 397–417.

8. Pardi G, Cetin I. Human fetal growth and organ development: 50 years of discoveries. *Am J Obstet Gynecol* 2006;**194**:1088–1099.

9. Meschia G. Placental respiratory gas exchange and fetal oxygenation. In Creasy RK, Resnik R, Iams JD, *et al.* (eds.) *Creasy & Resnik's Maternal Fetal Medicine: Principles and Practice*, 6th edn. Philadelphia, PA: Saunders-Elsevier, 2009, pp. 181–191.

10. Meschia G. Fetal oxygenation and maternal ventilation. *Clin Chest Med* 2011;**32**:15–19.

11. Erkkola R, Pirhonen J, Polvi H. The fetal cardiovascular function in chronic placental insufficiency is different from experimental hypoxia. *Ann Chir Gynaecol Suppl* 1994;**208**:76–79.

12. Fraser D, Jensen D, Wolfe LA, *et al.* Fetal heart rate response to hypocapnia and hypercapnia in late gestation. *J Obstet Gynaecol Can* 2008;**30**:312–316.

13. Roberts D, Dalziel SR. Antenatal corticosteroids for accelerating fetal lung maturation for women at risk of preterm birth. *Cochrane Database Syst Rev* 2006(**3**): CD004454.

14. Doyle LW, Crowther CA, Middleton P, Marret S, Rouse D. Magnesium sulphate for women at risk of preterm birth for neuroprotection of the fetus. *Cochrane Database Syst Rev* 2009(**1**): CD004661.

Pharmacology, pharmacokinetics, and management of the patient after overdose

Edward J. Hayes and Warwick D. Ngan Kee

Introduction

Knowledge of the way that pregnancy affects pharmacological response is essential to optimal management of the critically ill parturient. Pregnancy is a state of flux with the placental–fetal unit undergoing constant changes that affect both pharmacodynamics and pharmacokinetics of many drugs. Additionally, it is important to consider placental transfer and metabolism, and fetal effects and handling of drugs. The changes of pregnancy affect not only prescribed drugs but also impact the management of patients with overdose and patients intoxicated with illicit drugs.

When considering pharmacology in the parturient, it is important to note that, for practical and ethical reasons, experimental data are limited in quality and quantity and it often may not be valid to extrapolate animal data because of species differences. Therefore, some of the available knowledge may be based on theoretical considerations and application of basic principles. As a result, a comprehensive model that will predict response to most individual drugs is lacking. Furthermore, the dynamic physiological changes of pregnancy mean that dose adjustment may be necessary not only because of pregnancy but also according to the different stages of pregnancy.

Safety of drugs in pregnancy

Although some drugs have been proven safe and some are known to be harmful in pregnancy, there are many drugs for which insufficient data are available. The US Food and Drug Administration has introduced a classification system for use of drugs in pregnancy based on possible fetal risks (Table 14.1) [1]. However, because this system has limited ability to accurately and consistently convey risk and benefit, it is currently

under review and is likely to be changed or eliminated. Currently, the majority of drugs marketed in the USA are classified in category C (risks cannot be ruled out in humans) and although some drugs in this category may be harmful, there are many drugs that are not licensed for use in pregnancy because of insufficient data but are considered by clinicians as having benefits that outweigh potential risks; these drugs are sometimes used on an "off-label" basis.

One of the most important concerns when prescribing drugs is the potential for teratogenicity. Teratogenicity has traditionally referred to occurrence of structural defects in an embryo or fetus which was developing normally prior to exposure. Teratogenicity is determined according to specific criteria and may vary among species. The method of administration of drugs may be an important factor, as small, repeated, or sequential dosing may have a different effect to large bolus doses. The most sensitive time for drug exposure is considered to be during the period of organogenesis (3–8 weeks postconception or 35–70 days after the last menstrual period). However, drug exposure at later stages in pregnancy may also be associated with possible effects on morphology and function of the growing fetus, including growth restriction and developmental effects, as well as having potential effects during parturition and nursing. As an example, exposure to non-steroidal anti-inflammatory drugs in late pregnancy is associated with a risk of premature closure of the fetal ductus arteriosus [2]. Databases of drugs that are contraindicated in pregnancy are available online and are regularly updated [3]. In addition, pregnancy exposure registries exist for ongoing collection of data on use of medications and vaccines during pregnancy [1].

Note that although in general it is prudent to avoid drugs with known harmful effects during pregnancy, it

Maternal Critical Care: A Multidisciplinary Approach, ed. Marc Van de Velde, Helen Scholefield, and Lauren A. Plante.
Published by Cambridge University Press. © Cambridge University Press 2013.

Table 14.1. US Food and Drug Administration classification of drugs in pregnancy based on possible fetal risks

Category	Fetal risk
A	Adequate and well-controlled human studies have failed to demonstrate a risk to the fetus in the first trimester of pregnancy (and there is no evidence of risk in later trimesters)
B	Animal reproduction studies have failed to demonstrate a risk to the fetus and there are no adequate and well-controlled studies in pregnant women, *or* animal studies have shown an adverse effect but adequate and well-controlled studies in pregnant women have failed to demonstrate a risk to the fetus in any trimester
C	Animal reproduction studies have shown an adverse effect on the fetus and there are no adequate and well-controlled studies in humans, but potential benefits may warrant use of the drug in pregnant women despite potential risks
D	There is positive evidence of human fetal risk based on adverse reaction data from investigational or marketing experience or studies in humans, but potential benefits may warrant use of the drug in pregnant women despite potential risks
X	Studies in animals or humans have demonstrated fetal abnormalities and/or there is positive evidence of human fetal risk based on adverse reaction data from investigational or marketing experience, and the risks involved in use of the drug in pregnant women clearly outweigh potential benefits

Source: US Food and Drug Administration [1].

is essential to appreciate that these considerations should not prevent use of appropriate emergency drugs during maternal resuscitation.

Pharmacodynamics

It is well recognized that pregnancy affects the clinical response to many drugs that are used in the settings of critical care and anesthesia, although the mechanisms underlying these observations are less well defined. Studies in animals and humans have shown that requirement (minimum alveolar concentration) for inhalational anesthetics is decreased by approximately one quarter, from early pregnancy to the early puerperium. Requirements for intravenous induction agents such as thiopental and propofol are also reduced in pregnancy [4]. It has been suggested that these increases in drug sensitivity may be related to increased progesterone, based on animal research that showed that chronic progesterone administration decreased volatile anesthetic requirements. However, other factors may also contribute, such as increased endorphin response, and pharmacokinetic changes may also be a factor. In pregnancy, there is also increased sensitivity to local anesthetics. This is evidenced by in vitro studies that have demonstrated increased sensitivity of nerves from pregnant animals to block from local anesthetics and clinical evidence of increased spread of spinal and epidural anesthesia, although changes in spinal canal volume caused by epidural vein engorgement are thought to also contribute to the latter.

Pharmacokinetics

The major physiological changes that occur during pregnancy have important effects on pharmacokinetics of many drugs.

Absorption

Although it is thought that gastric emptying is delayed in pregnancy, evidence is inconsistent. Gastric emptying is also delayed during labor, by pain, and after administration of opioids. Intestinal motility is decreased in pregnancy, leading to prolongation of intestinal passage, which is greater in the second and third trimesters [5]. These changes may lead to enhanced absorption of slowly absorbed drugs and delayed absorption of well-absorbed drugs [5]. Although gastric secretion remains acidic during pregnancy, gastric pH is greater than in non-pregnancy because of a 40% reduction in hydrogen ion secretion and increased mucus production [6]. This may reduce the absorption of drugs that are weak acids by increasing their ionization, particularly for single doses. However, despite the above considerations, the overall effect of pregnancy on bioavailability of oral drugs is thought to be minor [7]. However, nausea and vomiting associated with pregnancy may be a significant physical impediment to oral drug absorption.

Increased cardiac output, tissue flow, and vasodilatation during pregnancy may enhance absorption of drugs administered subcutaneously, intramuscularly, epidurally, transvaginally, and via mucous membranes.

Minute ventilation is substantially increased during pregnancy from 7–8 weeks of gestation, which may enhance absorption from the lungs of drugs such as bronchodilators as well as pollutants and cigarette smoke. However, the effect on uptake of inhaled anesthetics is complex. Increased alveolar ventilation and reduced functional residual capacity favor a faster rise in the alveolar concentration of volatile anesthetics and faster induction, but this is countered by the increase in cardiac output during pregnancy, which increases drug removal from the lung and slows the rate of rise of alveolar partial pressure of volatile drugs. These effects of ventilation and cardiac output are more pronounced with more soluble agents.

Distribution

Many factors contribute to changes in drug distribution in pregnancy, including marked increases in total body water (approximately 8 L), extracellular fluid, and plasma volume (approximately 40% or 1.3 L); decreased concentration of plasma proteins; increased body fat; and increased cardiac output [8]. These fluid changes have substantial effects on distribution and elimination of drugs, especially those that are polar and water soluble. For example, hydrophilic drugs such as neuromuscular-blocking agents have a greater space in which to distribute, leading to increased calculated values of volume of distribution. This also results in a decrease in the peak plasma concentrations of hydrophilic drugs, although the clinical effect of this may be offset by changes in protein binding [7]. Body fat increases in pregnancy by approximately 3–4 kg, but although this increases the volume of distribution of lipophilic drugs, the effect of this is small relative to the large baseline value.

The plasma concentration of albumin is decreased by about 30% (from approximately 4.2 to 3.6 g/dL) during pregnancy, although this may reflect a dilutional effect of the increase in plasma volume [8]. Since the concentration of α_1-acid glycoprotein is relatively unaffected, this may represent a reduction in albumin synthesis or an increase in its catabolism [9]. The result is a decrease in protein binding of many weakly acidic and weakly basic drugs and a consequent increase in the free fraction of drug. Steroid and placental hormones may also displace some drugs from their protein-binding sites [7]. These changes in protein binding are important because the free fraction of drug is responsible for both drug activity and drug toxicity, and only the free fraction can cross the placenta. Although an increased free fraction of drug would be anticipated to increase drug action, this effect is offset by the fact that a greater proportion of the drug will be available for hepatic biotransformation and/or renal elimination; this increased clearance means that the overall clinical effect of increased free fraction is minimal for chronic administration of most drugs [6]. However, for drugs that are highly bound to albumin, such as anticonvulsants and serotonin reuptake inhibitors, there may be a significant increase in drug effect. Conversely, there is little effect for basic drugs that bind to α_1-acid glycoprotein, such as opioids, tricyclic antidepressants and beta-blockers.

Changes in plasma protein binding are also important for monitoring of therapeutic drugs when attention should be given to whether reference values and measured concentrations are for total drug or free drug. For example, phenytoin is approximately 90% bound to albumin but monitored concentrations are usually reported as total (bound plus free) values; therefore an adjustment should be made taking into account reduced albumin levels when adjusting doses in pregnant patients.

Transplacental transfer

The human placenta is described as hemochorial with a structure that places the fetal and maternal blood circulations in close proximity. Trophoblast covering the placental villous tree is the main barrier for most substances. Most substances cross the placenta by passive diffusion down a concentration gradient, the extent of which is determined by properties such as molecular weight, dissociation constant, lipid solubility, and the extent of plasma protein binding of the substance. Generally, non-ionized lipophilic molecules with molecular weights up to 600 Da cross the placenta. Some drugs with structural similarity to endogenous compounds may be transferred by nutrient transporters.

Drug efflux transporters

Transporter proteins that facilitate active transport of drugs and xenobiotics are found in the placenta. In particular, these include the large group of ATP-binding cassette (ABC) transporters, which include P-glycoprotein, breast cancer resistant protein, and multidrug resistance proteins [10,11]. In addition, there are ATP-dependent transporters in the solute carrier protein (SLC) family. These transporters require energy and are able to transfer drugs and other xenobiotics across the placental barrier against a concentration gradient in a fetus to maternal direction and thus limit fetal exposure to some drugs and toxins. For example, drugs that are substrates for these transporters include cytotoxics, protease inhibitors, antibiotics, opiods, and antiemetics [5]. Expression and activity of drug efflux transporters is influenced by gestational age and pregnancy-related hormones and growth factors [11]. Drug interactions are possible if substrates or inhibitors of transporters are coadministered, and drug-induced induction of downregulation of inhibitors may occur [11]. Theoretically, choosing a drug that is a substrate for drug efflux transporter protein may be advantageous since fetomaternal transfer will be facilitated, thereby limiting fetal drug exposure. Conversely, if the fetus is the target of pharmacotherapy, selection of a drug that is not a substrate would be preferred [5].

Metabolism

Pregnancy-induced changes in protein binding, hepatic blood flow, and drug-metabolizing enzymes have an important influence on the metabolism of drugs. However, the overall effect on drug activity varies since clearance may be enhanced for some drugs but inhibited for others. Furthermore, the overall effect of pregnancy-induced changes in metabolism may be complex for prodrugs, which require metabolism to an active form, and may also affect the formation and clearance of active and toxic metabolites of some drugs.

Protein binding

As highlighted above, a decrease in protein binding increases the free fraction of drug that is available for metabolism.

Hepatic blood flow

Despite the global increase in overall cardiac output during pregnancy, studies quantifying changes in hepatic blood flow have had conflicting results, probably reflecting different methodologies used as well as the possibility of reciprocal changes in the flows of hepatic arterial and portal venous blood flow, which contribute approximately 25% and 75% of total hepatic blood flow, respectively. Studies that utilized hepatic vein catheterization and the Fick principle with indocyanine green clearance found that hepatic blood flow did not increase in pregnancy. However, evaluation using Doppler ultrasonography found that total hepatic

blood flow in the third trimester was increased to about 160% of non-pregnancy values, but this was related to an increase in portal venous blood flow with no significant increase found in hepatic arterial blood flow [12]. This is significant because portal venous flow is responsible for the first-pass metabolism of drugs.

The increase in hepatic blood flow in pregnancy has a variable effect on drug metabolism. Theoretically, drugs with a high hepatic extraction ratio should be affected the most since their clearance is more dependent on blood flow than for drugs with a low ratio. However, results have been variable for some high extraction ratio drugs such as morphine, propranolol, and midazolam, suggesting that other factors are involved [13].

Hepatic biotransformation

Pregnancy affects hepatic biotransformation in an enzyme-specific manner. Increased concentration of various hormones including estrogen, progesterone, placental growth hormones, and prolactin exert regulatory effects on the expression of drug-metabolizing enzymes by activating nuclear receptors. The activity of enzymes involved with both phase I and phase II hepatic biotransformation may be altered in pregnancy. The activity of some isoenzymes may be increased while others are decreased; consequently, it is not possible to produce a general model and knowledge of the metabolic handling of individual drugs is necessary to understand the effect of pregnancy on clearance of specific drugs.

Phase I enzymes

The cytochrome P450 (CYP) mixed function oxidase system is the most important enzyme family involved in drug metabolism. It is a large family of membrane-bound heme proteins that is responsible for the metabolism of a large range of endogenous and exogenous compounds, including drugs, toxins, and other xenobiotics. There are a large number of different CYP isoenzymes and these are classified with numbers and letters that indicate their gene family, subfamily, and individual gene.

The CYP isoenzymes showing *increased* activity during pregnancy include CYP3A4, CYP2C9, CYP2D6, CYP2A6.

CYP3A4. This is the most important CYP isoenzyme, responsible for the metabolism of over 40% of all drugs. For example,

153

investigation of the pharmacokinetics of oral nifedipine in patients with pregnancy-induced hypertension showed a shorter half-life, more rapid clearance, and lower maximum plasma concentration compared with non-pregnant controls. This suggests that efficacy would be improved by reducing the dosing interval [14]. Studies in pregnant women with HIV infection have shown increased metabolism of the protease inhibitor antiretroviral drugs indinavir, saquinavir, ritonavir and lopinavir, suggesting that dosage adjustment during pregnancy should be considered. Increased clearance of and lower plasma concentrations were found for methadone during pregnancy, suggesting that increased doses may be required for preventing withdrawal symptoms in heroin addicts on methadone maintenance.

CYP2C9. The 4′-hydroxylation of phenytoin by CYP2CP is increased in pregnancy, resulting in a decrease in both total and free plasma concentrations. Careful monitoring and consideration of dosage adjustment is indicated to prevent loss of seizure control [13].

CYP2D6. Drugs reported to be metabolized by CYP2D6 include metoprolol, dextromethorphan, and many antidepressants used in pregnancy, including paroxetine, duloxetine, fluoxetine, and citalopram.

CYP2A6. Clearance of nicotine and cotinine, which are metabolized by CYP2A6, is increased during pregnancy.

The CYP isoenzymes showing *decreased* activity during pregnancy include CYP1A2 and CYP2C19.

CYP1A2. Metabolism of caffeine by CYP1A2 is decreased in pregnancy. Decreased metabolism of theophylline may require dosage reduction to avoid toxicity. This isoenzyme also metabolizes clozapine, cyclobenzaprine, olanzapine, and ondansetron [13].

CYP2C19. The metabolism of the antimalarial drug proguanil to the active metabolite cycloguanil is catalyzed by CYP2C19. Decreased concentration of ycloguanil in pregnancy may indicate the need for dosage increase [13]. Metabolism of nelfinavir to its hydoxylated active metabolite is also catalyzed by CYP2C19.

Phase II enzymes

The activity of phase II enzymes may also be altered during pregnancy.

Uridine diphosphate glucuronosyltransferases. This family of microsomal enzymes catalyzes covalent addition of glucuronic acid to lipophilic endogenous and exogenous compounds, which increases their water solubility and promotes excretion into bile or urine. Increased activity has been shown for the isoenzymes that metabolize drugs, including lamotrigine, lorazepam, and acetaminophen (paracetamol). This results in increased clearance; consequently, dosing adjustment may be required to maintain therapeutic plasma concentrations during pregnancy [13]. For example, seizure control was shown to deteriorate when there was inadequate adjustment of lamotrigine in pregnancy [15].

N-Acetyltranferase. This is the first drug-metabolizing enzyme for which genetic polymorphism was discovered. Studies suggest that its activity is decreased during pregnancy. It catalyzes *N*-acetylation of a number of drugs including isoniazid, dapsone, and sulfamethoxazole.

Extrahepatic metabolism

The small intestine contains almost all of the biotransformation enzymes present in the liver, although in smaller amounts. Phase I and phase II metabolism occurs in the intestine and is an important contributor to first-pass metabolism of drugs. However, little information is available to indicate whether pregnancy-associated enzyme changes in the intestine are quantitatively different to those in the liver. Similarly, many biotransformation enzymes are also present in the kidney. Plasma cholinesterase activity is decreased by about 30% in pregnancy, but this is not associated with a prolonged effect of succinylcholine, probably because of the offsetting effect of increased volume of distribution. The placenta also contains some biotransformation enzymes that may play a part in preventing entry of xenobiotics into the fetal circulation. Phase I enzymes are present, of which CYP1A1 and CYP2E1 have demonstrable metabolic activity, and some phase II enzymes are also present [13]. Although not reaching full activity until after birth, the fetal liver contains biotransformation enzymes but data are limited regarding their activity.

Phase II metabolism of drugs by the fetus may prolong fetal exposure to potentially toxic metabolites because the more water-soluble conjugates do not readily cross the placenta to the maternal circulation for elimination. If excreted in fetal urine they may be recycled in the fetus by swallowing and reabsorption by the intestine.

Elimination

Renal excretion depends on the glomerular filtration rate and tubular secretion and absorption. By the end of the first trimester, the glomerular filtration rate has increased by 50% or more, which is related to an increase in renal blood flow, decreased renal vascular resistance, and increased cardiac output. It continues to increase during pregnancy, although it has been shown to decrease in the last three weeks of gestation. The increase in glomerular filtration rate favors an increase in excretion of hydrophilic drugs and metabolites. Increased free fraction in pregnancy also contributes to greater glomerular filtration of drugs. Drugs that have been shown to exhibit an increase in renal excretion in pregnancy include lithium, atenolol, digoxin, and antibiotics such as penicillins, cephalosporins, aminoglycosides, and sulfonamides [5]. Little information is available on the effect of pregnancy on tubular secretion and absorption of drugs.

Increased alveolar ventilation will enhance elimination of volatile anesthestics.

Pharmacogenetics

Genotype of mother and fetus can affect individual susceptibility to some drugs. For example, fetuses with low levels of the enzyme epoxide hydrolase are more likely to manifest the fetal hydantoin syndrome than those with normal levels. Although genetic differences will contribute to variability of drug response regardless of whether the patient is pregnant, much of the research that has been done in this area has been performed in patients who are pregnant or postpartum [16]. Much recent research has focused on the effect of single nucleotide polymorphisms. For example, genetic variability of the β_2-adrenoceptor affects response and neonatal outcome when beta-2 agonists are used for tocolysis and also affects vasopressor requirement during spinal anesthesia for cesarean delivery. Genetic variability of the opioid mu-receptor has been shown to affect response to both intrathecal and systemic opioids. The ATP-binding cassette transporter proteins also display genetic polymorphisms [17].

Vasoactive drugs

During pregnancy, a generalized reduction in the response to endogenous and exogenous vasoconstrictors occurs. However, the relative refractoriness of the systemic and uteroplacental circulation varies for different agents. For example, there is decreased sensitivity and reduced vasoconstrictor response to epinephrine, norepinephrine, and phenylephrine [18]. Clinically, this means that increased doses of vasopressors may be required for a given effect, for example the maintenance of blood pressure during regional anesthesia for cesarean delivery [19]. Of note, the uterine circulation is more responsive than the systemic circulation to the vasoconstrictor effects of alpha agonists [18], which means that during periods of high catecholamine release (e.g. hemorrhage) or during therapeutic administration of vasopressors, uteroplacental perfusion is unlikely to be preferentially preserved. The potential for vasoconstriction in the uteroplacental circulation should be balanced against the benefits of increased perfusion pressure, both to the uteroplacental circulation and to the vital organs.

In contrast, although the vasopressor response to angiotensin II is also reduced in pregnancy, the uterine circulation is less responsive to this agent than the systemic circulation [20]. This is thought to be an adaptive response to pregnancy that contributes to the redistribution of cardiac output and the increase in uterine blood flow.

Overdose

The treatment of drug overdose in pregnancy presents a unique challenge because of changes in the pharmacodynamics and pharmacokinetics of drugs during the gravid state. In addition to the drug's maternal effects, it is important to consider placental transfer, metabolism, and fetal effects. The goal of therapy in an overdose during pregnancy is aimed at preserving maternal well-being while attempting to limit the risk to the fetus.

The most frequently used agents for self-inflicted poisoning during pregnancy are analgesics, antipyretics, and antirheumatics [21]. It is difficult to quantify the number of women who overdose on these agents during pregnancy because of the resistance of individuals to report or seek medical help after exposure.

Appreciating the limitations previously noted, an estimate of the incidence is provided by a recent review of attempted suicides reported in the State of California between 1991 and 1999. During that period, there were 2132 pregnancies complicated by attempted suicide (0.4 per 1000 pregnancies), and of these 86% were by ingestion of solid or liquid. Since the vast majority were purposeful ingestion of a substance, this cohort can be used to extrapolate an approximate incidence of overdose of 0.4 per 1000 pregnancies [22].

This cohort also allows an estimation of maternal and perinatal outcomes following an overdose. Women who overdose during pregnancy have higher rates of the obstetric complications, premature labor, cesarean delivery, or a blood transfusion [22]. If the woman undergoes delivery during her hospitalization for her attempted suicide, then the newborn is at increased risk for respiratory distress syndrome and neonatal and infant death [22].

Acetaminophen overdose

The most common agent used for an overdose during pregnancy is acetaminophen [23]. Acetaminophen is metabolized by the liver primarily to form non-toxic glucuronides and sulfates, which are excreted in the urine. However, the liver enzyme CYP2E1 metabolizes a small fraction to highly reactive oxides such as N-acetyl-p-benzoquinoneimine (NAPQI). This is quickly bound by glutathione and excreted in the urine when the recommended dose of acetaminophen has been ingested.

When a toxic dose of acetaminophen is ingested, the primary site of cellular injury is in the liver. The primary enzyme pathways become saturated and a higher percentage of acetaminophen is converted to NAPQI by CYP2E1. If the amount of the toxic metabolite NAPQI formed in the hepatocyte exceeds the binding capacity of glutathione, hepatocellular injury occurs [23]. This damage may not be limited to the maternal unit since acetaminophen crosses the placenta and, in a similar fashion, the fetal primary enzymatic pathways may also become saturated, leading to the formation of sufficient levels of NAPQI to cause hepatic injury in the fetus or neonate [23]. Appreciating the increased risk to both the fetus and mother, the current practice guideline for the American Association of Poison Control Centers recommends pregnant woman be sent to the hospital for evaluation if more than 4 g or 100 mg/kg of acetaminophen has been consumed within a 24 hour time period. This threshold for hospital evaluation is lower than the 10 g or 200 mg/kg consumed in 24 hours in the non-pregnant adult [24].

After the ingestion of a lethal dose of acetaminophen, the patient will experience three stages of clinical symptoms, which may culminate with her demise unless she seeks out medical therapy. The first phase begins within several hours of ingestion and lasts, on average, less than 12 hours. The gastrointestinal symptoms of anorexia, nausea, vomiting dominate, and the patient rarely presents in shock. Phase II is heralded by improving gastrointestinal symptoms but there is biochemical evidence of hepatic injury. Phase III begins on day 3 to 5 and is dominant by signs and symptoms of overt hepatic damage, with a third of patients progressing to fulminant hepatic failure. This will be seen clinically as coagulopathy with hepatic encephalopathy, which may progress to maternal and fetal death.

The treatment of acetaminophen overdose is aimed at decreasing the absorption of acetaminophen and protecting the hepatocytes from the toxic effects of the highly reactive metabolites. After initial assessment and stabilization, the patient should undergo gastrointestinal decontamination with activated charcoal. The use of activated charcoal has been shown to decrease the incidence of liver injury compared with that in individuals who did not undergo treatment, without affecting the efficacy of N-acetylcysteine given subsequently [25]. The N-acetylcysteine is given to bind NAPQI and, therefore, protect the maternal and fetal hepatocytes from the toxic metabolites produced from an overdose of acetaminophen. The protocol is presented in Box 14.1.

Iron

The second most common drug implicated in intentional overdose in pregnancy is iron. This mostly likely reflects its readily availability to the gravid patient. Following a toxic ingestion of iron, the patient may progress through four clinical stages. The first stage occurs within 6 hours of ingestion and is dominated by symptoms of gastrointestinal irritation: nausea, vomiting, or abdominal pain. Stage II follows, starting 6 hours after ingestion, during which the patient develops metabolic acidosis and increased capillary permeability, leading to hypotension. Stage III results from iron's direct cytotoxicity and manifests as hepatic, renal, and, in some cases, cardiac failure, which if untreated may lead to the patient's demise. For those patients who survive stage III, stage IV occurs weeks to

---

Box 14.1 Treatment of acetaminophen overdose
in pregnancy

Step 1. Limit absorption from the
gastrointestinal tract
Activated charcoal 1 g/kg up to 50 g

Step 2. Bind toxic metabolites in the circulation
1. Determine blood level of acetaminophen
2. Use *N*-acetylcysteine (NAC)

- able to tolerate oral NAC 140 mg/kg orally
  followed by 17 maintenance doses of 70 mg/
  kg every 4 hours
- oral cannot be tolerated; use loading dose of
  150 mg/kg intravenous over 60 minutes and
  then infuse at 12.5 mg/kg per hour for the first
  4 hours and 6.25 mg/kg per hour for the next
  16 hours

Step 3. Follow-up acetaminophen level
1. If the level during the initial period of 4 to 16
    hours is found to be predictive of no liver injury,
    the NAC can be stopped

Adapted from Heard and Dart, 2012 [26].

Box 14.2 Treatment of iron overdose in
pregnancy

Step 1. Hydration
Intravenous hydration with isotonic solution

Step 2. Elimination of residual iron tablets from
the gastrointestinal tract
Gastric lavage with normal saline or intestinal irrigation with polyethylene glycol electrolyte solution

Step 3. Bind iron in the circulation with
deforxamine
Deforoxamine is infused at a rate of 15 mg/kg per
hour until symptoms resolve, serum iron levels return
to normal, or vin rose urine if any resolves

Adapted from Tran *et al.*, 2000 [27].

---

months after the acute event and results in gastrointestinal scarring. Iron overdose in the pregnant
patient also increases the rate of the obstetric complications, spontaneous abortion, and preterm delivery.
The risk of adverse pregnancy outcome is not correlated to the dose ingested, reflected by serum levels, but
whether the patient progresses to stage III [27].

The principle behind the treatment of iron overdose
during pregnancy is to limit the amount of iron
absorbed from the gastrointestinal tract and to safely
eliminate it from the patient to prevent progression to
stage III. Gastric lavage with normal saline or intestinal
irrigation with polyethylence glycol electrolyte solution
is recommended to remove any residual iron tablets
and attempt to limit absorption, Deferoxamine is used
to bind and eliminate the excess iron once it has been
absorbed. Deferoxamine is an iron chelator, which on
binding the ferric iron results in the formation of ferrioxamine. Ferrioxamine is excreted renally and is
responsible for the vin rose urine frequently experienced by patients undergoing treatment. The drug has
not been associated with human malformations and
does not cross the placenta [27].

The indications for treatment with deferoxamine
after ingestion of iron overdose are as follows: patient
is symptomatic [2]; patient has ingested >20 mg/kg of
elemental iron [4]; or patient's serum iron is >4 mg/L
[5]. The treatment protocol is presented in Box 14.2.

Aspirin (acetylsalicylic acid) overdose

Aspirin's therapeutic window, 100–300 mg/L, is in
close proximity to its toxic range, >400 mg/L. A pregnant patient who has ingested a toxic amount of
aspirin usually presents with a classic triad of symptoms: hyperventilation, tinnitus, and gastrointestinal
symptoms such as nausea and vomiting. These symptoms may be quickly followed by changes in mental
status, resulting from three major mechanisms: direct
toxicity of salicylate species in the central nervous
system, cerebral edema, and neuroglycopenia [28].

When aspirin is ingested, it is quickly metabolized
to salicylate. The treatment of aspirin poisoning is to
use sodium bicarbonate to increase the systemic pH
and trap the salicylate ions in the blood, since charged
molecules cannot easily diffuse across the blood–brain
barrier into the central nervous system [28].
Alkalinization also traps salicylate anions within the
renal tubule, thus inhibiting reabsorption and enhancing excretion.

The treatment of aspirin overdose does not vary from
the non-pregnant state and is presented in Box 14.3.

Carbon monoxide intoxication in pregnancy

Carbon monoxide is formed by the burning of carbon-
containing compounds such as coal, wood, or
petroleum-based fuels. Since carbon monoxide is a

Box 14.3 Treatment of aspirin overdose in pregnancy

Step 1. Determine plasma salicylate level
1. Determine levels every 2 hours until declining

Note that levels may not rise until 6 hours after ingestion and may take up to 35 hours to peak

Step 2. Obtain blood gas every 2 hours
Until acid–base status stable or improving and avoid pH >7.6 because of excessive sodium bicarbonate

Step 3. Gastrointestinal decontamination
Activated charcoal 1 g/kg up to 50 g orally every 4 hours up to three doses

Step 4. Supplemental glucose
Glucose-containing intravenous solution should be given to aid patient with altered mental status, even if serum glucose concentration is normal

Step 4. Consider hemodialysis
Proceed to hemodialysis if one of the following is present

1. Profound altered mental status
2. Renal insufficiency that interferes with salicylate excretion
3. Plasma salicylate concentration >1 g/L

Step 5. Alkalinize maternal serum with sodium bicarbonate
1. Bolus of sodium bicarbonate 2 mEq/kg intravenous push
2. Maintance of 100–150 mEq sodium bicarbonate in 1 L 5% dextrose in water infusing at 250 mL/h

Based on Traub, 2010 [28].

Box 14.4 Treatment of carbon monoxide poisoning in pregnancy

Step 1. Obtain maternal carboxyhemoglobin level
Criterion for intensive care and treatment is a carboxyhemoglobin level of greater than 10% in a pregnant patient

Step 2. Determine if hyperbaric oxygen therapy is readily available
- If it is available, treat patient with 2 hours of hyperbaric oxygen administered at 2 atmospheres absolute [30]
- If hyperbaric oxygen is not available, treat patient with 100% oxygen through a face mask for five times the time it takes her levels to return to less than 5%; this allows for the longer elimination of carbon monoxide from the fetus [29]

---

tasteless, odorless, and colorless gas, exposed individuals may not appreciate that they have been poisoned. Carbon monoxide leads to tissue hypoxia because of its strong affinity for hemoglobin. It has 200 times higher affinity than oxygen and displaces the oxygen dissociation curve to the left, decreasing oxygen delivery to the tissue [29]. Carbon monoxide dissolves in maternal plasma and easily diffuses across the placental barrier, where it quickly binds with fetal hemoglobin. Carbon monoxide binds 2.5 to 3 times more aggressively to fetal hemoglobin than to adult hemoglobin, which results in its longer half-life of 7 hours in the fetus compared with 2 hours for the mother [29]. This higher affinity of fetal hemoglobin for carbon monoxide can be observed clinically in the difference

between the maternal mortality rate of 19–24% and fetal mortality rate of 36–67% after carbon monoxide poisoning [30]. The therapeutic approach in carbon monoxide poisoning is to deliver high-dose oxygen to displace carbon monoxide from the hemoglobin molecule. The treatment varies according to the delivery method available and is presented in Box 14.4.

References

1. US Food and Drug Administration. *List of Pregnancy Exposure Registries.* Silver Spring, MD: Food and Drug Administration (http://www.fda.gov/ScienceResearch/SpecialTopics/WomensHealthResearch/ucm134848.htm, accessed 5 December 2012).

2. Koren G, Florescu A, Costei AM, Boskovic R, Moretti ME. Nonsteroidal antiinflammatory drugs during third trimester and the risk of premature closure of the ductus arteriosus: a meta-analysis. *Ann Pharmacother* 2006;**40**:824–829.

3. Prescribing Reference. *Drugs Contraindicated in Pregnancy* [website]. London: Prescribing Reference, 2012 (http://www.empr.com/drugs-contraindicated-in-pregnancy/article/125914/#, accessed 5 December 2012).

4. Mongardon N, Servin F, Perrin M, *et al.* Predicted propofol effect-site concentration for induction and emergence of anesthesia during early pregnancy. *Anesth Analg* 2009;**109**:90–95.

5. Pavek P, Ceckova M, Staud F. Variation of drug kinetics in pregnancy. *Curr Drug Metab* 2009;**10**:520–529.

6. Loebstein R, Lalkin A, Koren G. Pharmacokinetic changes during pregnancy and their clinical relevance. *Clin Pharmacokinet* 1997;**33**:328–343.

7. Dawes M, Chowienczyk PJ. Drugs in pregnancy. Pharmacokinetics in pregnancy. *Best Pract Res Clin Obstet Gynaecol* 2001;**15**:819–826.

8. Mendenhall HW. Serum protein concentrations in pregnancy. I. Concentrations in maternal serum. *Am J Obstet Gynecol* 1970;**106**:388–399.

9. Frederiksen MC. Physiologic changes in pregnancy and their effect on drug disposition. *Semin Perinatol* 2001;**25**:120–123.

10. Vahakangas K, Myllynen P. Drug transporters in the human blood–placental barrier. *Br J Pharmacol* 2009;**158**:665–678.

11. Ni Z, Mao Q. ATP-binding cassette efflux transporters in human placenta. *Curr Pharm Biotechnol* 2011;**12**:674–685.

12. Nakai A, Sekiya I, Oya A, Koshino T, Araki T. Assessment of the hepatic arterial and portal venous blood flows during pregnancy with Doppler ultrasonography. *Arch Gynecol Obstet* 2002;**266**:25–29.

13. Hodge LS, Tracy TS. Alterations in drug disposition during pregnancy: implications for drug therapy. *Expert Opin Drug Metab Toxicol* 2007;**3**:557–571.

14. Prevost RR, Akl SA, Whybrew WD, Sibai BM. Oral nifedipine pharmacokinetics in pregnancy-induced hypertension. *Pharmacotherapy* 1992;**12**:174–177.

15. Petrenaite V, Sabers A, Hansen-Schwartz J. Individual changes in lamotrigine plasma concentrations during pregnancy. *Epilepsy Res* 2005;**65**:185–188.

16. Landau R, Kraft JC. Pharmacogenetics in obstetric anesthesia. *Curr Opin Anaesthesiol* 2010;**23**:323–329.

17. Sia AT, Sng BL, Lim EC, Law H, Tan EC. The influence of ATP-binding cassette sub-family B member-1 (ABCB1) genetic polymorphisms on acute and chronic pain after intrathecal morphine for caesarean section: a prospective cohort study. *Int J Obstet Anesth* 2010;**19**:254–260.

18. Magness RR, Rosenfeld CR. Systemic and uterine responses to alpha-adrenergic stimulation in pregnant and nonpregnant ewes. *Am J Obstet Gynecol* 1986;**155**:897–904.

19. Ngan Kee WD, Khaw KS, Ng FF. Prevention of hypotension during spinal anesthesia for cesarean delivery: an effective technique using combination phenylephrine infusion and crystalloid cohydration. *Anesthesiology* 2005;**103**:744–750.

20. Naden RP, Rosenfeld CR. Effect of angiotensin II on uterine and systemic vasculature in pregnant sheep. *J Clin Invest* 1981;**68**:468–474.

21. McClure CK, Patrick TE, Katz KD, Kelsey SF, Weiss HB. Birth outcomes following self-inflicted poisoning during pregnancy, California, 2000 to 2004. *J Obstet Gynecol Neonatal Nurs* 2011;**40**:292–301.

22. Gandhi SG, Gilbert WM, McElvy SS, *et al.* Maternal and neonatal outcomes after attempted suicide. *Obstet Gynecol* 2006;**107**:984–990.

23. Wilkes JM, Clark LE, Herrera JL. Acetaminophen overdose in pregnancy. *South Med J* 2005;**98**:1118–1122.

24. Dart RC, Erdman AR, Olson KR, *et al.* Acetaminophen poisoning: an evidence-based consensus guideline for out-of-hospital management. *Clin Toxicol* 2006;**44**:1–18.

25. Spiller HA, Krenzelok EP, Grande GA, Safir EF, Diamond JJ. A prospective evaluation of the effect of activated charcoal before oral *N*-acetylcysteine in acetaminophen overdose. *Ann Emerg Med* 1994;**23**:519–523.

26. Heard K, Dart R. Acetaminophen (paracetamol) poisoning in adults: treatment. *UpToDate*, Nov 2012 (http://www.uptodate.com/contents/acetaminophen-paracetamol-poisoning-in-adults-treatment, accessed 15 January 2013).

27. Tran T, Wax JR, Philput C, Steinfeld JD, Ingardia CJ. Intentional iron overdose in pregnancy: management and outcome. *J Emerg Med* 2000;**18**:225–228.

28. Traub SJ. Salicylate (aspirin) poisoning in adults. *UpToDate*, Jan 2013 (http://www.uptodate.com/contents/salicylate-aspirin-poisoning-in-adults accessed 29 January 2013).

29. Yildiz H, Aldemir E, Altuncu E, Celik M, Kavuncuoglu S. A rare cause of perinatal asphyxia: maternal carbon monoxide poisoning. *Arch Gynecol Obstet* 2010;**281**:251–254.

30. Elkharrat D, Raphael JC, Korach JM, *et al.* Acute carbon monoxide intoxication and hyperbaric oxygen in pregnancy. *Intensive Care Med* 1991;**17**:289–292.

Chapter 15

Shock

Sreedhar Gaddipati and Marcel Vercauteren

Introduction

While shock is commonly assumed to be synonymous with hypotension, shock actually represents the clinical manifestation of tissue dysoxia, resulting from a failure to sustain the oxygen demands of organs at the cellular level. At this level, the hypoxic cell will change its metabolism from aerobic to anaerobic glycolysis, leading to cellular accumulation of lactate, hydrogen ion, and inorganic phosphates. Other consequences of shock at the tissue level include altered membrane potentials by dysregulated ion channels, and cellular edema. Production of ATP is inhibited without a decrease in ATP consumption, which leads to mitochondrial dysfunction and damage, and eventually to apoptosis and release of intracellular contents into the extracellular space. The release of hydrogen ions and lactate leads to lactic acidosis: this has been used as a surrogate for inadequate tissue perfusion. However, dysfunction at the cellular level is a result of dysfunction at the circulatory level, manifested by inadequate or altered regional distribution of blood flow between organs and within organs, leading to a differential in injury either by severity or in number of systems involved. Progression of shock eventually leads to multisystem organ failure and death [1,2].

Clinically, shock may manifest as hypotension, tachycardia, altered mental status, delayed capillary refill, oliguria, and temperature changes in the skin or extremities. While most pregnant patients infrequently enter clinical states that predispose them to shock, the obstetrician must be prepared. Obstetricians most commonly encounter shock in the form of hemorrhage, but it is important to realize that shock can be classified in several types [3], and correction of the physiological derangement can correct the dysoxia at the tissue level before shock becomes irreversible.

> **Case 15.1 A 32-year-old primigravida presented to the hospital in preterm labor**
>
> A 32-year-old woman in her first pregnancy presented to the hospital in preterm labor, with her past medical history notable for quiescent Crohn's disease and a history of bowel obstruction. She received penicillin as is common for women in preterm labor. During labor, non-reassuring fetal heart patterns necessitated urgent delivery via cesarean section under general anesthetic. The procedure itself was uncomplicated except for intra-abdominal adhesions. Blood loss was estimated to be 1200 mL. On postoperative day 2, she complained of nausea and vomiting. She was made nil by mouth, continued on intravenous hydration, and monitored. Later in the afternoon, she was febrile, tachycardic (130 beats/min), and her abdominal distension had worsened. Antibiotics were restarted. Computed tomographic imaging with contrast was attempted but interrupted when she vomited the oral contrast agent. Upon return to the ward, she was hypotensive, shocky, and confused. The team considered hypovolemic, septic, and anaphylactoid etiologies for shock.
>
> She was taken to the operating room, where ileal perforation was found; she was then moved postoperatively to the intensive care unit, intubated and given vasopressors, pain relief, and antibiotics.

Classification of shock

Shock can be classified by etiology or hemodynamics.

> *Hypovolemic shock.* Shock from loss of circulating volume. Peripheral vasoconstriction is a compensatory response.
>
> *Cardiogenic shock.* Shock from cardiac dysfunction with low cardiac output: clinical or hemodynamic parameters show elevated filling pressures.

Maternal Critical Care: A Multidisciplinary Approach, ed. Marc Van de Velde, Helen Scholefield, and Lauren A. Plante. Published by Cambridge University Press. © Cambridge University Press 2013.

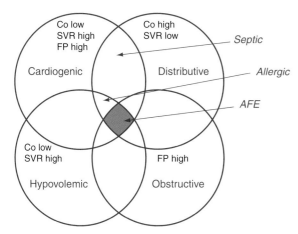

Figure 15.1. Different types of shock. AFE, amniotic fluid embolus; CO, cardiac output; FP, filling pressure; SVR, systemic vascular resistance.

Distributive (including septic) shock. Shock where vasodilatation is a hallmark feature; cardiac output is elevated and systemic vascular resistance is low.

Obstructive shock. Shock where obstruction to cardiac ejection, whether by vasoconstriction, occlusion, or by external compression, is the key feature.

These will be further described in this and other chapters but it is important to remember that there also may be features of several types of shock within one clinical entity (Figure 15.1).

In broad terms, shock is, ideally, recognized and evaluated before any alteration in mental status so that the patient's history and review of symptoms can aid in the differential diagnosis. When this is impossible, other sources must be relied upon, including information from relatives, prior medical records, and other medical personnel. Vital signs and physical examination can help to narrow the possible precipitant of the shock state. Laboratory testing and imaging can be of benefit, although again, depending on the progression of shock, the clinical picture may be mixed. Standard laboratory tests would include a complete blood count with differential, complete electrolyte panel including creatinine and blood urea nitrogen, liver function tests, amylase/lipase, troponin, indices of coagulation, arterial blood gases, toxicology screen, and serum lactate; these should provide a baseline of body functions and possibly provide clues for diagnosis and treatment. Additional testing such as blood cultures and urine culture should be obtained if there is suspicion

for infection. Imaging studies such as radiography, ultrasound, CT, or MRI may be helpful; electrocardiography or echocardiography can also be useful in diagnosis and directing therapy.

Hypovolemic shock

Tissue dysoxia in hypovolemic shock is precipitated by loss of circulating volume. In obstetrics, this is mainly but not exclusively caused by hemorrhage. A classic cause of hypovolemia in pregnancy is diabetic ketoacidosis. While diabetic ketoacidosis can occur in pregnancy at lower glucose levels than in the non-pregnant woman, it is a rare gravida who sustains such an osmotic diuresis that ends in cardiovascular compromise. Other rare causes of hypovolemic shock that may occur in pregnancy are adrenal insufficiency, extensive gastrointestinal losses by diarrhea and/or vomiting, burns over a sufficiently large surface area, and disorders leading to third-space accumulation of fluid, such as intestinal obstruction, severe pancreatitis, crush injuries, and peritonitis.

Hemorrhage can generally be divided into obstetric and non-obstetric causes. Causes of obstetric hemorrhage include placenta previa, placenta accreta, placental abruption, retained placenta, uterine atony, uterine inversion, trauma associated with delivery (lacerations, uterine rupture), and ectopic pregnancy. Non-obstetric causes of hemorrhage include hereditary bleeding diatheses (hemophilia, factor XI deficiency) and trauma. Once hemorrhage occurs, bleeding must be arrested before there is loss of clotting factors leading to disseminated intravascular coagulopathy. Obstetric hemorrhage is also covered in Chapter 39 and coagulopathy in Chapter 11. Classic studies of hemodynamic monitoring in normal pregnancy have allowed us to recognize changes that occur in pregnancy (Table 15.1) [4]. Cardiac output (CO) increases in pregnancy, because both stroke volume and heart rate increase: during pregnancy, prior to labor, CO rises by 50% [4]. Moreover, the proportion of CO directed to the uterus increases from 2% of output in the first trimester to 17% by term, so that blood flow to the uterus at term is approximately 450–650 mL/min. Labor diverts still more of the CO to the uterus (20–25%). During pregnancy, blood volume expands, plasma volume more so than red cell mass, which allows for blood loss at delivery and may serve to improve placental perfusion.

Hemorrhage has been staged into four classes (Table 15.2). Although these classes are based on a 70 kg man, they can still aid in recognition of the condition and in fluid management [5]. As hemorrhage progresses, heart rate is the first change, followed by peripheral vasoconstriction, then by hypotension and clinical signs of hypoperfusion.

The hemodynamic picture of hypovolemic shock is decreased preload and increased peripheral resistance.

Table 15.1. Hemodynamic parameters in non-pregnancy and term pregnancy

	Normal non-pregnant	Term pregnancy, not in labor
Cardiac output (L/min)	4.3 ± 0.9	6.2 ± 1.0
Heart rate (beats/min)	71 ± 10	83 ± 10
Systemic vascular resistance (dyne.s/cm^5)	1530 ± 520	1210 ± 266
Pulmonary vascular resistance (dyne.s/cm^5)	119 ± 47	78 ± 22
Central venous pressure (mmHg)	4 ± 3	4 ± 3
Pulmonary capillary wedge pressure (mmHg)	6 ± 2	8 ± 2
Serum colloid oncotic pressure (mmHg)	20.8 ± 1	18.0 ± 1.5
Left ventricular stroke work index	41 ± 8	48 ± 6

Source: adapted from Clark *et al.*, 1988 [4].

A pulmonary artery catheter would show low filling pressures and low CO; systemic venous resistance, a calculated variable, is high. Peripheral vasoconstriction preserves central perfusion and preload at the expense of peripheral tissues, and mixed venous oxygen saturation will decrease as more oxygen is unloaded to tissues.

Since the uterus has the capability of hemorrhaging 500 mL/min, there is an increased risk for shock to develop. Studies have shown that blood loss at delivery (classically defined averages are 500 mL for vaginal delivery and 1 L for cesarean section) is underestimated by obstetricians, and this failure to recognize and/or to communicate the situation to the rest of the medical team puts these women at risk [6]. Hemorrhage can be so brisk that despite the appropriate pharmacological and surgical techniques deployed in a timely fashion, shock may still result. As the emerging field of simulation in medicine matures, hemorrhage drills and improved team communication between obstetrician, obstetric anesthesiologist, nursing, and blood bank services may reduce the need for subsequent intensive care.

Treatment

As a first step in treating hemorrhage, intravenous fluid resuscitation is employed. Much has been debated on amounts of fluid to give, strategies for resuscitation (fixed versus restrictive versus goal-directed resuscitation), and type of fluid to be used. If using crystalloids, normal saline may be preferred in initial resuscitation, but excessive use of saline has been associated with hyperchloremic metabolic acidosis (normal anion gap metabolic acidosis). Normal saline may also be preferred in situations where fluid resuscitation is initiated

Table 15.2. Staging of hemorrhage

Parameter	Class I	Class II	Class III	Class IV
Blood loss (mL)	750	750–1500	1500–2000	>2000
Percentage circulating volume	15	15–30	30–40	>40
Heart rate (beats/min)	100	>100	>120	>140
Blood pressure	Normal	Decreased	Decreased	Decreased
Pulse pressure	Normal	Decreased	Decreased	Decreased
Capillary refill test (s)	2	>2	>2	>2
Respiration rate (per min)	14–20	20–30	30–40	>40
Urine output (mL/h)	>30	20–30	5–15	Negligible
Mental status	Slightly anxious	Mildly anxious	Anxious, confused	Lethargic
Replacement fluid	Crystalloid	Crystalloid	Crystalloid/blood	Crystalloid/blood

en route to a medical facility, and in the initial resuscitation for patients with diabetic ketoacidosis. Balanced electrolyte solutions (e.g. lactated Ringer's, PlasmaLyte) approximate the electrolyte composition of plasma while still being isotonic and are commonly utilized in the operating room. Excessive use of lactated Ringer's may be associated with metabolic alkalosis. However, excessive use of any of the isotonic crystalloids may alter platelet function, dilute coagulation factors and worsen coagulopathy, and contribute to the development of cardiac dysfunction, pulmonary edema, ileus, and abdominal compartment syndrome.

Hydroxyethyl starches (e.g. Hespan, Hextend) and albumin are also utilized in intravascular volume expansion, with the theoretical benefits resulting from colloidal solutions but having a higher likelihood of remaining intravascular: 20–30% of infused crystalloid volume remains intravascular compared with 70% with an albumin infusion. Despite a slightly longer presence in the intravascular space compared with saline (2–4 hours with albumin compared with <30 minutes with saline), albumin does not confer persistent improvement in intravascular oncotic pressure, and in clinical states of high permeability across capillary membranes (e.g. pre-eclampsia, burns, ongoing development of shock), albumin may then also enter the interstitium. There is neither increased nor decreased risk for pulmonary edema with albumin compared with crystalloid. Hydroxyethyl starches are better retained in the intravascular space than either crystalloid or albumin (100% of the volume remains intravascular over 24–36 hours) but they have been associated with renal toxicity and, in excessive use, may contribute to coagulopathy [3,7,8].

The specific cause of bleeding must be addressed. In postpartum hemorrhage caused by uterine atony, uterotonics (ergot alkaloids, prostaglandin E_1, E_2, $F_{2\alpha}$, and oxytocin) are employed to arrest bleeding. Occlusive and surgical management of hemorrhage includes intrauterine packing or an intracavitary balloon (e.g. Bakri balloon) to compress dilated spiral arteries, and suture techniques to compress and ligate vessels. Topical hemostatic sealants are increasingly employed in the surgical theater, and if the gravida is hemodynamically stable, selective arterial embolization by interventional radiology may arrest bleeding sufficiently to allow for coagulopathy to correct. Ultimately, hysterectomy is used as a life-saving technique. Current practice in massive transfusion is to replace packed red cells, fresh frozen plasma, and platelets in a 1:1:1 ratio.

Blood replacement is indicated for hemorrhagic shock that has either not responded or only responded transiently to initial fluid replacement, which suggests that blood loss is more profound than estimated. A restrictive approach to fluid management in uncontrolled hemorrhage has been studied in the prehospital management of major trauma, with the hypothesis that controlled hypotension that still maintains acceptable organ perfusion would be preferable to the demonstrated disadvantages of aggressive fluid replacement, namely inhibition of coagulation, hypothermia, and dilution of coagulation factors. This approach, while interesting, is unlikely to be applicable to the pregnant patient, where uteroplacental perfusion must be maintained for fetal reasons, but may possibly have a role in severe postpartum hemorrhage [9]. Goal-directed fluid management targets mean arterial blood pressure, systolic blood pressure, heart rate, urine output, or invasive hemodynamic parameters to monitor therapy.

The management of hypovolemic shock caused by hemorrhage [10,11] can be summarized in two stages: initial and secondary treatment.

Initial treatment

1. Assessment of airway management, breathing/respiratory effort, and circulation. If the patient is encountered before arrest, circulation will be the main focus.
2. Creation of an appropriate intravenous access (minimum 18G, preferably 16G, two sites cannulated at minimum).
3. Fluid resuscitation with 2 L crystalloid, wide open, warmed to 37°C. If there is no improvement in hypotension, then this is changed to blood replacement. If hemorrhage is massive (50% circulating volume within 3 hours, or whole blood volume in 24 hours), a massive transfusion protocol is initiated but overtransfusion should be minimized (hemocrit kept to <35%).
4. Provision of supplemental oxygen.

Secondary treatment

1. Provision of left lateral tilt to displace the gravid uterus and improve CO.
2. Consideration of invasive monitoring with central venous or pulmonary artery catheter in patients whose volume status does not respond to resuscitative measures, and whose central volume status is, therefore, unknown. Alternatively, non-

invasive monitoring (echocardiography, tissue hemoglobin oxygen saturation monitor) can be used. Pulmonary artery occlusion pressure or pulmonary capillary wedge pressure, a measure of central pressure, is actually a proxy for left ventricular end-diastolic volume, which can be measured directly with echocardiography.

3. Monitoring of the fetus is instituted *after* maternal condition has been stabilized, assuming delivery has not already occurred.
4. Urine output is monitored to assess end-organ perfusion.

Cardiogenic shock

Cardiogenic shock arises from cardiac dysfunction in the setting of normal intravascular volume, leading to decreased perfusion at the tissue level. Unless perfusion is corrected, ischemia at the cellular level further worsens pump function, leading to a decrease in stroke volume and in perfusion to the coronary arteries. Elevated left-sided filling pressures lead to pulmonary congestion and pulmonary edema, further contributing to hypoxia. This represents a downward spiral that leads to end-organ damage and death [12].

The causes of cardiogenic shock are multiple:

- infarction
- ventricular septal wall rupture
- rupture of papillary muscle or chordae tendinae (acute mitral regurgitation)
- rupture of free wall of left ventricle
- valvular dysfunction or obstruction
- outflow tract obstruction (e.g. idiopathic hypertrophic subaortic stenosis, left atrial myxoma)
- arrrhythmia
- pericardial effusion or tamponade
- myocarditis
- post-cardiopulmonary bypass
- cardiomyopathies
- left ventricular apical ballooning.

The most common cause is acute coronary syndromes, specifically acute myocardial infarction (MI). Most acute MIs are left ventricular infarction, but infarction at any location can lead to cardiogenic shock. Anterior wall infarction of > 40% of the left ventricle reliably causes cardiogenic shock, but smaller areas of infarction can lead to shock in a compromised heart (e.g. previously infarcted area, cardiomyopathy, right ventricular

infarct, or inferior infarct). Mechanical complications from acute MI can also lead to shock, such as ventricular septal wall rupture, ruptured papillary muscle or chordae tendinae leading to acute mitral regurgitation, and rupture of the free wall of the left ventricle.

In the setting of low CO, the patient will exhibit weakness and fatigue. If pulmonary congestion is part of the presentation, cough, dyspnea, orthopnea, and paroxysmal noctural dyspnea may also be present. Of note, pulmonary congestion may not be apparent on physical examination, nor is it usually associated with acute MI of the right ventricle or other causes of right ventricular pump failure. In the presence of right-sided pump failure, signs of systemic congestion may be noted, such as distended neck veins and edema; nonspecific symptoms of nausea and abdominal pain may also be present. Cardiac findings on examination may include S3 gallop. With compressive causes of cardiogenic shock (i.e. pericardial tamponade), clinical findings include muffled heart sounds, but in most cases of cardiogenic shock, chest radiography, and, crucially, rapid access to echocardiography will establish the cause and help to dictate the treatment.

While pulmonary artery catheterization is not required for a diagnosis of cardiogenic shock, it can aid in monitoring therapeutic interventions. Hemodynamic parameters characteristic of cardiogenic shock are severe depression of the cardiac index (<2.2 L/min per m^2) and sustained systolic arterial hypotension (<90 mmHg) despite an elevated filling pressure (>18 mmHg.) Systemic vascular resistance – a variable calculated from CO and mean arterial pressure – is elevated.

Treatment

Therapy for cardiogenic shock requires restoration of adequate coronary perfusion in order to minimize further myocardial depression and necrosis (Box 15.1). If acute MI is suspected, standard protocols for its treatment should be employed, such as aspirin, heparin, morphine, nitrates, and assessment for fibrinolytic therapy [13]. In the setting of cardiogenic shock, beta-blockade and angiotensin-converting enzyme (ACE) inhibitors should be avoided; ACE inhibitors would be contraindicated in pregnancy in any event. Intravenous fluid may be judiciously given to provide adequate preload and improve hypotension if present. In the setting of pulmonary edema, however, vasopressors rather than additional volume will be employed. Norepinephrine is a potent vasoconstrictive agent but also has mild inotropic effects and is an appropriate

Box 15.1. Approach to cardiogenic shock

Initial treatment
1. Assessment of airway management, breathing/respiratory effort, and circulation. Provide oxygenation and intravenous access
2. Assess cardiac status, presence of pulmonary edema, blood pressure. Obtain chest radiograph, electrocardiography, maternal echocardiography. Mechanical causes or compressive causes may warrant urgent surgical intervention
3. If acute myocardial infarction is suspected, initiate protocols for therapy
4. If low cardiac output noted in setting of hypotension, initiate vasopressor therapy. In the absence of pulmonary edema, may judiciously provide intravenous fluids. If no hypotension, initiate pure inotrope (e.g. dobutamine)
5. Once therapy has been initiated, assess the fetus, provide left lateral tilt to displace the gravid uterus to improve cardiac output

Secondary treatment
1. Consider invasive monitoring with pulmonary artery catheterization in patients with cardiogenic shock, particularly where there is poor response to vasopressor therapy. Pulmonary artery catheterization or echocardiography can be used to assess effectiveness of treatment
2. Move to cardiac catheterization if appropriate, consider intra-aortic balloon pump to minimize progression of ischemia

first choice. Dopamine has chronotropic and inotropic effects, but at higher infusion rates will stimulate α-adrenoceptors and produce vasoconstriction. Although either medication is appropriate, studies have noted a higher arrhythmogenic potential with dopamine, and there may be increased mortality with dopamine in cardiogenic shock. Dobutamine is not used in hypotension because of its potential to cause vasodilation. Milrinone, a phosphodiesterase inhibitor, also has inotropic effects, and while it may have a lower arrhythmogenic potential, it too can potentiate hypotension. Lastly, levosimendan has properties similar to dobutamine with inotropic and vasodilatory effects without chronotropic effects [14].

If shock is refractory to medical management, placement of an intra-aortic balloon pump may be crucial in stabilizing the patient, thus decreasing the likelihood of progression of ischemia and shock. Its use is primarily a bridge to definitive therapy (stenting or bypass surgery), but there are case reports of its use in pregnancy to prolong pregnancy. An intra-aortic balloon pump is not appropriate for aortic regurgitation or aortic dissection. Whether a left ventricular assist device is also meant to be a bridge to therapy versus a destination (i.e. the device as a definitive therapy) is beyond the scope of this chapter.

In pregnancy, acute MI is a still a rare event, occurring in 2.8 to 6.2 per 100 000 pregnancies. Risk factors in pregnancy include age >35 years, hypertension, diabetes, and obesity. Although pregnancy has not traditionally been thought to increase the risk, recent data suggest that pregnancy may increase the risk for acute MI by three- to four-fold. In a series from 1985, two thirds of the acute MIs in pregnancy occurred in the third trimester, and mortality was higher in the third trimester compared with the earlier two (45% versus 23%) [14]. More recent studies have suggested a 5–7% fatality rate. Since mortality is known to be higher if delivery occurs within the first 2–3 weeks after the MI, delivery should be avoided if possible during this time, but tocolytics would be ill-advised. If needed, fibrinolytic therapy can be used, with the caveat that there is a risk for bleeding. Postpartum use of fibrinolytic therapy is riskier than antepartum use because of the potential for hemorrhage, although if utilized 8 hours after delivery, the risk may be lower than otherwise feared.

Distributive shock

While distributive shock is not as familiar to obstetricians as hemorrhage, distributive shock is indeed possible in parturients. This type of shock is marked by normal or increased CO but pathologically dilated peripheral circulation. Anaphylactic shock falls into this category. Sepsis also is generally a distributive shock, although a mixed picture may also be seen. As septic shock is addressed in Chapter 31, it will not be covered here.

Distributive shock may occur after induction of general anesthesia and would be characterized by a moderate decrease in arterial blood pressure; but this is not common among parturients. Arterial blood pressure and CO may also fall after neuraxial techniques as a physiological consequence of sympathetic blockade, and this may be pronounced among obstetric patients. Third, distributive shock may occur through anaphylactic or hypersensitivity reactions to substances to which the parturient is exposed during the surgical and anesthetic procedure. This section will focus exclusively on allergic reactions and their diagnosis and management.

Allergic reactions

An anaphylactic reaction is an immediate type hypersensitivity reaction to a substance or drug, causing acute life-threatening symptoms in two or more organ systems. Immunoglobulin E (IgE) antibodies are involved in more than 70% [15]. The reaction is independent of the pharmacological actions and the dose of the substance or drug. The term *anaphylaxis* is used when IgE antibodies are involved. An *anaphylactoid* reaction is clinically indistinguishable from an anaphylactic reaction but is not mediated by IgE. Therefore, the distinction can only be made after investigation [16–18]. In the clinical situation, the term "suspected anaphylactic reaction" should be used. However, since in the literature there is confusion about the terminology, some have suggested abandoning the term anaphylactoid all together: anesthesiologists treat the syndrome regardless of the definition.

During anesthesia, many different drugs are used in rapid succession: not only anesthetics but also antibiotics, colloids, local anesthetics, non-steroidal anti-inflammatory drugs, and so on. In addition, the patient is exposed to materials such as latex and skin preparation solutions. Since most drugs given during anesthesia are given intravenously and in bolus, they bypass the body's primary immune filters and present high concentrations of antigen directly to the mast cells and basophils. So it is difficult to say which drug caused the suspected reaction, or whether a reaction was the result from the additive side effects of several drugs injected simultaneously.

Pathophysiology

In a "classical" anaphylactic reaction, previous contact with the drug is necessary. Nevertheless, reactions are possible after first contact with a substance, which is attributed to cross-sensivity with related substances present in some medications, cosmetics, bacteria, or ambient air. On first exposure to an antigen, B-lymphocytes produce IgE antibodies, which bind to high-affinity receptors on the surface of mast cells and the basophils. On second exposure, the antigen causes bridging of two adjacent IgE antibodies, resulting in degranulation of the mast cells and the basophils [16,18,19].

Mediators can be divided into three groups, depending on the time they are liberated after stimulation of the mast cell and the basophil. There is an immediate release of preformed mediators such as histamine, tryptase, heparin, and eosinophil and neutrophil chemotactic factors. Within minutes, newly synthesized inflammatory mediators from the cell membrane are liberated: leukotrienes via the lipoxygenase pathway, prostaglandins via the cyclooxygenase pathway, and platelet activating factor. Finally, for several hours, cytokines are produced and liberated [16,18–20].

The effects of these mediators are decreased myocardial contractility, increased heart rate, coronary and pulmonary vasoconstriction, peripheral vasodilatation, increased hepatic venous resistance with pooling of blood in the splanchnic system, increased permeability (with up to 40% loss of intravascular fluid), smooth muscle contraction in the bronchi and the gastrointestinal tract, increased mucus production, stimulation of sensory nerve endings, and attraction of other inflammatory cells. In addition, these mediators and inflammatory cells activate the coagulation, the complement, and the kinin–kallikrein pathways [16,18–20].

In an anaphylactoid reaction, IgE antibodies are not involved. Previous contact with the drug is not required. The mechanism of mast cell and basophil degranulation is either non-immunological histamine release or immunological (immunoglobulins G or M) or non-immunological complement activation with the production of anaphylatoxins [16,18,19]. Anaphylatoxins increase vascular permeability, contract smooth muscle and attract, aggregate, and activate leukocytes and platelets [19]. This may cause pulmonary leukostasis and even worsen pulmonary hypertension.

Non-immunological or direct histamine release will primarily affect the mast cells; the most important mediator is histamine, which is liberated in a dose-dependent fashion [19]. The clinical effects are usually mild [21]. Most drugs release histamine from the mast cell of the skin, which is harmless. However, some other drugs, such as atracurium and propofol, also release histamine from the lung mast cell. Only atracurium releases histamine from the mast cell of the heart.

Differential diagnosis

Based upon simulation sessions, it appears that anesthesiologists require at least 10 minutes before making a correct diagnosis of an anaphylactic reaction [22]. In clinical circumstances, this may become even more difficult, particularly when a patient with known allergy is pretreated with drugs such as antihistamines or steroids. During anesthesia, several other possibilities may mimic an allergic reaction. Some substances do not cause an instant reaction after administration, such as latex, antibiotics, and local anesthetics. In obstetric anesthesia, the most important situations causing hypotension, which may be confused with anaphylaxis, are local anesthetic-induced sympathetic blockade, local anesthetic toxicity, vasovagal reaction, high or total spinal block, neuraxial opioid-induced side effects, and pulmonary embolism.

Obstetric patients may sustain different types of embolic complication. Rates of venous thromboembolism, including pulmonary embolus, are increased (see Chapter 25.)

Air embolism is caused by the entrance of air via the placental uterine bed, facilitated by the exteriorization of the uterus during cesarean section. Fortunately, the amount of air entering the pulmonary circulation is usually limited and unnoticed, though the possibility must be kept in mind.

The most devastating event complicating the differential diagnosis of anaphylaxis is amniotic fluid embolism (see Chapter 40). The diagnosis of this life-threatening complication is most commonly made by exclusion or, sometimes, alas, at autopsy. As serum tryptase levels have been found to be increased [23,24], the difficulty in distinguishing amniotic fluid embolism from anaphylaxis is not surprising. In fact, a proposed synonym for this entity is "anaphylactoid syndrome of pregnancy."

General epidemiology

The incidence of an anaphylactic reaction during anesthesia is estimated to be between 1:3500 and 1:20 000 [15,16]. Adult females are more likely to be affected [15]. There is a geographical variation in incidence, being lower in the USA and South Africa and higher in France and New Zealand [16]. However, it is difficult to calculate the exact incidence because of inaccuracies in recognizing and reporting anaphylactic reactions and differences in the definition and investigation of an anaphylactic reaction. Death from a suspected anaphylactic reaction is between 3 and 5% [15–18].

An allergy network in France (Groupe d'Etudes des Réactions Anaphylactoïdes Peranesthésiques) [15,17] recently reported a nationwide survey over 8 years and following more than 2000 referrals: 72% of the reactions were IgE mediated; females were involved three times more than males; and 58% was caused by neuromuscular-blocking drugs, followed by latex and antibiotics.

Obstetric epidemiology

Although anaphylactic reactions have been reported for all types of substance used during anesthesia, the obstetric literature contains only a limited number of such reactions during childbirth.

Obstetric patients may be relatively protected because of the tendency to employ regional rather than general anesthetic techniques and the avoidance of polypharmacy where possible in anesthesia.

The most common substances to which a patient admitted for labor or surgical delivery is exposed are induction agents, muscle relaxants, analgesic substances, latex, antibiotics, oxytocic drugs, and histamine receptor antagonists.

Although the overall incidence of anaphylactic reactions during anesthesia is highest following the use of neuromuscular-blocking agents [15–18], reporting of such reactions in the obstetric literature is rather sparse. Most probably, the low incidence in obstetric anesthesia is attributable to the low number of general anesthesia procedures undertaken nowadays. Succinylcholine is still considered the mainstay for rapid sequence induction, and the few reports on anaphylaxis to neuromuscular-blocking agents during cesarean section are exclusively related to succinylcholine. Mechanisms may be either a true anaphylaxis or direct histamine release from mast cells.

Amongst the neuromuscular-blocking agents, there is a strong female predominance of anaphylactic reactions, with a female to male ratio ranging from 2:1 to 8:1. The antigenic determinant is probably the quaternary ammonium ion, which is abundantly present in drugs, cosmetics, and household products, thus facilitating an anaphylactic reaction on first exposure to the neuromuscular-blocking agent. There is controversy about the increased use of rocuronium in some countries (France and Norway) compared with other neuromuscular-blocking agents [15]. As rocuronium can be antagonized now very quickly with sugammadex, it may replace succinylcholine for rapid sequence intubation during cesarean section, thus undoubtedly resulting in the appearance sooner or later of anaphylactic reactions.

The most commonly reported allergic reactions during delivery are related to antibiotics and latex.

Latex causes IgE-mediated reactions. Symptoms occur 30–60 minutes after the start of the exposure. As there may be no relationship with any drug administration, the diagnosis of an allergic reaction is seldom made promptly, causing a significant delay in the start of accurate treatment. Patients with atopy, asthma, spina bifida, spinal cord injury, allergy to tropical fruits, multiple prior surgical procedures, or who are themselves healthcare workers, are at risk for an anaphylactic reaction to latex [16–18]. The incidence of latex allergy has been declining as latex-free rooms and equipment are becoming more accessible. Nevertheless, latex allergy is actually the most frequently reported reaction in obstetric anesthesia. Patients at risk should be first to have their operation in the morning. Recent literature has suggested that parturients may be more at risk for latex allergy than females operated for non-obstetric reasons [21]. Any allergic reaction occurring at a long interval after any drug administration should raise suspicion that latex is responsible.

Antibiotics may induce several types and clinical manifestations of allergy; common culprits are ampicillin, penicillin, ceftriaxone, and cefazolin. A recent review found an incidence of 2.9 per 100 000 deliveries [25].

Colloids have been found to be superior to crystalloids in preventing hypotension during cesarean section under neuraxial, mainly spinal, techniques Dextrans, gelatins, and starches may be administered. Dextrans have fallen out of favor because of the potential to cause anaphylaxis and coagulopathy. Gelatins have also largely been abandoned because of an allergic potency as high as 1 in 300 [26]. Starches may be considered a safer alternative as allergy seems to occur in fewer than 1 in 2500 patients, but allergic reactions are still possible [26]. There seem to be no major differences with respect to the risk of an allergic reaction among starches of a comparable molecular weight, or starches made from corn versus potato.

Reactions to local anesthetics are also generally rare. The risk is higher for esters (e.g. chloroprocaine, tetracaine) than for amide substances (e.g. bupivacaine, ropivacaine). Of 205 patients referred to an allergy clinic for a suspected anaphylactic reaction to local anesthetics, only four had a true anaphylactic reaction and four had delayed allergic reactions [22]. Most of the alleged allergic reactions were noticed in dentistry practice and caused by toxicity and/or epinephrine, vasovagal reactions, or reactions to the preservatives (e.g. methylparaben or bisulfites). In obstetric anesthesia, only three cases have been reported with proven allergy for

bupivacaine. In patients at high risk for such a reaction, infiltration with diphenhydramine 0.5–1% has been proposed for repair of episiotomy as this substance appears to have weak anesthetic properties [11].

When a parturient claims to be allergic to a certain local anesthetic, a provocative challenge with an alternative agent should be performed. For ropivacaine and levobupivacaine, no adverse reactions consistent with hypersensivity has been reported in obstetric anesthesia over more than a decade of use.

Allergic reactions have been reported to uterotonic drugs, which are universally used on maternity units [25]. Since these substances are mostly in the hands of the obstetrician, the anesthesiologist may not be present at the moment the reaction occurs. Oxytocin may also cause bronchospasm directly *without* immunological involvement, making an immediate correct diagnosis difficult.

Surprisingly, anaphylactoid reactions have been found to occur with ranitidine, a histamine H_2 receptor antagonist used for aspiration prophylaxis prior to cesarean section This is of particular concern because histamine H_2 receptor antagonists are often recommended as as a secondary treatment option when anaphylaxis occurs.

Anaphylactic reactions to opioids are extremely rare. Non-immunological histamine release, however, is rather frequent, particularly with codeine, morphine, and meperidine, rarely used now during labor or cesarean section. The mast cells of the skin, more than in other organs, are extremely sensitive to opioids and will precipitate reactions, which are generally harmless. Although allergy to the fentanyl analogues is ignorable, one obstetric case has been described of an allergic reaction to neuraxial administration of fentanyl.

Finally, other solitary cases of anaphylaxis have been reported in obstetric patients, attributed to diclofenac, iron, ethylene oxide (used for equipment sterilization), propofol, and metabisulfite (within a local anesthetic–epinephrine combination). No allergic reactions have been reported to thiopental, etomidate, or ketamine, the most widely used induction agents for general anesthesia for cesarean section.

Symptoms and diagnosis

In more than 90% of cases, symptoms start within minutes after exposure to the inciting agent; latex, antibiotics, and local anesthetics, however, may be exceptions in that symptoms may be delayed even for

Table 15.3. Clinical manifestations of a suspected anaphylactic or anaphylactoid reaction

Organ system	Symptom	Sign	Specific sign during anesthesia
Cutaneous	Itching	Goose-flesh Rash, erythema, flushing Urticaria Periorbital and perioral edema	
Respiratory	Lump in the throat Hoarseness Dysphonia Dyspnea	Stridor (laryngeal edema) Wheezing (bronchospasm) Pulmonary edema Cyanosis	Difficult to ventilate ↑ Peak airway pressure ↓ Oxygen saturation ↑ End-tidal carbon dioxide
Cardiovascular	Angina Light-headedness Faintness	Tachycardia Hypotension–cardiac arrest Dysrhythmias	↓ End-tidal carbon dioxide ↑ Hematocrit
Gastrointestinal	Nausea Abdominal pain	Vomiting Diarrhoea	

hours. Anaphylactic (IgE-mediated) and anaphylactoid (non-IgE-mediated) reactions are clinically indistinguishable, although the symptoms and signs of anaphylactic reactions tend to be more severe [3]. The involved target organs are the skin and the respiratory, cardiovascular, and gastrointestinal systems (Table 15.3). The full range of clinical manifestations does not occur in every patient [16,18,19].

The incidence of cardiac arrest is about 10%. Cutaneous symptoms may be recognized in 70% of the patients. In the 30% in which cutaneous symptoms are absent, they may have been missed, particularly if patients were anesthetized or under drapes; the incidence of cutaneous symptoms is higher outside the anesthesia setting. Bronchospasm is the most prominent feature in 20%, and is almost inevitable in patients with pre-existing asthma. For obvious reasons, gastrointestinal features are uncommon during anesthesia. The most common initial features during anesthesia are absence of pulse, oxygen desaturation, difficulty in ventilating the lungs, and flushing.

Factors that increase the severity of the reaction are a history of asthma, use of beta-adrenergic blocking drugs, and neuraxial anesthesia. All of these states are associated with a reduced efficiency of the endogenous catecholamine response.

Treatment

The goals of management of anaphylaxis are interrupting contact with the responsible drug, modulating the effects of the released mediators, and preventing further mediator production and release [16–19].

Box 15.2 summarizes the management of a suspected anaphylactic reaction.

The initial therapy consists of discontinuing the administration of the suspected trigger to prevent further activation of mast cells and basophils and stopping or minimizing administration of agents that may further aggravate hemodynamic instability. Endotracheal intubation should be performed immediately if the airway appears to be at risk (e.g. stridor, edema of the face or upper airway). To compensate for intravascular fluid loss, intravenous crystalloids are administered. Although colloids may be given, they may cause or worsen anaphylaxis, and because of increased membrane permeability they may leak out of the intravascular compartment. Leg elevation will increase the circulating volume by more than 0.5 L.

The cornerstone of successful therapy is epinephrine [16,18,23]. Epinephrine counteracts some of the effects of mediator release: stimulation of α_1-adrenoceptors directly constricts capacitance and resistance blood vessels; stimulation of β_1-adrenoceptors increases myocardial contractility; and stimulation of β_2-adrenoceptors dilates the bronchioles, decreases hepatic venous resistance (and as a consequence increases venous return) and increases cyclic AMP in the mast cells basophils, thereby decreasing mediator release. Because of its β-adrenoceptor effects, epinephrine is more useful than the pure alpha-adrenergic agonists (e.g. norepinephrine). The dose of intravenous epinephrine depends on the severity of symptoms. If the patient is hypotensive, boluses of 5 to 10 µg are given every 1 to 2 minutes. In the case of cardiovascular collapse, boluses up to 100 µg are administered every minute together

---

Box 15.2. Management of a suspected anaphylactic reaction

Initial therapy
1. Stop administration of the agent, call for help; interrupt ongoing procedures such as surgery
2. Give 100% oxygen and assess and secure the airway
3. Initiate volume expansion; elevate legs
4. Give epinephrine (norepinephrine) 5–100 µg intravenous; use closed chest cardiac compressions if pulseless

Secondary therapies
The following may be considered:

1. Histamine H_1 receptor antagonists, e.g. promethazine 50 mg intramuscular
2. Histamine H_2 receptor antagonists, e.g. ranitidine 50 mg intravenous
3. For persistent hypotension, norepinephrine infusion with starting dose 2–4 µg/min
4. For refractory bronchoconstriction, nebulization of bronchodilators (salbutamol or albuterol)
5. Corticosteroids: hydrocortisone 5 mg/kg intravenous

---

with closed chest cardiac compressions. A higher dose is needed during anesthesia than in the non-anesthesia setting, because both general and regional anesthesia impair the sympathetic response. Patients taking beta-blockers are more resistant to the effects of epinephrine and show unopposed α-adrenoceptor effects. Glucagon, 1–5 mg intravenously, increases intracellular cyclic AMP independent of the β-adrenoceptors and may be helpful in patients taking beta-blockers. Patients taking antidepressants (tricyclic antidepressants, monoamine oxidase inhibitors) or cocaine are more sensitive to the effects of epinephrine. Mortality in anaphylaxis increases if epinephrine is delayed or given inappropriately, and in patients with asthma or cardiovascular disease.

Histamine H_1 receptor antagonists (e.g. promethazine) compete with histamine at the receptor sites. The use of histamine H_2 receptor antagonists is controversial because they may induce or aggravate bronchoconstriction through unblocked histamine H_1 receptor activity. Corticosteroids are of limited usefulness in acute anaphylaxis because they require 12–24 hours to work.

Treatment considerations in the parturient

In order to increase venous return, parturients with severe hypotension should be turned into the left lateral position unless emergency delivery of the fetus is warranted or cardiac massage is mandatory.

Severe hypotension in a pregnant woman, as in life-threatening anaphylaxis, raises the question of whether to use vasopressors. In situations with a bad neonatal outcome following an anaphylactic reaction in the mother, it is not possible to determine whether neonatal morbidity or death was the consequence of the cardiovascular collapse, the hypoxia resulting from bronchial constriction, drugs used in the treatment of this event, or a combination of all these elements. The placenta and umbilical cord have no compensatory mechanisms when perfusion is endangered. The blood flow to the placenta is mainly dependent on the maternal systolic blood pressure and CO as placental blood vessels are almost maximally dilated in normal pregnancy. As a consequence, maternal hypotension will be directly translated into less uteroplacental perfusion. However, when treating hypotension, care should be taken to ensure that raising the maternal blood pressure is not achieved at the expense of significant constriction of the uterine arteries, which supply the circulation reaching the fetus. Ephedrine, still the most commonly used vasopressor in obstetric anesthesia, is a direct acting adrenergic agonist and an indirect sympathomimetic. Despite its general vasoconstrictive effects, the uterine vessels may be selectively spared unless high doses are given. However, for the treatment of anaphylactic shock, even high doses may fail to correct hypotension. Small doses of 10–20 µg epinephrine, as recommended for treating moderate anaphylactic reactions, result in a 30–40% reduction of uterine blood flow, at least in normotensive subjects. In hypotension, the restoration of blood pressure may be the paramount effect. An uneventful fetal outcome has been reported after a low-dose infusion of epinephrine for 4 hours [24]. If bronchoconstriction is the sole symptom, direct intratracheal administration may be considered so as to reduce the systemic effects of epinephrine upon uteroplacental perfusion.

Similarly, phenylephrine, a selective alpha-adrenergic agonist, has constrictive effects upon the fetal blood supply, but doses up to 100 µg may not compromise neonatal outcome because the increase of maternal blood pressure may outweigh the increased resistance of the uterine vasculature. Although in resistant cases the use of norepinephrine has been suggested, in parturients this option may be of concern because of both heightened uterine vasoconstriction and increased uterine tone. Less experience exists with amnirone and milrinone, which both have inotropic and vasodilatory effects. These may only be useful in patients with decreased CO caused by heart failure.

Investigation of a suspected anaphylactic reaction

The goals of the investigation [16,17] are to:

- determine the nature of the reaction
- identify the responsible drug and
  - determine if there is cross-reactivity between the culprit drug and other substances
  - select substances that are probably safe for future procedures.

Investigations start with a detailed clinical history, including the previous medical, drug, and anesthetic history; previous allergies; the drugs used before and during the suspected anaphylactic reaction; the severity of the symptoms; and the timing of the suspected trigger in relation to the symptoms. Further investigation may consist of immediate and delayed tests. The purpose of immediate testing is to try to determine whether the reaction is immune mediated, while the delayed tests seek to identify the responsible agent.

Immediate or intraoperative testing

Immediate testing, such as levels of histamine or mast cell tryptase, is geared toward ascertaining whether the reaction is immune mediated. Unfortunately, the half-life of the mediators is short, and resuscitation rather than testing is the priority. Resuscitation is the same whether the reaction is IgE mediated or not.

Delayed or postoperative testing

Delayed testing is typically done by skin tests 4–6 weeks after the suspected anaphylactic reaction, and is beyond the scope of this chapter. Radioallergosorbent testing is available for specific IgE antibodies in serum and is done in vitro. Finally, because of the risk of life-threatening reactions, challenge tests are not used except for local anesthetics.

Summary

Anaphylactic and anaphylactoid reactions are clinically indistinguishable. The most incriminated agents

in obstetric anesthesia are antibiotics, succinylcholine, and latex. Treatment consists of instant interruption of contact with suspected trigger, 100% oxygen, airway support including intubation, volume expansion, and vasopressors where necessary. Further investigation is mandatory to find the responsible drug and to make future healthcare interactions safer.

Obstructive shock

A fourth type of shock is obstructive shock, in which there is mechanical or pressure obstruction to emptying of the ventricles. This may be embolic, as in pulmonary embolus (Chapter 25) or amniotic fluid embolus (Chapter 40) or constrictive, as in pericardial tamponade.

Although this is very rare, pericardial effusion, possibly resulting in life-threatening tamponade, may be caused by infection (bacterial or viral), trauma (including myocardial perforation following central vein catheterization), MI, hypothyroidism, intracardiac space-occupying lesions, carcinomatous neoplastic effusion, autoimmune disease, end-stage renal disease, or may be idiopathic. It is not an "all-or-none" phenomenon as symptoms may be very variable. Most important symptoms consist of dyspnea/ orthopnea, chest pain, tachycardia, and hypotension/ shock. Diagnosis is suggested by jugular vein distention, pulsus paradoxus, pericardial friction rub, and right ventricular failure (particularly with pericardial constriction in case of chronic inflammation). The effusate may be serous, suppurative, hemorrhagic, or serosanguineous. Treatment consists of pericardiocentesis, preferentially under echocardiographic guidance [27].

Mixed shock types

There are several clinical entities where, because of progression of the clinical state, more than one type of shock is manifested. Septic shock may have a distributive component (through activation of the systemic inflammatory response system), a hypovolemic component (i.e. hemorrhage in coagulopathy), a cardiogenic component (myocardial dysfunction in the systemic inflammatory response syndrome and with toxins associated with septicemia), and an obstructive component in septic embolism (see Chapter 31). Although amniotic fluid embolism has been classically considered to cause shock by obstructing the pulmonary vascular system, pathophysiology in humans suggests vasospasm in the pulmonary vasculature and, therefore, right as well as left ventricular failure. Amniotic fluid embolism has also been called "anaphylactoid syndrome of pregnancy" and has features of both cardiogenic and distributive shock, plus – because coagulopathy also occurs in this syndrome – hypovolemic shock may be superimposed (see Chapter 40).

Fetal/maternal considerations

While many articles that address the need for intensive care for the gravida, few provide a detailed accounting of shock in pregnancy. Although the likelihood of the gravida entering a shock state is, fortunately, low, it is important for all members of the care team to realize that first and foremost, the woman is the primary focus of care and their important patient. This fact is sometimes lost even for the obstetrician, and while the fetus is also of clinical importance, its needs should never supersede those of the mother, and it should only become the primary patient once it clear that resuscitative measures are futile.

To this extent, therapies and treatment that have been reviewed in this chapter should not be withheld from a gravid patient; the state of pregnancy should never penalize a woman nor relegate her to second class status.

References

1. Antonelli M, Levy M, Andrews PJ, et al. Hemodynamic monitoring in shock and implications for management. [International Consensus Conference, Paris, France, 27–28 April 2006.] Intensive Care Med 2007;33:575–590.

2. Germain S; Wyncoll D; Nelson-Piercy, C. Management of the critically ill obstetric patient. Curr Obstet Gynaecol 2006;16:125–133.

3. Moranville MP, Mieure KD, Santayana EM. Evaluation and management of shock states: hypovolemic, distributive, and cardiogenic shock. J Pharm Pract. 2011;24:44–60.

4. Clark SL, Cotton DB, Lee W, et al. Central hemodynamic assessment of normal term pregnancy. Am J Obstet Gynecol 1989;161:1439–1442.

5. American College of Surgeons Committee on Trauma. Advanced Trauma Life Support for Doctors: Student Course Manual, 8th edn. Chicago, IL: America College of Surgeons, 2008.

6. Dildy GA III, Paine AR, George NC, Velasco C. Estimating blood loss: can teaching significantly improve visual estimation? Obstet Gynecol 2004;104:601–606.

7. Cotton BA, Guy JS, Morris JA, Abumrad NN. The cellular, metabolic, and systemic consequences of aggressive fluid resuscitation strategies. Shock 2006;26:115–121.

8. Devlin JW, Barletta JF. Albumin for fluid resuscitation: implications of the saline versus albumin fluid evaluation. Am J Health Syst Pharm 2005;62:637–642.

9. Nolan J. Fluid replacement. Br Med Bull 1999;55:821–843.

10. Shields LE, Smalarz K, Reffigee L, et al. Comprehensive maternal hemorrhage protocols improve patient safety and reduce utilization of blood products. Am J Obstet Gynecol 2011;205:368.e1–8.

11. Fujitani S, Baldisseri MR. Hemodynamic assessment in a pregnant and peripartum patient. Crit Care Med 2005;33:S354–S361.

12. Patel AK, Hollenberg SM. Cardiovascular failure and cardiogenic shock. Semin Respir Crit Care Med 2011;32:598–606.

13. Anderson JL, Adams CD, Antman EM, et al. ACC/AHA 2007 guidelines for the management of patients with unstable angina/non-ST-Elevation myocardial infarction: a report of the American College of Cardiology/American Heart Association Task Force on Practice Guidelines (Writing Committee to Revise the 2002 Guidelines for the Management of Patients With Unstable Angina/Non-ST-Elevation Myocardial Infarction) developed in collaboration with the American College of Emergency Physicians, the Society for Cardiovascular Angiography and Interventions, and the Society of Thoracic Surgeons endorsed by the American Association of Cardiovascular and Pulmonary Rehabilitation and the Society for Academic Emergency Medicine. J Am Coll Cardiol 2007;50:e1–e157.

14. Hankins GD, Wendel GD, Leveno KJ, Stoneham J. Myocardial infarction during pregnancy: a review. Obstet Gynecol 1985;65:139–146.

15. Mertes PM, Laxenaire MC, GERAP. Anaphylactic and anaphylactoid reactions occurring during anaesthesia in France. Seventh epidemiologic survey (January 2001-December 2002). Ann Fr Anesth Reanim 2004;23:1133–1143.

16. Hepner DL, Castells MC. Anaphylaxis during the perioperative period. Anesth Analg 2003;97:1381–1395.

17. Mertes PM, Alla F, Tréchot P, for the Groupe d' etudes des reactions anaphylactoides perianesthésiques. Anaphylaxis during anesthesia in France: an 8-year national survey. J Allergy Clin Immunol 2011;128:366–373.

18. Levy J. The allergic response. In Barash P, Cullen B, Stoelting R (eds.) *Clinical Anesthesia*, 5th edn. Philadelphia, PA: Lippincott Williams & Wilkins, 2006, pp. 1298–1312.

19. Jacobsen J, Lindekaer A, Ostergaard H, *et al.* Management of anaphylactic shock evaluated using a full-scale anaesthesia simulator. *Acta Anaesthesiol Scand* 2001;**45**, 315–331.

20. Farrar SC, Gherman RB. Serum tryptase analysis in a woman with amniotic fluid embolism. A case report. *J Reprod Med* 2001;**46**:926–928.

21. Draisci GD, Zanfini BA, Nucera E, *et al.* Latex sensitization. A special risk for the obstetric population? *Anesthesiology* 2011;**114**:565–569.

22. Fisher MM, Bowey CJ. Alleged allergy to local anaesthetics. *Anesth Intensive Care* 1997;**25**:611–614.

23. Gei AF, Pacheco LD, Vanhook JW, Hankins GD V. The use of continuous infusion of epinephrine for anaphylactic shock during labor. *Obstet Gynecol* 2003;**102**:1332–1335.

24. Harper NJN, Dixon T, Dugue P, *et al.* Suspected anaphylactic reactions associated with anaesthesia. *Anaesthesia* 2009;**64**:199–211.

25. Mulla ZD, Ebrahim MS, Gonzales JL. Anaphylaxis in the obstetric patient: analysis of a statewide hospital discharge database. *Ann Allergy Asthma Immunol* 2010;**104**:55–59.

26. Laxenaire MC, Charpentier C, Feldman L. Anaphylactoid reactions to colloid plasma substitutes: incidence, risk factors, mechanisms. A French multicenter prospective study. *Ann Fr Anesth Reanim* 1994;**13**:301–310.

27. Ristic AD, Seferovic PM, Ljubic A, *et al.* Pericardial disease in pregnancy. *Herz* 2003;**28**:209–215.

Chapter 16

Brain death and somatic support

Sarah Armstrong and Roshan Fernando

Brain death in pregnancy

"Brain death" describes the irreversible loss of brain-stem function in a patient receiving artificial organ support that delays the onset of cardiac arrest and somatic death [1]. It is a concept legally recognized in most countries. Brain death is ultimately followed by somatic death, often within days, and it is generally considered futile and, therefore, unethical to continue to support vital organ function once a diagnosis of brain death has been made [2]. In the case of a pregnant woman, the mother and fetus may be considered as two distinct organisms and consideration should be given to the appropriateness of continuing maternal somatic support to prolong gestation to attain fetal viability [3]. The incidence of brainstem death in pregnant women is, fortunately, very low and there are only around 30 case reports of extended life support after brain death in pregnancy in the literature. Suddaby *et al.* [4] found that of 252 brain-dead patients, only 5 (2.8%) involved pregnant women between 15 and 45 years of age.

Fetal viability and the extent of maternal somatic support

The likelihood of a successful outcome for the fetus depends primarily on the duration of time required for the fetus to attain viability. It is clear that the nearer the pregnancy to term, the more likely the chance of fetal survival. A gestational age of 32 weeks is commonly considered to be a reasonable time for delivery in this context in order to achieve a good chance of survival with a low risk of handicap [5]. The upper physiological limit to the prolongation of somatic function in the absence of brainstem function is not known. In a UK study, median time to cardiac arrest following

brainstem death in non-pregnant patients was 3.5–4.5 days [6] and in their series of 1200 brain-dead non-pregnant patients, Jennett and Hessett were unable to find a single case of somatic survival beyond 14 days [7]. The longest reported duration of successful maternal somatic support following brain death to date is 107 days [8]. In this case, maternal somatic function remained relatively stable up until delivery of the infant at approximately 32 weeks, when organ support was discontinued. At present, there is no clear lower limit to the gestational age from which the pregnancy should be supported. It has been suggested that attempts to prolong maternal somatic function are futile in all cases where the pregnancy is less than 16 weeks of gestation at the time of maternal brain death, as this approaches the maximum duration of sustained maternal somatic function to date. This has not been extended in 15 years of case reports, despite dramatic advances in organ support therapies in the interim [3]. There are three reported cases in the literature where maternal organ donation was carried out after successful delivery of the fetus and the role of the mother as a potential organ donor should also be borne in mind [9–11]. In the review by Suddaby *et al.* of 252 brainstem-dead potential donors [4], five of seven pregnant women functioned as organ donors for 20 transplant recipients.

The mechanism of maternal death may be a key factor in the determination of fetal outcome. The fetal central nervous system may be affected by any hypoxic or metabolic insults that resulted in maternal brainstem death. Maternal pathophysiological processes may be present in the fetus or may compromise placental function (such as maternal thrombocytosis) as may any drug therapy given to the mother between the onset of the fatal illness and maternal brainstem death [12]. These factors must

Maternal Critical Care: A Multidisciplinary Approach, ed. Marc Van de Velde, Helen Scholefield, and Lauren A. Plante.
Published by Cambridge University Press. © Cambridge University Press 2013.

all be taken into consideration when deciding on the likely success of maintaining maternal somatic function after brainstem death.

Medical management of brain death in pregnancy

Prolongation of maternal somatic function constitutes experimental care where the physician must consult case reports [2,8,13,14] and reviews [15] and extrapolate from experiences in sustaining organ function after brain death to facilitate organ donation [16]. During extended life support, patients are likely to follow a relatively predictable course of complications, including sepsis, hemodynamic instability, panhypopituitarism, loss of temperature regulation, metabolic instability, and eventual cardiac arrest.

Specific attention should be paid to mechanical ventilation in pregnant patients. Carbon dioxide elimination in the fetus is facilitated in pregnancy by a progesterone-induced increase in tidal volume and respiratory rate, while an increase in renal bicarbonate excretion compensates for hypocarbia [17]. Ventilation should maintain arterial partial pressure of carbon dioxide and oxygen within the normal pregnancy physiological ranges.

Cardiovascular instability most commonly presents as hypotension, which should be treated by optimizing intravascular fluid status and colloid oncotic pressure within physiological ranges [18]. Vasopressors such as dopamine or dobutamine may be required, and adrenocortical failure should be considered in hypotension unresponsive to these measures. Invasive and minimally invasive hemodynamic monitoring such as the lithium-dilution cardiac output method or the pulse-contour continuous cardiac output method may be considered to guide treatment. Labetalol, methyldopa, beta-blockers, prazosin, calcium channel blockers, and/or hydralazine may be used for treatment of hypertension in pregnancy. Angiotensin-converting enzyme inhibitors and angiotensin receptor blockers should be avoided as they can cause fetal renal tubular dysgenesis, oligohydramnios, and fetal death [19].

Pituitary failure may mandate hormonal replacement with thyroxine and corticosteroids. Diabetes insipidus may occur, which should be treated with aggressive fluid replacement and vasopressin in non-pregnant patients. In pregnancy, vasopressin should be used with caution because it may have a detrimental effect on uterine blood flow and in one case report initiated premature uterine contractions [20,21]. Adrenal insufficiency requires treatment with systemic steroids, and prednisolone or methylprednisolone have been recommended because they do not cross the placenta readily, thus minimizing fetal exposure [22]. Glucose intolerance is common and may require insulin therapy.

Maternal thermodynamic instability may be particularly problematic to manage, manifesting as hypothermia or hyperthermia. Active and passive measures may be required to maintain temperature homeostasis. Pregnant women are hypercoagulable and this is exacerbated following brainstem death by flaccid paralysis and immobility. They are at a high risk of venous thrombosis, and prophylaxis using fractionated or unfractionated heparin should be considered. Warfarin should be avoided because of its potential teratogenic effects on the fetal skeletal and central nervous systems [3].

Maternal seizures may occur before brainstem death and anticonvulsants are commonly required for their control. Issues of possible teratogenesis with anticonvulsant drugs are irrelevant once organogenesis is complete, that is, after the first trimester. As with all drugs used in pregnancy it is necessary to establish both the benefits and risks of the treatment as well as the potential risk of the untreated condition on the fetus.

Nutritional support should be initiated early and preferably via the enteral route. Special attention should be paid to the management of gastroesophageal reflux in the context of pregnancy and of the reduced motility of the gastrointestinal tract in brain-dead patients. The basal energy expenditure and nutritional requirements of a brainstem-dead pregnant woman are thought to be around 75% of a healthy pregnant woman's requirements, and expenditure and nutritional supplementation should be tailored to this [23].

Three main sources of sepsis may complicate prolonged somatic support, including ventilator-associated pneumonia, urinary tract infections from indwelling catheters, and infection of intravascular catheters. These may be by organisms resistant to a wide variety of antibacterial agents. It has been suggested that these infections should be treated with the most effective agent available, regardless of any potential effect on the fetus [24–26]. Strict asepsis, including isolation of the maternal body, has been recommended to reduce the risk of infection [3].

Fetal and neonatal considerations

The gestational age and the condition of the fetus are the most important factors affecting perinatal outcome [16]. Most case reports have described daily fetal monitoring using cardiotocography or non-stress testing. It has also been suggested that serial ultrasound examinations should be performed to evaluate the fetoplacental unit, amniotic fluid, and fetal growth [27–29].

Conclusions

Brainstem death in the pregnant patient is a tragic but fortunately rare event that involves complex medical, ethical, and legal issues. The goal of extended maternal somatic support is to attempt to facilitate fetal maturation in order to deliver a healthy, viable infant. The likelihood of a successful outcome determines whether extended maternal somatic support after brain death should be attempted. It has been suggested that a dialogue involving the immediate family, the wishes of the mother (whether expressed or implied), and advice from appropriate legal external and multidisciplinary medical experts is central to resolving this issue. From a medical point of view, the management of the brainstem-dead mother should follow standard guidelines and recommendations for organ preservation alongside an awareness of the physiological and pharmacological implications of pregnancy.

References

1. Pallis CHD (ed.). *From Brain Death to Brainstem Death*, 2nd edn. London: BMJ Press, 1996.

2. Field DR, Gates EA, Creasy RK, Jonsen AR, Laros RK Jr. Maternal brain death during pregnancy. Medical and ethical issues. *JAMA* 1988;**260**:816–822.

3. Farragher RA, Laffey JG. Maternal brain death and somatic support. *Neurocrit Care* 2005;**3**:99–106.

4. Suddaby EC, Schaeffer MJ, Brigham LE, Shaver TR. Analysis of organ donors in the peripartum period. *J Transpl Coord* 1998;**8**:35–39.

5. Slattery MM, Morrison JJ. Preterm delivery. *Lancet* 2002;**360**:1489–1497.

6. Jennett B, Gleave J, Wilson P. Brain death in three neurosurgical units. *BMJ* 1981;**282**:533–539.

7. Jennett B, Hessett C. Brain death in Britain as reflected in renal donors. *BMJ* 1981;**283**:359–362.

8. Bernstein IM, Watson M, Simmons GM, *et al*. Maternal brain death and prolonged fetal survival. *Obstet Gynecol* 1989;**74**:434–437.

9. Beguin F. [Introduction: maternal cerebral brain death.] *Arch Gynecol Obstet* 1993;**253**(Suppl):S1–S3.

10. Nettina M, Santos E, Ascioti KJ, Barber MA. Sheila's death created many rings of life. *Nursing* 1993;**23**:44–48.

11. Lane A, Westbrook A, Grady D, *et al*. Maternal brain death: medical, ethical and legal issues. *Intensive Care Med* 2004;**30**:1484–1486.

12. Farragher R, Marsh B, Laffey JG. Maternal brain death: an Irish perspective. *Ir J Med Sci* 2005;**174**:55–59.

13. Feldman DM, Borgida AF, Rodis JF, Campbell WA. Irreversible maternal brain injury during pregnancy: a case report and review of the literature. *Obstet Gynecol Surv* 2000;**55**:708–714.

14. Finnerty JJ, Chisholm CA, Chapple H, Login IS, Pinkerton JV. Cerebral arteriovenous malformation in pregnancy: presentation and neurologic, obstetric, and ethical significance. *Am J Obstet Gynecol* 1999;**181**:296–303.

15. Powner DJ, Bernstein IM. Extended somatic support for pregnant women after brain death. *Crit Care Med* 2003;**31**:1241–1249.

16. Esmaeilzadeh M, Dictus C, Kayvanpour E, *et al*. One life ends, another begins: management of a brain-dead pregnant mother. A systematic review. *BMC Med* 2010;**8**:74.

17. Bhatia P, Bhatia K. Pregnancy and the lungs. *Postgrad Med J* 2000;**76**:683–689.

18. Dictus C, Vienenkoetter B, Esmaeilzadeh M, Unterberg A, Ahmadi R. Critical care management of potential organ donors: our current standard. *Clin Transplant* 2009;**23**(Suppl 21): 2–9.

19. Koren G, Pastuszak A, Ito S. Drugs in pregnancy. *N Engl J Med* 1998;**338**, 1128–1137.

20. Hauksson A, Akerlund M, Melin P. Uterine blood flow and myometrial activity at menstruation, and the action of vasopressin and a synthetic antagonist. *Br J Obstet Gynaecol* 1988;**95**:898–904.

21. Dillon WP, Lee RV, Tronolone MJ, Buckwald S, Foote RJ. Life support and maternal death during pregnancy. *JAMA* 1982;**248**:1089–1091.

22. van Runnard Heimel PJ, Franx A, *et al*. Corticosteroids, pregnancy, and HELLP syndrome: a review. *Obstet Gynecol Surv* 2005;**60**:57–70; quiz 73–54.

23. Rivera-Alsina ME, Saldana LR, Stringer CA. Fetal growth sustained by parenteral nutrition in pregnancy. *Obstet Gynecol* 1984;**64**:138–141.

24. Christensen B. Which antibiotics are appropriate for treating bacteriuria in pregnancy? *J Antimicrob*

Chemother 2000;**46**(Suppl 1):29–34; discussion 63–25.

25. Korzeniowski OM. Antibacterial agents in pregnancy. *Infect Dis Clin North Am* 1995;**9**:639–651.

26. Einarson A, Shuhaiber S, Koren G. Effects of antibacterials on the unborn child: what is known and how should this influence prescribing. *Paediatr Drugs* 2001;**3**:803–816.

27. Webb GW, Huddleston JF. Management of the pregnant woman who sustains severe brain damage. *Clin Perinatol* 1996;**23**:453–464.

28. Lawson EE. Antenatal corticosteroids-too much of a good thing?, *JAMA* 2001;**286**:1628–1630.

29. Lewis DD, Vidovich RR. Organ recovery following childbirth by a brain-dead mother: a case report. *J Transpl Coord* 1997;**7**:103–105.

Chapter

17

Airway management

Felicity Plaat and Alison MacArthur

Introduction

Maternal mortality is regarded as a major indicator of the quality of healthcare of a nation, and inadequate airway management remains a significant cause of anesthetic-related mortality in the obstetric population. Failure to intubate the trachea of a pregnant woman is associated not only with maternal morbidity and mortality but also, potentially, with fetal demise or compromise. The aftermath may profoundly affect family members (particularly those who may have witnessed the event) and medical and nursing staff.

Airway issues in the pregnant woman

The problems in the pregnant woman are universal: physiological changes during pregnancy lead to a reduction in time from onset of apnea to oxygen desaturation and to an increased likelihood of regurgitation from a full stomach. There is also increased difficulty with visualization at intubation. The specific challenges in obstetric airway management in North America reflect the increasing comorbidities of the obstetric population associated with advancing age and obesity, and the way care is delivered within the North American system. The increased concerns for medicolegal risk and, potentially, a service setting where not all anesthesia providers are physicians and other salient factors.

Although the higher incidence of failed tracheal intubation compared with the non-pregnant state is well documented, it has been recently disputed [1]. Nevertheless, recent prospectively collected cohort studies from Australia and New Zealand confirm the increased risk of morbidity associated with the obstetric airway compared with women who are not pregnant [2]. Most cases are unanticipated, occur in emergency situations, and frequently outside "office"

hours. The incidence of failed intubation is in the region of eight times that in the non-obstetric population [3]. The use of cuffed endotracheal tubes followed publication of work by Mendelson in the1950s on aspiration pneumonia [4].

The unfortunate and paradoxical consequence of this change of practice in the UK was an *increase* in anesthetic-related maternal mortality from failed intubation and failure to oxygenate (Figure 17.1). Between 1970 and 1972, there were 32 direct anesthesia deaths in the UK, although by 2000–2002 this number had fallen to six. In the earlier period, most of the deaths were related to general anesthesia, whereas in the latter, *all* were associated with general anesthesia and three were from unrecognized esophageal intubation. Although guidelines for the management of failed intubation were introduced [5], there is still lack of consensus over the specific drill to be used in obstetrics and a variety are currently in use [6]. Established algorithms used in the wider setting fail to address the obstetric airway [7].

Subsequent developments in airway management have been driven by the safety imperative. In the UK, the challenges have included changes in medical training and practice that have led to a decrease in the airway management experience of British-trained anesthesiologists. Use of general anesthesia has decreased from 83% of cesarean sections in the 1990s to 23% in 2011. Exposure of trainees to obstetric general anesthesia has reduced by a third in some units [8]. With the reduction in use of general anesthesia in the USA, there has been a corresponding reduction in maternal mortality by a factor of 17 between 1985 and 1990 [9].

Why is the pregnant airway more difficult? Comparison of the airway at 12 and 38 weeks of gestation revealed a 14% increase in the incidence

Maternal Critical Care: A Multidisciplinary Approach, ed. Marc Van de Velde, Helen Scholefield, and Lauren A. Plante.
Published by Cambridge University Press. © Cambridge University Press 2013.

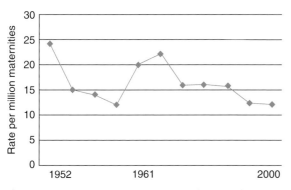

Figure 17.1. Maternal anesthetic-related death rates in the UK.

of patients with grade IV Mallampati scores [10]. Labor and delivery have also been shown to be associated with worsening Mallampati scores, although the effects of the observed changes on ease of intubation have not been determined [11]. It has been suggested that pharyngeal edema might account for some of these changes. Progesterone-induced edema of the airways, tongue, cords, face, and neck may be exacerbated by pregnancy-induced hypertension, oxytocin infusion, and a Trendelenberg position during labor. Valsalva maneuvers associated with pushing in the second stage of labor may cause laryngeal edema.

During pregnancy, body weight increases by 10 to 20 kg. North American anesthesiology providers must face what has become an "endemic" problem of obesity amongst women in their reproductive years. Most North American studies estimate that >20% of the pregnant population has a body mass index (BMI) of >30 kg/m² prior to pregnancy [12], and 5% may have a BMI of >40 [13]. The accompanying comorbidities include obstructive sleep apnea, type 2 diabetes mellitus, pregnancy-induced hypertension, and the increased likelihood of an operative delivery. In North America, it has become common for most maternity centers delivering women with a BMI >40 to refer them for an antenatal anesthesia consultation. The prevalence of obesity (BMI ≥30) in the general population in the UK has increased markedly since the early 1990s. In 2004, 24% women over 16 were obese and a national cohort study gave an estimated prevalence of morbid obesity (BMI >50) of 87 per 100 000 maternities [14]. A report on maternal mortality in the UK made the specific recommendation that "morbidly obese women should not be anesthetised by trainees without direct supervision" and "management by consultant anesthesiologists is essential and difficulties

with airway management and intubation should be anticipated" [15]. In a recent UK nationwide audit of major complications of airway management, 75% of obstetric patients were obese and half had significant medical conditions [16].

Management

An antenatal visit allows the airway to be evaluated and discussion to be held with the parturient about the use of invasive monitors such as invasive arterial blood pressure monitoring and the use of continuous positive airway pressure devices during and after labor and delivery. Women with BMI >50 require particular antenatal planning as laboring beds and operating tables must be able to operate at their weight and have sufficient width to contain them. Preparation for these patients and identification of their arrival at time of delivery helps to minimize circumstances of preventable airway mishaps.

Obese parturients may well benefit from early regional anesthesia, including placement of an epidural catheter in the intrathecal space should inadvertent dural puncture occur [17]. The establishment of functioning regional anesthesia has long been controversial in the face of potential airway difficulties; however, the likelihood of converting to a general anesthetic is less with a good functioning epidural or intrathecal catheter. Ultrasound identification of midline spinous processes when bony landmarks are not palpable may improve success, and testing mechanisms, such as the Tsui test, can help to confirm the location of catheters [18]. Contraindications to regional anesthesia techniques, such as established maternal hemorrhage, can be minimized by adequate preparation and early communication with obstetric colleagues [19].

A recent development in the management of the airway in the obese patient is the use of the so-called "ramped" position. The trunk, neck, and head are aligned so that the sternal notch and external auditory meatus are at the same level (Figure 17.2). A towel roll or folded blanket under shoulders and head compensates for the exaggerated flexion caused by postcervical fat. Specifically designed wedges are also available. Laryngoscopy and intubation are facilitated, and the head-up position provides some protection against aspiration, should regurgitation occur. Respiratory mechanics are also improved (better diaphragmatic excursion on inspiration), delaying the onset of hypoxia [20].

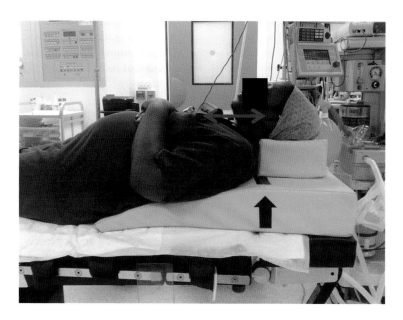

Figure 17.2. Ramped position for airway optimization.

In addition of the problems created by obesity, other prevalent conditions that increase the likelihood of operative delivery, and thus a potential for sudden general anesthesia induction, are increasing maternal age; chronic maternal diseases such as pre-existing hypertension, acquired or congenital cardiac diseases; or lack of adequate antenatal care in indigent populations such as poor communities of urban cities or native Indian populations in the rural areas of Canada and the USA [19,21].

With evidence that these comorbidities are increasing amongst pregnant women and that the overall cesarean delivery rate increased to 32.3% in 2008 in the USA [22] and 26.3% in 2006 in Canada, the absolute number of general obstetric anesthetics administered in North America may actually be increasing. However, one center in Canada has reported the reverse trend [23].

Although all units have guidelines, a recent survey in the UK found that in 50% of failed intubation in obstetrics, there was failure to follow these guidelines [24]. Nevertheless, the need for guidelines is indisputable as the potential for administering an emergency general anesthetic to a parturient will always exist and the anesthesiologist will need to provide safe and rapid general anesthesia for all parturients who require it [25]. No one algorithm has proven to be superior to another.

Figure 17.3 illustrates the algorithm taught to anesthesia residents at Mount Sinai Hospital during their obstetric anesthesia rotation in the event of a difficult obstetric airway following induction of general anesthesia prior to delivery. Important points in the algorithm to comment on include the second intubation attempt and the attempts to establishing a supraglottic airway. During the second intubation attempt, manoeuvers to improve visualization should be incorporated quickly as oxygen desaturation below 90% mandates manual ventilation. Such manoeuvers include use of videoscope devices, improving position of patient's head's sniffing position, and use of different laryngoscope blades or bougie. Once two attempts have been made without success, it is critical to quickly focus on adequate oxygenation and ventilation of the parturient. The choice of laryngeal mask airway is between the classic or the ProSeal laryngeal mask airway, the latter offering an advantage if a patient has a full stomach but can be more difficult for an inexperienced user to place. Again the priority is establishment of adequate gas exchange, and both are suitable. Lastly, in consideration of carrying on with a cesarean delivery with a supraglottic airway, the parturient is usually allowed to breathe spontaneously as long as gas exchange is adequate. This may be difficult with an obese parturient or one with significant cardiopulmonary compromise. Muscle relaxation is generally not advocated after the initial induction dose of succinylcholine and must only be considered when weighing the risk of airway device dislodging compared with improving ventilation with paralysis.

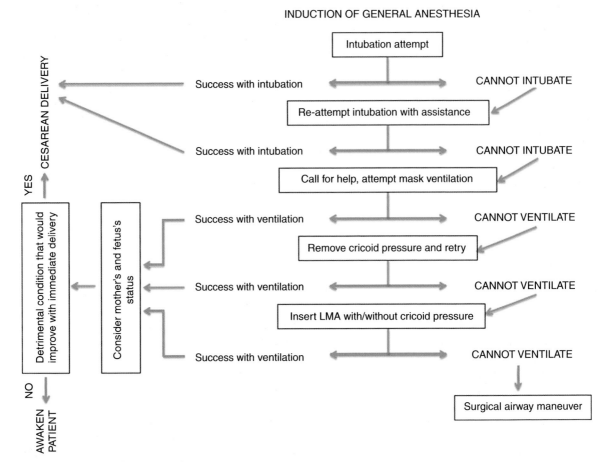

INDUCTION OF GENERAL ANESTHESIA

Figure 17.3. Protocol for a failed intubation.

From a 20-year study of a homogeneous population in eastern Canada delivering at a university teaching hospital, investigators reported a remarkably low incidence of failed intubations amongst their delivery population and a declining number of general anesthetics for cesarean delivery. The key to their success was summarized in the leading editorial by one of Canada's distinguished obstetric anesthesiologists, Dr. Joanne Douglas [26]. She succinctly identified the factors important in the unexpectedly low incidence of difficult and failed intubations and diminishing number of general anesthetics: "24-hour in-house service by obstetric anaesthesiologists, the opportunity for airway assessment either antepartum or early in labour, and appropriate planning, including avoidance of GA in patient with a predicted difficult airway". Both the total number and the proportion of general anesthetics in the Canadian study were noted to decline over the 20 years. The incidence of general anesthetics in later years

of this study (1999–2003; 2.6%) compares with the 1 year rate during 2005–2006 of the Australian study (2.2%). Another explanation for the Canadian study's falling incidence of general anesthesia and accuracy of intubation visualization was the retrospective study design. Misclassification is more likely with a retrospective study than with a prospective study, as was the Australian, resulting in underestimation of the population incidence. Only 17% of women's anesthetic charts contained information on airway evaluations, and the women were primarily a Caucasian population, with potentially less difficult intubations compared with the mixed ethnicity population examined in Australia.

Perhaps the main factor responsible for a higher incidence of difficulties in airway management is that general anesthesia is generally reserved for extreme obstetric emergencies: certainly the overwhelming majority of reported deaths is associated with emergency cesarean sections. All the obstetric cases reported to the national UK audit of airway management complications were out of hours. In 50%, general anesthesia had not been planned but was attempted perioperatively, with obvious implications for the ease of intubation. In the emergency situation, conditions for airway management may be worsened by lack of attention to positioning, poorly applied cricoid pressure, and pressure of time leading to inadequate oxygenation.

In a recent audit, the main cause of death was aspiration of gastric contents, and this was a non-fatal complication in one of the obstetric patients [16]. Although gastric acidity prophylaxis (with histamine H_2 receptor blockers, proton pump inhibitors, prokinetic drugs, and/or non-particulate antacids) is reported to be routine by 98% of UK units prior to emergency cesarean section, a decreasing number of units routinely give it to high-risk women in labor [27]. The short duration of action of non-particulate antacids such as sodium citrate needs to be borne in mind. In the UK, only a very small minority of units advised a nil by mouth policy for women in labor, and in some a light diet is actively encouraged [28]. The use of a large-bore orogastric tube to empty the stomach before extubation has been recommended. Extubation should be delayed until the patient is able to protect her own airway.

A survey from the south of England covering a period of 5 years also found that the majority of cases were emergencies and all had been in the hands of non-consultant grade anesthesiologists [24]. This highlights the problem of remote supervision of trainees, particularly as a significant proportion of UK maternity units are separate from general inpatient facilities. This separation of facilities also highlights the need for properly trained assistance for the anesthesiologist. Management of patients recovering from general anesthesia is also an area for concern: although in the UK, midwives in recovery units manage the majority of obstetric patients, such management is not a core competency of the midwifery training program. Furthermore, the majority of midwives do not undertake nursing training prior to midwifery. The decline in the use of general anesthesia means that even those who have received appropriate training may find it challenging to maintain those skills.

However, only a third of obstetric units in the UK undertake difficult intubation training. Although simulation is well established in general medical education, it has only recently begun to be utilized in obstetric anesthesia. In two obstetric patients with major airway complications, the reporters commented on the lack of awareness and/or help from the non-anesthetic staff present. Skills and drills courses devoted to obstetric emergencies that include advanced airway skills and management are now available across the UK. By providing the opportunity for multidisciplinary training they may go some way to solving such problems.

In North America, a corresponding challenge is the presence of non-physician providers in some obstetric anesthesia settings. In a health services review of anesthesia-provider models, representing over one million women delivering across six states, certified registered nurse anesthesiologists were present in approximately 60% of labor and delivery units. They commonly provided services along with physician–anesthesia providers [29]. Only 23% of the labor and delivery units had services provided only by certified registered nurse anesthesiologists. The study was unable to demonstrate any increased risk of maternal complications on discharge summaries related to anesthesia by provider type based upon codes in the *International Statistical Classification of Diseases and Related Health Problems* (ICD) [30]. A specific review of malpractice claims against nurse anesthesiologists between 1990 and 1996 indicated that 19/41 (46%) were for general anesthesia (compared with 17% in similar time period for anesthesiologists) [31]. The severity of injury in the 19 claims involving general anesthesia were higher than regional techniques and included difficult or failed intubation (7/19) and esophageal intubation (1/19). The incidence of airway difficulties for certified registered nurse anesthesiologists was higher than that reported for anesthesiologists (16/73) [32]. Changes in practice may not be as quickly adopted amongst nurse anesthesiologists but further study will need to confirm whether an increased risk for obstetric airway emergencies exists amongst certified registered nurse anesthesiologists.

The use of supraglottic airways in the management of the obstetric airway is undergoing evaluation. The role in establishing an airway lost during a "can't intubate, can't ventilate" situation is established, but the type of device used is not. As oxygenation/ventilation as rapidly as possible is needed in this situation, some argue that the device with which the anesthesiologist has most experience should be used. In the UK, this is the classic laryngeal mask airway. However since aspiration is a specific concern in the obstetric population, there are a growing number who recommend that a second-generation device should be used that would provide protection against aspiration and aid insertion of a definitive airway. The use of such a device, the ProSeal laryngeal mask airway has been described in 3000 cesarean sections. Cricoid pressure was applied during insertion of the airway and obstetricians were warned to apply gentle fundal pressure to limit intra-abdominal pressure. All the patients, however, were receiving elective surgery. The authors of the national survey recommend that obstetric anesthesiologists should become familiar with the use of such devices. Which device should be used, particularly where waking the patient up is not an option [16]? The ProSeal has been found to be easy to insert, providing a better seal and more effective ventilation than a standard laryngeal mask airway, with the potential for gastric drainage and protection against aspiration. It has been used during emergency cesarean section, with release of cricoid pressure after insertion and ventilatory pressures between 26 and 35 cmH_2O with no evidence of air leak. A gastric tube was easily passed on the first attempt [33]. Awake flexible fiberoscopic intubation is another recommended skill, although far from universal amongst UK anesthesiologists [34]. A recent UK survey found that although all obstetric units had a "difficult airway trolley," the equipment available varied [35].

A high failure rate with emergency cannula cricothyroidotomy was a feature of both obstetric and non-obstetric cases in the national audit. This was attributed to lack of familiarity with the equipment, lack of training, and lack of practice. Some of the skills and drills courses described above do teach such advanced airway management techniques, which could go some way to addressing this problem. In the UK, the McCoy laryngoscope (Figure 17.4) has overtaken the polio blade in popularity. The role of videolaryngoscopy is yet to be defined, although an increasing number of units are adding such equipment to their difficult intubation trolleys (F. Plaat, personal communication). In one survey of failed and difficult intubation in obstetrics, the most commonly used additional piece of equipment initially used was a gum elastic bougie [36].

There is lack of consensus over the optimum method of preoxygenation, particularly in an emergency. When eight vital capacity breaths were compared with a standard 3 minute preoxygenation, no differences in maternal oxygenation or fetal

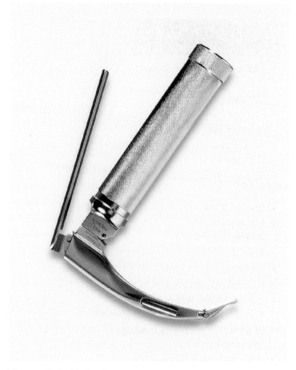

Figure 17.4. McCoy laryngoscope.

outcome were detected. Eight vital capacity breaths taken over 1 minute were associated with better outcomes than four vital capacity breaths over 30 seconds [37].

Rapid sequence induction, with cricoid pressure and intubation, remain the initial management plan of choice for all obstetric cases in the UK. The view of the larynx achieved with one-handed cricoid pressure is significantly better than when two-handed cricoid pressure is applied and the latter is no longer recommended [38].

Succinylcholine is still the relaxant of choice, although high-dose rocuronium, with reversal by sugammadex, has been described for cesarean section [39].

As to the specific difficult airway equipment suggested for obstetric units, most academic units in the USA and Canada have a separate cart in or near the delivery operating room [40,41].

Suggested equipment to maintain in the difficult airway cart is compiled from University of Toronto, Mount Sinai Hospital labor and delivery unit and delivery units in Nashville, Tennessee and the Mayo Clinic (Box 17.1). An excellent review of the equipment is provided by Mhyre and Healy for aids to improve laryngoscopy and supraglottic devices [25].

Box 17.1. Suggested contents of obstetric difficult airway equipment cart

- Fiberoptic bronchoscope that fits 6.0 ETT and light source
- Glidescope
- Laryngeal masks: classic in sizes 2, 3, 4; Pro-Seal in 3, 4; intubating laryngeal airway mask in 3, 4
- Jet ventilation apparatus as kit or components
- Cricothyroidotomy apparatus
- Retrograde intubation apparatus
- Airways: oral and nasal in various sizes
- Endotracheal cuffed tubes, sizes 5.0–7.0
- Laryngoscope blades: No. 4 MacIntosh, Nos. 3 and 4 Miller blades
- Short handle for laryngoscope
- Antisialogogues, defogging agents
- Guedel airways for oral fiberoptic intubation
- Lidocaine 2% spray/jelly/ointment, lidocaine 4% liquid, atomizer, tongue depressors
- Light wand, gum elastic bougie, endotracheal tube exchangers
- Infusion pump for sedation

The important feature is that all colleagues providing anesthesia coverage in labor and delivery must have available the equipment options they would choose to improve the intubating conditions of a second attempt: different laryngoscope blade or videolaryngoscope or surgical airway devices (cricothyroidotomy equipment or kit). In addition, the maintenance of this cart requires specific personnel and scheduling, as is done with the cardiac arrest equipment.

Medical legal concerns are greater in North America than most other developed countries, with an average of $600 000 paid on behalf of anesthesiologists for claims of outcomes such as maternal death and brain damage [32]. Reviews of the insurance claims resulting in litigation have provided insight into changing obstetric anesthesia practice patterns. Amongst recent reviews of North American claims involving obstetric anesthetic services, the proportion of general anesthetic-related claims has fallen as have the number of claims resulting from esophageal intubations or inadequate oxygenation/ventilation [32].

This is a direct result of the publications in the early 1990s reporting that general anesthesia was associated with greater maternal mortality and morbidity.

Practice patterns have changed and regional anesthesia has predominated in most larger delivery units in North America. It is reassuring that occurrences of maternal hypoxic injury appear to be more infrequent than in the past, regardless of whether this has been propelled by the litigious medicolegal climate or improved practice methods.

References

1. Goldszmidt E. Is there a difference between the obstetric and non-obstetric airway? In Halpern SH, Douglas MJ (eds.) *Evidence Based Obstetric Anesthesia*. Oxford: Blackwell, 2007, pp. 225–236.

2. McDonnell NJ, Paech MJ, Clavisi OM, for the ANZCA Trials Group. Difficult and failed intubation in obstetric anaesthesia: an observational study of airway management and complications associated with general anaesthesia for caesarean section. *Int J Obstet Anesth* 2008;**17**:292–297.

3. Barnardo PD, Jenkins JG. Failed tracheal intubation in obstetrics: a 6-year review in a UK region. *Anaesthesia* 2000;**55**:685–694.

4. Mendelson CL. The aspiration of stomach contents into the lungs during obstetric anesthesia. *Am J Obstet Gynecol* 1946;**52**:191–205.

5. Tunstall ME. Failed intubation drill. *Anaesthesia* 1976;**31**:850.

6. Obstetric Anaesthetists' Association. *Failed Intubation Guidelines* (website). London: Obstetric Anaesthetists' Association (http://www.oaa-anaes.ac.uk/content.asp?ContentID=357, accessed 29 January 2013).

7. Henderson JJ, Popat MT, Latto IP, Pearce AC. Difficult Airway Society guidelines for the management of the unanticipated difficult intubation. *Anaesthesia* 2004;**59**:675–694.

8. Hawthorne L, Wilson R, Lyons G, Dresner M. Failed intubation revisited. *Br J Anaes* 1996;**76**:680–684.

9. Hawkins JL, Koonin LM, Palmer SK, Gibbs CP. Anesthesia-related deaths during obstetric delivery in the United States, 1979–1990. *Anesthesiology* 1997;**86**:277–284.

10. Pilkington S, Carli F, Dakin MJ, *et al.* Increase in Mallampati score during pregnancy. *Br J Anaesth* 1995;**74**:638–642.

11. Bhavani-Shankar K, Bulich LS, Kafiluddi R, *et al.* Does labor and delivery induce airway changes? *Anesthesiology* 2000;**93**:A1072.

12. Shin YK, Dietz PM, England L, Morrow B, Callaghan WM. Trends in pre-pregnancy obesity in nine states, 1993–2003. *Obesity* 2007;**15**:986–993.

13. Ogden CL, Carroll MD, Curtin LR, *et al.* Prevalence of overweight and obesity in the United States, 1999–2004. *JAMA* 2006;**295**:1549–1555.

14. Knight M, Kurinczuk JJ, Spark P, Brocklehurst P. Extreme obesity in pregnancyin the United Kingdom. *ObstetGynecol* 2010;**115**:989–997.

15. Lewis G (ed.) *Saving Mothers' Lives: Reviewing Maternal Deaths to Make Motherhood Safer, 2003–2005. The Seventh Report on Confidential Enquiries into Maternal Deaths in the United Kingdom.* London: CEMACH, 2007.

16. Quinn A, Bogod D. Obstetrics. In Cook T, Woodall N, Frerk C (eds.) *Major Complications of Airway Management in the UK:4th National Audit Project.* London: Royal College of Anaesthetists and Difficult Airway Society, 2011, pp. 181–187.

17. Brodsky JB, Mariano ER. Regional anaesthesia in the obese patient: lost landmarks and evolving ultrasound guidance. *Best Pract Res Clin Anaesthesiol* 2011;**25**:61–72.

18. Tsui BC, Gupta S, Finucane B. Determination of epidural catheter placement using nerve stimulation in obstetric patients. *Reg Anesth Pain Med* 1999;**24**:17–23.

19. Lilker S, Meyer RA, Downey KN, Macarthur AJ. Anesthesia considerations for placenta accreta. *Int J Obstet Anesth* 2011;**20**:288–292.

20. Ogunnaike BO, Jones SB, Jones DB, *et al.* Anesthetic considerations for bariatric surgery. *Anesth Analg* 2002;**95**:1793–1805.

21. Luo ZC, Wilkins R, Platt RW, Kramer MS. Fetal and infant health study group of the Canadian Perinatal Surveillance System. *Paediat Perinat Epidemiol* 2004;**18**:40–50.

22. Cabacungan ET, Ngui EM, McGinley EL. Racial/ethnic disparities in maternal morbidities: a statewide study of labor and delivery hospitalizations in Wisconsin. *Matern Child Health.* 2012;**16**:1455–1467.

23. Canadian Institute for Health Information. *Giving Birth in Canada: Regional trends from 2001–2002 to 2005–2006.* Ottawa: Canadian Institute for Health Information, 2007.

24. Rahman K, Jenkins JG. Failed tracheal intubation in obstetrics: no more frequent but still badly managed. *Anaesthesia* 2005;**60**:168–171.

25. Mhyre JM, Healy D. The unanticipated difficult intubation in obstetrics. *Anesth Analg* 2011;**112**:648–652.

26. Douglas MJ, Preston RL. The obstetric airway: things are seldom as they seem. *Can J Anesth* 2011;**58**:494–498.

27. Royal College of Obstetricians and Gynaecologists. *The National Sentinel Caesarean Section Audit.* London: RCOG Press, 2001.

28. O'Sullivan G, Liu B, Hart D, *et al.* Effect of food intake during labour on obstetric outcome, a randomised controlled trial. *Br Med J* 2009;**358**:784.

29. Needleman J, Minnick AF. Anesthesia provider model, hospital resources, and maternal outcomes. *Heath Res Educ Trust* 2009;**44**:464–482.

30. World Health Organization. *The International Statistical Classification of Diseases and Related Health Problems*, 9th revision. Geneva: World Health Organization, 2002.

31. Crawforth K. The AANA Foundation Closed Malpractice Claims study: Obstetric anesthesia. *AANA J* 2002;**70**:97–104.

32. Davies JM, Posner KL, Lee LA, Cheney FW, Domino KB. Liability associated with obstetric anesthesia. *Anesthesiology* 2009;**110**:131–139.

33. Awan R, Nolan JP, Cook TM. Use of Proseal laryngeal mask airway for airway maintainence during emergency Caesarean section after failed tracheal intubation. *Br J Anaesth* 2004;**92**:144–146.

34. Popat MT, Srivastava M, Russell R. Awake fibreoptic intubation skills in obstetric patients: a survey of anaesthetists in the Oxford region. *Int J Obstet Anesth* 2000;**9**:78–82.

35. Bullough AS, Carraretto M. A United Kingdom national obstetric intubation equipment survey. *Int J Obstet Anesth.* 2009;**18**:342–345.

36. Obstetric Anaesthetists' Association. *Pencil-Point*, Spring 2005 (http://www.oaa-anaes.ac.uk/assets/_managed/editor/File/Pencilpoint/21_2005_pencilpoint.pdf, accessed 29 January 2013).

37. Chiron B, Sauvagnac X, Gaillard S, *et al.* Preoxygenation and parturient patient: a comparison of three techniques. *Eur J Anesthesiol* 2001;**18**:111–112.

38. Cook TM. Cricoid pressure, two hands better than one. *Anaesthesia* 1996;**51**:365–368.

39. Pühringer FK, Kristen P, Rex C. Sugammadex reversal of rocuronium-induced neuromuscular block in Caesarean section patients: a series of seven cases. *Br J Anaesth* 2010;**105**:657–660.

40. Vasdev GM, Harrison BA, Keegan MT, Burkle CM. Management of the difficult and failed airway in obstetric anesthesia. *J Anesth* 2008;**22**:38–48.

41. Rasmussen GE, Malinow AM. Toward reducing maternal mortality: the problem airway in obstetrics. *Int Anesthesiol Clin* 1994;**32**:83–101.

Chapter 18

Mechanical ventilation

Paul E. Marik, David Grooms, and Malachy O. Columb

Introduction

Fortunately, the admission of the critically ill obstetric patient to the intensive care unit (ICU) is an infrequent event. Even more reassuring is that the mortality rates are much lower for obstetric patients than for matched non-pregnant women (2.3% compared with 14.7%) [1]. The requirement for endotracheal intubation and mechanical ventilation is the most common indication for admission to ICU. The most common reason for mechanical ventilation is hypoxic respiratory failure (type I respiratory failure). In addition, patients with hypercarbic respiratory failure (type II respiratory failure) who have failed non-invasive modes of ventilation (NIV) require endotracheal intubation and mechanical ventilation. With the development, refinement, and popularization of non-invasive positive pressure ventilation as a primary mode of ventilatory support (continuous positive airway pressure (CPAP) and bilevel positive airway pressure (Bi-PAP)), many patients who previously would have required intubation and mechanical ventilation are now treated with NIV [2–4]. The most common indications in the general population for NIV are an acute exacerbation of chronic obstructive pulmonary disease and acute cardiogenic pulmonary edema. Use of NIV is generally inappropriate for patients with severe respiratory failure caused by pneumonia, aspiration pneumonitis, asthma, or acute lung injury. These acute conditions are more likely to affect the obstetric patient, who is also likely to be at increased risk of gastroesophageal reflux and aspiration pneumonitis with NIV. This chapter will initially deal with issues related to mechanical ventilation in general and then consider those relevant to the obstetric patient.

General issues with mechanical ventilation

The most common indications for intubation and mechanical ventilation are:

- hypoxic respiratory failure
  - deliver a high fraction of inspired oxygen (Fio_2)
  - reduce shunt
  - apply positive end-expiratory pressure (PEEP)
- hypercapnic respiratory acidosis
  - reduce the work of breathing and thus prevent respiratory muscle fatigue
  - maintain adequate alveolar ventilation
- unprotected or unstable airways (e.g. coma)
  - secure the airway
  - reduce the risk of aspiration
  - maintain adequate alveolar ventilation
- other: to facilitate procedure (bronchoscopy), bronchial suctioning.

Mechanical ventilation is not without risks. The complications associated with mechanical ventilation are discussed below.

It should be recognized that intubation eliminates the respiratory protective reflexes (patient cannot cough effectively) and interferes with the mucociliary escalator; these effects significantly increase the risk for the development of pneumonia (ventilator-associated pneumonia). In addition, mechanical ventilation is never a curative intervention but rather provides ventilatory assistance while the underlying disorder improves. Consequently, the decision to initiate mechanical ventilation is often difficult, and the clinician should weigh the risks and benefits of the

Maternal Critical Care: A Multidisciplinary Approach, ed. Marc Van de Velde, Helen Scholefield, and Lauren A. Plante.
Published by Cambridge University Press. © Cambridge University Press 2013.

intervention. It is also important to recognize that positive pressure ventilation is potentially lethal in patients with severe pulmonary hypertension. The decision to intubate and initiate mechanical ventilation is essentially one of clinical judgment and should be based on a number of factors including the respiratory rate, heart rate, blood pressure, signs of respiratory distress (nasal flaring, use of accessory muscles, use of abdominal muscles, grunting, etc.), arterial blood gas analysis (ABG; for arterial partial pressure of carbon dioxide (Pa_{CO_2}) and oxygen (Pa_{O_2}), pH), and/or pulse oximetry, as well as the patient's comorbidities, acute medical problem, and the likely response to medical interventions.

In recent years, a convincing body of evidence has accumulated that the "traditional" modes of mechanical ventilation frequently caused the disease we were trying to treat: acute lung injury. A landmark study published by the Acute Respiratory Distress Syndrome Network in 2000 demonstrated that a strategy of volume-control (VC) continuous mandatory ventilation (CMV), otherwise referred to as assist/control ventilation, using a low tidal volume (V_T) of 6 mL/kg predicted body weight (PBW), coupled with limiting end-inspiratory alveolar pressure (plateau pressure) to ≤ 30 cm H_2O, was associated with a significant reduction in 28-day all-cause mortality compared with ventilation with traditional V_T (12 mL/kg PBW) in patients with acute lung injury and acute respiratory distress syndrome (ARDS) [5]. Such an approach, called the "lung protective strategy," is now considered the standard of care and applies to all mechanically ventilated patients, not just those with ARDS [6–8]. It is important to use PBW and not actual body weight for these calculations in order to normalize V_T to lung size, since lung size depends most strongly on height and sex. The use of V_T based on PBW is particularly important in obese and pregnant patients as lung volumes do not increase in size with these conditions, and, in fact, decrease. For example, a person who ideally weighs 70 kg and who then gains 35 kg has essentially the same lung size as she did at her previous weight of 70 kg: she should not receive ventilation with a higher V_T because of the weight gain. The PBW should be calculated for all patients undergoing mechanical ventilation. The formula for women is:

$$PBW\ (kg) = 45.5 + 0.91\ (\text{height (cm)} - 152.4)$$

Alveolar overdistention has been shown to damage normal as well as injured lungs. A number of studies have demonstrated that large V_T values are

independently associated with increases in inflammatory biomarkers and the development of acute lung injury in patients who did not have acute lung injury at the onset of mechanical ventilation [9–12]. A recent population-based cohort study suggested that ARDS is mainly a healthcare-related syndrome: 67% developed ARDS after hospital admission, and of those who did not have ARDS at admission, more than half had had a recent interaction with the heathcare system such as recent hospitalization [13]. The strongest evidence for the benefit of a "protective lung ventilation" strategy in patients without acute lung injury comes from a randomized clinical trial in postoperative patients [14]. Intubated, mechanically ventilated patients in a surgical ICU were randomly assigned to mechanical ventilation with a V_T of 12 or 6 mL/kg PBW. The incidence of pulmonary infection was lower and durations of intubation and ICU stay were shorter for patients randomly assigned to the lower V_T strategy, suggesting that morbidity may be decreased. Regardless of the mode of mechanical ventilation and the underlying medical condition, the V_T of all patients undergoing mechanical ventilation should not exceed 6–8 mL/kg PBW, and this V_T should be coupled with a plateau pressure <30 cmH$_2$O.

Ventilator variables and modes of ventilation

Current nomenclature related to mechanical ventilation is outdated and confusing. For example, the 8th edition of *Mosby's Respiratory Care Equipment* lists 56 unique names for ventilator mode labels [15]. However, when analyzing the targeting schemes (the feedback control system the ventilator uses to deliver a specific ventilatory pattern) in detail, only about 25 of these modes are "unique" and identifiable using six basic targeting schemes. Standardization of terminology is urgently needed [16,17].

The clinician should be familiar with a number of modes of ventilation, all of which have specific indications. Standard ventilator terminology and variables are listed in Table 18.1 while initial (default) ventilator settings are listed in Table 18.2. Ventilator phase variables are illustrated in Figure 18.1.

The most common mode of mechanical ventilation in the ICU is VC-CMV and this can be considered a "default mode" (Figure 18.2).

Pressure-controlled (PC) CMV (also termed pressure control ventilation) is equally considered as

Table 18.1. Ventilator terminology and parameters

Term	Definition
Fio_2	Fraction of inspired oxygen, i.e. the percentage of oxygen in the air the patient is breathing
Pco_2	Partial pressure carbon dioxide ($Paco_2$, arterial)
Po_2	Partial pressure oxygen (Pao_2, arterial; Pao_2, alveolar)
Rate	Respiratory rate or number of breaths per minute
V_T	Tidal volume, the volume of each breath (usually in mL)
Sensitivity	How responsive the ventilator is to the patient's efforts
Peak flow	The maximum flow rate used to deliver each breath to the patient (usually in L/min)
Inspiratory time	The time spent in the inspiratory phase of the ventilatory cycle
I:E ratio	The ratio of inspiratory time to expiratory time; the sum of inspiratory time and expiratory time is the total cycle time
Flow pattern	The shape of the inspiratory flow profile representing the breath type or patient effort; it can be square wave, sinusoidal, or decelerating
Mode	A predetermined pattern of patient–ventilator interaction; the mode can be described at various levels of detail, e.g. just specifying the control variable (volume or pressure), adding the breath sequence (e.g. volume- or pressure-controlled continuous mandatory ventilation, pressure-controlled intermittent mandatory ventilation) and finally including the targeting scheme (e.g. pressure-controlled continuous spontaneous ventilation with adaptive pressure targeting)
CMV	Continuous mandatory ventilation; a breath sequence that does not allow spontaneous breaths between mandatory breaths
CSV	Continuous spontaneous ventilation; a breath sequence consisting of only spontaneous breaths
Cycling	The change from inspiration to expiration
Expiration	The phase of a breath from the start of expiratory flow to the start of inspiratory flow
IMV	Intermittent mandatory ventilation; a breath sequence that allows spontaneous breaths to occur between mandatory breaths
Inspiration	The phase of a breath from the start of inspiratory flow to the start of expiratory flow
Target	A predetermined goal of ventilator output such as inspiratory pressure, tidal volume, inspiratory flow, or minute ventilation
Targeting scheme	A model of the relationship between operator inputs and ventilator outputs to achieve a specific ventilatory pattern; the targeting scheme is a key component of a mode description
Mandatory breath	A breath for which inspiration is machine triggered and/or machine cycled
Spontaneous breath	A breath for which inspiration is both patient triggered and patient cycled
Trigger	To start inspiration; triggering may be machine initiated (e.g. by a preset frequency) or patient initiated (e.g. by sensing an inspiratory effort using a pressure or flow signal)
PEEP	Positive end-expiratory pressure (usually measured in cmH_2O)

a default/standard mode, particularly in ICUs that have a highly involved respiratory therapy presence and a protocol in which the exhaled V_T is closely monitored (Figure 18.2).

Continuous spontaneous ventilation (also termed pressure-support ventilation (PSV)), where the breath sequence consisting of only spontaneous breaths, or CPAP is commonly used in ventilator-dependent patients with chronic respiratory failure (Figure 18.3) [16] and is a level 1, evidence-based recommendation for ventilator liberation (weaning). Because the word "assist" describes the elevation of airway pressure above baseline during inspiration, PSV breath types are assisted, whereas CPAP breaths are unassisted.

Intermittent mandatory ventilation (IMV) with volume control (VC-IMV) is also known as synchronized IMV (SIMV; the addition of the letter "S" is no longer necessary because all modern ventilators can be patient triggered) has a limited role, mainly in patients with asthma and those with unresolved respiratory alkalosis.

Table 18.2. Initial (default) ventilator settings[a]

	Description
Initial setting	
Mode	Volume-controlled CMV (also known as assist/control ventilation) or pressure-controlled CMV
V_T	8 mL/kg predicted body weight
Rate	6–12/min
PEEP	5 cmH$_2$O
Fio$_2$	1.0 (100%)
Flow rate	40–80 L/min
Waveform	Decelerating
Settings dynamically adjusted according to plateau pressures	keep 30 cmH$_2$O (unless stiff chest wall disorder is present, e.g. kyphoscoliosis, morbid obesity, increased abdominal pressures, neuromuscular disease)
Arterial hemoglobin saturation/pulse oximetry	92–96%
pH and Pco$_2$	
Intrinsic PEEP	
Flow and pressure waveforms	

[a] See Table 18.1 for definitions.

- **A Trigger**
  - Patient (assisted)
  - Machine (controlled)
- **B Limit**
  - Flow
  - Pressure
- **C Cycle**
  - Volume
  - Time

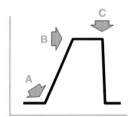

Figure 18.1. Ventilator phase variables.

It is the only mode of ventilation not recommended for the ventilator liberation process [16] (Figure 18.4).

Use of PC-CMV and airway pressure release ventilation (APRV) should be considered in patients with severe ARDS who have "failed" conventional low V_T ventilation in the VC-CMV mode. In some centers, APRV is considered the default mode for acute lung injury/ARDS as well as for cardiogenic pulmonary edema [18]. Airway

pressure release ventilation is a useful mode in patients with atelectasis and reduced chest wall compliance.

Ventilator variables

Table 18.1 outlines the various variables, which are discussed further below.

Cycling

Ventilators have traditionally been classified according to the cycling method (i.e. termination of inspiration). However, modern ventilators have microprocessors that allow them to function in many different modes with enormous versatility. Therefore cycling is either machine or patient cycled. Machine cycling is required if the patient is unable to change the inspiratory time with inspiratory or expiratory efforts or changes to the respiratory system time constant; types of machine cycling include volume and time cycling.

> *Volume cycled.* The ventilator delivers fresh gas until the preselected volume of gas is delivered. Alveolar pressure is proportional to respiratory system elastance and inversely proportional to compliance. Airway pressure is a function of volume and flow for a given elastance and resistance.
>
> *Time cycled.* Inspiration continues for a preset interval, with exhalation beginning when this time interval has elapsed, regardless of airway pressure or volume delivered.

Patient cycling refers to the influence of the patient on changing inspiratory time by making changes in inspiratory or expiratory effort, or respiratory system time constant. Pressure and flow cycling are examples of patient cycling.

> *Pressure cycled.* Inspiration continues until a predetermined peak airway pressure is reached. The V_T is variable (from breath to breath) and depends on pulmonary time constant, inspiratory time, and flow rate.
>
> *Flow cycled.* Inspiration continues until the inspiratory flow decays to a preset value (usually a preset flow rate or a percentage of the peak inspiratory flow rate).

Ventilator trigger variables

With all modes of mechanical ventilation, a predetermined threshold must be reached by the patient or the ventilator before the ventilator will deliver gas flow. In

Volume ventilation   Pressure ventilation

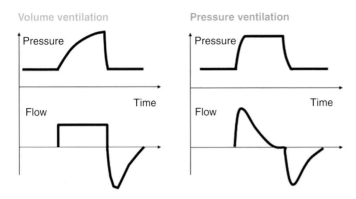

Figure 18.2. Volume- and pressure-limited ventilation.

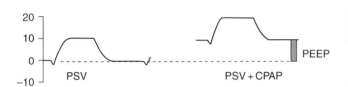

Figure 18.3. Pressure support ventilation (PSV) and continuous positive airway pressure (CPAP). PEEP, positive end-expiratory pressure.

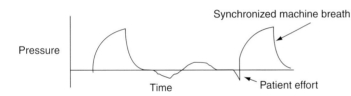

Figure 18.4. Synchronized intermittent mandatory ventilation.

spontaneously breathing patients, pressure and flow triggering are the most commonly used trigger variables. With pressure triggering, a set negative pressure (relative to PEEP) must be attained for the ventilator to deliver fresh gas into the inspiratory circuit. This is commonly set at −2 cmH₂O. The higher (more negative) the trigger sensitivity, the harder the patient has to work to trigger a breath. With flow triggering, the patient must inspire a predetermined inspiratory flow rate (usually between 1 and 4 L/min) to start inspiration. During the initial phase of inspiration, the patient is able to inspire fresh gas, which is supplied from a base flow that circulates continuously throughout the inhalation and exhalation circuit. The initial demand for flow is satisfied by the base flow, while at the same time generating the inspiratory flow signal according to the set flow sensitivity. In both the healthy subject and in the intubated patient, the inspiratory muscle work has been demonstrated to be significantly higher with pressure-triggered CPAP (without PSV) than with flow-triggered CPAP. However, pressure support of 5 cmH₂O has been demonstrated to reduce the

inspiratory muscle work of pressure-triggered CPAP to a level comparable with that of flow-triggered CPAP. The goal of the bedside clinician is to reduce the trigger sensitivity as much as possible in an attempt to minimize the patient work to trigger without creating inadvertent ventilator auto-triggering.

Inspiratory to expiratory ratio

Some ventilators allow the operator to set the inspiratory to expiratory ratio directly. Other ventilators allow adjustment of the ratio by altering the flow rate, respiratory rate, and inspiratory time or percentage (including an inspiratory pause). For most adults, a normal inspiratory to expiratory ratio of 1:2 or 1:3 is used. In patients with chronic obstructive lung disease and asthma, longer ratios (>1:4) are necessary to allow the lungs time to exhale to resting functional residual capacity (FRC) and to avoid hyperinflation. Patients who are hypoxemic secondary to ARDS require increased mean airway pressure to increase the FRC and allow more surface area for gas transfer to occur. This can be achieved using either PEEP or inverse ratio

191

Table 18.3. Common modalities of mechanical ventilation

Common mode terminology	Breathing pattern	Mandatory breaths			Patient-initiated breaths			Advantage	Disadvantage
		Trigger	Target	Cycle	Trigger	Target	Cycle		
Assist/control	VC-CMV	T, P, F	F, V	V	NA	NA	NA	Consistent V_T	Prone to flow dysychrony
Pressure control	PC-CMV	T, P, F	P	T	NA	NA	NA	Improved flow synchrony	Inconsistent V_T delivery
Pressure-regulated volume control	VC-CMV	T, P, F	F, V, P	T	NA	NA	NA	Auto-pressure control adjustment to sustain consistent V_T	Pressure control reduction when inspired V_T > delivered V_T
Synchronized intermittent mandatory ventilation	VC-IMV, PC-IMV	T, P, F	F, V, P	V, T	P, F	P	F	Allows spontaneous breathing	Longer weaning times and breath type mismatching
Continuous positive airway pressure	PC-CSV	NA	NA	NA	P, F	P	P	Improved synchrony	Hemodynamic compromise
Pressure-support ventilation	PC-CSV	NA	NA	NA	P, F	P	F, P	Improved synchrony	Inconsistent V_T delivery
Airway pressure release ventilation	PC-CSV	T	P	T	P, F	P	F	Can sustain mean airway pressure with lower plateau pressure	Inconsistent V_T delivery

CMV, continuous mandatory ventilation; F, flow; IMV, intermittent mandatory ventilation; P, pressure; PC, pressure controlled; T, time; V, volume; VC, volume controlled; V_T, tidal volume.

ventilation. In addition, studies have demonstrated that prolonging inspiration can result in a more homogeneous distribution of ventilation within abnormal lungs. When the inspiratory to expiratory ratio is increased to 1:1 or more, the inspiratory pressure is maintained for a longer period of time, but the peak inspiratory pressure does not increase.

Common modes of mechanical ventilation

The most common modes of mechanical ventilation are given in Table 18.3.

Volume-controlled continuous mandatory ventilation

In the VC-CMV mode, the ventilator delivers a preset V_T, inspiratory flow pattern, flow rate, and inspiratory time, within a machine- or patient-triggered breath (Figure 18.2). In this mode, the control parameter is V_T, which also implies flow control. The inspiratory pressure will fluctuate from breath to breath. In the patient who does not spontaneously initiate a breath, a set frequency determines the rate of mandatory breath delivery. In the spontaneously breathing patient, if the

patient effort is detected before the next time-triggered mandatory breath is scheduled to be delivered, the ventilator will deliver the breath to the patient. The set rate also serves as a back-up rate in the event of apnea. Unless the patient is ventilated using a mode that allows her to dictate her own frequency (in which the mandatory breath delivery is not based on a time cycle,) this mode will always deliver ventilation at the set frequency.

Pressure-controlled continuous mandatory ventilation

The PC-CMV mode delivers a preset pressure and inspiratory time within a machine- or patient-triggered breath. The control parameters are pressure and time. Both V_T and inspiratory flow will vary for each breath as determined by respiratory system mechanics and patient inspiratory effort. As the lungs are filled, the inspiratory flow decreases (decelerating wave) in order to maintain a constant pressure. The point at which inspiratory flow decays to zero represents completed filling of the lung at the preset pressure. This inspiratory waveform has been shown to result in a more homogeneous distribution of gas flow in patients with ARDS. Improved patient comfort and lower work of breathing have been observed in spontaneously breathing patients with the use of PC-CMV in comparison to VC-CMV [19,20].

Volume-controlled and pressure-controlled intermittent mandatory ventilation

When using a mode that provides an IMV breath sequence, the patient may be given two different breath types: (1) a mandatory volume-controlled or pressure-controlled breath, or (2) a spontaneous breath that may be assisted (e.g. with pressure support) or unassisted (pressure does not rise above PEEP during inspiration). The original clinical intent was to partition ventilatory support between assisted and unassisted breaths. Historically, this was an evolutionary milestone in mechanical ventilation, as it was the first breath sequence of its kind to allow patients to breathe spontaneously through the ventilator circuit at a V_T and acute lung injury that he/she determined according to need. Although it is perceived to "synchronize" with the patient's respiratory efforts (i.e. SIMV), this was later realized to be untrue, as synchrony is based on the ventilator's frequency of breath detection, satisfying inspiratory flow demand, and ability to cycle into exhalation, which are now present in most modes of ventilation (see Figure 18.4).

Continuous mandatory ventilation

The acronym CMV has been used by ventilator manufacturers to define a variety of modes of ventilation and has blurred the historical distinction between CMV and IMV [17]. With CMV (commonly known as assist/control ventilation), all breaths are mandatory unless there is provision for spontaneous breaths during mandatory breaths (i.e. using a so-called active exhalation valve). *The defining characteristic of CMV is that spontaneous breaths are not permitted between mandatory breaths because an inspiratory effort after a mandatory breath triggers another mandatory breath.* Typically, CMV provides a preset mandatory breath frequency in the case of apnea, but the actual breathing frequency at any time is a function of the patient's inspiratory efforts (the actual frequency is usually higher than the set frequency).

Continuous spontaneous ventilation with pressure support ventilation

The development of PSV (classified as a type of pressure-controlled continuous spontaneous

ventilation) was intended to reduce the work of spontaneous breathing in the IMV and CPAP modes (Figure 18.3). With pressure support, each breath is patient triggered, pressure targeted, and flow cycled, This is different from a PC-CMV breath, for which breaths are patient or machine triggered, pressure targeted, and time cycled. Therefore, this breath type allows the patient to have a more flexible inspiratory time. Use of PSV also compensates for the inherent impedance of the ventilator circuit and endotracheal tube, enabling the patient to establish a more natural breathing pattern. A PSV of 5–10 cmH_2O will overcome the resistance of the ventilator circuit and endotracheal tube. With PSV, the patient controls the rate, volume, and duration of each breath.

Airway pressure release ventilation

The time-triggered, pressure-targeted, time-cycled APRV mode of ventilation allows unrestricted spontaneous breathing throughout the entire ventilatory cycle (Figure 18.5). It is an alternative approach to the "open-lung" ventilation strategy [21]. Although recruitment maneuvers may be effective in improving gas exchange and compliance, these effects are not sustained, and APRV may be viewed as a nearly continuous recruitment maneuver [22]. The ventilator maintains a high-pressure setting for the bulk of the respiratory cycle, which is followed by a periodic release to a low pressure [23]. The periodic releases aid in carbon dioxide elimination. The release periods at low pressure are kept short (0.2–1.0 seconds) in order to induce a level of intrinsic auto-PEEP, which prevents alveolar derecruitment and enhances spontaneous breathing during the high-pressure period [21,24]. The advantages of APRV over VC-CMV include an increase in mean alveolar pressure with alveolar recruitment, improved patient/ventilator synchrony, the hemodynamic and ventilatory benefits associated with spontaneous breathing, and the reduced requirement for sedation.

Positive end-expiratory pressure

Use of PEEP provides an end-expiratory pressure above atmospheric pressure (Figure 18.3). The mean airway pressure increases in proportion to the level of PEEP. In patients with pulmonary edema, PEEP shifts the pressure–volume inflation curve toward normal, increasing compliance, recruiting alveoli, and increasing FRC. Use of PEEP also decreases the left

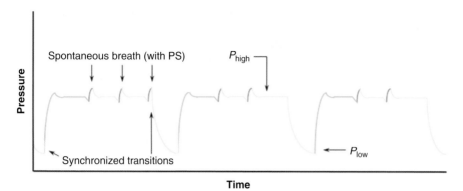

Figure 18.5. Airway pressure-release ventilation.

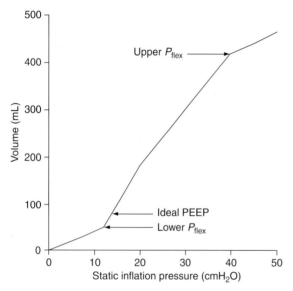

Figure 18.6. Static pressure–volume curve showing upper and lower inflection points (flex). PEEP, positive end-expiratory pressure.

ventricular transmural pressure gradient and tension, thus decreasing afterload. It is also thought that PEEP redistributes lung water. In patients with a large (>30%) shunt, increasing Fio_2 has little effect on Pao_2: increased PEEP is required to increase Pao_2 in patients with a large shunt. It should be noted that although PEEP is "good" for left ventricular function, it may cause cardiovascular collapse in patients with severe right ventricular dysfunction. Some clinicians use "physiological" or prophylactic PEEP (5 cmH$_2$O) to prevent atelectasis/pneumonia. Manzano *et al.* [25] randomized 131 mechanically ventilated patients with normal chest radiograph and Pao_2/Fio_2 >250 to receive mechanical ventilation with 5–8 cmH$_2$O PEEP or no PEEP. Ventilator-associated pneumonia was detected in 16 (25.4%) patients in the control

group and 6 (9.4%) in the PEEP group. The number of patients who developed hypoxemia was significantly higher in the control group (34 of 63; 54%) than in the PEEP group (12 of 64; 19%).

Increased PEEP (>5 cmH$_2$O) is primarily used in patients with pulmonary edema (cardiogenic and non-cardiogenic) and a large intrapulmonary shunt who become refractory to increasing Fio_2. The optimal method of setting PEEP in patients with ARDS is controversial. Excessive PEEP will overinflate compliant lungs and increase ventilation/perfusion mismatching as well as reducing cardiac output. However, inadequate PEEP may result in airway collapse at the end of expiration, leading to the cyclic opening and closing of alveolar units, which may further perpetuate lung injury. The goal is to set PEEP at a level that does not overdistend healthy alveoli but at the same time does not let diseased airways collapse. The term "open lung approach" has been used to describe this method of ventilation [26]. It has been reported that a mean PEEP of 15 cmH$_2$O is required to sustain alveolar opening at end-expiration in patients with ARDS [26]. While the beneficial effects of a low tidal volume strategy is largely accepted, the role of PEEP as part of the "lung protective strategy" is more controversial [27–29]. A meta-analysis demonstrated a trend towards improved mortality with high PEEP, with the pooled cumulative risk of 0.90 (95% confidence interval, 0.72–1.02; $p = 0.077$) [30]. "Best PEEP" can be estimated by plotting a static pressure–volume curve measuring airway pressure at each incrementally higher tidal volume (Figure 18.6). This curve classically demonstrates an upper and lower inflection point, representing respiratory system opening and overdistention. The level of PEEP should be set above the lower inflection point such that the sum of the PEEP and the inspiratory pressure should be 30 cm H_2O (a plateau pressure up to 35 cmH_2O may be acceptable) or the upper inflection point. Should an inflection point not be present on the pressure–volume curve, or it is not possible to perform this maneuver, the initial PEEP should be set between 10 and 15 cmH_2O.

Ideally, both V_T and PEEP should be adjusted according to transpulmonary pressures (airway pressure minus pleural pressure) to maintain oxygenation while minimizing both repeated alveolar collapse (negative end-expiratory transpulmonary pressure) and alveolar overdistension (high end-inspiratory transpulmonary pressure). While pleural pressure is very difficult to measure clinically, it can be estimated using esophageal manometry [31].

Monitoring patients undergoing mechanical ventilation

All patients receiving mechanical ventilation should be monitored by pulse oximetry. Analysis of ABGs should be performed during the initial ventilator adjustments and then when clinically indicated. The arterial hemoglobin saturation, as measured by pulse oximetry, provides adequate information for managing most ventilated patients. Patients with carbon dioxide retention and those with complex metabolic derangements generally require regular ABG analyses. It is not necessary to perform an ABG analysis after every ventilator change. In fact, studies have demonstrated that obtaining a routine ABG following completion of a spontaneous breathing trial did not affect extubation decision making and that outcomes were similar to those who did not receive routine ABG measurements [32,33]. Routine ABG analysis following a spontaneous breathing trial is not recommended unless clinically indicated. All the ventilator parameters, including plateau pressure, mean airway pressure, V_T, and minute volume, should be monitored periodically. A chest radiograph should be performed after intubation and repeated as clinically indicated. Routine daily chest radiographs are not cost-effective [34].

Mechanical ventilation during pregnancy

In the era before the H1N1 influenza pandemic, ARDS was reported to account for as many as 19% of obstetric ICU admissions, with a maternal mortality as high as 44% [35–38]. The commonest causes of ARDS included community-acquired pneumonia (particularly in patients with HIV infection), aspiration pneumonitis, septic abortion, and eclampsia/pre-eclampsia [35–38]. The H1N1 influenza virus has a predilection to cause severe ARDS in pregnant patients [39]. Consequently, the number of pregnant patients admitted to the ICU with severe respiratory failure increased dramatically during the pandemic of 2009.

The clinical criteria for intubating a pregnant patient are similar to those in non-pregnant patients and include increased work of breathing, mental status deterioration, hemodynamic instability, and inability to protect the airway or manage secretions [40]. Blood gas criteria for intubation may vary depending on the gestational age of the pregnancy, but later in pregnancy, which is when most cases of ARDS in pregnancy occur, a normal $Paco_2$ should be interpreted as a sign of impending respiratory failure. Inability to maintain a Pao_2 of >70 mmHg (9 kPa), or a blood oxygen saturation of >95%, with conservative therapy should also be interpreted as a sign of respiratory compromise requiring intubation [40].

The physiological changes of pregnancy have a significant impact on the pathophysiology of ARDS. The mechanical effect of pregnancy causes a decrease in chest wall compliance, particularly in late pregnancy [41]. This compounds the decrease in lung compliance associated with ARDS, causing a significant fall in total compliance. The FRC and residual volume decrease with advancing pregnancy [41]. These changes increase the risk of alveolar collapse, particularly in the dependent areas of the lung. Although a Pao_2 of 55 mmHg (7.5 kPa) and an oxygen saturation of 88% is well tolerated in non-pregnant patients with ARDS, "classic teaching" states that fetal oxygenation requires a Pao_2 of >70 mmHg (9 kPa), which corresponds to a maternal oxygen saturation of approximately 95% [40,42].

There are no published studies that have investigated a low V_T ventilatory strategy in pregnant women with ARDS and such a strategy may result in severe lung derecruitment. Furthermore, because of the increased oxygen demands, a low V_T ventilatory strategy may be unable to maintain adequate arterial oxygenation. Permissive hypercapnia has not been studied in pregnancy. Theoretically, maternal respiratory acidosis could lead to fetal acidosis, a shift of the fetal oxyhemoglobin dissociation curve to the right, and consequently impaired oxygenation of fetal hemoglobin. An animal model suggested that maternal hypercapnia

195

(Pa_{CO_2} >60 mmHg (8 kPa)) may lead to increased uterine vascular resistance and decreased uteroplacental blood flow [43]. However, good pregnancy outcomes have been reported with the use of permissive hypercapnia in a few pregnant patients with status asthmaticus [44]. Observational data on the higher V_T ventilation technique that predated the current standard suggest that pregnant women with ARDS are even more susceptible to barotrauma than the non-pregnant population [36,38]. This may have been because of the higher airway pressures required to deliver a set V_T because of the decreased extra-thoracic compliance. These data suggest that in pregnant patients undergoing a low V_T ventilatory strategy, esophageal manometry may be essential to optimize PEEP and V_T. In patients who have "failed" a low V_T ventilatory strategy, APRV should be considered. In fact, APRV may be an ideal ventilatory mode in pregnant patients with severe ARDS, as the increased mean alveolar pressure with short release time will recruit collapsed dependent lung while preventing overdistension of ventilated alveoli. We have previously reported two pregnant patients with life-threatening ARDS who were successfully managed with APRV [45]. We believe that APRV should be considered as an alternative ventilatory strategy in pregnant patients with severe ARDS. During the H1N1 influenza outbreak, many patients failed "conventional" modes of ventilation and required inhaled nitric oxide, high-frequency oscillatory ventilation, and/or extracorporal membrane oxygenation [39,46,47].

Sedation is crucial to achieve optimal ventilation, particularly with a low V_T strategy, which is often poorly tolerated. However, the safety of continuous sedative usage in pregnant patients is not known [48] (see also Chapters 14 and 18). Use of APRV has the distinct advantage of requiring minimal sedation.

Positioning of the mechanically ventilated patient in the flexed 30° head-up position has been promoted to reduce the risk of gastroesophageal reflux and aspiration and the subsequent development of ventilator-associated pneumonia. Although there is no specific guidance in mechanically ventilated obstetric patients, there is some recent evidence of the benefit of a 30° head-up position in improving FRC in awake pregnant subjects, where FRC increased significantly by 188 mL in changing from the supine position [49]. It also was noticeable in this study that there was a trend to less benefit in increasing FRC with increasing body mass index. Nevertheless, there may be some benefits to be gained in possibly avoiding derecruitment. Although position of the pregnant woman does cause significant changes in cardiac index and other hemodynamic variables [50,51], in practice these are small and not likely to affect overall cardiorespiratory efficiency, although direct aorto-caval compression should of course be avoided.

Shortly after beginning care for a pregnant woman with ARDS, fetal assessment should take place and plans for possible delivery should be made. These plans are influenced by the gestational age of the fetus, fetal status, maternal status, and the gestational age at which the treating institution can support a preterm infant, which is often 24–26 weeks for larger centers [40]. As is often the case in the management of the critically ill pregnant women, difficult decisions have to be taken in circumstances when optimal management of the mother may reduce the chance of a good fetal outcome.

Non-invasive ventilation in pregnancy

Non-invasive ventilation can be delivered nasally or by face mask, using either a conventional mechanical ventilator or a machine designed specifically for this purpose. There are two major modes of supplying NIV support: CPAP and BiPAP. Use of CPAP provides continuous positive pressure throughout the respiratory cycle; recruits underventilated alveoli by increasing lung volume at the end of expiration, resulting in improved gas exchange; and is also effective in decreasing work of breathing compared with unsupported ventilation.

The advantages of NIV include improved patient comfort; reduced need for sedation; and avoidance of the complications of endotracheal intubation, including upper airway trauma, sinusitis, and nosocomial pneumonia. Furthermore, airway defense mechanisms and speech and swallowing are left intact, and the patient remains alert and communicative. Non-invasive ventilation has been used successfully to treat acute respiratory failure in postoperative patients and in those with pulmonary edema, chronic obstructive pulmonary disease, and obstructive sleep apnea. It has also been used to facilitate weaning from ventilation support. There is very little experience worldwide with the use of NIV in pregnancy [52]. Gastric distension and vomiting with NIV are more likely in the pregnant patient because of the reduced tone of the lower esophageal sphincter. A careful trial of NIV may be appropriate in selected patients with respiratory failure that is likely to be rapidly reversible. The patient should understand the risks involved and be highly cooperative. High inspiratory pressures should be avoided, with a low threshold for endotracheal intubation.

Conclusions

This chapter has dealt with mechanical ventilator strategies in general and for the critically ill pregnant patient in particular. It has also the range of terminologies that abound and the respiratory physiology that underpins these. The indications for, and modes of, mechanical ventilation for the population of patients in critical care are similar to those for the obstetric patient. The 2009 H1N1 influenza pandemic and the particular susceptibility of pregnancy in such circumstances reinforce the need to appraise the rationale for mechanical ventilation in such patients. Finally, APRV as a ventilatory paradigm, in particular, may be particularly useful in the pregnant patient with pneumonits, acute lung injury, or ARDS.

References

1. Harrison DA, Brady AR, Rowan K. Case mix, outcome and length of stay for admissions to adult, general critical care units in England, Wales and Northern Ireland: the Intensive Care National Audit & Research Centre Case Mix Programme Database. *Crit Care* 2004;**8**:R99–R111.

2. International Consensus Conference in Intensive Care Medicine. Noninvasive positive pressure ventilation in acute respiratory failure. *Am J Resp Crit Care Med* 2001;**163**:283–191.

3. Garpestad E, Brennan J, Hill NS. Noninvasive ventilation for critical care. *Chest* 2007;**132**:711–720.

4. Weng CL, Zhao YY, Liu QH, *et al.* Meta-analysis: noninvasive ventilation in acute cardiogenic pulmonary edema. *Ann Intern Med* 2010;**152**:590–600.

5. Acute Respiratory Distress Syndrome Network. Ventilation with lower tidal volumes as compared with traditional tidal volumes for acute lung injury and the acute respiratory distress syndrome. *N Engl J Med* 2000;**342**:1301–1308.

6. Girard TD, Bernard GR. Mechanical ventilation in ARDS: a state-of-the-art review. *Chest* 2007;**131**:921–929.

7. Wheeler AP, Bernard GR. Acute lung injury and the acute respiratory distress syndrome: a clinical review. *Lancet* 2007;**369**:1553–1565.

8. Malhotra A. Low-tidal-volume ventilation in the acute respiratory distress syndrome. *N Engl J Med* 2007;**357**:1113–1120.

9. Gajic O, Frutos-Vivar F, Esteban A, *et al.* Ventilator settings as a risk factor for acute respiratory distress syndrome in mechanically ventilated patients. *Intensive Care Med* 2005;**31**:922–926.

10. Wrigge H, Zinserling J, Stuber F, *et al.* Effects of mechanical ventilation on release of cytokines into systemic circulation in patients with normal pulmonary function. *Anesthesiology* 2000;**93**:1413–1417.

11. Zupancich E, Paparella D, Turani F, *et al.* Mechanical ventilation affects inflammatory mediators in patients undergoing cardiopulmonary bypass for cardiac surgery: a randomized clinical trial. *J Thorac Cardiovasc Surg* 2005;**130**:378–383.

12. Gajic O, Dara SI, Mendez JL, *et al.* Ventilator-associated lung injury in patients without acute lung injury at the onset of mechanical ventilation. *Crit Care Med* 2004;**32**:1817–1824.

13. Shari G, Kojicic M, Li G, *et al.* Timing toset of acute respiratory distress syndrome: A population-based study. *Resp Care* 2011;**56**:576–582.

14. Lee PC, Helsmoortel CM, Cohn SM, *et al.* Are low tidal volumes safe? *Chest* 1990;**97**:430–434.

15. Cairo JM, Pilbeam SP. *Mosby' Respiratory Care Equipmen*, 8th edn. St. Louis, MO: Mosby-Elsevier, 2009.

16. Boles JM, Bion J, Connors A, *et al.* Weaning from mechanical ventilation. *Eur Resp J* 2007;**29**:1033–1056.

17. Chatburn RL. Classification of ventilator modes: update and proposal for implementation. *Resp Care* 2007;**52**:301–323.

18. Habashi NM. Other approaches to open-lung ventilation: airway pressure release ventilation. *Crit Care Med* 2005;**33**:S228–S240.

19. Kallet RH, Campbell AR, Alonso JA, *et al.* The effects of pressure control versus volume control assisted ventilation on patient work of breathing in acute lung injury and acute respiratory distress syndrome. *Resp Care* 2000;**45**:1085–1096.

20. Campbell RS, Davis BR. Pressure-controlled versus volume-controlled ventilation: does it matter? *Resp Care* 2002;**47**:416–424.

21. Myers TR, MacIntyre N. Does airway pressure release ventilation offer important new advantages in mechanical ventialtor support? *Resp Care* 2007;**52**:452–458.

22. Hemmila MR, Napolitano LM. Severe respiratory failure: advanced treatment options. *Crit Care Med* 2006;**34**:S278–S290.

23. Rose L, Hawkins M. Airway pressure release ventilation and biphasic positive airway pressure: a systematic review of definitional criteria. *Intensive Care Med* 2008;**34**:1766–1773.

24. Neumann P, Golisch W, Strohmeyer A, *et al.* Influence of different release times on spontaneous breathing pattern during airway pressure release ventilation. *Intensive Care Med* 2002;**28**:1742–1749.

25. Manzano F, Fernandez-Mondejar E, Colmenero M, *et al.* Positive-end expiratory pressure reduces incidence of ventilator-associated pneumonia in nonhypoxemic patients. *Crit Care Med* 2008;**36**:2225–2231.

26. Amato MB, Barbash CS, Medeiros DM, *et al.* Beneficial effects of the "Open lung approach" with low distending pressures in acute respiratory distress syndrome: A prospective randomized study on mechanical ventilation. *Am J Resp Crit Care Med* 1995;**152**:1835–1846.

27. Meade MO, Cook DJ, Guyatt GH, *et al.* Ventilation strategy using low tidal volumes, recruitment maneuvers, and high positive end-expiratory pressure for acute lung injury and acute respiratory distress syndrome: a randomized controlled trial. *JAMA* 2008;**299**:637–645.

28. Brower RG, Lanken PN, MacIntyre N, *et al.* Higher versus lower positive end-expiratory pressures in patients with the acute respiratory distress syndrome. *N Engl J Med* 2004;**351**:327–336.

29. Mercat A, Richard JC, Vielle B, *et al.* Positive end-expiratory setting in adults with acute lung injury and acute respiratory distress syndrome. A ramdomized controlled trial. *JAMA* 2008;**299**:646–655.

30. Phoenix SI, Paravastu S, Columb M, *et al.* Does a higher positive end expiratory pressure decrease mortality in acute respiratory distress syndrome? A systematic review and meta-analysis. *Anesthesiology* 2009;**110**:1098–1105.

31. Talmor D, Sarge T, O'Donnell CR, *et al.* Esophageal and transpulmonary pressures in acute respiratory failure. *Crit Care Med* 2006;**34**:1389–1394.

32. Salam A, Smina M, Gada P, *et al.* The effect of arterial blood gas values on extubation decisions. *Resp Care* 2003;**48**:1033–1037.

33. Pawson SR, DePriest JL. Are blood gases necessary in mechanically ventilated patients who have successfully completed a spontaneous breathing trial? *Resp Care* 2004;**49**:1316–1319.

34. Hejblum G, Chalumeau-Lemoine L, Ioos V, *et al.* Comparison of routine and on-demand prescription of chest radiographs in mechanically ventilated adults: a multicentre, cluster-randomised, two-period crossover study. *Lancet* 2009;**374**:1687–1693.

35. Vasquez DN, Estenssoro E, Canales HS, *et al.* Clinical characteristics and outcomes of obstetric patients requiring ICU admission. *Chest* 2007;**131**:718–724.

36. Mabie WC, Barton JR, Sibai BM. Adult respiratory distress syndrome in pregnancy. *Am J Obstet Gynecol* 1992;**167**:950–957.

37. Perry KG Jr., Martin RW, Blake PG, *et al.* Maternal mortality associated with adult respiratory distress syndrome. *South Med J* 1998;**91**:441–444.

38. Catanzarite V, Willms D, Wong D, *et al.* Acute respiratory distress syndrome in pregnancy and the puerperium: causes, courses, and outcomes. *Obstet Gynecol* 2001;**97**:760–764.

39. Jamieson DJ, Honein MA, Rasmussen SA, *et al.* H1N1.2009 influenza virus infection during pregnancy in the USA. *Lancet* 2009;**374**:451–458.

40. Cole DE, Taylor TL, McCullough DM, *et al.* Acute respiratory distress syndrome in pregnancy. *Crit Care Med* 2005;**33**:S269–S278.

41. Unterborn J. Pulmonary function testing in obesity, pregnancy, and extremes of body habitus. *Clinics Chest Med* 2001;**22**:759–767.

42. Oram MP, Seal P, McKinstry CE. Severe acute respiratory distress syndrome in pregnancy. Caesarean section in the second trimester to improve maternal ventilation. *Anaesth Intensive Care* 2007;**35**:975–978.

43. Walker AM, Oakes GK, Ehrenkranz R, *et al.* Effects of hypercapnia on uterine and umbilical circulations in conscious pregnant sheep. *J Appl Physiol* 1976;**41**:727–733.

44. Elsayegh D, Shapiro JM. Management of the obstetric patient with status asthmaticus. *J Intensive Care Med* 2008;**23**:396–402.

45. Hirani A, Plante LA, Marik PE. Airway pressure release ventilation in pregnant patients with ARDS: a novel strategy. *Resp Care* 2009;**54**:1405–1408.

46. Oluyomi-Obi T, Avery L, Schneider C, *et al.* Perinatal and maternal outcomes in critically ill obstetrics patients with pandemic H1N1 Influenza A. *JOGC* 2010;**32**:443–447.

47. Ang LT, Gandhi K, Qin YH. Respiratory failure in pregnant women infected by Swine-Origin influenza A (H1N1). *Aust N Z J Obstet Gynaecol* 2010;**50**:294–296.

48. Tajchman SK, Bruno JJ. Prolonged propofol use in a critically ill pregnant patient. *Ann Pharmacother* 2010;**44**:2018–2022.

49. Hignett R, Fernando R, McGlennan A, *et al.* A randomized crossover study to determine the effect of a 30{degrees} head-up versus a supine position on the

functional residual capacity of term parturients. *Anesth Analg* 2011;**113**:1098–1102.

50. Armstrong S, Fernando R, Columb M, *et al.* Cardiac index in term pregnant women in the sitting, lateral, and supine positions: an observational, crossover study. *Anesth Analg* 2011;**113**:318–322.

51. Armstrong S, Fernando R, Columb M. Minimally and non-invasive assessment of maternal cardiac output: go with the flow! *Int J Obstet Anesth* 2011;**20**:330–340.

52. Banga A, Khilnani GC. Use of non-invasive ventilation in a pregnant woman with acute respiratory distress syndrome due to pneumonia. *Indian J Chest Dis Allied Sci* 2009;**51**:115–117.

Chapter

19

Sedation and pain management

Thierry Girard

Introduction

There are several reasons why critically ill patients might need analgesia and/or sedation in the intensive care unit (ICU). Analgesia aims to prevent, treat, and manage pain during a stay in the ICU. Analgesia is obviously needed for postoperative pain, for pain following trauma, or for painful procedures performed in the ICU. Sedation aims to provide anxiolysis to the patient and to prevent agitation. Sedation might be needed because the patient is agitated, frequently as an accompaniment to mechanical ventilation, or to improve neurological outcome in patients with intracranial pathologies. Analgesia and sedation should be dosed according to the needs of the patient. The correct dosage for analgesia and sedation is not easily determined and as many as half of the patients on the ICU can be oversedated [1]. There are a number of different scoring systems to evaluate analgesia and sedation in ICU patients. One of the better validated scores is the Richmond Sedation and Agitation Score (Table 19.1). In general, sedation of patients in ICU is used much more restrictively now than in the past. Analgesia is by far the more important component, and sufficient analgesia can reduce or eliminate the need for sedation. Even in intubated and mechanically ventilated patients, there is a clear tendency now towards much less sedation than previously. Sedation in ICU is associated with delirium and prolonged ICU stay. If patients need sedation, then – with the exception of severe intracranial pressure or brain damage – it should be interrupted on a daily basis and the patient given the opportunity to arouse. Caution is also required for renal or hepatic failure as this might influence the depth of analgesia and sedation and might prolong the action of many sedative or analgesic drugs.

Since pregnancy also affects pharmacokinetics and dynamics of many drugs, knowledge of these changes is required to correctly use these drugs in pregnancy. Chapter 14 has more in-depth information on this topic. Almost none of the drugs used for analgesia and sedation in the ICU have been extensively investigated in pregnant patients; however, many of these drugs are used during anesthesia and there is literature about anesthesia of the pregnant patient [2,3]. From these studies it is known that none of these drugs seems to have a teratogenic effect [2]. There is a small increase in miscarriage and preterm delivery among women who underwent surgery and anesthesia during pregnancy, but this seems to be unrelated to the drugs used.

Analgesia

Whenever possible, a regional anesthetic technique should be chosen for pain control [4]. Intravenous drugs cross the placenta and have the potential to influence the fetus. In contrast, continuous infusion of local anesthetics, as used for regional techniques, leads to minimal plasma concentrations. Thoracic epidural analgesia is a very effective analgesic technique for patients with rib fractures. Peripheral nerve blocks can be used for patients with trauma to the upper or lower extremities. Inadequately controlled pain leads to a generalized stress response, with secondary effects on circulation, metabolism, oxygen consumption, and immune function. In patients with whom communication is possible, the numeric rating scale is a valuable tool to measure pain. The scale uses a 0 (no pain) to 10 (worst pain) scale and has been validated in critically ill patients. Appropriate pain control can eliminate the need for sedation in patients in ICU. Non-steroidal anti-inflammatory agents are useful drugs to provide

Table 19.1. Richmond agitation–sedation score

Score	Term	Description
+4	Combative	Overtly combative or violent; immediate danger to staff
+3	Very agitated	Pulls on or removes tube(s) or catheter(s) or has aggressive behavior towards staff
+2	Agitated	Frequent non-purposeful movement or patient–ventilator dyssynchrony
+1	Restless	Anxious or apprehensive but movements not aggressive or vigorous
0	Alert and calm	
−1	Drowsy	Not fully alert but has sustained (>10 seconds) awakening, with eye contact, to voice
−2	Light sedation	Briefly (10 seconds) awakens with eye contact to voice
−3	Moderate sedation	Any movement (but no eye contact) to voice
−4	Deep sedation	No response to voice, but any movement to physical stimulation
−5	Unarousable	No response to voice or physical stimulation

analgesia but should be avoided from the third trimester onwards as they can cause premature closure of the ductus arteriosus.

The drugs most frequently used for pain control are opioids. All opioids increase vagal tone and can, therefore, decrease fetal heart rate and reduce fetal heart rate variability. These effects are pharmacological and are not signs of adverse effects on the fetus. However, as a result, one of the signs of acute fetal distress is no longer helpful to assess the fetus during ICU stay. Repetitive or continuous application of drugs can lead to a substantial accumulation. It is, therefore, important to keep metabolic pathways and the presence or absence of active metabolites in mind. Accumulation of lipophilic drugs in adipose tissue can also lead to significant prolongation of drug half-life. Particularly in lipophilic drugs, half-life is very much dependent on the duration of infusion. Therefore the term "context-sensitive half-life" is of great importance. This describes the half-life of a drug based on the duration of infusion. The half-lives of diazepam, thiopental, and fentanyl increases rapidly with increasing duration of infusion. A very

notable exception is remifentanil. Remifentanil is a synthetic opioid that is hydrolyzed by plasma esterases independent of liver or renal function. Remifentanil has a reliably short half-life that is not dependent on the duration of infusion. This constant context-sensitive half-life, favors remifentanil for prolonged analgesia [5]. However, some short-acting opioids, particularly remifentanil, have been shown to be involved in opioid-induced hyperalgesia. Opioid-induced hyperalgesia is a "paradoxical" reduction in pain threshold in patients who have received opioids. There seems to be an involvement of the N-methyl-D-aspartate (NMDA) receptors, and ketamine, which is an antagonist of NMDA, decreases opioid-induced hyperalgesia. As a result, patients who have received remifentanil might experience more severe pain, particularly when remifentanil was given during a longer period [6].

Probably the most commonly used opioid for analgesia in the ICU is fentanyl. Fentanyl has a potency approximately 100 times higher than morphine. Fentanyl is a lipophilic drug and the context-sensitive half-life is, therefore, not constant. The main advantage of fentanyl is that elimination is mostly independent of organ function and there is – in contrast to morphine – no active metabolite.

Morphine and diamorphine are also used, and commonly used, in certain areas. Extrapolating from studies on labor analgesia, meperidine (pethidine) and the mixed agonist/antagonist agents nalbuphine and butorphanol may be used during pregnancy. These will seldom be relevant for the critically ill pregnant patient, however, as these drugs are not much used in the ICU.

Summary

Appropriate analgesia is of great importance in ICU patients. Fentanyl is the most frequently used drug for this purpose but can lead to a substantial "overhang" after prolonged administration. Remifentanil is a promising alternative with a stable context-sensitive half-life. However, additional options such as morphine are also excellent choices for sedation. As mentioned above, adequate analgesia can frequently reduce the need for sedation.

Sedation

Agitation is the most frequent reason to sedate the patient, and the drug of choice is usually midazolam. Midazolam is lipophilic and accumulates in adipose tissue, leading to an inconstant context-sensitive half-life. Clearance of midazolam is dependent on cytochrome P450 and is reduced in pathological liver dysfunction. Elimination of the active metabolite 1-hydroxymidazolam glucuronide is dependent on renal function. Apart from their accumulation, the main disadvantage of benzodiazepines is a withdrawal syndrome and a high incidence of delirium following sedation. These side effects delay extubation and prolong ICU stay. Flumazenil can be used as reversal agent. However its effects on pregnancy are unclear.

There is a growing trend to use propofol in ICU sedation. Propofol has the advantage of less accumulation and, therefore, has a more stable context-sensitive half-life. Although propofol seems to be an almost ideal sedative, there is concern about the propofol infusion syndrome. The etiology is not known in detail, but fatty acid metabolism and mitochondrial function seem to be involved [7]. Propofol infusion syndrome was first described in children under prolonged sedation (>48 hours) with high doses of propofol. Propofol infusion syndrome has a high mortality and there is no specific therapy. Although most frequently described in children, there are also reports of its occurrence in adults. Because propofol does cross the placenta, it may not be a wise choice for long-term (>24 hours) sedation of pregnant patients. This recommendation is absolutely arbitrary, as there are no data and no official recommendation on the use of propofol for ICU sedation in pregnant patients. It is unclear if there is a fetal form of the propofol infusion syndrome.

Another and more recently introduced drug for ICU sedation is the alpha-2 agonist dexmedetomidine. Dexmedetomidine has both sedative and analgesic properties and the short half-life is another advantage. Dexmedetomidine is associated with less delirium when compared with benzodiazepines for ICU sedation. Dexmedetomidine has not yet been investigated in pregnant patients and can, therefore, not be recommended.

Volatile anesthetics are frequently used for anesthesia in pregnant patients. More recently, volatile anesthetics have also been used for sedation in the ICU. They are delivered through the AnaConDa device. The main advantage is the lack of substantial accumulation. There are, however, no safety records on usage of volatile anesthetics over prolonged periods in pregnant women.

Other drugs

Although muscle relaxants are often used in ICU to facilitate mechanical ventilation, they are not absolutely required and in many instances, they are redundant. Since they cross the placenta, a cautious approach reducing their use is a good idea. However, when they are required, (cis)atracurium is our personal preference because of its unique pharmacokinetic profile (Hoffman degeneration not requiring enzymatic breakdown).

Conclusions

Analgesia and sedation are frequently used in ICU patients. Adequate analgesia is more important and can reduce the need for sedation. Whenever possible, a regional anesthesia technique should be used for analgesia. Accumulation is a major problem in long-term sedation and analgesia. It is, therefore, recommended that sedation and analgesia are interrupted on a daily basis and the patient allowed to awaken. Scoring systems should be used to quantify the level of both analgesia and sedation. There are little to no data about sedation and analgesia of the pregnant patient. From the data available, remifentanil and fentanyl seem to be reasonable choices for analgesia, as is midazolam for sedation. Propofol is commonly used but it is unclear if the drug is safe for prolonged sedation (>24 hours).

References

1. Jackson DL, Proudfoot CW, Cann KF, Walsh TS. The incidence of sub-optimal sedation in the ICU: a systematic review. *Crit Care* 2009;**13**:R204.
2. Van de Velde M. Nonobstetric Surgery during Pregnancy. In Chestnut DH, Polley LS, Tsen LC, Wong CA (eds.) *Obstetric Anesthesia*, 4th edn. Philadelphia, PA: Mosby-Elsevier, 2009, pp. 337–360.
3. Reitman E, Flood P. Anaesthetic considerations for non-obstetric surgery during pregnancy. *Br J Anaesth* 2011;**107**(Suppl 1):i72–i78.
4. Wu CL, Raja SN. Treatment of acute postoperative pain. *Lancet* 2011;**377**:2215–2225.
5. Ullman R, Smith LA, Burns E, Mori R, Dowswell T. Parenteral opioids for maternal pain relief in labor. *Cochrane Database Syst Rev* 2010(**9**):CD007396.
6. van Gulik L, Ahlers SJGM, van de Garde EMW, *et al.* Remifentanil during cardiac surgery is associated with chronic thoracic pain 1 yr after sternotomy. *Br J Anaesth* 2012;**109**:616–622.
7. Vasile B, Rasulo F, Candiani A, Latronico N. The pathophysiology of propofol infusion syndrome: a simple name for a complex syndrome. *Intensive Care Med* 2003;**29**:1417–1425.

Chapter 20

Nutrition

Michael P. Casaer, Jean T. Cox, and Sharon T. Phelan

Introduction

Women of reproductive age are generally healthy. However, because of direct complications of pregnancy (e.g. pre-eclampsia with hypertensive events or hyperemesis gravidarum), indirect complications of pregnancy (e.g. worsening cardiac disease, community-acquired pneumonia, urosepsis), or unrelated pathology (e.g. trauma, burns, cancer), approximately 1% of pregnant women may require intensive care unit (ICU) admission, with a fetal mortality rate up to 32% and maternal mortality rate of 12–20%. Sepsis-related multiple organ failure is the leading cause of maternal death, followed by intracranial hemorrhage [1]. Often women admitted to an ICU are unable to maintain their normal diet and nutritional intake. Maternal basal metabolism and nutrient oxidation is increased by inflammation and infection. Critical illness catabolism, however, provides a high flux of endogenous nutrients through proteolysis and lipolysis. This induced tissue breakdown, mediated by catecholamines, cortisol, interleukins, glucagon and others, is not effectively suppressed by enhanced nutritional intake [2,3]. Although a fetus can tolerate a day or two of minimal nutrient intake, prolonged malnourishment may have significant impact on both the woman and her fetus and further complicate the disease that initially prompted the ICU admission. To aid in the nutritional care of such patients, this chapter will outline typical nutritional needs for a pregnant woman, review some of the unique issues of administering adequate nutrition for the benefit of the maternal–fetal dyad, and will provide an overview of some of the more common clinical situations. While recommendations on optimal feeding during pregnancy are supported by robust data from adequately powered randomized controlled trials [4–6] and epidemiological analyses mainly focused on the child's well-being [7,8], critical care nutrition is largely based on association, assumption, and rather small methodologically weaker randomized controlled trials [9]. Evidence to guide nutrition in the pregnant critically ill patient is not available. The main message, therefore, is to prevent micronutrient deficiencies, avoid hypo- and hyperglycemia, and to hesitate before initiating aggressive therapy not supported by reliable scientific evidence.

Maternal nutritional requirements for a pregnancy

In general, calorie, protein, vitamin, and mineral requirements during pregnancy are increased over non-pregnant needs as the mother has increased demands herself and is nourishing a very metabolically active growing fetus. On average, a normal pregnant women needs approximately 300 kcal more per day to meet demands of a singleton pregnancy, particularly during the last half of the pregnancy, when up to an additional 450 kcal/day may be required. The increase in both maternal and fetal tissue enhances the oxygen requirements and the basal metabolic rate by 15–20%. If a patient is undernourished, she will need another 300 kcal more from early in the pregnancy and even more later because of the greater fetal requirements.

The infant is dependent on glucose for its primary energy source so it will effectively take glucose from the mother regardless of her nutritional status. Additional glucose requirements at term may be over 30 g/day. However, hyperglycemia is as problematic as hypoglycemia. Hyperglycemia promotes fetal macrosomia, anomalies (if present during organogenesis), and premature aging of the placenta through toxic effects of hyperglycemia on placental and fetal blood vessels. Each of these can result in a complicated pregnancy and/or delivery. Ideally blood sugar should be in the range 70–120 mg/dL (3.9–6.5 mmol/L)

Maternal Critical Care: A Multidisciplinary Approach, ed. Marc Van de Velde, Helen Scholefield, and Lauren A. Plante.
Published by Cambridge University Press. © Cambridge University Press 2013.

consistently throughout the day to optimally meet the needs of both individuals.

Free fatty acids, especially the essential ones, are needed for the development of the fetal central nervous system. The essential fatty acids linoleic acid and alpha-linolenic acid are precursors of arachidonic acid and docosahexanoic acid, respectively, and are particularly important in brain and blood vessel development. The placenta is very effective in transferring these free fatty acids. The presence of the hormone human placental lactogen promotes lipolysis of maternal adipose tissue, thereby increasing the amount of free fatty acids in maternal serum later in pregnancy. Moreover, mobilization of this maternal caloric source protects more of the maternal glucose for the fetal growth. The presence of human placental lactogen, however, makes pregnant women somewhat insulin resistant and can precipitate gestational diabetes or worsen pre-existing diabetes. Lipid intake should account for 20–25% of the non-protein calories to meet the essential fatty acid requirements.

Protein requirements are initially about 60 g/day (approximately 1 g/kg maternal weight) for the average woman. This needs to be increased by about 20% as the pregnancy progresses into the second and third trimesters [10]. The protein sources should be balanced and primarily of high biological value. Because of changes in maternal physiology, monitoring status by serum protein levels and urea nitrogen excretion may not work well [10].

With adequate nutrition, the expected weight gain during a typical singleton pregnancy in an average weight woman is around 25–35 pounds (11.5–16.0 kg). Women who enter a pregnancy markedly underweight (body mass index (BMI) <18.5 kg/m^2) or as very young adolescents will often benefit from a weight gain in the range 28–40 pounds (12.5–18 kg). Women entering pregnancy already obese (BMI ≥30) may be advised to gain only 11–20 pounds (5–9 kg) [11]. The important point for the provider is that actual weight gain is only a proxy of nutritional status. A woman can gain an "appropriate" amount of weight with a very nutritionally inadequate diet. This can be even more problematic in the ICU where fluid shifts, edema, and other confounders may make maternal weight an ineffective way to assess nutrient intake. Weight gain recommendations will vary based on maternal status going into the pregnancy. Clearly, poorly nourished and underweight women or women with a multiple gestation are more at risk of fetal compromise through nutritional issues

during pregnancy. They also have less reserve in the event of a major medical complication. It is important to remember that obese women may be calorically oversupplied but commonly have poor nutritional intake of protein, vitamins, and key minerals. There is a tendency to assume that an obese woman (pregnant or not) is in less need of nutritional assessment and that she might benefit from fasting. This is a poor assumption and can cause harm to both the woman and her fetus.

Fetal implications of poor maternal nutrition

To compound these concerns, it is becoming more apparent that the environment that a fetus experiences in utero has long-term effects on its health and survival [12]. Inadequate maternal nutrition may be associated with a low infant birth weight and is significantly correlated with later development of adult diseases such as cardiovascular disease, stroke, obesity and type 2 diabetes mellitus, even when adjusting for lifestyle factors. This is thought to be a consequence of upregulation in utero by the fetal "thrifty genes" [13]. Maternal obesity also significantly increases (by 30%) fetal and neonatal adiposity, which increases risk of obesity in the child in later life. If poor fetal growth is caused by maternal starvation, there may be neurological impairment [14]. Other increasing populations at risk for nutritional problems are women with bariatric surgery or those with significant underlying eating disorders. A provider needs to understand the impact of the surgical intervention for absorption in the setting of bariatric surgery – Roux-en-Y (malabsorption) versus a banding (restrictive) procedure. In either there is a risk of nutritional deficiencies, particularly iron, folate, calcium, vitamins A, B$_{12}$, and K. In the setting of severe eating disorders, the deficiency can be prolonged and severe with not only nutritional concerns but also severe metabolic derangements that can seriously compromise maternal and fetal status.

Nutritional considerations during critical illness

The first step is to stabilize the patient as quickly as possible from the initial insult. Ultimately, the extent of the initial insult and the rapid stabilization of the mother has more impact on the patient and the fetus than the management of the specific issues of pregnancy-related nutrition. However, once the woman is stabilized, consideration must be quickly given to the need for nutritional support during the remainder of the ICU and hospital stay. This involves determining whether current intake meets the nutritional needs of the patient, given her medical status, along with the requirements of the pregnancy. If not, the best method to achieve this balance needs to be determined considering the indicated dietary restrictions of the mother (e.g. liver failure may require decreased protein intake) and how best to provide the additional nutrients. Although this can be accomplished through oral intake, tube feeding, or intravenous nutrition, there are significant advantages and risks to each modality in a critically ill pregnant woman. The risk–benefits of each mode need to be considered prior to implementation.

The optimal energy and nutrient intake would be the one resulting in improved clinical outcome during critical illness. Unfortunately, different energy doses have never been adequately compared in the critically ill population even outside of pregnancy, let alone in the critically ill pregnant patient. Indirect calorimetry is considered to be the gold standard to determine energy requirements in the critically ill. This uses respiratory gas exchange to estimate the caloric consumption. Since gas exchange is key to the calculations, any interference such as oxygen supplementation, unstable cardiovascular status, fever, and other medical complications will compromise the estimate. Also interventions such as chest drains, high inspiratory oxygen fraction, renal replacement therapy, and so on add to measurement errors with this method [15]. Enhanced nutrition itself increases measured energy expenditure values [16]. More fundamentally, there is no reason to assume that the amount of energy being burned is an indication of the amount of energy that should be given to the critically ill patient. As mentioned above, much of this will be drawn from muscle and adipose tissue, and this flux of endogenous nutrients will not stop when exogenous nutrition is added [2,3]. The first pilot trial comparing nutrition guided by indirect calorimetry to standard formula calculation-based nutrition showed more complications and prolonged organ failure but an unexplained decrease in hospital mortality with indirect calorimetry [17]. However, energy calculations – traditionally the Harris–Benedict formula with adjustments for pregnancy and particular medical conditions – are also not recommended, since they confer a degree of precision that evidence does not support.

Administering nutrients to patients in intensive care

General considerations

The goal of optimized nutrition during critical illness is to improve outcome by attenuating catabolism. It is, however, unclear if enhanced nutrition can suppress catabolism. Indeed, the driving force behind catabolism in the critically ill is not the decreased intake of food but the inflammatory response [2,3,18]. International guidelines on nutrition in the (non-pregnant) critically ill adult agree, however, that enteral nutrition should be initiated as soon as possible in order to prevent nutritional debt from accumulating [19,20]. Large observational trials indeed showed an association between inadequate nutrition early during critical illness and increased morbidity, even mortality [21,22]. Although these data are a good basis for hypothesis generation, they are not enough for guiding therapy. This is true for all observational data but in particular for nutrition and recovery; they are closely linked, making it impossible to draw conclusions on causality. Interestingly, very few studies have randomized critically ill patients to nutrition versus no-nutrition or delayed nutrition, the only approach that could detect whether enhanced feeding is beneficial. These trials suggested reduced mortality with feeding but even their meta-analyses were 10-fold underpowered [23]. Recent randomized trials comparing minimal versus closer to target enteral nutrition showed no benefit at all with higher intakes [24,25]. In two large cluster randomized studies implementing nutrition guidelines, while the first study demonstrated shortened hospital stay in the intervention hospitals, the second found no improvement of clinical outcome despite enhanced nutrition [26]. European and American/Canadian guidelines disagree on the initiation of parenteral nutrition (PN) when enteral nutrition (EN) is not sufficient. The first advise considering PN within 48 hours in order to prevent nutritional deficit to accumulate, the latter prefer tolerating hypocaloric feeding for up to 1 week [19,27].

The EPaNIC trial recently compared the impact of early initiation of PN to supplement insufficient EN up to nutritional target (early PN group) to withholding parenteral nutrition during the first week in ICU (late PN group), accepting in the latter approach that an important nutritional deficit would build up over the first week of critical illness. Patients in both groups received parenteral micronutrients until adequate EN was achieved. The EPaNIC trial is the first randomized controlled trial on nutrition in (non-pregnant) critically ill patients with enough power to detect or rule out clinically meaningful differences in outcome. Of a total of 4640 patients, 2312 patients were allocated to the early PN group and 2328 to the late PN group. All analyzes were on an intention-to-treat basis and defined in a previously published statistical analysis plan [28,29].

Unexpectedly, the EPaNIC trial showed a clear benefit from late PN. Recovery of organ functions was enhanced and the incidence of new infections was reduced from 26.2 to 22.8% ($p = 0.04$). Time to alive discharge from the ICU was the primary efficacy endpoint. The likelihood of being discharged earlier in the late PN group was 1.06 (95% confidence interval (CI), 1.00–1.13; $p = 0.04$) compared with early PN in a Cox proportional hazard analysis corrected for type and severity of disease. Use of late PN also shortened median hospital stay by 2 days (hazard ratio, 1.06; 95% CI, 1.00–1.13; $p = 0.04$) without affecting functionality at hospital discharge and it reduced mean healthcare-related costs during hospitalization per patient by €1110 ($p = 0.04$). The beneficial effect of late PN was even more pronounced in patients with a contraindication for EN at ICU admission even though in these patients the intervention came down to almost no feeding.

Other similar studies have been submitted for publication or are ongoing and will help to further guide our view on what is optimal for patients unable to feed themselves because of critical illness. Unfortunately, there are no large-scale studies addressing this issue in pregnant ICU patients.

Enteral feeding. This is probably less dangerous than PN since it is less invasive and utilizes the normal physiology of the gastrointestinal tract, thereby precluding the administration of high doses of macronutrients. The gastrointestinal tract also modulates the absorption of many nutrients such as calcium, iron, and magnesium, thus avoiding toxic excess [30]. This, in turn, makes it easier to maintain maternal homeostasis, particularly normoglycemia. The first pass through the portal system is a crucial step in the regulation of glucose and amino acid metabolism. The use of enteral feeding may help to maintain bowel function and mucosal integrity, thus potentially preventing bacterial translocation to the bloodstream and remote organs. By

avoiding PN, EN reduces the risk of infections and eventually thrombosis. Although oral intake is least invasive, many patients are too weak or mentally unable to deal with the effort to effectively swallow adequate volumes. This can be overcome with the use of tube feeding. Nasogastric tube feeding can provide concentrated nutritional sources but still depends on an intact and functional intestinal system. The rate of the infusion may require careful titration of flow rates. These flow rates may need to be modified in pregnancy to minimize the risk of reflux and aspiration, which can be greater because of the upward displacement of the stomach and relaxation of the esophageal–gastric sphincter. This may be further influenced by medications being used or the underlying medical/trauma insult that prompted the admission. When determining flow rates, the normal slower emptying rate of the maternal stomach and slower intestinal transit time must be taken into consideration. Continuous feeding with periodic checks of residual volume to guide the rate of infusion may help to avoid gastric distention and the associated risk of regurgitation [30], although checking gastric residual volume has not proven to be beneficial in the general ICU population [31]. Contraindications to enteral feedings include gastrointestinal obstruction, fistulas, or bleeds; ileus; and severe diarrhea.

Parenteral nutrition. Many of the pathologies requiring ICU admission will compromise gastrointestinal function through hypotensive shock, septic shock, ileus from bowel injury, or surgery. Whether, how, and when these patients benefit from intravenous nutrition through a peripheral or central line is debated. Nevertheless, this approach allows the gastrointestinal system to be bypassed while still providing adequate calories and essential nutrients for maternal and fetal support. However total parenteral nutrition has (TPN) numerous risks in addition to the basic risks of a central line. Pregnant women are immunologically suppressed, which may make them less responsive when exposed to an infectious insult. The combination of pregnancy, medical insult with ICU admission, and an invasive line increases the risk of maternal sepsis significantly [10,30,32]. In some review studies, up to one third of pregnant patients on TPN experience an infectious complication and over 66% require treatment for infections, thromboembolism, or both. The increased incidence of infections with early PN as compared with hypocaloric feeding has been discussed above [29]. The relative insulin resistance of the maternal physiology makes control of glucose levels challenging. Although the infant can tolerate hypoglycemia in the mother, being able to selectively transport glucose across the placenta, hyperglycemia is problematic [33]. The detrimental effects of hyperglycemia include polyhydramnios, fetal macrosomia, fetal hepatomegaly, fetal cardiomegaly, congenital anomalies (if occurring during the first trimester), and perinatal death. Maternal hyperglycemia causes fetal hyperglycemia, which, in turn, increases insulin release in the fetus and subsequent increased fetal oxygen demands. If these demands are not met, the fetus can become hypoxic and acidotic. Since hyperglycemia itself can reduce perfusion of the placenta, placental insufficiency is a significant risk in the setting of a critically ill patient.

The challenge for the clinician will, therefore, be to balance the well-known PN-related risks in a setting where transient (~1 week) hypocaloric feeding might have unpredictable consequences for mother and child. Vigilant monitoring for signs of evident macronutrient deficiency when choosing to withhold PN seems advisable. The focus should be directed towards hypoglycemia since hypoalbuminemia, ketones, and electrolyte abnormalities can be caused either by the disease process or by nutritional problems. Spontaneous hypoglycemia (in the absence of insulin administration) should prompt administration of at least some parenteral nutrition.

Many of the commercial solutions for either EN or TPN are not designed for pregnancy and commonly do not have adequate iron, trace elements, and vitamins for the requirements of the maternal–fetal dyad. The actual recommendations for each nutrient vary by country and professional organizations. Table 20.1 represents the US recommendations. Close monitoring of liver

Table 20.1. Selected nutritional recommended intakes for the healthy non-pregnant and pregnant women in the USA

Nutrient	Non-pregnant recommended, daily	Pregnant recommended, daily	Maximum supplementation for pregnancy[a]	Special considerations, daily
Protein (g)	46	71		~1 g/kg maternal weight
Carbohydrates (g)	130	175		
Fat (g)				
Total	ND	ND		
Linoleic acid (g)	12	13		
Alpha-linolenic acid (g)	1.1	1.4		
Vitamins				
A (retinol) (µg)	700	770	3000	Excessive levels may increase fetal anomalies
C (mg)	75	85	2000	Deficiencies associated with premature rupture of membranes
D (µg)	15	15	100	Increased recently
E (mg)	15	15	1000	Low birth weight or growth restriction with low levels
K (µg)	90	90	ND	Bleeding in fetus can cause injury; may require intramuscular supplementation
B_1 (thiamine) (mg)	1.1	1.4	ND	

Table 20.1. *(cont.)*

Nutrient	Non-pregnant recommended, daily	Pregnant recommended, daily	Maximum supplementation for pregnancy[a]	Special considerations, daily
B$_2$ (riboflavin) (mg)	1.1	1.4	ND	
B$_3$ (niacin) (mg)	14	18	35	
B$_6$ (mg)	1.3	1.9	100	
Folate (μg)	400	600	1000	Deficiency impairs cell division and protein synthesis, giving megaloblastic anemia in mother and neural tube defect and low birth weight in infant
B$_{12}$ (μg)	2.4	2.6	ND	
Minerals				
Iron (mg)	18	27	45	Deficiency more common in pregnancy and/or obesity; may be associated with low birth weight
Calcium (mg)	1000	1000	2.5	Teenagers may need up to 1300 mg/day; deficiency associated with decreased fetal bone density
Copper (μg)	900	1000	10 000	Both increased zinc intake (for wound healing or to improve immune response) and iron intake can depress copper levels
Iodine (μg)	150	220	1100	Usually not a problem because of the use of iodine antiseptic preparations
Magnesium (mg)	310	350	350, as supplements	Deficiency from renal loss or gastrointestinal loss through malabsorption
Selenium (μg)	55	60	400	
Zinc (mg)	8	11–12	40	Needed for DNA, immunological response, and wound healing; deficiency often after trauma or prolonged total parenteral nutrition; associated with fetal intrauterine growth retardation

ND, not determined.
[a] The maximum refers to daily routine use maximums and not therapeutic levels.
Source: adapted from Otten *et al.*, 2006 [34].

function tests, iron, ferritin, vitamin B$_{12}$, folate, thiamine, and trace elements are indicated. A recent article outlined recommended serum levels at different times during pregnancy and can be used as a reference as needed [35] (Table 20.2). Non-pregnant laboratory values are often inappropriate. For example, when monitoring triglyceride and lipid levels, it must be realized that during pregnancy these levels are commonly increased by 40% or more.

Although peripheral intravenous administration might have fewer complications, it rarely can achieve the nutrient loads of calories, protein, and fats required by the maternal–fetal dyad without excessive fluid load. Sometimes multiple approaches to nutritional supplementation may be necessary simultaneously.

The key issue is that attention must be given to ongoing nutritional assessment and support within 24–48 hours of admission to an ICU, or sooner once

Table 20.2. Selected laboratory studies by trimester of pregnancy compared with non-pregnant women

Common laboratory tests	Non-pregnant	Pregnant[a]		
		First trimester	Second trimester	Third trimester
Albumin (g/dL)	4.1–5.3	3.1–5.1	2.6–4.5	2.3–4.2
Protein, total (g/dL)	6.7–8.6	6.2–7.6	5.7–6.9	5.6–6.7
Creatinine (mg/dL)	0.5–0.9	0.4–0.7	0.4–0.8	0.4–0.9
Cholesterol, total (mg/dL)	<200	141–210	176–299	219–349
Triglycerides (mg/dL)	<150	40–159	75–382	131–453
Vitamin A (retinol) (μg/dL)	20–100	32–47	35–44	29–42
Vitamin C (mg/dL)	0.4–1.0	ND	ND	0.9–1.3
25-Hydroxyvitamin D (ng/mL)	14–80	18–27	10–22	10–18
Vitamin E (alpha-tocopherol) (μg/mL)	5–18	7–13	10–16	13–23
Folate, serum (ng/mL)	5.4–18.0	2.6–15.0	0.8–24.0	1.4–20.7
Vitamin B_{12} (pg/mL)	279–966	118–438	130–656	99–526
Thiamine (ng/mL)	44–52	24–40	24–42	23–45
Hemoglobin (g/dL)	12–15.8	11.6–13.9	9.7–14.8	9.5–15.0
Hematocrit (%)	35.4–44.4	31.0–41.0	30.0–39.0	28.0–40.0
Ferritin (ng/mL)	10–150	6–130	2–230	0–116
Iron, serum (μg/dL)	41–141	72–143	44–178	30–193
Calcium, total (mg/dL)	8.7–10.2	8.8–10.6	8.2–9.0	8.2–9.7
Copper (μg/dL)	70–140	112–199	165–221	130–240
Magnesium (mg/dL)	1.5–2.3	1.6–2.2	1.5–2.2	1.1–2.2
Phosphate (mg/dL)	2.5–4.3	3.1–4.6	2.5–4.6	2.8–4.6
Selenium (μg/L)	63–160	116–146	75–145	71–133
Zinc (μg/dL)	75–120	57–88	51–80	50–77
Creatinine, 24 hour clearance (mL/min)	91–130	69–140	55–136	50–166

ND, not determined.
These are only generalizations to serve as a guide. They are derived through combinations of data reviews and direct patient evaluations during pregnancy of healthy women without major medical confounders.
Sources: adapted from Abbassi-Ghanavati, *et al.*, 2009 [32]; Baker, *et al.*, 2002 [35].

the pregnant patient is stabilized. In all patients not adequately fed by mouth, micronutrients (in particular selenium) should be administered; EN should be attempted and blood glucose fluctuations should be avoided. It is probably safe to give 200–400 kcal of parenteral glucose 5% plus potassium and phosphorus until some EN is achieved. The goal for nutrition in the pregnant patient is not simply to maintain the mother's status but also to build a fetus. The decision when to opt for more enhanced EN methods, such as postbulbar feeding, or gastroprokinetics (e.g. metoclopramide or erythromycin) and when to initiate PN in order to obtain these goals should be taken cautiously.

Specific situations that prompt admission to intensive care

The situations that prompt admission to ICU can be direct complications of pregnancy or unrelated to the pregnancy but still impact the pregnancy.

Complications of pre-eclampsia with renal, neurological, or liver compromise

Patients with pre-eclampsia or eclampsia are at significant risk for adult respiratory distress syndrome (ARDS), cardiac dysfunction, seizure, and/or stroke. Eclampsia is a multiorgan disease that causes vascular bed spasm with marked third spacing of fluid, hemo-concentration, and ischemic changes in liver and kidneys; it may even precipitate disseminated intravascular coagulation or neurological events. Although pre-eclampsia or eclampsia tend to be self-limiting, with resolution shortly after birth, the complicating events (renal failure, intracerebral bleeding, liver failure, or ARDS) can result in a long complicated hospital stay. Since delivery often happens about the same time as the need for ICU admission, the nutritional concerns relative to the fetus are often not an issue in the ICU. In the situation where the obstetric plan is to provide antenatal steroids prior to delivery, a pregnant patient may be admitted to ICU for a few days. In the setting of pre-eclampsia, fluid management is difficult and aims to allow maintenance of fluid perfusion of organs while not precipitating ARDS.

In the setting of pre-eclampsia and eclampsia, withholding PN for up to 1 week while attempting to start some EN will probably be the safest option. The risk for prolonged fetal underfeeding is low and early recovery of gastrointestinal function is very likely.

Sepsis

Because of the downregulation of the immune system, pregnant patients are more at risk from sepsis, particularly urosepsis and pneumonia [1]. Sepsis, like other inflammatory conditions, is a catabolic state. An inflammatory state differs from what is typically seen in chronic starvation. With starvation, there are initial physiological mechanisms that tend to protect lean muscle mass in the non-pregnant adult. The inflammatory state, however, is characterized by early and not suppressible muscle breakdown [2,3]. It is unclear if this is the same or worse in the pregnant patient and if nutrition can attenuate the consequences for mother and child. In the setting of shock, blood flow is directed from the gastrointestinal tract to the central nervous and cardiac systems. Consequently, perfusion of the gastrointestinal mucosa is compromised and this may result in ischemic injury because the intestines have a high metabolic rate; this, in turn, increases the risk of intestinal bacteria getting into the circulation. Some recommend that the mucosal pH is followed to track this problem but there are no studies to see if this is useful in the pregnant patient. These are the patients who are most likely to have a prolonged stay with insufficient EN while still carrying a child, but they are also more likely to suffer from the complications of early PN. Our general recommendation still holds: to try some EN with background 200–400 kcal glucose and micronutrients, and maintain close monitoring for hypo- and hyperglycemia.

Burns

Extensive burns result in a very serious metabolical burden for all patients. Nutritional needs for the mother alone may double, not accounting for possible increasing fetal needs. Unfortunately, predictive formulas for patients with burns are not very reliable because of huge individual variability [36]. Therefore, the risks of over- or underfeeding should be feared. For this reason, indirect calorimetry may be the best method to estimate needs. Moreover, patients with extended burn wounds have increased losses of all micronutrients in the wound secretions. Central and peripheral line access may also be compromised and the risk for catheter-related bloodstream infection increased. Nutritional consultation and intervention is needed early in care. Ideally, severely burned pregnant patients should be taken care of by an experienced burn team with input from the maternal–fetal medicine team.

Multiple trauma: hypovolemia with extensive soft tissue and bony injury

In the setting of extensive trauma, there can be major fluid shifts and third spacing. In pregnancy, these shifts can often be hard to assess. These changes make maternal weight irrelevant as a tool to assess nutritional status. Detailed evaluation and assessment of needs must be done proactively and followed with laboratory testing for ketones, which increase when caloric needs are met by increased lipolysis, nitrites, and other abnormalities. Given blood loss-induced anemia and the impact of altered (upregulated) hepcidin, appropriate iron supplementation can be difficult to ascertain.

Adult respiratory distress syndrome provoked by sepsis, shock, or infections

The commonly occurring respiratory acidosis of ARDS results in hyperkalemia, which, in turn, causes hypophosphatemia and can trigger muscle weakness. This can be problematic with the pregnant woman's need to "breathe for two." Also, these patients tend be critically ill for a longer time (median 18 days; interquartile range, 10–20) in community-acquired pneumonia [1], so the option to accept a short period of moderately hypocaloric feeding until physical recovery and spontaneous feeding occurs becomes rather unrealistic. Luckily, these patients most often do tolerate some EN.

Cardiac decompensation

Given the 40% increase in vascular volume during pregnancy, women with cardiac disease characterized by a fixed output, may decompensate during pregnancy. This poses the challenge of meeting nutritional needs while not fluid overloading the mother. In patients on successful EN, energy-dense nutrition can be considered, with increased caution for overfeeding and for glycemic dysregulation during and after nutrition pauses.

Renal failure

Pregnant patients with renal failure will often require additional protein and calorie intake, particularly in the setting of dialysis. Whether positive nitrogen balances improve outcome for the mother–fetal dyad is unclear. The often cited study investigating this issue in non-pregnant adults demonstrated that improved nitrogen balance with enhanced protein intake did not improve outcome [37]. To provide the additional nutrients without fluid overloading the patient who is not yet on dialysis will be challenging. Continuous renal replacement therapy simplifies fluid management but can result in increased losses of macro- and micronutrients [38].

Cancer and other chronic diseases

Severe chronic disease can contribute both to poor nutritional status and marked anemia. In cancer this can result from both treatment with chemotherapy or radiation and suppressed erythropoietin response from long-standing cancer. This can be further complicated in the pregnant patient because of the nausea and vomiting common in pregnancy.

Severe hyperemesis

Patients with severe hyperemesis typically are not admitted to ICU but they can get severe electrolyte imbalance and, through chronic malnutrition, need aggressive but careful nutritional support. These patients need thiamine and typically vitamin B_6 early in their care since introduction of high levels of only glucose as a calorie source may precipitate a refeeding syndrome, including Wernicke's encephalopathy. Use of TPN is fraught with septic risks, as seen readily in the medical literature, and can even result in death from sepsis. Since most of these patients have an intact intestinal system, TPN should be used as a last resort when pharmaceutical interventions and tube feeding are unable to maintain nutrient intake.

Generalized issues of nutritional concerns in the intensive care setting

Refeeding syndrome is a dangerous complication of nutrition therapy initiated after a period of starvation. Indeed, starvation is characterized by gluconeogenesis, protein catabolism, and losses of water, vitamins, and minerals. The time frame in which this develops can be variable, depending on patient's nutritional status prior to the event that prompted the ICU admission, the metabolic demands of the event (i.e. sepsis versus pre-eclampsia), and nutritional intake. Upon initiation of nutrition, often with glucose initially, blood insulin and cell glucose uptake increase, resulting in increased thiamine utilization and eventually thiamine deficiency. This increased glucose intake, in turn, increases intracellular transport of magnesium, and potassium, resulting in hypophosphatemia, hypomagnesemia, and hypokalemia. The hypophosphatemia can lead to severe if not fatal cardiopulmonary dysfunction, convulsions, and altered mental status [30]. This is the situation experienced by the patient with severe hyperemesis, severe eating disorders, pancreatitis, cancer, or prolonged hospitalization without attention to nutritional status. In one study [39], up to one third of ICU patients demonstrated refeeding hypophosphatemia. Such at-risk patients need to be monitored for complications by following laboratory results for hypophosphatemia, hypokalemia, and hypomagnesemia as well as for the other nutrients already discussed. Electrolytes may need to be followed more frequently when initially refeeding, but once the patient is stabilized monitoring may be decreased to every 1–3 days depending on the underlying medical situation.

During pregnancy, the vascular volume must increase by 40%, which requires increased production of red blood cells. For this reason, iron deficiency-related anemia is common in pregnancy, particularly in the latter half of gestation. Anemia is common in the setting of chronic inflammatory diseases (cancer, irritable bowel syndrome, congestive heart failure) as well as in sepsis and renal failure. Anemia in the critically ill patient is a reflection of both inflammation and iron deficiency. This is thought to result from a series of events including shortened red blood cell life span, inadequate erythropoietin response to the severity of anemia, erythroid cells not being as receptive to erythropoietin, and inhibited red cell proliferation and differentiation. Through a complicated pathway, this leads to low serum iron and decreased transferrin saturation despite normal or high ferritin [40]. To complicate the situation further, a liver-derived peptide that is a negative regulator of iron stores, hepcidin, has now been described. Typically, it is suppressed by erythropoiesis and iron deficiency and upregulated with iron overload [41]. Inflammatory processes or stress pathways will increase hepcidin levels. Hepcidin works by decreasing iron absorption across the gastrointestinal tract and the release of iron from the reticuloendothelial system. There is no information currently available on how pregnancy affects this process [41].

Because ferritin synthesis is induced by inflammation independently of iron stores, increased ferritin concentration does not necessarily indicate adequate iron stores. However, most critically ill patients have varying degrees of iron-deficiency anemia. The typical estimated blood loss from blood draws in an intensive care setting is over 125 mL/day. Nutritional sources are typically low in iron. Thus in the setting of high ferritin levels, iron status must be determined more by serum iron, hypochromic microcytic red blood cells, and a low reticulocyte count for the level of anemia [40].

Folate deficiency determination by assessment of mean corpuscular volume is very insensitive, particularly in the setting of iron deficiency. Folate deficiency is a reflection of the folate balance over many months. Folate determination needs to be done by direct measurement of folate in serum or plasma. This is a very sensitive assessment of recent folate intake and utilization [42].

Vitamin B_{12} status is also challenging in pregnancy. In pregnancy, low serum cobalamin does not accurately reflect tissue levels even when <150 ng/L. Functional biomarkers such as serum methylmalonic acid and serum total homocysteine reflect an accumulation of unmetabolized precursors because of the lack of adequate vitamin B_{12}. However, these markers are also limited as they will be changed also by folate deficiency and become uncoupled from vitamin B_{12} status with advanced gestation. Patients with a prior good nutritional status are unlikely to have vitamin B_{12} deficiency. However in the setting of an ICU admission, particularly with chronic disease, weekly supplementation is likely a reasonable approach.

Supplementation

Carbohydrates are typically given as dextrose, which yields about 4 kcal/g. However, when this is metabolized it uses more oxygen, generates increased carbon dioxide production, and can increase lipogenesis, which may worsen the status of an ICU patient, particularly those with cardiopulmonary problems [10].

Fat emulsions can provide a denser source of calories (9 kcal/g). The metabolism of fats uses less oxygen and produces less carbon dioxide while providing essential fatty acids for fetal brain development, nerve myelination, and lung surfactant. The emulsions used are commonly infused for only 12 hours per day. This gives a higher concentration gradient to improve placental passive diffusion. There is a great deal of debate among intensivists regarding the best fat emulsion to use (fish oil, olive oil, etc.). This should be a discussion between the ICU physicians and the obstetrician, with input from the nutritionist.

Protein requirements during pregnancy are significantly increased in the average gravida, as a source of both energy (4 kcal/g) and amino acids for tissue formation. Animal experiments have found that protein deficiency results in the pregnant animal losing weight. The earlier the deficiency the more severe the adverse effects, including fetal pup mortality and morbidity, including growth restriction. However, a significant protein deficiency often is accompanied by a marked decrease in calories and other nutrients. The specific effects of protein deficiency in the setting of adequate calorie and micronutrient supplementation in the critically ill gravida is unclear [30]. There will be decreased protein synthesis as well as decreased serum albumin, transferrin, prealbumin, and binding globulins. Given that albumin is also decreased in the inflammatory response, it may not be the best marker for nutritional status in the acutely ill patient, particularly the pregnant patient. Monitoring of protein status is challenging, particularly during pregnancy when both nitrogen balance and creatinine clearance are markedly altered. Most commercially available amino acid products seem to be adequate to support fetal growth [10].

Water supplementation during an ICU stay can be challenging. Although the total body water content of a woman during pregnancy increases by 8 to 9 L, this translates only to 30–50 mL more fluid/day of pregnancy. However, because of increased urine output and pulmonary losses from tachypnea of pregnancy, fluid demands in pregnancy are clearly increased beyond this. In the setting of trauma, burns, or sepsis, the baseline needs for water are greatly increased in pregnancy and those must be accommodated. In contrast, fluid restriction may be necessary to prevent exacerbation of cardiopulmonary status in those with either

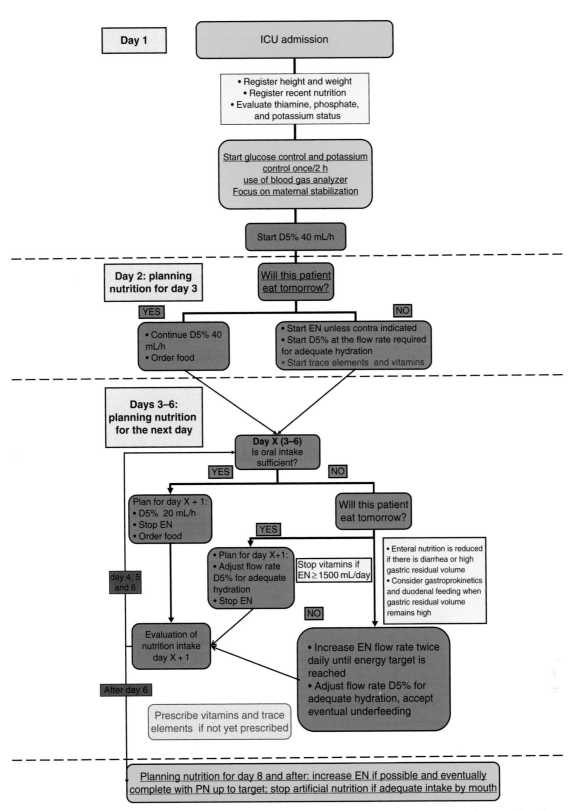

Figure 20.1. A dynamic early nutrional assessment and management protocol. EN, enteral nutrition; PN, parenteral nutrition; D5%, dextrose 5% (sodium chloride and potassium phosphate are added to this solution according to the plasma levels and renal function).

213

Box 20.1. Suggestions for monitoring nutritional supplementation in pregnancy during hospitalization

- Daily weight: being careful to interpret this in light of third spacing
- Fluids and calories: intake and output
- Urine for glucose and ketones: these are marginal for evaluating for the development of diabetes because of the increased glomerular filtration rate and typically high-sugar/high-carbohydrate intake in ICU. Urine glycosuria should be verified with serum measurements since pregnant women will lose sugar at a normal serum level because of the greater kindney clearance
- Blood sugars: every 6–12 hours once stabilized and as often as every 1–2 hours when initiating supplementation; measure during critical illness with a blood gas analyzer
- Daily electrolytes: calcium, phosphate, magnesium
- Liver function tests and albumin: every 2–3 days; albumin is typically low in pregnancy
- Nitrogen balance: calculate at least weekly
- Fundal height: measure every 1–2 weeks
- Antenatal testing with amniotic fluid index: if pregnancy greater than 28 weeks, consider frequent testing; the maternal–fetal medicine team can guide the frequency, which may be from twice daily to twice weekly
- Fetal ultrasound: every 3–4 weeks for interval growth

prolonged organ failure. The initial focus for nutritional supplementation should be to optimize the micronutrients, avoid hypo- or hyperglycemia, and maintain an appropriate fluid balance (Figure 20.1). As the situation stabilizes, then efforts towards adequate macronutrients and calories can be undertaken, while avoiding refeeding syndrome, avoiding overfeeding, and balancing the iatrogenic complications of aggressive EN or PN against the risks of underfeeding (Box 20.1). This is often best done with the guidance of a professional trained in the complexities of nutrition therapy.

Key points

- Stabilize the condition of the mother first. The best thing for the fetus is a good maternal cardiopulmonary status. Keep maternal status and well-being paramount.
- There is no need to rush to provide adequate macronutrients if micronutrients are provided early. The fetus can handle a few days as needed to stabilize the mother.
- Try to use enteral supplementation as much as feasible since it has fewer risks.
- Realize that pregnant women have a different physiology and so nutritional needs and laboratory testing will vary from a non-pregnant patient.
- Try to avoid hypo- or hyperglycemia. Measure glucose frequently by blood gas analyzer.
- Upon initiation of feeding after fasting, be aware of the refeeding syndrome: give potassium, thiamine, and phosphate.
- Acknowledge that many of the recommendations for critical care nutrition in the pregnant woman are extrapolated from non-pregnant patients or are "expert" opinion with little serious research in support.
- A team approach is best, with an intensivist, nutritionist, and obstetrician/perinatologist being actively involved.

congestive heart failure or ARDS. Practically, titration based on diuresis, hemodynamics, peripheral and wound circulation, and evolution of creatinine clearance appears the only option for fluid management.

Conclusions

During normal pregnancy, metabolic needs are increased and glucose and lipid homeostasis are altered dramatically. Prolonged macro- and micronutrient deficiencies compromise the future for mother and child. Unfortunately, the biochemical and physical assessment of nutritional status is complicated by pregnancy, and the nutritional needs of the critically ill obstetric patient are unknown.

Avoidance of iatrogenic harm should be the first concern in this setting since enhanced nutrition has not yet proven to benefit outcome in the ICU and might increase the incidence of infections and

References

1. Vasquez DN, Estenssoro E, Canales HS, *et al.* Clinical characteristics and outcomes of obstetric patients requiring ICU admission. *Chest* 2007;**131**:718–724.

2. Tappy L, Berger M, Schwarz JM, *et al.* Hepatic and peripheral glucose metabolism in intensive care patients receiving continuous high- or low-carbohydrate enteral nutrition. *JPEN J Parenter Enteral Nutr* 1999;**23**:260–267.

3. Muller TF, Muller A, Bachem MG, Lange H. Immediate metabolic effects of different nutritional regimens in critically ill medical patients. *Intensive Care Med* 1995;**21**:561–566.

4. Fawzi WW, Msamanga GI, Urassa W, *et al*. Vitamins and perinatal outcomes among HIV-negative women in Tanzania. *N Engl J Med* 2007;**356**:1423–1431.

5. Kusin JA, Kardjati S, Houtkooper JM, Renqvist UH. Energy supplementation during pregnancy and postnatal growth. *Lancet* 1992;**340**:623–626.

6. Osrin D, Vaidya A, Shrestha Y, *et al*. Effects of antenatal multiple micronutrient supplementation on birthweight and gestational duration in Nepal: double-blind, randomised controlled trial. *Lancet* 2005;**365**:955–962.

7. Black RE, Allen LH, Bhutta ZA, *et al*. Maternal and child undernutrition: global and regional exposures and health consequences. *Lancet* 2008;**371**:243–260.

8. Bhutta ZA, Ahmed T, Black RE, *et al*. What works? Interventions for maternal and child undernutrition and survival. *Lancet* 2008;**371**:417–440.

9. Doig GS, Simpson F, Sweetman EA. Evidence-based nutrition support in the intensive care unit: an update on reported trial quality. *Curr Opin Clin Nutr Metab Care* 2009;**12**:201–206.

10. Phelan JP, Maryn KA. Hyperalimentation. In Belfort M (ed.) *Critical Care Obstetrics*, 5th ed. Chichester, UK: John Wiley, 2010, pp. 181–187. Blackwell.

11. Rasmussen KM, Yaktine AL for the Food and Nutrition Board. *Weight Gain During Pregnancy Reexamining the Guidelines*. editors. Washington, DC: National Academies Press, 2009.

12. Gluckman PD, Hanson MA, Cooper C, Thornburg KL. Effect of in utero and early-life conditions on adult health and disease. *N Engl J Med* 2008;**359**:61–73.

13. Simmons R. Epigenetics and maternal nutrition: nature v. nurture. *Proc Nutr Soc* 2011;**70**:73–81.

14. Bishop PJ, Sedlak EB. Pregnancy. In Cresci G (ed.) *Nutrition Support for the Critically Ill Patient: A Guide to Practice*. Boca Raton, FL: Taylor & Francis, 2005, pp. 359–370.

15. Branson RD, Johannigman JA. The measurement of energy expenditure. *Nutr Clin Pract* 2004;**19**:622–636.

16. Cankayali I, Demirag K, Kocabas S, Moral AR. The effects of standard and branched chain amino acid enriched solutions on thermogenesis and energy expenditure in unconscious intensive care patients. *Clin Nutr* 2004;**23**:257–263.

17. Singer P, Anbar R, Cohen J, *et al*. The tight calorie control study (TICACOS): a prospective, randomized, controlled pilot study of nutritional support in critically ill patients. *Intensive Care Med* 2011;**37**:601–609.

18. Jeevanandam M, Young DH, Schiller WR. Influence of parenteral nutrition on rates of net substrate oxidation in severe trauma patients. *Crit Care Med* 1990;**18**:467–473.

19. Martindale RG, Mcclave SA, Vanek VW, *et al*. Guidelines for the provision and assessment of nutrition support therapy in the adult critically ill patient: Society of Critical Care Medicine and American Society for Parenteral and Enteral Nutrition: Executive Summary. *Crit Care Med* 2009;**37**:1757–1761.

20. Kreymann KG, Berger MM, Deutz NE, *et al*. ESPEN guidelines on enteral nutrition: intensive care. *Clin Nutr* 2006;**25**:210–223.

21. Dvir D, Cohen J, Singer P. Computerized energy balance and complications in critically ill patients: an observational study. *Clin Nutr* 2006;**25**:37–44.

22. Villet S, Chiolero RL, Bollmann MD, *et al*. Negative impact of hypocaloric feeding and energy balance on clinical outcome in ICU patients. *Clin Nutr* 2005;**24**:502–509.

23. Doig GS, Heighes PT, Simpson F, Sweetman EA, Davies AR. Early enteral nutrition, provided within 24 h of injury or intensive care unit admission, significantly reduces mortality in critically ill patients: a meta-analysis of randomised controlled trials. *Intensive Care Med* 2009;**35**:2018–2027.

24. Ibrahim EH, Mehringer L, Prentice D, *et al*. Early versus late enteral feeding of mechanically ventilated patients: results of a clinical trial. *JPEN J Parenter Enteral Nutr* 2002;**26**:174–181.

25. National Heart, Lung, and Blood Institute Acute Respiratory Distress Syndrome (ARDS) Clinical Trials Network. Initial trophic vs full enteral feeding in patients with acute lung injury: the EDEN randomized trial. *JAMA* 2012;**307**:795–803.

26. Doig GS, Simpson F, Finfer S, *et al*. Effect of evidence-based feeding guidelines on mortality of critically ill adults: a cluster randomized controlled trial. *JAMA* 2008;**300**:2731–2741.

27. Singer P, Berger MM, Van den Berghe G, *et al*. ESPEN guidelines on parenteral nutrition: intensive care. *Clin Nutr* 2009;**28**:387–400.

28. Casaer MP, Hermans G, Wilmer A, Van den Berghe G. Impact of early parenteral nutrition completing enteral nutrition in adult critically ill patients (EPaNIC trial): a study protocol and statistical analysis plan for a randomized controlled trial. *Trials* 2011;**12**:21.

29. Casaer MP, Mesotten D, Hermans G, *et al*. Early versus late parenteral nutrition in critically ill adults. *N Engl JMed* 2011;**365**:506–517.

30. Hamaoui E, Hamaoui M. Nutritional assessment and support during pregnancy. *Gastroenterol Clin North Am* 1998;**27**:89–121.

31. Ridley EJ, Davies AR. Practicalities of nutrition support in the intensive care unit: the usefulness of gastric residual volume and prokinetic agents with enteral nutrition. *Nutrition* 2011;**27**:509–512.

32. Abbassi-Ghanavati M, Greer LG, Cunningham FG. Pregnancy and laboratory studies: a reference table for clinicians. *Obstet Gynecol* 2009;**114**:1326–1331.

33. Mackenzie IM, Whitehouse T, Nightingale PG. The metrics of glycaemic control in critical care. *Intensive Care Med* 2011;**37**:435–443.

34. Otten JJ, Hellwig JP, Meyers LD. *Dietery Reference Intakes (DRI): the Essential Guide to Nutrient Requirements.* Washington, DC: National Academies Press, 2006.

35. Baker HB, DeAngelis B, Holland B, *et al.* Vitamin profile of 563 gravidas during trimesters of pregnancy. *J Am Coll Nutr* 2002;**21**:33–37.

36. Dickerson RN, Gervasio JM, Sherman JJ, *et al.* A comparison of renal phosphorus regulation in thermally injured and multiple trauma patients receiving specialized nutrition support. *JPEN J Parenter Enteral Nutr* 2001;**25**:152–159.

37. Scheinkestel CD, Kar L, Marshall K, *et al.* Prospective randomized trial to assess caloric and protein needs of critically ill, anuric, ventilated patients requiring continuous renal replacement therapy. *Nutrition* 2003;**19**:909–916.

38. Casaer MP, Mesotten D, Schetz M. Bench-to-bedside review: metabolism and nutrition. *Crit Care* 2008;**12**:222.

39. Chiarenza L, Pignataro A, Lanza V. Refeeding syndrome in early pregnancy. Case report. *Minerva Anestesiol* 2005;**71**:803–808.

40. Munoz M, Garcia-Erce JA, Remacha AF. Disorders of iron metabolism. Part 1: molecular basis of iron homoeostasis. *J Clin Pathol* 2011;**64**:281–286.

41. Sihler KC, Raghavendran K, Westerman M, Ye W, Napolitano LM. Hepcidin in trauma: linking injury, inflammation, and anemia. *J Trauma* 2010;**69**:831–837.

42. Wheeler S. Assessment and interpretation of micronutrient status during pregnancy. *Proc Nutr Soc* 2008;**67**:437–450.

Chapter 21

Monitoring the critically ill gravida

Emily Gordon, Lauren A. Plante, and Clifford S. Deutschman

Introduction

One of the most important functions of any intensive care unit (ICU) is to enable patients to arrive at specific, goal-directed endpoints of care. The exact nature of this care plan is individualized based on the character of the patient, the disease process, the unit, and the ICU team; to ensure that care is proceeding along the desired trajectory requires objective data. These data are most often provided by monitors – devices that measure specific physiological variables. Collection of data over time allows for minute-to-minute assessment of trends in a patient's physiological state. Intensivists, physicians specially trained in critical care medicine, and other members of the ICU care team may have in-depth knowledge of monitors not available to the practitioner, who does not use them on a daily basis. It is important that these non-intensivists understand the utility, indications/contraindications, and basic interpretation of the information provided by the monitors currently in use.

Non-invasive monitors do not require significant intrusion into a patient's body. The most commonly encountered non-invasive monitors are electrocardiography (ECG), pulse oximetry, blood pressure measurement by manometry, urine output, pulse oximetry and end-tidal carbon dioxide monitoring. Invasive monitors are those which require encroachment on a patient's body such as cannulation of vessels, insertion of neurological monitors, or insertion of pressure monitors.

Non-invasive monitoring

Electrocardiography

Monitoring with ECG is vitally important in the ICU and many other settings. It is inexpensive, non-invasive and, once a certain level of competence is achieved, relatively easy to interpret. It provides real-time data, details beat-to-beat variability in rate and rhythm, and alerts to the possibility of myocardial ischemia.

Most ECG monitors display two leads, most often II and V5. Lead II allows for close monitoring of P waves (to detect atrial arrhythmias) while lead V5 is highly sensitive to ischemic changes.

Ischemia monitoring typically is accomplished using an ST segment monitoring system. The computer initially creates a template of the patient's normal QRS complex and imprints the QRS complexes and the J point. This allows the computer to "memorize" the location of an isoelectirc point just before the QRS and a similar point in the ST segment 60–80 millisecond after the J point [1]. The distance between horizontal lines drawn through each of these points is determined and compared with the same distance in subsequent complexes. A deviation of >2 mm suggests ischemia.

Sphygmomanometry: non-invasive blood pressure monitoring

The mercury manometer remains the standard for blood pressure measurement. A cuff placed above an artery is inflated to a pressure that occludes the artery and then slowly released while the examiner listens with a stethoscope. The appearance of Korotkoff sounds indicates the systolic pressure while the loss of these sounds denotes the diastolic.

Automated blood pressure cuffs are now utilized in most locations. These devices inflate the cuff to a pressure that occludes the artery before releasing the pressure. As the pressure decreases, a piezo-electric crystal measures arterial waveforms distal to the deflating cuff. The return of oscillations corresponds to the systolic pressure. The point of maximal oscillations is found at the mean pressure while the diastolic blood pressure is denoted by a loss of oscillations [2]. As one

Maternal Critical Care: A Multidisciplinary Approach, ed. Marc Van de Velde, Helen Scholefield, and Lauren A. Plante.
Published by Cambridge University Press. © Cambridge University Press 2013.

would suspect based on the mechanism, the mean pressure is the most accurate of the three numbers obtained. However, most automated blood pressure units have not been validated for accuracy in pregnancy, and some have been found to underestimate blood pressure in women with pre-eclampsia compared with intra-arterial measurements [3]; consequently, caution may be advised in this population.

Urine output

It is customary to measure the amount of urine produced within a specific time period in the critically ill patient. The underlying assumption is that urine production reflects renal perfusion, which, in turn, is a function of the adequacy of blood volume. This number, however, is easily misinterpreted. The production of urine at 0.5 mL/kg body weight is often felt to be "adequate." This number reflects "normal physiology." When eating a normal diet, the normal individual produces approximately 12 Osm of nitrogenous waste in a 24 hour period, or about 500 mOsm/h. The maximal ability to concentrate the urine is about 1200 mOsm/mL. Thus,

$$500 \text{ mOsm/h per kg/1200 mOsm/mL}$$
$$= 0.42 \text{ mL/h per kg}$$

This value is close to the 0.5 mL/h per kg body weight that is taken as the norm. However, many factors present in both pregnant and critically ill patients may alter this number. First, diet is variable – nitrogenous load may increase, decrease, or be unchanged. Second, and most importantly, metabolism, and thus nitrogen production, is characteristically increased in pregnancy, increasing the denominator. Third, maximal concentration of the urine is decreased in pregnancy and by the capillary leak and redistribution of renal blood flow found in critically ill patients. These changes decrease the denominator. Finally, a slight change in renal function may have immense effects on the value of renal function. For example,

- if 1 L/min fluid is filtered and the kidney is 99.9% efficient, the net result is production of 1 mL/min urine
- if the kidney is slightly damaged so that it becomes only 99% efficient, 10 mL urine will be produced in that same minute
- if a 90% decrease in filtration is then imposed on this slightly damaged system, it will result in

production of 1 mL/min urine, the same as would occur in the "normal" kidney.

This example clearly illustrates the limitations inherent in relying on UOP as a monitor in isolation of other measures.

Pulse oximetry

Pulse oximeters detect the absorption of light across a tissue bed, most often a finger, containing pulsatile blood flow. Red (660 nm) and infrared (940 nm) light is absorbed by oxygenated and deoxygenated hemoglobin, respectively [4,5]. The percentage of oxygenated blood can be calculated based on the relative absorption at each wavelength [6] (Figure 21.1). The heart rate also can be detected. Monitoring the saturation of hemoglobin provides some assurance that a patient is receiving an adequate supply of oxygen. Oxygen saturation measured by pulse oximetry is denoted by the term Sp_{O_2}.

A number of factors can interfere with accurate determination of Sp_{O_2} by pulse oximetry. The algorithm used to determine saturation is not fully accurate at arterial values $(Sa_{O_2}) <70\%$ [7] or when the venous values (Sv_{O_2}) and Sa_{O_2} differ by <3%. Dyshemoglobinemia, such as occurs when there are high levels of carboxyhemoglobin or methemoglobin [8]), and sluggish flow also limit accuracy. Anemia itself does not affect the accuracy of Sp_{O_2} measurements [9,10]. Dark skin tone [11] or the presence of fingernail polish [12,13] also affect readings.

Pulse oximetry is probably most useful in any patient receiving supplemental oxygenation in the ICU setting. It may also be used to determine responses to therapeutic intervention. The accuracy of pulse oximetry at moderate to high levels of arterial oxygen partial pressure (Pa_{O_2}) and hemoglobin has been validated in multiple studies [14]. The measures become less reliable as each of these variables decrease. Pulse oximeter is superior to periodically obtaining arterial blood gases because it is less expensive, non-invasive, better tolerated by patients, able to instantaneously detect significant hypoxemic episodes, and has virtually no potential for harm. Clearly, oximetry does not provide other measurements that can be obtained with arterial blood gas analysis, such as pH, arterial carbon dioxide partial pressure (Pa_{CO_2}), additional chemistry, and hematology results. In addition, while pulse oximetry is able to detect episodes of hypoxemia in the postoperative setting, its use has never been shown to alter morbidity or mortality [15–18].

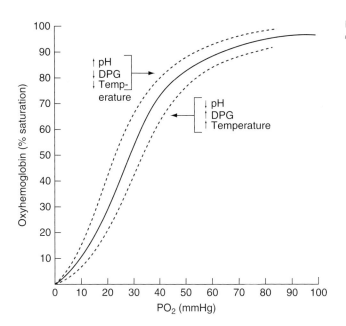

End-tidal carbon dioxide

The end-tidal carbon dioxide ($ETco_2$) measurement is used to assess the patient's ventilatory status. In essence, it functions as a surrogate for $Paco_2$ [19]. In general, the measurement is plotted continuously against time, although some monitors will plot $ETco_2$ as a function of expired volume, a more useful measurement. Monitoring is based on infrared light absorption at 4300 nm by exhaled carbon dioxide in the airway. Carbon dioxide analyzers can be placed in the expiratory limb of ventilator tubing or on specialized nasal cannulas. Infrared carbon dioxide detectors have a rapid response and can measure changes in carbon dioxide during a single exhalation. The measurement is useful in the management of sedation, chronic obstructive pulmonary disease, bronchospasm, narcotic administration, some drug overdoses, and hypo/hyperventilation. It is particularly useful to confirm appropriate placement of an endotracheal tube [19–21]. Measurement of $ETco_2$ has been found to be more reliable than other methods in detecting esophageal intubation [22].

The Pco_2 at the onset of exhalation is minimal because the gas in the upper airways is the first to leave the lungs. As exhalation continues, the carbon dioxide rises steadily until it reaches a plateau and it remains there until inhalation commences. If the lungs are normal, then the Pco_2 at the end of exhalation is close to the Pco_2 in end-capillary (arterial) blood [23].

The gradient between the aveolar carbon dioxide ($Paco_2$) and the $ETco_2$ is typically <5. In general, differences between $Paco_2$ and $ETco_2$ reflect the amount of dead space. Therefore, disorders such as chronic obstructive pulmonary disease or obstructive sleep apnea, which increase dead space, limit the reliability of the measurement. Both anatomical and physiological dead space contribute to the discrepancy. It has been assumed that this gradient is constant as long as the patient's condition remains unchanged. In the face of disease processes that vary over time, changes in exogenous ventilation, and/or mode of support or fluid therapy, the gradient between $Paco_2$ and $ETco_2$ may change very quickly. Changes in patient management that affect gas exchange (i.e. changes in ventilator settings) also may change this gradient, which will have to be recalculated.

There is a progesterone-induced increase in minute ventilation seen soon after conception. This change leads to a 40% increase in minute ventilation in the second trimester and this results in a baseline $Paco_2$ of 27–32 mmHg [24]. The development of respiratory alkalosis is countered by a compensatory decrease in serum bicarbonate (Table 21.1).

Invasive monitoring

Intra-arterial blood pressure monitoring

Intra-arterial blood pressure monitoring is indicated when there is a need for tight blood pressure control,

Table 21.1. Arterial blood gas measurements[a]

	Antepartum	Postpartum
pH	7.43 ± 0.027	7.41 ± 0.013
Arterial partial pressure of CO_2 (mmHg)	30.4 ± 2.7	35.3 ± 3.1
Arterial partial pressure of O_2 (mmHg)	102 ± 5	95 ± 7

[a] Arterial blood gas values from measurements reported in Templeton and Kelman, 1976 (25), obtained in semirecumbent position with 15°pelvic tilt at 38 weeks of gestation and 5 weeks after delivery.

a potential for rapid, unheralded changes in blood pressure with adverse consequences, or a need to titrate inotropic and/or vasoactive medications. Common clinical scenarios requiring monitoring include hypertensive crisis, acute respiratory failure, shock (hemorrhagic, distributive, cardiogenic), pre-eclampsia, and massive blood loss.

Virtually any artery other than the carotid can be cannulated for invasive arterial monitoring. Most common sites are the radial arteries, but use of the ulnar, brachial, axillary, dorsalispedis, or femoral artery is not uncommon. Care must be taken when using an end-artery such as the brachial or an artery close to the cerebral circulation (axillary) where inadvertent air or particulate embolism imposes a risk of neurological injury.

Accurate arterial blood pressure monitoring requires a continuous column of fluid from the cannula to the transducer. Air bubbles or particulate matter will dampen the system [26]. This defect should have only a minor effect on mean blood pressure but can radically alter systolic and diastolic pressures. The pulsation in the vasculature acts as an underdamped second-order harmonic oscillator. Consequently, the observed waveform often is biphasic, the result of measuring both forward and reflected flow.

The only absolute contraindication to arterial cannulation is distal ischemia. Relative contraindications include blood diathesis, current anticoagulant use, and thrombolytic agents. Site-specific indications include full-thickness burns, presence of vascular prosthesis, infection at the proposed site of placement, or severe arterial disease with distal ischemia.

Complications of arterial cannulation included thrombosis/distal ischemia, bleeding, or infection at the site of insertion. Following radial artery cannulation, the rate of distal ischemia approaches 0.1% [27]. Most other complications are related to equipment failure or misinterpretation of data.

Central venous pressure

Central venous pressure (CVP) is measured by placing a catheter into or near the right atrium or vena cava. The validity of the measurement, however, depends on the proximity to these major structures; the greater the distance from the right atrium, the less accurate the measurement, even if the column of fluid separating the catheter from the right atrium is uninterrupted. Practically speaking, the numerical value of measured venous pressure is significantly affected by the extramural pressure. In the abdomen or extremities, this may be nil or positive. However, in the chest of a spontaneously breathing (not mechanically ventilated) patient, the pressure is most often zero (at end inspiration) or negative (during inspiration) and only becomes positive when expiration is active or occurs against a closed glottis (Valsalva maneuver) These normal pressures. change with the use on mechanical ventilation or ventilator-support modes. In addition, valvular insufficiency may alter the waveform and make identification of the actual plateau pressure difficult. Thus, the absolute value of the CVP must be interpreted with caution.

The importance of measuring CVP lies in the belief that this number is an index of preload or venous return to the heart and, therefore, is predictive of stroke volume or overall volume status. These theories are of questionable validity because they are based on a number of potentially erroneous assumptions. First, the assumption that this pressure is related to volume, either the volume of blood entering the right heart or the total blood volume, requires that there be a consistent, predictable, reproducible *linear* relationship between pressure and volume. In both the right ventricle and the entire vascular system, which is constructed not of rigid pipes but of compliant vessels whose caliber changes as pressure changes, alterations in pressure or volume will alter the pressure–volume relationship. In addition, because preload on the left side of the heart is left ventricular end-diastolic volume, the assumption that CVP reflects preload in the left ventricle requires that the pressure measured in the right ventricle or superior vena cava be proportional to the pressure in the left ventricle. This, in turn, mandates that the column of fluid connecting the left ventricle to the right atrium or superior vena cava be continuous and arising from a single source. Neither is true – valves and a profuse vascular tree that may expand or contract continuously separate CVP from the pressure in the left ventricle, and the return to the left atrium arises not just from the pulmonary circulation but also from the bronchial and

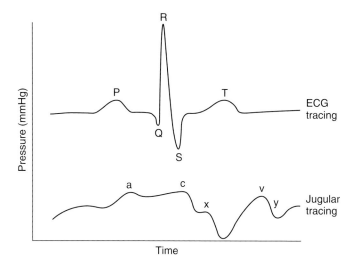

Figure 21.2. Coorelation of jugular pressure trace changes with the electrocardiograph (ECG). The a wave results from increased atrial pressure during right atrial contraction and it correlates with the P wave on the ECG. The c wave is caused by a slight elevation of the tricuspid valve into the right atrium during early ventricular contraction and correlates with the end of the QRS segment. The x descent is probably caused by the downward movement of the ventricle during systolic contraction and it occurs immediately before the T wave. The v wave arises from the pressure produced when the blood filling the right atrium comes up against a closed tricuspid valve and it occurs as the T wave is ending. The y descent wave is produced by the tricuspid valve opening in diastole with blood flowing into the right ventricle and it occurs prior to the P wave.

thebesian circulations. This argument again mandates that CVP be interpreted cautiously.

Catheters for CVP measurement can be placed at many different sites. These include the internal jugular vein, subclavian vein, femoral vein, and antecubital veins. The internal jugular route is often preferred because it is technically simpler to perform and is less likely to result in arterial puncture because the nearby carotid artery can be palpated and both the vein and artery are easily visualized using ultrasonography, which reduces complications. Further, if the artery is inadvertently perforated it is simple to apply direct pressure and thus control bleeding. In contrast, the subclavian vein is technically more challenging, not as amenable to ultrasound identification, and, if the artery is entered, control of the arterial bleeding is more difficult. However, some studies suggest that catheters placed in the subclavian vein may have the lowest risk of infection [28–30]. Placement via the femoral route should be reserved for urgent/emergency situations where internal jugular or subclavian placement is difficult or contraindicated. Because of its remote location, the pressure measured in the femoral vein may not be a good approximation of right atrial pressure. The femoral vein is a poor choice in the pregnant patient because of difficulty in maintaining sterility and the potential for interference with obstetric procedures. Placement via the antecubital site requires that the catheter be threaded centrally. This approach has recently gained popularity for long-term use. However, the length of the catheter increases the risk for thrombosis and may make rapid administration of fluids problematic.

The CVP waveform is directly related to the cardiac cycle and, therefore, to the ECG (Figure 21.2). Alterations in the CVP waveform can be seen in a number of pathological conditions, such as tricuspid regurgitation (large v waves) and cardiac arrhythmias.

Other indications for central line placement include the infusion of medications that must be given centrally, rapid administration of fluids, administration of parenteral nutrition, and administration of vasoactive medications.

There are no absolute contraindications to central line insertion, but relative contraindications may include anatomical abnormalities, previous injury to the vessel, bleeding diathesis or coagulopathy, a patient's inability to tolerate the procedure if awake, the potentially dire consequences of a pneumothorax in some patients, or superior vena cava syndrome.

The risks associated with central venous cannulation include vascular rupture, hemorrhage, pneumothorax, thrombosis, catheter-related infection, and arterial puncture during placement. Vascular erosion is seen most commonly with left internal or external jugular cannulation [31]. The most common complication is inadvertent puncture of the internal carotid artery. In a large meta-analysis, the rate of pneumothorax associated with internal jugular catheterization was 1.3% versus 1.5% with subclavian vein cannulation [32]. Long-term complications include migration of the catheter [33,34] and infection (line sepsis). The rates of infection have decreased dramatically since the institution of guidelines for the prevention of catheter-related infections [30,35]. The National Nosocomial Infection Surveillance system reports the rate of central venous catheter-related infection as approximately 3.2–4.0 per 1000 catheter days in medical–surgical ICUs [36]. While the risk of catheter-associated bacteremia has been reported to be as high as 3–8%, recent studies utilizing improved sterile technique and catheter technologies have reported rates below 2% [35,37].

Pulmonary artery catheter

The pulmonary artery catheter (PAC) is inserted via a central vein and, directed by a balloon inflated at its tip, is advanced through the tricuspid valve, the right ventricle, and the pulmonary valve into the outflow tract of the right ventricle. Using appropriately placed transducers, direct measurements of pressure can be made from the right atrium, right ventricle, and pulmonary artery. The balloon may be inflated in the pulmonary artery until flow is stopped. A transducer distal to the balloon then records the pressure in the pulmonary artery, presumably unaffected by inflow. This has been termed the "wedge," "pulmonary capillary wedge," or "pulmonary artery occlusion" pressure. It may be taken as an index of left ventricular end-diastolic pressure, which, in turn, is used as an approximation of left ventricular end-diastolic volume: in other words, left ventricular preload. As noted above in the discussion of CVP, these assumptions are not well justified because of changes in the pressure–volume relationship and because of the presence of collateral circulation that interferes with the continuity of the fluid column separating the left ventricle from the PAC tip in the pulmonary artery [37,38]. Therefore, use of the wedge pressure as a gauge of preload is problematic. Fortunately, most PACs in use today also are equipped with a thermistor that, using thermodilution, allows measurement of right ventricular stroke volume. Software included in the module used for pressure transduction collects stroke volume values for several minutes and averages them to determine the output (in L/min) from the right heart. Because, over time, the output from the left heart must equal that of the right, this permits determination of cardiac output. The combination of pressure and cardiac output measurements provides a very powerful tool for assessing the effects of changes in volume status or cardiac contractility and in the use of vasoactive medications. In addition, most PACs contain an electrode to measure mixed Svo_2. This value, coupled with Sao_2 value obtained from an arterial sample or transcutaneously, allows for the calculation of oxygen extraction, which has been taken as an index of the adequacy of perfusion. Finally, data from the PAC have been used to calculate values invented to describe important physiological parameters. Thus, pulmonary and systemic vascular resistance are calculated by dividing the pressure gradient across the vascular bed by the cardiac output. In theory, this provides an index of "vascular tone," that is, a description of the extent to which these beds are constricted or dilated. However, a change in cardiac output alone can alter pulmonary and systemic vascular resistance without any change in the vasculature itself. Therefore, once again, these numbers must be interpreted with caution. Combining oxygen content or extraction with cardiac output permits calculation of oxygen delivery and consumption.

Clinically, PACs are most helpful in two settings. The first involves clarification of a clinically confusing picture, for example unexplained hypotension. The PAC allows differentiation of hypovolemia (such as may occur in hemorrhage) from vasodilatation (often present in sepsis), from primary cardiac dysfunction. The first is characterized by a low cardiac output, the second by high cardiac output/stroke volume in the face of an overly dilated vasculature, and the last by persistently low cardiac output/stroke volume despite resuscitation. All will require fluid administration, but the PAC may help to determine the type of fluid required, the tests needed for source identification, the indications for other therapeutic interventions (i.e. blood products, antibiotics, inotropes), and the endpoints of resuscitation. The PAC measurement also is quite useful in determining fluid needs, particularly during active resuscitation. Consequently, fluid challenges can be attempted until cardiac output/stroke volume no longer changes. This finding usually indicates that preload has been optimized and that other approaches to improving tissue perfusion, such as inotropic agents or vasodilators, are necessary. Finally, the PAC may be useful in identifying elevated pulmonary artery pressures and thus right heart outflow obstruction and in minimizing fluids in patients with respiratory distress.

Clark *et al.* [39] examined hemodynamic parameters during pregnancy and postpartum. These data demonstrate that the obstetric patient has increases in cardiac output and decreases in both systemic and pulmonary vascular resistance (Table 21.2). Consequently, the normal hemodynamic picture in pregnancy resembles that of sepsis.

Table 21.2. Normal cardiovascular and arterial blood gas values for women at term and postpartum[a]

	Antepartum	Postpartum
Cardiac output (L/min [±SD])	6.2 ± 1.0	4.3 ± 0.9
Heart rate (beats/min [±SD])	83 ± 10	71 ± 10
Mean arterial pressure (mmHg [±SD])	90 ± 6	86 ± 7
Systemic vascular resistance (dyne.s/cm^5 [±SD])	1210 ± 266	1530 ± 520
Pulmonary vascular resistance (dyne.s/cm^5 [±SD])	78 ± 22	119 ± 47.0
Colloid osmotic pressure (mmHg [±SD])	18.0 ± 1.5	20.8 ± 1.0
Pulmonary capillary wedge pressure (mmHg [±SD])	7.5 ± 1.8	6.3 ± 2.1

The cardiovascular values from Clark *et al.,* 1989 [39] were obtained in left lateral recumbent position at 36–38 weeks of gestation and 11–13 weeks after delivery.

The complications associated with PAC insertion include those associated with placing central venous access – bleeding, arterial puncture, pneuomthorax, air embolism – and those associated specifically with the PAC itself – arrhythmias, air embolism from balloon rupture, entanglement in and damage to cardiac structures, valvular insufficiency, pulmonary infarction secondary to pulmonary artery occlusion, thrombosis, pulmonary infarction, and pulmonary artery rupture. Most of these are easily reversed (arrhythmias by repositioning of the catheter) or exceedingly rare (pulmonary artery rupture). The risk of pulmonary artery rupture has been reported to be 0.1–0.2% [40–42].

Although the PAC has been used in obstetric patients, especially in patients with severe pre-eclampsia in which fluid management is difficult, use has been declining, probably as a reflection of the general rate of decline in use in recent years [43–45].

Minimally invasive techniques for hemodynamic monitoring

Pulse contour methods determine cardiac output semi-invasively using standard arterial access and facilitate monitoring of many physiological parameters, including cardiac output, volumetric preload, extravascular lung water, afterload, contractility, and volume responsiveness. Monitoring is achieved through the insertion of an arterial cannula into the femoral, axillary, or brachial arteries. The pulse contour cardiac output method utilizes both transpulmonary thermodilution and arterial pulse contour analysis principles.

Pulse contour analysis provides beat-to-beat parameters obtained from the arterial pressure waveform. The technique is capable of computing a single stroke volume from a single pulse after calibration with an initial transpulmonary thermodilution measurement. The rise and fall of the blood pressure curve is based upon the distensibility of an individual patient's arteries. Stroke volume will vary depending on when it is assessed during the ventilatory cycle, and this is represented by the stroke volume variation. This parameter is seen as a surrogate for preload responsiveness but it is only accurate in mechanically ventilated patients who are in sinus rhythm and it is seen as a surrogate for preload responsiveness. The pulse contour cardiac output monitor may give inaccurate measurements in patients with arrhythmias, intracardiac shunts, aortic aneurysms, aortic stenosis, rapid temperature changes, pneumonectomy, significant lung embolism, or during extracorporeal circulation.

Given that volume status and responsiveness is one of the most difficult assessments to make in the ICU, the stroke volume variation, pulse pressure variation, and volumetric preload can assist the ICU physician in making this determination. Studies showing that pulse pressure variation is an accurate indicator of fluid responsiveness in septic, mechanically ventilated patients [46] or that it is a good predictor of cardiac output response in patients after a coronary artery bypass graft have been difficult to replicate although these measures appeared to be more valuable than CVP and pulmonary artery occlusion pressure in these patients [47]. In a prospective clinical study of patients with septic shock, volumetric preload calculated from the pulse contour cardiac output monitor was found to be a better index of cardiac preload than CVP in a prospective clinical study [48]. There are case reports detailing use of pulse contour cardiac output or pulse contour wave analysis during cesarean section in patients with pre-eclampsia [49,50], and this might be extrapolated to ICU management in pregnancy.

This technology's greatest value may lie in the ability to acquire hemodynamic data without right heart catheterization. Measurements rely upon assessment of the dilution of a lithium bolus administered through a via central or peripheral venous catheter and measured at an arterial catheter (pulse contour cardiac output monitor or a LiDCO cardiac sensor system). The lithium dilution technique has also been used in pregnancy [51] as the total lithium dose is very small and teratogenesis is not of concern past the first trimester.

Intracranial pressure monitoring

Continuous, clinically useful intracranial pressure (ICP) monitoring was initially developed for patients with traumatic brain injury [52], where it has been shown to give prognostic information and assist in management decisions; it has also been suggested that it improves outcomes [53–55]. It has since been used in a number of other settings, including subarachnoid hemorrhage, hepatic encephalopathy, encephalitis, and stroke. Monitoring of ICP in the critically ill patient can be invaluable as the signs and symptoms of increased ICP are unreliable in this setting [56].

The indications for ICP monitoring following traumatic brain injury have been addressed by the Brain Trauma Foundation. Patients should be considered for ICP monitoring if they have a Glasgow Coma Score of ≤8 or an abnormal CT scan: that is, they may have contusions, hematomas, edema, or compressed ventricles [57].

The physiological basis for monitoring ICP is based on two separate but related mechanisms that contribute to cerebral ischemia. The ischemic brain will swell, eventually filling the cranial vault and causing herniation of brain tissue into the area surrounding the brainstem or out of the foramen magnum into the spinal canal, damaging the primitive brain that controls most autonomic function [58].

In the first putative mechanism, it is postulated that an ischemia-induced elevation in the pressure in the brain parenchyma that exceed about 18 mmHg will lead to venous collapse, which will increase brain swelling by obstructing outflow. The net result is further ischemia and ultimately herniation. Intraparenchymal pressure is most often approximated by ICP. This theory explains why treatment of raised ICP is usually initiated at pressures between 15 and 20 mmHg. In practice, it is not known to what extent venous collapse contributes to the progression of brain injury.

The second justification for measuring ICP lies in the relationship between cerebral perfusion pressure, the difference between the mean blood pressure and some "downstream" pressure, and cerebral blood flow. To avoid ischemia, normal, intact brain tissue is perfused at a relatively constant flow rate. In normal brain, vasoconstriction and vasodilatation assure minimal variation in blood flow across a range of blood pressures. In the injured brain, this relationship may be attenuated or altogether abolished, and flow to the brain becomes dependent on cerebral perfusion pressure. The downstream pressure used to calculate cerebral perfusion pressure is either the venous pressure, most often the CVP, or the pressure within the brain itself, most often approximated by the ICP, whichever is higher [59]. If cerebral perfusion pressure falls, blood flow becomes insufficient and ischemia develops. This again increases swelling and the risk of herniation. If cerebral perfusion pressure becomes elevated and cerebral blood flow rises, pressure itself (from an increase in blood volume within the fixed cranial vault) may directly damage the brain or lead to herniation. Therefore, the mainstay of treatment for injured brain is control of ischemia, pressure damage, and herniation by limiting ICP or optimizing cerebral perfusion pressure. The Brain Trauma Foundation recommend a minimum cerebral perfusion pressure of 60 mmHg [59].

There are four general types of systems used to monitor ICP: ventriculostomies (ventricular catheter), subarachnoid bolts, fiberoptic sensors, and catheter tip strain gauges.

The ventriculostomy is a hollow cannula placed into one of the lateral cerebral ventricles and connected to a fluid-filled signal transduction system that can generate an electric signal. It can be inserted at the bedside and used for both diagnosis – measuring ICP – and therapy, that is drainage of cerebrospinal fluid. Graphing pressure over time generates a waveform that can provide information about dynamic cerebrovascular responses. Most often, the mean pressure is calculated and that number is taken as the ICP.

Ventriculostomies can become infected; most centers report infection rates between 1 and 10%. Hemorrhage during catheter placement occurs 1–2% of the time and rarely requires surgical exploration. Placement can be technically challenging as there may be significant difficulty in locating small, compressed or shifted ventricles.

A subarachnoid bolt is screwed into a small burr hole in the skull. The dura at the tip of the device is punctured, placing cerebrospinal fluid in continuity with the fluid-filled hollow core of the bolt and the attached transduction system. In contrast to ventriculostomy, the subarachnoid bolt cannot be used to drain fluid. Readings from subarachnoid bolts tend to be lower than those from a ventriculostomy. Placement of a subarachnoid bolt carries a very low complication rate. Damage to the brain itself is rare, but intracerebral hematoma secondary to a placement mishap can occur.

Fiberoptic ICP monitors involve placement of a miniature transducer into the cerebrospinal fluid (either ventricular or subarachnoid) or even into brain tissue itself. Fiberoptic cables carry a light that is projected onto a mirror at the catheter tip. The extent to which the light is displaced is a function of ICP [60]. This monitor does not require fluid-filled systems, removing a potential source of dampening and thus error. As with all invasive devices, there is risk of infection, but it is significantly less than that observed in other systems because of the absence of fluid in the device. The incidence of complications such as hemorrhage and infection is also less than in other ICP monitors.

A catheter tip strain-gauge catheter consists of a solid-state pressure sensor in a titanium box that is placed at the tip of a long, thin, flexible nylon tube. The transducer tip consists of a microchip with diffuse piezoresistive strain gauges, connected to wires that traverse the length of the tube [61].

Brain tissue oxygenation

Brain tissue oxygenation can be measured via a small microcatheter inserted into the frontal white matter. Normal brain tissue oxygen tension has been estimated to be 40 mmHg [62–66]. Lower values putatively suggest increased oxygen extraction to compensate for reduced delivery(i.e. reduced cerebral blood flow). Use of these measurements is controversial. True normal values are not really known. It is unclear what information on global or focal brain injury can be derived from a measurement made in one discrete region of the brain that may or may not be injured. The value of trending also is unsubstantiated. There are no studies evaluating the relationship between changes in brain tissue oxygenation and outcome, nor is it clear that intervention to alter this oxygenation is beneficial. Thus, measurement of brain tissue oxygenation is, at this time, of unknown value.

Fetal monitoring

Fetal monitoring, in practice, is generally limited to the generation and interpretation of fetal heart rate patterns obtained through Doppler ultrasound. Unless membranes are ruptured and the woman is in labor, the signal is obtained transabdominally. The fetal heart rate signal is displayed over time as an irregular line, in which the interval between events in the cardiac cycle is recorded. The original method of measuring fetal heart rate was using a direct fetal ECG and displaying the R-R interval, but this required direct fetal access in the form of a stainless steel electrode screwed into the fetal scalp.

Interpretation of the fetal heart rate tracing or cardiotocograph is second nature to obstetricians, but will be unfamiliar to most other physicians in the ICU setting. The underlying principle is that the intact fetal central nervous system will manifest a balance between sympathetic and parasympathetic influences, but hypoxemia or acidemia can effect a number of changes in the tracing [67]. General signs indicative of the *absence* of metabolic acidemia in the fetus include cardioaccelerations, either spontaneous or provoked by acoustic stimulation, and the presence of normal baseline fetal heart rate variability (Figure 21.3). While these are signs of fetal health, their absence does not indicate fetal compromise: fetal sleep cycles or maternal medications may vitiate them. The presence of decelerations in the tracing suggests some interruption of the oxygen transfer pathway between maternal lungs and fetal central nervous system, but in the absence of significant metabolic acidemia, fetal injury remains unlikely. It is important to note here that fetal heart rate patterns are better understood in labor than in the antepartum setting, and that electronic fetal heart rate monitoring was introduced more than 50 years ago without randomized trials.

Extrapolation to the antepartum setting is common, although largely unsupported by randomized trials [68]. The "non-stress test" refers to the fetal heart rate tracing obtained in the absence of uterine contractions (which inevitably interrupt fetoplacental perfusion.) If fetal well-being is questioned on the basis of the fetal heart rate trace, further information can be obtained through real-time ultrasound, looking for parameters of fetal activity. The components of the biophysical profile include fetal tone, fetal movements, fetal breathing, and an assessment of amniotic fluid. With the exception of amniotic fluid, these parameters are also subject to alteration depending on maternal medications. Opioid or sedative drugs that cross the placenta – and that would be most of them – will also suppress fetal activity.

Despite the absence of good-quality data demonstrating a benefit from antenatal fetal heart rate monitoring or cardiotocography [69], current medicolegal practice in the USA at least holds obstetricians to this

(a) (b)

(c)

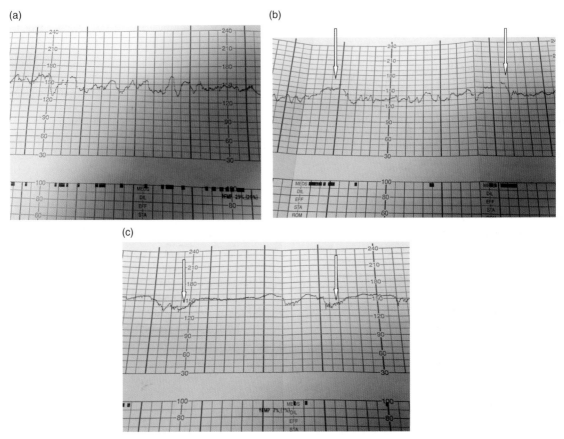

Figure 21.3. Examples of fetal heart rate tracings. The lower channel for uterine contractions (tocodynamometry or tocometry) is not shown here. (a) Average baseline variability (normal, no concerns about fetal status). (b) Average baseline variability with accelerations (arrowed): normal, no concerns about fetal status. (c) Minimal variability (less than 5 beats/min) plus decelerations (arrowed): requires further assessment and perhaps correction of modifiable factors.

standard for mothers or fetuses perceived to be at increased risk. Consequently, it would be expected to be deployed for pregnant patients in the ICU, at least in the third trimester. Practice may vary from intermittent to continuous monitoring. The tracings generated should be interpreted by physicians or nurses with expertise in the area. Diminished fetal heart rate variability or the presence of decelerations may, in the ICU setting, reflect maternal acid–base status, hypotension, electrolyte disturbances, hypoxemia, or medication, and may respond to correction of the underlying maternal condition in many cases. An argument can be made that the fetal heart rate tracing in this setting is an indicator of uteroplacental perfusion in the same way that the maternal ECG is an indicator of coronary perfusion.

Variability refers to the jiggle in the tracing in labor, this may be obtained from a direct fetal ECG,

obtained from an electrode screwed into the fetal scalp, and variability reflects the R-R intervals in the cardiac cycle. In the case of external fetal monitoring, which would be the rule in the ICU, the auditory events of the cardiac cycle, obtained by Doppler, are autocorrelated for calculation and display. *Accelerations* are deflections significantly above baseline (by 10 or 15 beats/min, depending on gestational age;); and *decelerations* refer to deflections significantly below baseline. *Variable decelerations* are visually abrupt in both onset and recovery and are thought to reflect umbilical cord compression. Gradual, symmetrical, uniform deceleration is unusual except in labor; when they occur at the time of contractions they are attributed to baroreceptor stimulation as the fetal head is compressed, while those that occur after contractions are believed to represent diminished uteroplacental perfusion.

References

1. Clements FM, Bruijn NP. Noninvasive cardiac monitoring. *Crit Care Clin* 1998;**4**:435–454.

2. Borrow KM, Newberger JW. Non-invasive estimation of central aortic pressure using indirect systolic, diastolic and mean brachial artery pressure with simultaneous direct ascending aortic pressure measurements. *Am Heart J* 1982;**103**:879.

3. Shennan AH, Halligan AWF. Measuring blood pressure in normal and hypertensive pregnancy. *Balliere Clin Obstet Gynecol* 1999;**13**:1–26.

4. Jubran A. Pulse oximetry. In Tobin MJ (ed.) *Principles and Practice of Intensive Care Monitoring*. New York: McGraw-Hill, 1998, pp. 261–287.

5. Wukitisch MW, Peterson MT, Tobler DR, Pologe JA. Pulse oximetry: analysis of theory, technology, and practice. *J Clin Monit* 1988;**4**:290–301.

6. McGough EK, Boysen PG. Benefits and limitations of pulse oximetry in the ICU. *J Crit Illness* 1989;**4**:23.

7. Jubran A, Tobin MJ. Reliability of pulse oximetry in titrating supplemental oxygen therapy in ventilator-dependent patients. *Chest* 1990;**97**:1420–1425.

8. Barker SJ, Badal JJ. The measurement of dyshemoglobins and total hemoglobin by pulse oximetry. *CurrOpinAnaesthesiol* 2008;**21**:805–810.

9. Jay GD, Highes L, Renzi FP. Pulse oximetry is accurate in acute anemia from hemorrhage. *Ann Emerg Med* 1994;**24**:32–35.

10. Ortiz FO, Aldrich TK, Nagel RL, et al. Accuracy of pulse oximetry in sickle cell disease. *Am J Resp Crit Care Med* 1999;**159**:447–451.

11. Zeballos RJ, Weisman IM. Reliability of noninvasive oximetry in black subjects during exercise and hypoxia. *Am Rev Resp Dis* 1991;**144**:1240–1244.

12. Cote CJ, Goldstein EA, Fuchsman WH, Hoaglin DC. The effect of nail polish on pulse oximetry. *Anesth Analg* 1989;**67**:683–686.

13. Hinkelbein J, Genzwuerker HV, Sogl R, Fiedler F. Effect of nail polish on oxygen saturation determination by pulse oximetry in critically ill patients. *Resuscitation* 2007;**72**:82–91.

14. Emergency Care Research Institute. Next generation pulse oximetry. *Health Devices* 2003;**32**:49–103.

15. Moller JT, Pederson T, Rasmussen LS, et al. Randomized evaluation of pulse oximetry in 20 802 patients. I: Design, demography, pulse oximetry failure rate and overall complication rate. *Anesthesiology* 1993;**78**:436–444.

16. Moller JT, Johannessen NW, Espersen K, et al. Randomized evaluation of pulse oximetry in 20,802 patients. II: Perioperative events and postoperative complications. *Anesthesiology* 1993;**78**:445–453.

17. Pederson T. Does perioperative pulse oximetry improve outcome? Seeking the best available evidence to answer the clinical question. *Best Pract Res Clin Anaesthesiol* 2005;**19**:111–123.

18. Pederson T, Moller AM, Pederson BD. Pulse oximetry for perioperative monitoring: systemic review of randomized, controlled trials. *Anesth Analg* 2003;**96**:426–431.

19. Hoffman RA, Ershowsky PF, Krieger BP. Determination of auto-PEEP during spontaneous and controlled ventilation by monitoring changes in end-expiratory thoracic gas volume. *Chest* 1989;**96**:613–616.

20. Birmingham PK, Cheney FW, Ward RJ. Esophageal intubation: a review of detection techniques. *Anesth Analg* 1986;**65**:886–891.

21. Vaghadia H, Jenkins LC, Ford RW. Comparison of end-tidal carbon dioxide, oxygen saturation and clinical signs for the detection of oesophageal intubation. *Can J Anaesth* 1989;**36**:560–564.

22. Knapp S, Kofler J, Stoiser B, et al. The assessment of four different methods to verify tracheal tube placement in the critical care setting. *Anesth Analg* 1999;**88**:766–770.

23. Loeb RG, Santos WC. Monitoring ventilation. In Hanowell LH, Waldron RJ (eds.) *Airway Management*. Philadelphia, PA: Lipincott-Raven, 1996, pp. 15–37.

24. Campbell LA, Klocke RA. Implication for the pregnant patient. *Am J Resp Crit Care Med* 2001;**163**:1051–1054.

25. Templeton A, Kelman GR. Maternal blood-gases, (P_{AO_2}–P_{aO_2}), physiological shunt and VD/VT in normal pregnancy. *Br J Anaesth* 1976;**48**:1001–1004.

26. Shinozaki T, Deane RS, Mazuzan JE. The dynamic responses of liquid filled catheter systems for direct measurements of blood pressure. *Anesthesiology* 1980;**53**:498.

27. Scheer BV, Perel A, Pfeiffer UJ. Clinical review: complications and risk factors of peripheral arterial catheters used for haemodynamic monitoring in anaesthesia and intensive care medicine. *Crit Care* 2002;**6**:198–204.

28. Merrer J, De Jonghe B, Golliot F, et al. Complications of femoral and subclavian venous catheterization in critically ill patients: a randomized controlled trial. *JAMA* 2001;**286**:700.

29. Raad I. Intravascular-catheter-related infections. *Lancet* 1998;**351**:893.

30. O'Grady NP, Alexander M, Dellinger EP, et al. Guidelines for the prevention of intravascular catheter-related infections. *Am J Infect Control* 2002;**30**:476.

31. Duntley P, Siever J, Korwes ML, et al. Vascular erosion by central venous catheter. Clinical features and outcomes. *Chest* 1992;**101**:1633.

32. Ruesch S, Walder B, Tramer MR. Complications of central venous catheters: internal jugular versus subclavian access – a systematic review. *Crit Care Med* 2002;**30**:454.

33. Curelaru I, Linder LE, Gustavsson B. Displacement of catheters through internal jugular veins with neck flexion and extension. A preliminary study. *Intensive Care Med* 1980;**6**:179.

34. Wojciechowski J, Curelaru I, Gustavsson B, *et al.* "Half-way" venous catheters. III. Tip displacements with movements of the upper extremity. *Acta Anaesthesiol Scand* 1985;**81**:36.

35. Raad II, Hohn DC, Gilbreath BJ, *et al.* Precention of central venous catheter-related infections by using maximal sterile barrier precautions during insertion. *Infect Control Hosp Epidemiol* 1994;**15**:231.

36. National Nosocomial Infection Surveillance System: National Nosocomial Infection Surveillance (NNIS) system report, data summary from January 1992 through June 2004; issued October 2004. *Am J Infect Control* 2004;**32**:470.

37. Maki DG, Cobb L, Garman JK, *et al.* An attachable silver-impregnated cuff for prevention of infection with central venous catheters: a prospective randomized multicenter trial. *Am J Med* 1988; **85**: 307.

38. Pinsky MR. Clinical significance of pulmonary artery occlusion pressure. *Intensive Care Med* 2003;**29**:175–178.

39. Clark SL, Cotton DB, Lee W, *et al.* Central hemodynamic assessment of normal term pregnancy. *Am J Obstet Gynecol* 1989;**161**:1439–1442.

40. Damen J, Bolton D. A prospective analusis of 1400 pulmonary artery catheterizations in patients undergoing cardiac surgery. *Acta Anaesthesiol Scand* 1986;**14**:1957.

41. McDaniel DD, Stone JG, Faltas AN, *et al.* Catheter induced pulmonart artery hemorrhage: diagnosis and management in cardiac operations. *J Thorac Cardiovasc Surg* 1981;**82**:1.

42. Shah KB, Roa TL, Laughlin S, *et al.* A review of pulmonary artery catheterization in 6245 patients. *Anesthesiology* 1984;**61**:271.

43. Carlin A, Alfirevic Z. Physiological changes of pregnancy and monitoring. *Best Pract Res Clin Obstet Gynecol* 2008;**22**:801–823.

44. Koo KY, Sun JCJ, Zhou Q, *et al.* Pulmonary artery catheters: evolving rates and reasons for use. *Crit Care Med* 2011;**39**:1613–1618.

45. Vincent J-L. So we use less pulmonary artery catheters: but why? *Crit Care Med* 2011;**39**:1820–1822.

46. Michard F, Boussat S, Chemla D, *et al.* Relation between respiratory changes in arterial pulse pressure and fluid responsiveness in septic patients with acute circulatory failure. *Am J Resp Crit Care Med* 2000;**162**:134–138.

47. Kramer A, Zygun D, Hawes H, *et al.* Pulse pressure variation predicts fluid responsiveness following coronary artery bypass surgery. *Chest* 2004;**126**:1563–1568.

48. Michard F, Alaya S, Zarka V, *et al.* Global end-diastolic volume as an indicator of cardiac preload in patients with septic shock. *Chest* 2003;1900–1908.

49. Dyer RA, Piercy JL, Reed AR, *et al.* Hemodynamic changes associated with spinal anesthesia for cesarean delivery in severe preeclampsia. *Anesthesiology* 2008;**108**:802–811.

50. Archer TL, Heitmyer TD. Perioperative hemodynamics obtained by pulse contour wave analysis facilitated the management of a patient with chronic hypertension, renal insufficiency, and superimposed preeclampsia during cesarean delivery. *J Clin Anesth* 2010;**22**:274–279.

51. Armstrong S, Fernando R, Columb M. Minimally and non- invasive assessment of maternal cardiac output: go with the flow! *Int J Obstet Anesth* 2011;**20**:330–340.

52. Vries JK, Becker DP, Young HF. A subarachnoid screw for monitoring intracranial pressure. Technical note. *J Neurosurg* 1973;**39**:416–419.

53. Gopez JJ, Meagher RH, Narayan RK. When and how should I monitor intracranial pressure? In Valadka AB, Andrews BT (eds.) *Neurotrauma*. New York: Thieme, 2005, pp. 53–57.

54. Marmarou A, Anderson RL, Ward JD, *et al.* Impact of ICP instability and hypotension on outcome in patient with severe head injury. *J Neurosurg* 1991;**75**:S59–S66.

55. Rosner MJ, Rosner SD, Johnson AH. Cerebral perfusion pressure: management protocol and clinical results. *J Neurosurg* 1995;**83**:949–962.

56. Feldman Z, Narayan RK. Intracranial pressure monitoring: techniques and pitfalls. In Cooper PR, Golfinos JG (eds.) *Head Injury*, 4th edn. New York: McGraw-Hill, 2000, pp. 265–292.

57. Brain Trauma Foundation, American Association of Neurologic Surgeons, Joint Section on Neurotrauma and Critical Care. Management and prognosis of severe traumatic brain injury: Part 1. Guidelines for the management of severe traumatic brain injury. Indications for intracranial pressure monitoring. *J Neurotrauma* 2000;**17**:47–69.

58. Maramou A, Signoretti S, Fatouros PP, *et al.* Predominance of cellular edema in traumatic brain swelling in patients with severe head injuries. *J Neurosurg* 2000;**104**:720–730.

59. Brain Trauma Foundation. *The American Association of Neurologic Surgeons, the Congress of Neurological Surgeons, the Joint Section on Neurotrauma and Critical Care: Update Notice, Guidelines for the Management of Severe Traumatic Brain Injury: Cerebral Perfusion Pressure*. New York, Brain Trauma Foundation, 2003.

60. Barnett G, Chapman P. Insertion and care of intracranial pressure monitoring devices. In Ropper A, Kennedy S (eds.) *Neurological and Neurosurgical Intensive Care*. Rockville, MD, Aspen, 1998, pp. 000–000.

61. Turtz A. Intracranial monitoring. In Parillo JE, Dellinger, RP (eds.) *Critical Care Medicine: Principles of Diagnosis and Management in the Adult*. Philadelphia, PA: Mosby-Elsevier, 2008, pp. 281–288.

62. Maas AI, Fleckenstein W, de Jong DA, *et al.* Monitoring cerebral oxygenation: experimental studies and preliminary clinical results of continuous monitoring of cerebrospinal fluid and brain tissue oxygen tension. *Acta Neurochirurg Suppl* 1993;**59**:50–57.

63. Meixensberger J, Dings J, Kuhnigk H, *et al.* Studies of tissue P_{O_2} in normal and pathological human brain cortex. *Acta Neurochirurg Suppl* 1993;**59**:58–63.

64. van den Brink WA, Haitsma IK, Avezaat CJ, *et al.* Brain parenchyma/P_{O_2} catheter interface: a histopathological study in the rat. *J Neurotrauma* 1998;**15**:813–824.

65. Leniger-Follert E. Oxygen supply and microcirculation of the brain cortex. *Adv Exp Med Biol* 1985;**191**:3–19.

66. Hoffman WE, Carbel FT, Edelman G, *et al.* Brain tissue oxygen pressure, carbon dioxide pressure and pH during ischemia. *Neurol Res* 1996;**18**:54–56.

67. Stout MJ, Cahill AG. Electronic fetal monitoring: past, present and future. *Clin Perinatol* 2011;**38**:127–142.

68. American College of Obstetricians and Gynecologists. *Practice Bulletin 9: Antepartum Fetal Surveillance*. Washington, DC: American College of Obstetricians and Gynecologists, 1999, updated 2012.

69. Grivell RM, Alfirevic Z, Gyte GML, Devane D. Antenatal cardiotocography for fetal assessment. *Cochrane Database Syst Rev* 2010(1):CD007863.

Chapter 22

Imaging issues in maternal critical care

Melina Pectasides, Filip Claus, and Susanna I. Lee

Introduction

Radiological imaging of the critically ill pregnant woman poses many challenges and constraints unique to this patient population. Correct choice of an imaging examination must take into account not only the clinical scenario but also the potential effects of radiation exposure and intravenous contrast agent administration to both the mother and the fetus. Unfortunately, the appropriate indications, safety concerns, and diagnostic performance associated with the multitude of radiological studies represent a knowledge gap for many physicians. Among physicians and the public as a whole, the perception of fetal risk associated with imaging is generally higher than the actual risk. Moreover, in the intensive care unit (ICU) setting, a missed or delayed diagnosis usually poses a much greater risk to the woman and her pregnancy than the hazards of a radiological examination.

Close consultation between the clinical team and the radiologist is essential to optimize the choice and performance of the radiological examination. Seamless communication is required to expedite addressing the diagnostic dilemma while minimizing the risk to either the mother or the fetus. This chapter describes the various imaging modalities and the safety concerns associated with each when used during pregnancy or in the immediate postpartum period. The relative advantages and disadvantages of imaging modalities are discussed in the context of specific clinical scenarios relating to maternal critical care.

Effects of radiation on the fetus

The radiation effects to the fetus are categorized into deterministic and stochastic effects (Box 22.1). Deterministic effects are non-stochastic, dose related and are seen above a baseline threshold dose. Examples of deterministic effects include pregnancy loss, growth restriction, mental retardation, and organ malformation. In contrast, stochastic effects are possible at any level of radiation exposure with no minimum threshold and with the likelihood increasing with dose. In pregnancy, stochastic effects primarily refer to risk of childhood cancer. The type and severity of deterministic effects and the likelihood of stochastic effects vary with gestational age at the time of exposure and with radiation dose delivered to the uterus [1].

The American College of Radiologists practice guidelines for imaging pregnant patients, issued in 2010, provided a summary of induced deterministic radiation effects in utero at various gestational ages and radiation exposures [2]. This summary suggests that risks are unlikely at doses smaller than 100 mGy. At doses above 100 mGy, the risks for deterministic effects such as developmental deficits start to appear but remain low until doses exceed 150–200 mGy. As for stochastic effects, the data are not consistent, but it has been estimated that fetal radiation dose of 100 mGy increases the risk for childhood cancer, particularly leukemia, by 0.1%. The risk of childhood cancer becomes negligible at doses of less than 50 mGy [1,3].

Fetal radiation dose from almost all diagnostic imaging examinations falls well below clinically negligible doses. Examinations where the fetus is not directly in the radiation beam would administer much less than 1 mGy. When the fetus is directly in the radiation beam, such as pelvic radiography or abdominopelvic CT, the fetus will be exposed to the highest doses but, nevertheless, these are estimated to still fall below the 50 mGy threshold. When outcomes are evaluated, the offspring of women exposed to major radiological studies in pregnancy do not appear to be at higher risk of childhood malignancy than the children of unexposed mothers [4].

Maternal Critical Care: A Multidisciplinary Approach, ed. Marc Van de Velde, Helen Scholefield, and Lauren A. Plante.
Published by Cambridge University Press. © Cambridge University Press 2013.

Imaging modalities

Plain radiography and fluoroscopy

Plain radiographic studies in which the uterus is not included in the field of view (e.g. head, neck, chest, and limbs) expose the fetus to scattered radiation only and the dose is negligible:

- non-abdominal plain radiographs: negligible
- abdominopelvic plain radiograph: well below 50 mGy [1]
- fluoroscopic procedures: more variable and substantial, unlikely to exceed 100 mGy [5].

Even for plain radiographic studies of the abdomen and pelvis, where the uterus is included in the field of view, the typical fetal dose is estimated at 2–3 mGy [1]. With fluoroscopic procedures, the fetal dose is more variable and more substantial but is highly unlikely to exceed the threshold of 100 mGy for deterministic and stochastic effects [5].

Ultrasound

Ultrasound (US) is often the first imaging modality in evaluating the pregnant patient for abdominopelvic pathologies. It can be performed at the bedside and can reliably evaluate the gallbladder, kidneys, and the urinary bladder, while simultaneously evaluating the gestation. It also detects moderate to large amounts of free intraperitoneal fluid. Because of its limited field of view and low soft tissue contrast, US is less reliable in detecting hepatic, pancreatic, splenic, appendiceal, and adnexal pathologies. Ultrasound evaluates bowel

poorly and is unreliable in detecting abscesses, hematomas, and free air. Consequently, in the context of high clinical suspicion of these pathologies, referring the patient directly to CT or MRI, particularly in practice settings where these modalities are readily available, may allow a faster diagnosis.

No biological effects have been documented from diagnostic US examinations in the pregnant patient, despite widespread use over several decades. With Doppler, the risks to the fetus from heat and cavitation exists and, therefore, it should be used judiciously, keeping the exposure time and acoustic output to the lowest level possible [6].

Computed tomography

Computed tomography is fast, reliable, and affords a large field of view; consequently, it is considered the first-line imaging modality for many indications in non-pregnant adults. The fetal radiation dose with CT is:

- when not directly imaging the fetus (e.g. head, chest, neck): negligible
- abdominopelvic CT, typically about 20 to 35 mGy and rarely exceeds 50 mGy [7].

In pregnancy, the potential effects of fetal radiation exposure should be factored into the risk–benefit analysis when considering ordering an abdomino-pelvic scan:

- seek radiological consultation to maintain diagnostic image quality while minimizing fetal dose
- avoid repeat examinations.

Therefore, the physician should understand what types of CT examination have the potential to deliver biologically significant radiation doses to the fetus.

Fetal radiation exposure during non-abdominal CT scans is minimal. Scans of the head, cervical spine, and extremities can be performed safely regardless of gestation age. For a chest CT examination, the fetal dose is also negligible if the fetus is not included in the field of view. The maximum fetal dose from a chest CT is estimated to be less than 1 mGy [7,8].

With abdominopelvic CT, where the uterus is directly imaged by the radiation beam, fetal dose can be more substantial, ranging between 20 and 35 mGy [7]. Here, close consultation with a radiologist is advised to insure that the examination is tailored to address the diagnostic question while minimizing radiation dose. The radiologist can optimize such variables as scanning parameters, patient positioning, and choice of contrast to insure patient safety without sacrificing diagnostic accuracy. While a single CT pass through the abdomen and pelvis confers negligible fetal radiation dose, multiple consecutive examinations or acquisitions through the uterus during the same examination should be avoided as fetal dose can then exceed 50 mGy [9].

Magnetic resonance imaging

An MRI scan can be used to assess a number of maternal and fetal diseases quickly with high image quality, multiplanar capability, and a large field of view without raising radiation concerns. Pelvic MRI has been in use for more than 20 years with no evidence of adverse effects to the fetus in both clinical and laboratory investigations [10]. Nevertheless, safety concerns regarding potential heating effects of radiofrequency pulses and acoustic injury to the fetus have not been completely dispelled [11]. While no fetal harm has been reported with 1.5 T magnetic field strength, little experience has been reported at higher field strengths. Given the lack of evidence indicating any adverse effects, MRI for the pregnant patient is considered of equivalent safety regardless of gestational age and should not be delayed or deferred for safety concerns if clinically indicated [10].

Disadvantages of MRI include limited access to the scanner itself or to radiologist expertise to implement and interpret the examinations in some practice settings. Most examinations require the patient to lie still in an enclosed high field strength magnet for up to 20–40 minutes. In the critically ill patient, monitoring and supportive-care equipment that are compatible with high field strength magnets are required. In the conscious patient, concerns such as claustrophobia or inability to cooperate with the scanning procedure can hinder successful image acquisition.

Nuclear medicine

Fetal radiation dose during nuclear medicine studies depends upon the maternal uptake and excretion of the radiopharmaceutical, placental permeability, fetal distribution, and tissue affinity, and also on the half-life, dose, and type of radiation emitted. The fetal radiation exposure:

• for the most commonly performed nuclear medicine studies is well below the level of concern [12]

• can be reduced by maternal hydration and frequent voiding, which reduces fetal exposure from its proximity to radionuclides excreted into the maternal bladder.

However, the long scanning times render this approach less suitable for the critically ill patient.

The most commonly performed diagnostic nuclear medicine studies use technetium-99m, which has a short half-life [12] and delivers a fetal radiation dose far below the threshold of concern. Bone scans deliver approximately 5 mGy, thyroid scans 0.2 mGy, and lung ventilation/perfusion scans 0.37 mGy to the fetus [1,13]. The few data available on the use of ^{18}F-fluorodeoxyglucose positron emission tomography studies during pregnancy suggest that the radiation dose to the fetus is small, ranging from 1.1 to 2.43 mGy [14].

An important disadvantage of several nuclear medicine studies is the long scanning time, upwards of 30 minutes and up to several hours, which renders them less suitable for the critically ill patient.

Contrast agents in pregnancy and lactation

Table 22.1 summarizes the contrast agents used in pregnancy and lactation.

Iodinated contrast agents

Iodinated contrast agent administered to a pregnant woman crosses the placenta, resulting in possible fetal thyroid depression by exposure to free iodine [16]. While such an effect has never been directly demonstrated [18], infants of mothers who received iodinated contrast during pregnancy should be tested for hypothyroidism, already a standard neonatal screening procedure in the USA. No evidence suggesting that iodinated contrast is teratogenic or carcinogenic has been reported. Given the lack of definitive evidence of adverse effect, they are considered a category B drug (i.e. no evidence of fetal risk in human and/or animal studies [15]) by the US Food and Drug Administration. Hence, the chance of fetal harm should be considered remote when iodinated contrast is used in pregnancy.

Gadolinium

Gadolinium contrast agents administered to a pregnant woman cross the placenta and enter the fetal circulation, are filtered via the fetal kidneys, and

Table 22.1. Contrast agents in pregnancy and lactation

Agent	Features
Iodinated contrast for CT and fluoroscopy	Category B drug, i.e. can be used in pregnancy as long as there is appropriate clinical indication [15] Crosses the placenta and ingested by the fetus Administer contrast if it will improve diagnostic yield and so minimize need for repeat imaging with ionizing radiation Theoretical concern of transient fetal hypothyroidism with in utero exposure; therefore, maternal exposure during pregnancy requires that neonates be screened for hypothyroidism [16]
Gadolinium-based contrast for MRI	Category C drug, i.e. should not be used routinely in pregnant patients [15] Crosses the placenta and is ingested by the fetus Administer only if non-contrast imaging proves inconclusive and if the contrast images are likely to yield diagnostic information that will benefit the mother or fetus
Lactation	Breastfeeding after maternal intravenous contrast administration would result in the infant absorbing <0.05% of the permitted dose [17] Cessation of breastfeeding is thought to be unnecessary to insure infant safety [15–17] Active expression and discarding of breast milk for 24 hours after intravenous contrast administration is the only method to insure no infant exposure

excreted into the amniotic fluid, where they may remain for an indeterminate time. To date, no adverse effects to the human fetus have been reported. However, because the potential effects of fetal absorption of gadolinium contrast agents have not been fully explored, most practices refrain from using it routinely in pregnancy. Because MRI without contrast administration affords a high degree of tissue contrast, intravenous contrast should only be given if, after review of the non-contrast-enhanced images, the radiologist deems that this is necessary and likely to aid in addressing the diagnostic question. Since there have been no adequate studies of the effects of gadolinium in pregnancy, it is considered a category C drug (i.e. risks cannot be ruled out in humans) by the US

Food and Drug Administration [15]. Hence, gadolinium should be used in pregnancy only if the potential benefits are thought to outweigh possible fetal risks.

Lactation

Following intravenous administration, very low levels of iodinated or gadolinium-based contrast agents are excreted in breast milk and ingested by the infant. After oral ingestion, very small amounts are absorbed into the bloodstream of the neonate. Because this represents <0.05% of the permitted pediatric dose [17], cessation of breastfeeding is thought to be unnecessary to insure infant safety. However, active expression and discarding of breast milk for 24 hours after intravenous contrast administration, recommended by the manufacturers of intravenous contrast agents, is the only method to insure that the infant incurs no exposure [15,16].

Clinical scenarios

Deep venous thrombosis and pulmonary embolus

Venous thrombosis most commonly occurs in the lower extremities (Table 22.2). However, pregnant patients are also at risk for pelvic, hepatic, mesenteric, and gonadal venous thrombi [19]. For evaluation of the lower extremities, vascular US with compression and Doppler is the preferred examination as it demonstrates sensitivity and specificity of 94% [20], and a positive result leads to systemic anticoagulation and renders additional testing for pulmonary embolus unnecessary [21]. However, because of its limited field of view, US has a limited role in the detection of pelvic vein thrombosis. Rather, CT venography or MR venography should be used as both demonstrate high sensitivities and specificities (>90%) [22]. Intravenous contrast is required for CT venography and it will also involve fetal ionizing radiation exposure. Use of MR venography avoids fetal ionizing radiation and can be performed without intravenous contrast administration utilizing time-of-flight pulse sequences [23].

When pulmonary embolus is suspected in a patient with chest pain or dyspnea, plain chest radiograph is usually the first imaging study performed. Its purpose is not to detect pulmonary embolus but to exclude alternative diagnoses (e.g. pneumothorax, pneumonia, pulmonary edema, rib fracture) that may account for the symptoms. Pulmonary embolus can be diagnosed using CT pulmonary angiography (Figure 22.1) or

Table 22.2. Pulmonary embolus

Modality	Advantages	Disadvantages
Chest radiography	Negligible fetal ionizing radiation	Does not directly detect pulmonary embolus
	Available at bedside	
	Enabled diagnosis of non-embolic causes of pulmonary symptoms	
CT	Negligible fetal ionizing radiation [24]	Intravenous contrast required
	High (99%) negative predictive value	Higher maternal radiation dose than nuclear medicine scan
	Enabled diagnosis of non-embolic causes of pulmonary symptoms	20% indeterminate results [25]
	Short (usually <5 minutes) scanning time	
Nuclear medicine	Negligible fetal ionizing radiation [24]	Long (usually >30 minutes) scanning time
	High (100%) negative predictive value	20% indeterminate results [25]
	Lower maternal radiation dose than chest CT	

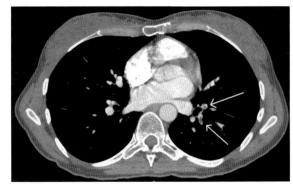

Figure 22.1. Pulmonary embolus. A CT pulmonary angiogram in a 38-year-old pregnant woman at 10 weeks of gestation who presented with sudden onset of dyspnea on exertion, chest tightness, and palpitations. The angiogram shows filling defects (arrows) representing embolic thrombi in branches of the left pulmonary artery.

ventilation/perfusion nuclear medicine scan. Both deliver negligible (<1 mGy) fetal radiation dose and demonstrate high (>99%) negative predictive value [24], with approximately 20% rate of indeterminate results in the pregnant patient [25]. The advantages of CT are the rapid image acquisition time and the potential for identifying alternative diagnoses. The advantages of the nuclear medicine scan are lower radiation dose to the maternal breast and the avoidance of intravenous iodinated contrast.

Acute abdomen

In pregnant patients with acute non-specific abdominal pain, the imaging examination most readily available is a plain abdominal radiograph (Table 22.3). This can be performed at the bedside and can quickly assess for severe bowel obstruction or free intraperitoneal air, conditions that would warrant urgent surgical

evaluation and possible intervention. Unfortunately, the radiograph is insensitive for detecting all other intra-abdominal pathologies. Ultrasound is also available at the bedside, can reliably evaluate the gestation, the gallbladder, kidneys, and the urinary bladder and detect free intraperitoneal fluid. It is less reliable in detecting hepatic, pancreatic, splenic, appendiceal, and adnexal pathologies. Ultrasound provides poor evaluation of the bowel and it is unreliable in detecting abscesses, hematomas, and free air. Computed tomography provides a thorough and accurate evaluation of the solid organs, bowel, and vessels and it reliably detects abscesses, hematomas, and free air. In non-pregnant patients, with no fetal radiation safety considerations, this would be the preferred imaging modality for this indication. Magnetic resonance imaging also evaluates solid organs, gestation, adnexa, and vessels well and can accurately diagnose a wide variety of acute pathologies including appendicitis, adnexal torsion, cholecystitis, abscess, and hematomas [26]. However, MRI is less sensitive than CT in the detection of free air and occult bowel pathologies.

Appendicitis

Diagnosis of appendicitis in pregnancy is particularly challenging because of the unpredictable location of the appendix and the underlying physiological leukocytosis (Table 22.4). Graded compression US, available at the bedside, can be used. However, because its accuracy is determined by several factors, including operator experience, patient body habitus, and depth of the imaging target, a wide range of test

Table 22.3. Acute abdomen

Modality	Advantages	Disadvantages
Plain radiography	Available at bedside	Fetal ionizing radiation
	Evaluates for free air and bowel obstruction	Insensitive for detecting all other intra-abdominal pathologies
Ultrasound	No ionizing radiation	Limited bowel evaluation
	Available at bedside	Unreliable in detecting abscess, hematoma and free air
	Evaluates gestation, gallbladder, kidneys, and bladder well	Limited field of view in evaluating adnexa
CT	Typically <10 minutes scanning time	Fetal ionizing radiation
	Evaluates solid organs, bowel, and vessels well	Intravenous contrast needed for optimal test performance
MRI	Reliably detects abscess, hematoma, and free air	Limited availability of technology and/ or expertise
	Evaluates solid organs, vessels, gestation, and adnexa well [26]	Requires patient to lie still in an enclosed high field strength magnet for approximately 20–40 minutes
	Reliably detects abscess and hematoma	Less reliable than CT for detecting bowel pathologies and free air

Table 22.4. Appendicitis

Modality	Advantages	Disadvantages
Ultrasound	No ionizing radiation	Highly variable test performance; reported sensitivity of 67–100% [27,28]
	Available at bedside	Up to 50% of normal appendices not visualized
CT	Reproducibly high accuracy, 95–100% [30]	Fetal ionizing radiation
	>99% normal appendices visualized	
MRI	No ionizing radiation	Limited availability of technology and/or expertise
	High accuracy 100% sensitive, 94% specific [28,29]	Requires patient to lie still in an enclosed high field strength magnet for approximately 30–60 minutes
	~80% normal appendices visualized	

performance (sensitivities of 67–100%) has been reported. Furthermore, US fails to visualize up to 50% of normal appendices, making it a poor choice for excluding appendicitis [27,28]. Several studies have shown MRI (Figure 22.2) to have very high sensitivity (100%) and specificity (94%) and it visualizes the normal appendix in over 80% of patients [28,29]. The imaging protocol involves administration of a bowel-darkening oral contrast agent (ferumoxsil) but no intravenous contrast. A CT with intravenous contrast diagnoses appendicitis with sensitivity and specificity approaching 100% [30] and, in the non-pregnant patient, is usually the preferred imaging modality.

Renal colic and urosepsis

Urolithiasis, obstructive hydronephrosis, pyelonephritis, and cystitis can cause abdominal pain and lead to life-threatening complications of urosepsis (Table 22.5). Plain radiographs can detect urinary calculi, albeit with a lower sensitivity and fetal radiation dose than CT. With US, secondary findings of urinary obstruction such as hydronephrosis can be confidently detected [19]. However, late in pregnancy, distinguishing hydronephrosis from physiological dilatation remains a diagnostic challenge. Ultrasound is unreliable in identifying obstructing stones and is insensitive for detecting complications of ureteral obstruction such as pyelonephritis, abscess, or urinoma. Low-dose CT without intravenous contrast (Figure 22.3) reproducibly demonstrates high sensitivity and specificity (>90%) for detecting and measuring the size of obstructing stones while subjecting the fetus to negligible doses of radiation [1]. However, intravenous contrast is necessary for optimal assessment for complications. Hydronephrosis and hydroureter can also be clearly visualized with MRI, which can often differentiate them from physiological dilatation. It also reliably detects complications. However, MRI is insensitive for directly visualizing

Table 22.5. Renal colic and urosepsis

Modality	Advantages	Disadvantages
Plain radiography	Available at bedside	Fetal ionizing radiation
	Can detect radiopaque stones	Less sensitive than CT for stone detection
		Insensitive for detecting complications of ureteral obstruction, e.g. pyelonephritis, abscess, urinoma
Ultrasound	No ionizing radiation	Highly variable test performance in detecting obstructing stones
	Available at bedside	Insensitive for detecting complications of ureteral obstruction, e.g. pyelonephritis, abscess, urinoma
CT	Reproducibly high sensitivity and specificity of >90% for detecting obstructing stone [1]	Fetal ionizing radiation
	Reliably detects complications of ureteral obstruction, e.g. pyelonephritis, abscess, urinoma	Intravenous contrast needed to detect complications of ureteral obstruction
MRI	No ionizing radiation	Limited availability of technology and/or expertise
	Reliably detects complications of ureteral obstruction, e.g. pyelonephritis, abscess, urinoma	Requires patient to lie still in an enclosed high field strength magnet for approximately 20–40 minutes
		Does not detect stones

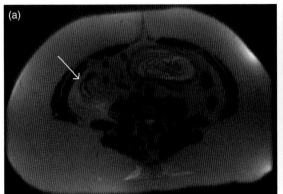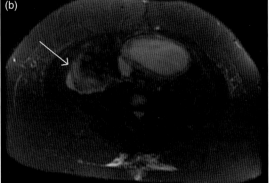

Figure 22.2. Appendicitis. Pelvic MRI without intravenous contrast in a 23-year-old pregnant woman at 15 weeks of gestation who presented with epigastric to right lower quadrant pain. T_2-weighted (a) and inversion recovery (b) sequences demonstrate a distended, fluid-filled appendix (arrow), with periappendiceal inflammation and fluid.

calculi and assessing their size. Sonographic guidance is preferred above conventional fluoroscopy or CT guidance for percutaneous nephrostomy catheter placement.

Trauma

Trauma is a major cause of maternal and fetal mortality, and imaging choices in this setting should be prioritized for fast and accurate diagnosis:

- CT of head, cervical spine, and chest; plain radiography of cervical spine and chest if CT not available

- US of the abdomen and pelvis: assess gestation, detect hemoperitoneum, and signs of gross solid organ injury
- CT of the abdomen and pelvis with intravenous contrast: detect vascular, bone, bowel, and most solid organ injuries, including placental abruption.

In the pregnant patient with suspected major injuries, choice of examination is the same as in the non-pregnant woman, with the acquisition parameters modified to minimize fetal radiation dose while maintaining adequate image quality. In examinations where the fetus is not directly within the field of view, such as

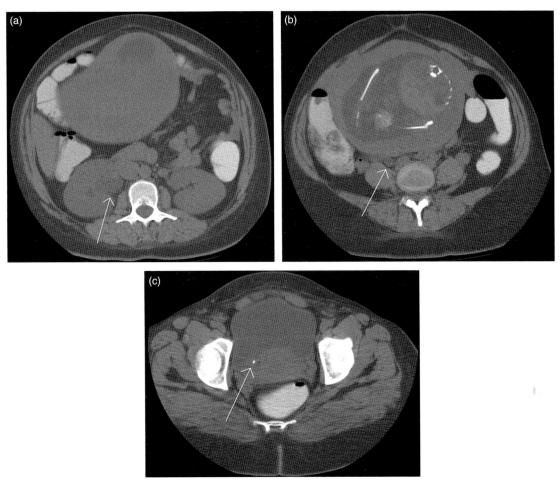

Figure 22.3. Obstructive urolithiasis. Abdominopelvic CT without intravenous contrast in a 34-year-old woman at 27 weeks of gestation who presented with right-sided abdominal pain, fever and elevated white blood count. The scans demonstrate right-sided hydronephrosis (arrow) (a), hydroureter (arrow) (b), and a stone at the ureterovesical junction (arrow) (c).

chest and cervical spine radiography and chest, cervical spine, and head CT, radiation dose to the fetus is negligible and should not be part of the risk–benefit analysis for appropriate imaging choice.

For abdominopelvic imaging, US, rapidly performed at the bedside, is best suited to triage the unstable patient. It assesses the gestation and evaluates for intraperitoneal free fluid and major solid organ injury. The sensitivity of US for hemoperitoneum is highest in the first trimester but is overall lower in the pregnant than in the non-pregnant patient [31]. In addition, solid organ injuries without associated hemoperitoneum are often missed, while bowel, retroperitoneal, bladder, and bony pelvic injuries go undetected [32].

The most accurate and cost-efficient tool for abdominopelvic evaluation of any major trauma patient, including the pregnant woman, is CT (Figure 22.4) [33]. Examination can be performed rapidly, even in unconscious or uncooperative patients, and it can be tailored to minimize fetal radiation dose to negligible levels. The large field of view allows the physician to comprehensively define the extent of intra- and extraperitoneal injuries to bones and soft tissues. Intravenous contrast administration is necessary, particularly for detection of life-threatening arterial vascular extravasation, solid organ laceration, and small volumes of free, low-density fluid, which may be the only finding of significant injury to the bowel [34]. While MRI performs similarly in diagnosing traumatic injuries, its limited availability and long examination times make it an impractical tool for evaluating most major trauma patients [21].

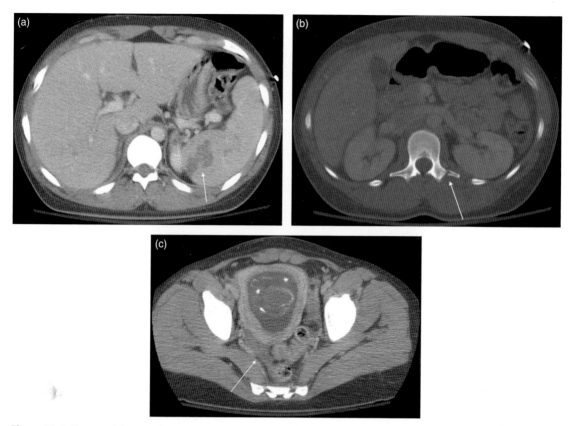

Figure 22.4. Trauma. Abdominopelvic CT with intravenous contrast in a 32-year-old woman at 18 weeks of gestation following a major motor vehicle accident. The scans demonstrate a splenic laceration (arrow) (a), fracture of the left transverse process of L1 vertebral body (arrow) (b), and blood in the pelvis (arrow) (c).

In the context of motor vehicle accidents, assaults or falls, special emphasis should be placed on the risk of an acute placental abruption. In this condition, large blood loss can potentially lead to fetal and maternal death. Although US is a good modality to screen for placental abnormalities, it lacks sensitivity to detect abruption, particularly in the second and third trimester. Therefore CT evaluation is strongly recommended in patients with an acute abdomen who suffered abdominal trauma (Figure 22.5) [35].

Ectopic pregnancy

An ectopic pregnancy (implantation of the embryo outside the uterine cavity) occurs most commonly in the fallopian tube, but it may occur anywhere in the abdomen. Tubal, ovarian, and cervical implantations are not viable and bear a risk of potential life-threatening internal hemorrhage. Early symptoms are non-specific, such as pain in the lower abdomen or vaginal bleeding, and are progressive if there is severe internal bleeding,

including shoulder pain and cramping. An elevated human beta-chorionic gonadotropin (>1.500 IU/L) in the absence of an intrauterine pregnancy is highly indicative for an ectopic implantation. Transvaginal and transabdominal US are the imaging modalities of choice to screen tubal pregnancies, although MRI can be used as an adjunct to US in stable clinical conditions [36]. Detection of tubal pregnancy on CT is rare (Figure 22.6), and is typically reported in the clinical context of an acute abdomen without any suspicion of pregnancy. The presence of an ectopic gestational sac is a highly specific imaging sign, but this is generally obscured by foci of bleeding. In advanced abdominal pregnancies (primary or secondary after tubal rupture), MRI is a valuable tool to screen for placental implantation into abdominal viscera or parasitization of major vessels. Patients presenting with advanced abdominal pregnancies are diagnostically challenging and require experienced obstetric surgical care because of the high incidence of complications such as severe internal bleeding.

Pre-eclampsia

Pre-eclampsia, eclampsia, and HELLP (hemolysis, elevated liver enzymes, low platelets) syndrome represent common reasons for admission in the maternal ICU (Table 22.6). The role of imaging in these patients is not for primary diagnosis but for detecting and assessing the extent of complications.

Evidence for extravasation of fluid can be seen with chest radiography as pleural effusions and pulmonary edema, or with US as ascites or pleural effusion. Hepatic complications of organomegaly, fatty infiltration, hemorrhage (progressing to rupture), and infarction (progressing to necrosis) can be seen with US, CT, or MRI, with increasing reliability with each successive modality (Figure 22.7). Findings indicating cerebrovascular complications of posterior reversible encephalopathy syndrome are detected with greater sensitivity with MRI than CT [37].

Table 22.6. Pre-eclampsia, eclampsia, and the HELLP syndrome

Complication	Examination
Fluid extravasation	Pleural effusion: chest plain radiograph or US Ascites: US of abdomen and pelvis
Hepatic complications	Organ enlargement fatty infiltration, hemorrhage, infarcts, and necrosis: evaluate with US, CT, or MRI
Cerebrovascular complications	Posterior reversible encephalopathy syndrome: MRI is more sensitive than CT [35]

US, ultrasound.

Obstetric hemorrhage

Postpartum hemorrhage may result from uterine atony, genital tract lacerations, abnormal placentation, pseudoaneurysms, arteriovenous malformations, retained products of conception, and surgical complications [38].

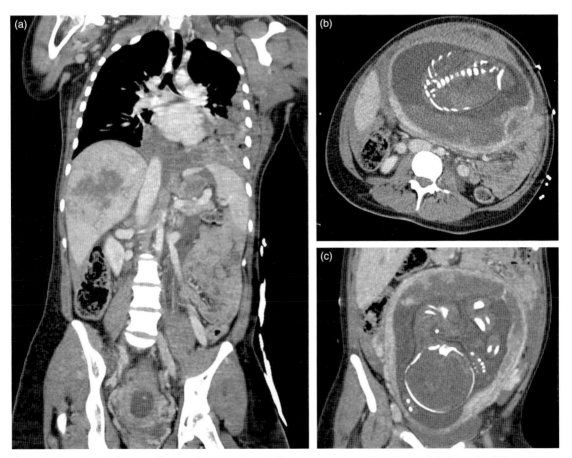

Figure 22.5. Placental abruption. Computed tomography with intravenous contrast of the chest and abdomen in a 25-year-old woman at 30 weeks of gestation who had a serious car accident. The scans show a left-sided lung contusion and a hepatic laceration (a) and absent perfusion in over 75% of the placenta (b,c). The fetus died within 6 hours after the accident.

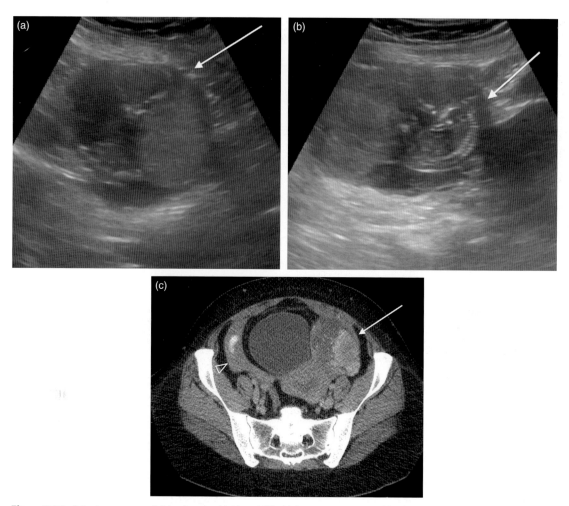

Figure 22.6. Ectopic pregnancy. Pelvic ultrasound (a,b) and CT with intravenous contrast (c) in a 40-year-old woman with acute abdominal pain. (a,b) Ultrasound demonstrates a left adnexal ectopic pregnancy (white arrows) with positive fetal heart rate and crown–rump length consistent with a 12-week gestation. (c) Confirmation of the ruptured left adnexal ectopic pregnancy (white arrow) with presence of blood within the gestational sac and in the peritoneum (white arrowhead). Laparoscopic investigation confirmed the presence of a left-sided tubal pregnancy.

If conservative measures and balloon tamponade of the uterus fail to control the hemorrhage, then pelvic arterial embolization under fluoroscopy (Figure 22.8) should be included as the next step of management [39]. It should be considered before surgical alternatives, because ligation of the uterine arteries renders subsequent attempt at embolization more challenging, while the failure to stop the hemorrhage with embolization does not preclude surgery [40].

Pelvic arterial embolization should be considered as the first-line therapy for postpartum hemorrhage if uterine balloon tamponade fails. Absence of contrast extravasation is frequent on angiography. The angiographer should nevertheless proceed with embolizing the uterine arteries or the anterior divisions of the internal iliac arteries bilaterally. Pelvic arterial embolization has an approximately 90% success rate in controlling postpartum hemorrhage [41,42]. Repeat embolization may be performed if bleeding persists.

Pelvic arterial embolization starts with catheterization of the internal iliac artery and angiography, which may or may not demonstrate active extravasation. Extravasation is frequently not visualized, especially with uterine atony [41]. This may be because there is diffuse bleeding from the uterine bed that does not exceed the 1 mL/min required for angiographic detection, there is intermittent bleeding, or there is arterial spasm secondary to the angiogram itself. Even if no

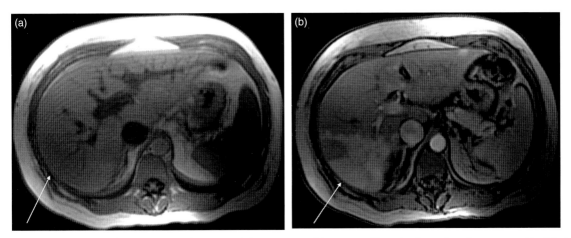

Figure 22.7. Hepatic infarct in HELLP syndrome. Liver MRI in a 36-year-old woman at 20 weeks of gestation who presents with clinical suspicion of HELLP syndrome and right upper quadrant pain. The scan demonstrates an ill-defined hypoattenuating area within the right lobe of the liver (arrow) on the T_1-weighted sequence (a), which shows perfusional abnormality after intravenous contrast administration (b).

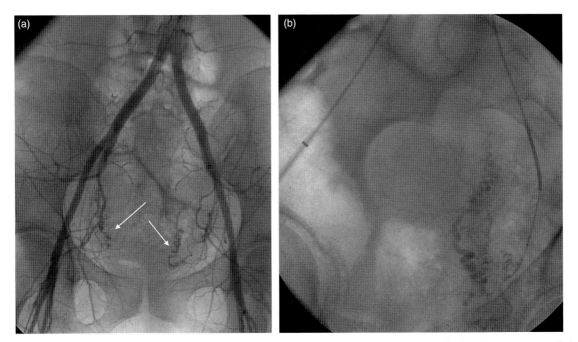

Figure 22.8. Postpartum hemorrhage. (a) Pelvic arteriography in a 37-year-old woman with postpartum bleeding that was not controlled with a uterine tamponade balloon, demonstrating bilateral enlarged uterine arteries (arrows) without evidence of active extravasation. (b) Bilateral uterine artery embolization with Gelfoam was successful in achieving hemostasis.

bleeding site is identified, embolization of bilateral uterine arteries or of the anterior divisions of internal iliac arteries is performed. Gelatin sponge is most commonly used as the embolic agent, which provides temporary occlusion with recanalization in 3–6 weeks [38,42]. The procedure demonstrates an approximately 90% success rate in controlling postpartum hemorrhage [43,44]. Repeat embolization may be performed, with attention to accessory arteries supplying the uterus or vagina.

Postpartum sepsis

In patients with postpartum sepsis, the most common etiology is endometritis, occurring more frequently following cesarean section (Table 22.7). Findings with US are variable and non-specific as there is significant overlap in the appearance of the normal and infected postpartum endometrium. The endometrial cavity may contain fluid and air postpartum [45,46], with the latter seen up to 3 weeks after delivery [47].

Table 22.7. Postpartum sepsis

Etiology	Examination
Endometritis	Considerable overlap in imaging findings between the normal and infected postpartum endometrium
	CT or MRI used to detect complications, e.g. myonecrosis or abscess
	Image-guided drainage is a treatment option for abscess
Retained products of conception	US with Doppler is the initial examination for diagnosis
	MRI with intravenous contrast can be used to differentiate retained products of conception from hematoma

US, ultrasound.

Therefore, US findings should be correlated with the clinical evaluation in this setting. Complications of endometritis such as myonecrosis or abscesses can be detected with CT (Figure 22.9) or MRI. Administration of intravenous contrast significantly improves diagnostic accuracy with either modality. Image-guided aspiration and drainage of an abscess can be performed as a less invasive alternative to surgery.

The initial imaging examination to detect retained products of conception is US, which will identify an intracavitary mass of heterogeneous echotexture (Figure 22.10) [45]. Doppler US can be helpful in distinguishing retained products from a hematoma as the former can be hypervascular. However, failure to visualize elevated blood flow does not eliminate the possibility of retained products [46]. Use of CT will not reliably distinguish these entities, as both can be seen as dense masses. If necessary, MRI with intravenous contrast can aid in resolving this diagnostic dilemma, as a hematoma will demonstrate T_1-weighted hyperintensity and enhance minimally, whereas retained products will appear T_1-weighted isointense and enhance avidly.

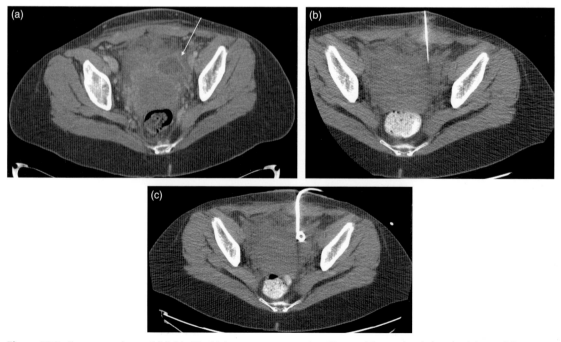

Figure 22.9. Postpartum abscess. (a) Pelvic CT with intravenous contrast in a 33-year-old woman with fever and dysuria following cesarean section demonstrates a fluid collection with a thick enhancing wall (arrow) anterior to the bladder. (b,c) A needle (b) followed by a catheter (c) was placed into the cavity under CT guidance to achieve abscess drainage and avoid surgical debridement.

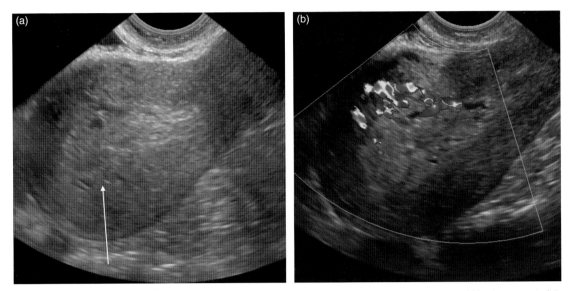

Figure 22.10. Retained products of conception. Transvaginal ultrasound in a 29-year-old woman with vaginal bleeding 2 weeks following termination at 16 weeks of gestation. (a) Ultrasound demonstrates hyperechoic heterogeneous material within the uterine cavity. (b) Doppler imaging showed increased vascular flow. This was confirmed to be retained products of conception after dilatation and curettage.

Conclusions

In referring a maternal critical care patient for a radiology examination, the first question posed should be whether the results of the imaging study are likely to direct or alter patient management. If not, imaging should not be undertaken, as it consumes valuable time and resources that would be better directed toward treatment. If, however, imaging is likely to be helpful, the modality should be chosen with care to insure fetal and maternal safety, to maximize the likelihood of yielding an accurate result, and to minimize the number of examinations and associated delayed diagnosis should the initial choice prove suboptimal or indeterminate.

References

1. McCollough CH, Schueler BA, Atwell TD, *et al.* Radiation exposure and pregnancy: when should we be concerned? *Radiographics* 2007;**27**:909–917; discussion 917–918.

2. American College of Radiology. *Practice Guideline 26: Imaging Pregnant or Potentially Pregnant Adolescents and Women with Ionizing Radiation.* Washington, DC: American College of Radiology, 2010.

3. American Congress of Obstetricians and Gynecologists Committee on Obstetric Practice. Committee Opinion. No. 299, September 2004 (replaces No. 158, September 1995). Guidelines for diagnostic imaging during pregnancy. *Obstet Gynecol* 2004;**104**:647–651.

4. Ray JG, Schull MJ, Urquia ML, *et al.* Major radiodiagnostic imaging in pregnancy and the risk of childhood malignancy: a population-based cohort study in Ontario. *PLoS Med* 2010;7:e1000337.

5. Parry RA, Glaze SA, Archer BR. The AAPM/RSNA physics tutorial for residents. Typical patient radiation doses in diagnostic radiology. *Radiographics* 1999;**19**:1289–1302.

6. Abramowicz JS, Kossoff G, Marsal K, Haar Ter G, International Society of Ultrasound in Obstetrics and Gynecology Bioeffects and Safety Committee, Executive Board of the International Society of Ultrasound in Obstetrics and Gynecology. Safety Statement, 2000 (reconfirmed 2003). International Society of Ultrasound in Obstetrics and Gynecology. *Ultrasound Obstet Gynecol* 2003;**21**:100.

7. Hurwitz LM, Yoshizumi T, Reiman RE, *et al.* Radiation dose to the fetus from body MDCT during early gestation. *AJR Am J Roentgenol* 2006;**186**:871–876.

8. Doshi SK, Negus IS, Oduko JM. Fetal radiation dose from CT pulmonary angiography in late pregnancy: a phantom study. *Br J Radiol* 2008;**81**:653–658.

9. Goldberg-Stein S, Liu B, Hahn PF, Lee SI. Body CT during pregnancy: utilization trends, examination indications, and fetal radiation doses. *AJR Am J Roentgenol* 2010;**196**:146–151.

10. Shellock FG, Crues JV. MR procedures: biologic effects, safety, and patient care. *Radiology* 2004;**232**:635–652.

11. De Wilde JP, Rivers AW, Price DL. A review of the current use of magnetic resonance imaging in

pregnancy and safety implications for the fetus. *Prog Biophys Mol Biol* 2005;**87**:335–353.

12. Schaefer C, Meister R, Wentzeck R, Weber-Schoendorfer C. Fetal outcome after technetium scintigraphy in early pregnancy. *Reprod Toxicol* 2009;**28**:161–166.

13. Winer-Muram HT, Boone JM, Brown HL, *et al.* Pulmonary embolism in pregnant patients: fetal radiation dose with helical CT. *Radiology* 2002;**224**:487–492.

14. Takalkar AM, Khandelwal A, Lokitz S, Lilien DL, Stabin MG. ^{18}F-FDG PET in pregnancy and fetal radiation dose estimates. *J Nucl Med* 2011;**52**:1035–1040.

15. Segal A, Ellis J. *Manual on Contrast Media,* version 6. Washington, DC: American College of Radiology, 2008.

16. Webb JAW, Thomsen HS, Morcos SK, for the Contrast Media Safety Committee of European Society of Urogenital Radiology. The use of iodinated and gadolinium contrast media during pregnancy and lactation. *Eur Radiol* 2005;**15**:1234–1240.

17. Lee I, Chew FS. Use of IV iodinated and gadolinium contrast media in the pregnant or lactating patient: self-assessment module. *AJR Am J Roentgenol* 2009;**193**(Suppl):S70–S73.

18. Atwell TD, Lteif AN, Brown DL, *et al.* Neonatal thyroid function after administration of IV iodinated contrast agent to 21 pregnant patients. *AJR Am J Roentgenol* 2008;**191**:268–271.

19. Cappell MS, Friedel D. Abdominal pain during pregnancy. *Gastroenterol Clin North Am* 2003;**32**:1–58.

20. Goodacre S, Sampson F, Stevenson M, *et al.* Measurement of the clinical and cost-effectiveness of non-invasive diagnostic testing strategies for deep vein thrombosis. *Health Technol Assess* 2006;**10**:1–168, iii–iv.

21. Patel SJ, Reede DL, Katz DS, Subramaniam R, Amorosa JK. Imaging the pregnant patient for nonobstetric conditions: algorithms and radiation dose considerations. *Radiographics* 2007;**27**:1705–1722.

22. Ho VB, van Geertruyden PH, Yucel EK, *et al.* ACR Appropriateness Criteria on suspected lower extremity deep vein thrombosis. *J Am Coll Radiol* 2011;**8**:383–387.

23. Durán-Mendicuti A, Sodickson A. Imaging evaluation of the pregnant patient with suspected pulmonary embolism. *Int J Obstet Anesth* 2011;**20**:519.

24. Shahir K, Goodman LR, Tali A, Thorsen KM, Hellman RS. Pulmonary embolism in pregnancy: CT pulmonary angiography versus perfusion scanning. *AJR Am J Roentgenol* 2010;**195**:W214–W220.

25. Revel M-P, Cohen S, Sanchez O, *et al.* Pulmonary embolism during pregnancy: diagnosis with lung scintigraphy or CT angiography? *Radiology* 2011;**258**:590–598.

26. Oto A, Ernst RD, Ghulmiyyah LM, *et al.* MR imaging in the triage of pregnant patients with acute abdominal and pelvic pain. *Abdom Imaging* 2009;**34**:243–250.

27. Andreotti RF, Lee SI, Choy G, *et al.* ACR Appropriateness Criteria on acute pelvic pain in the reproductive age group. *J Am Coll Radiol* 2009;**6**:235–241.

28. Pedrosa I, Zeikus EA, Levine D, Rofsky NM. MR imaging of acute right lower quadrant pain in pregnant and nonpregnant patients. *Radiographics* 2007;**27**:721–743; discussion 743–753.

29. Israel GM, Malguria N, McCarthy S, Copel J, Weinreb J. MRI vs. ultrasound for suspected appendicitis during pregnancy. *J Magn Reson Imaging* 2008;**28**:428–433.

30. Lazarus E, Mayo-Smith WW, Mainiero MB, Spencer PK. CT in the evaluation of nontraumatic abdominal pain in pregnant women. *Radiology* 2007;**244**:784–790.

31. Richards JR, Ormsby EL, Romo MV, Gillen MA, McGahan JP. Blunt abdominal injury in the pregnant patient: detection with US. *Radiology* 2004;**233**:463–470.

32. Lowdermilk C, Gavant ML, Qaisi W, West OC, Goldman SM. Screening helical CT for evaluation of blunt traumatic injury in the pregnant patient. *Radiographics* 1999;**19**:S243–S255; discussion S256–S258.

33. Wieseler KM, Bhargava P, Kanal KM, *et al.* Imaging in pregnant patients: examination appropriateness. *Radiographics* 2010;**30**:1215–1229; discussion 1230–1233.

34. Rhea JT, Garza DH, Novelline RA. Controversies in emergency radiology. CT versus ultrasound in the evaluation of blunt abdominal trauma. *Emerg Radiol* 2004;**10**:289–295.

35. Wei S, Helmy M, Cohen A. CT evaluation of placental abruption in pregnant trauma patients. *Emerg Radiol* 2009;**16**:365–373.

36. Levine D. Ectopic pregnancy. *Radiology* 2007;**245**:385–397.

37. Bartynski WS, Boardman JF. Distinct imaging patterns and lesion distribution in posterior reversible encephalopathy syndrome. *AJNR Am J Neuroradiol* 2007;**28**:1320–1327.

38. Salazar GMM, Petrozza JC, Walker TG. Transcatheter endovascular techniques for management of obstetrical and gynecologic emergencies. *Tech Vasc Interv Radiol* 2009;**12**:139–147.

39. Lee JS, Shepherd SM. Endovascular treatment of postpartum hemorrhage. *Clin Obstet Gynecol* 2010;**53**:209–218.

40. Gonsalves M, Belli A. The role of interventional radiology in obstetric hemorrhage. *Cardiovasc Intervent Radiol* 2010;**33**:887–895.

41. Tourné G, Collet F, Seffert P, Veyret C. Place of embolization of the uterine arteries in the management of post-partum haemorrhage: a study of 12 cases. *Eur J Obstet Gynecol Reprod Biol* 2003;**110**:29–34.

42. Ganguli S, Stecker MS, Pyne D, Baum RA, Fan C-M. Uterine artery embolization in the treatment of postpartum uterine hemorrhage. *J Vasc Interv Radiol* 2011;**22**:169–176.

43. Ratnam LA, Gibson M, Sandhu C, *et al.* Transcatheter pelvic arterial embolisation for control of obstetric and gynaecological haemorrhage. *J Obstet Gynaecol* 2008;**28**:573–579.

44. Doumouchtsis SK, Papageorghiou AT, Arulkumaran S. Systematic review of conservative management of postpartum hemorrhage: what to do when medical treatment fails. *Obstet Gynecol Surv* 2007;**62**:540–547.

45. Zuckerman J, Levine D, McNicholas MM, *et al.* Imaging of pelvic postpartum complications. *AJR Am J Roentgenol* 1997;**168**:663–668.

46. Nalaboff KM, Pellerito JS, Ben-Levi E. Imaging the endometrium: disease and normal variants. *Radiographics* 2001;**21**:1409–1424.

47. Wachsberg RH, Kurtz AB. Gas within the endometrial cavity at postpartum US: a normal finding after spontaneous vaginal delivery. *Radiology* 1992;**183**:431–433.

Chapter

23

Cardiovascular disease

Els Troost and Meredith Birsner

Introduction

Up to 4% of all pregnancies are complicated by cardiovascular disease and the number of patients presenting with cardiac problems during pregnancy is increasing. Knowledge about the hemodynamic burden of pregnancy and the risks associated with cardiovascular disease are of pivotal importance for the counseling and management of pregnancy in these patients. Ideally, counseling should start before a pregnancy is undertaken in order to have all possible factors corrected to reduce the risks and to allow women to have a full understanding about the possibilities and limitations of their childbearing potential.

Epidemiology

The spectrum of cardiovascular disease presenting during pregnancy is evolving and differs according to geographical conditions. While in non-Western countries rheumatic heart disease still accounts for approximately 75% of cases, the pattern of cardiovascular disease during pregnancy is quite different in Europe and North America, where rheumatic lesions are reported in only 15 to 20% of cases. Thanks to major advances in the diagnosis and management, both interventional and surgical, of patients with congenital heart disease, their outcomes have greatly improved over the last decades so that many of these women reach childbearing age and wish to become pregnant. As such, cardiovascular disease during pregnancy in Western women presents a wide spectrum of congenital heart disease, accounting now for more than 50% of lesions during pregnancy [1]. Cardiomyopathies and coronary artery disease during pregnancy are rare conditions but carry a high risk of cardiac morbidity. Because of the increasing age at first pregnancy and increased global

cardiovascular risk associated with Western lifestyle and diet, the prevalence of well-known cardiovascular risk factors such as diabetes, obesity, hypercholesterolemia, and hypertension is increasing and they complicate more pregnancies.

Unfortunately, cardiac disease has become the major cause of indirect (non-obstetric) maternal death in the UK and accounts for about 15% of pregnancy-related mortality in Western countries: this is mainly a result of an increase in acquired conditions such as ischemic heart disease [2]. Indeed, in some US series, the leading cause of transfer from the obstetric service to the intensive care unit (ICU) is maternal cardiac disease, and the proportion of maternal mortality attributable to cardiovascular conditions is rising [3,4]. Aortic dissection, peripartum cardiomyopathy, and severe left ventricular dysfunction also contribute to significant morbidity and mortality among pregnant women. According to the seventh triennial Confidential Enquiries into Maternal and Child Health (CEMACH) report, which records and examines all maternal deaths during pregnancy and within the first postpartum year in the UK, insufficient access to specialized care seems to be significantly contributing to the death of these women as these conditions often occur acutely and dramatically in women with no previously known heart disease [2]. This calls for improving early recognition and management of these vulnerable patients, ideally through multidisciplinary assessment.

Cardiac risk estimation of pregnancy

The risk of pregnancy depends on the functional status of the patient prior to pregnancy as well as the specific cardiac lesion and generally increases with increasing disease complexity.

Maternal Critical Care: A Multidisciplinary Approach, ed. Marc Van de Velde, Helen Scholefield, and Lauren A. Plante.
Published by Cambridge University Press. © Cambridge University Press 2013.

Table 23.1. Predictors of maternal cardiovascular events according to the CARPREG study

Risk factor	Feature
Prior cardiac event	Heart failure or pulmonary edema Transient ischemic attack or stroke Symptomatic arrhythmia
Functional class/cyanosis	NYHA class >II Oxygen saturation <90%
Reduced systemic ventricular function	Ejection fraction <40%
Left heart obstruction	Aortic valve area <1.5 cm^2 Peak left ventricular outflow tract gradient >30 mmHg Mitral valve area <2 cm^2
Risk score	
0 risk factors	5%
1 risk factor	27%
2 risk factors	75%

NYHA, New York Heart Association.
Source: based on Siu et al., 2001 [5].

Table 23.2. Predictors of maternal cardiovascular events according to the ZAHARA and Khairy et al. studies

ZAHARA risk factors	Khairy *et al.* risk factors
History of arrhythmias	Severe pulmonary regurgitation
Use of cardiac medication before pregnancy	Reduced subpulmonary ejection fraction
Baseline NYHA class III or IV	Smoking history
Left heart obstruction (peak instantaneous gradient at aortic valve >50 mmHg)	
Moderate or severe systemic atrioventricular valve regurgitation	
Moderate or severe subpulmonary atrioventricular valve regurgitation	
Mechanical valve prosthesis	
Cyanotic heart disease, repaired or unrepaired	

NYHA, New York Heart Association.
Source: based on Drenthen et al., 2010 [6]; Khairy et al., 2006 [7].

Functional risk assessment

Several risk scoring systems have been developed and represent easily identifiable hemodynamic predictors for maternal and/or fetal risk. The Cardiac Disease in Pregnancy (CARPREG) study [5] was the first risk index (Table 23.1) to predict maternal and fetal risk during pregnancy. The index was based on a prospective enrollment of 599 pregnancies among a population of women with acquired or congenital heart disease or primary rhythm abnormalities.

This risk score has been validated in other studies and is commonly used for risk stratification. In 2010, the ZAHARA study [6] and in 2006 Khairy et al. [7] retrospectively analyzed the outcome of pregnancies of women with congenital heart disease and were able to identify additional independent predictors of maternal cardiac complications including New York Heart Association (NYHA) functional class >II, left heart obstructive lesions, left ventricular dysfunction, and arrhythmias; the authors emphasized the risk score calculation had highest utility in pre-pregnancy risk assessment (Table 23.2). High-risk conditions such as Marfan disease, severe aortopathy, and pulmonary arterial hypertension could not be identified by these studies as independent predictors of worse outcome but as these women are counseled against pregnancy,

they are often under-represented in such studies. In the USA and Europe, the most widely used functional assessment in cardiac patients is that of the NYHA, a fluid classification system that allows movement from one class to another as symptoms change. Introduced in 1928 and revised most recently in 1994 to augment functional capacity with objective assessment, it is used in clinical trials not only as an outcome measure but also as an inclusion or exclusion criterion (Table 23.3) [8].

Lesion-specific risk assessment

Data that are lesion specific are based on retrospective series but provide additional information when considering pregnancy in an individual patient with underlying cardiac disease. The modified World Health Organization (WHO) classification divides specific cardiovascular lesions into four groups according to the severity of the lesions and concomitant morbidity and mortality [9–11]. Class I carries no additional risks compared with the general population, whereas class II holds a small increased risk of maternal morbidity and mortality. Class III comprises conditions with significantly increased risk of maternal morbidity and mortality. For class IV conditions,

Table 23.3. New York Heart Association classification

Class	Features
I	No limitations Ordinary physical activity does not cause fatigue, breathlessness, or palpitation
II	Slight limitation of physical activity Comfortable at rest Ordinary physical activity causes fatigue, breathlessness, angina pectoris, or palpitation
III	Marked limitation of physical activity Comfortable at rest Less than ordinary physical activity causes fatigue, breathlessness, angina pectoris, or palpitation
IV	Inability to do any physical activity without discomfort Symptoms of heart failure are even present at rest

Source: Criteria Committee for the New York Heart Association [8].

pregnancy is contraindicated as the estimated maternal mortality risk exceeds 10% (Table 23.4). Van Mook and Peeters [12] developed a lesion-specific risk stratification in which low-risk patients had 1% mortality risk, medium-risk patients had 5–15% mortality risk, and the highest risk patients, including those with lesions such as severe pulmonary hypertension or NYHA class III or IV symptoms, had a 25–50% mortality risk.

General issues for the cardiologist

Pregnancy counseling and follow-up

Prepregnancy counseling

Prepregnancy counseling of the woman with cardiovascular disease desiring pregnancy should include the following [10,13]:

- frank assessment of underlying disease severity and functional status
- history of previous events
- most recent echocardiography and cyclo-ergospirometry with measurement of transcutaneous oxygen saturation
- magnetic resonace imaging (MRI) and/or cardiac catheterization where needed
- basic natriuretic peptide and its *N*-terminal prohormone (NT-proBNP) levels pre-pregnancy can be helpful

- possibility of maternal complications antepartum and postpartum; discuss hemodynamic effects of pregnancy and associated maternal and fetal risk with patient and partner
- appropriate referral to maternal–fetal medicine subspecialist
- referral for pre-pregnancy intervention to reduce risks in those with, for example, severe left heart obstruction, marfan syndrome with dilated aortic root, symptomatic valvular lesions
- risks to the fetus: neonatal complications, including premature birth, small-for-gestational-age birth weight, respiratory distress syndrome, intraventricular hemorrhage, fetal and neonatal death, increased risk of congenital heart disease when mother has congenital heart disease [14]
- medication adjustment to limit exposure to teratogens and allow safe breastfeeding
- initiation of prenatal vitamins
- genetic counseling when a chromosomal disorder or familial inheritance pattern is suspected; genetic testing may also be useful in cardiomyopathies and/or rhythm disturbances (channelopathies)
- expectation of family size
- need for fetal echocardiography
- place of delivery and need for intrapartum maternal and fetal monitoring
- route of delivery and need for analgesia
- medications in breastmilk
- contraceptive planning postpartum.

Cardiac medications that are contraindicated in breastfeeding mothers include procainamide, propafenone, amiodarone, and statins [15].

Patients should be counseled against pregnancy in conditions of irreversible high-risk conditions with estimated maternal mortality risk of >10% and should be offered termination services in these situations as well as for those involving an undesired pregnancy.

Pregnancy follow-up

Joint care with a dedicated obstetric team is necessary and the following should be ensured:

- all patients: clinical and echocardiographic follow-up at each patient visit to allow timely recognition of hemodynamically significant alterations that could complicate the further pregnancy course
- low-risk lesions (WHO class I): gynecological and obstetric follow-up at a locoregional center is

Table 23.4. World Health Organization classification of cardiovascular lesions

Class	Risk level	Lesions
I		
Class I: uncomplicated small/mild lesions	Very low	Mild pulmonary stenosis Restrictive ventricular septal defect Restrictive patent ductus arteriosus Mild mitral valve prolapse
Class I: succesfully repaired simple lesions	Very low	Corrected atrial septal defect, ventricular septal defect, patent ductus arteriosus Corrected anomalous pulmonary venous return
Class II lesions (if otherwise well and uncomplicated)	Low to moderate	Unoperated atrial septal defect Repaired tetralogy of Fallot Most arrhythmias
Class II/III lesions (depending on individual)	Moderate to high	Mild left ventricular impairment (ejection fraction ≥40%) Hypertrophic cardiomyopathy Native or tissue valve disease not considered class IV Repaired coarctation Marfan syndrome without aortic dilatation Aorta <45 mm in bicuspid aortic valve-associated aortic disease
Class III	High	Mechanical valve Systemic right ventricle Fontan circulation Unrepaired cyanotic heart disease Aortic dilatation 40–45 mm in Marfan syndrome Aortic dilatation 45–50 mm in bicuspid aortic valve-associated aortic disease Other complex congenital heart disease
Class IV	Very high risk, pregnancy contraindicated	Pulmonary arterial hypertension of any cause Severe systemic ventricular dysfunction (ejection fraction 30%, NYHA class III or IV) Previous peripartum cardiomyopathy with any residual impairment of left ventricular function Severe left heart obstruction Aortic dilatation >45 mm in Marfan syndrome Aortic dilatation >50 mm in bicuspid aortic valve-associated aortic disease Native severe coarctation

NYHA, New York Heart Association classification.
Source: World Health Organization, 1994 [9].

possible; cardiac check-up is desirable before and once or twice during pregnancy

- WHO class II lesions: cardiac check-up before and follow-up during each trimester of pregnancy is necessary; delivery at a locoregional center is possible in an uncomplicated pregnancy
- WHO class III conditions: cardiac check-up before and surveillance bimonthly or even monthly during pregnancy is advised; delivery at a highly specialized or tertiary center in a context of multidisciplinary management has to be planned
- WHO class IV conditions: termination is often advised, but if pregnancy is undertaken, tight

follow-up on a monthly or bimonthly basis and/or hospitalization for close surveillance is warranted.

Diagnosis of heart failure during pregnancy

Diagnosis of heart failure symptoms during pregnancy can be quite challenging, as pregnancy itself introduces hemodynamic changes that can mimic symptoms and clinical signs of heart failure. Pre-existing cardiac disease often elicits clinically significant signs during the second trimester of pregnancy as the hemodynamic pregnancy-related changes reach a peak. If heart failure occurs, management should be as for non-pregnant patients, with prescription of diuretics to relieve congestion, and beta-blockers for afterload reduction and modulation of sympathomimetic tone. Furosemide and hydrochlorothiazide can be used, but overuse should be avoided as these medications can decrease placental blood flow. Aldosterone antagonists have been labeled as category 4 by the US Food and Drug Administration because of antiandrogenic effects documented in rats. Angiotensin-converting enzyme inhibitors and angiotensin-receptor blockers are contraindicated during pregnancy because of fetotoxicity. Because data on eplerenone and aliskiren are insufficient, these products are actually not prescribed for pregnant women. Bed rest and restriction of physical activities should be prescribed for severe disabling symptoms.

Timing and mode of delivery

Women with significant cardiac conditions, WHO class III or IV, should deliver at a tertiary care center. For most conditions, a vaginal delivery with good analgesia and low threshold for assisted second stage is preferred because this is associated with less blood loss and abrupt hemodynamic changes than a cesarean section. Valsalva maneuver during labor, however, increases intrathoracic pressure, leading to decreased venous return, decreased preload, and, therefore, decreased cardiac output. These maternal pushing efforts can be limited when a vaginal delivery is accomplished with vacuum, ventouse, or forceps. The choice to deliver via cesarean section is usually made based on obstetric factors. There are few maternal cardiac indications for delivery by cesarean section: these include patients with Marfan syndrome, aortic root dilatation, aortic dissection or aneurysm, severe pulmonary hypertension or Eisenmenger syndrome, and uncontrolled heart failure. Patients taking oral anticoagulation at onset of labor may also require a cesarean because of the risk of fetal intracranial hemorrhage associated with vaginal delivery. In some centers, severe aortic stenosis and a mechanical prosthetic heart valve combined with unfavorable obstetric factors that could predict prolonged labor are also considered for cesarean delivery, although no consensus exists today in literature [10,16,17].

Women should labor in left lateral decubitus position to increase venous return, with supplemental oxygen if necessary. Close monitoring, possibly in a cardiac intensive care setting with capability of advanced cardiac monitoring during the immediate postpartum phase, must be stressed, as important

changes in circulating volume and fluid shifts in the first 24 hours following delivery predispose women with structural heart disease for development of heart failure. Additional treatment with diuretics may be necessary. Labor induction can proceed by the usual techniques; however, bolus administration of oxytocin can have potent cardiovascular side effects in vulnerable patients because it induces a 30% decrease in mean arterial pressure, a 50% decrease in systemic vascular resistance, and, therefore, can increase cardiac output by as much as 50% [18,19]. These potential deleterious side effects were highlighted in the CEMACH Report in the UK [2]. Therefore, bolus administration should be avoided in women at high risk who would not tolerate profound tachycardia and hypotension (e.g. lesions with a fixed cardiac output such as obstructive and stenotic left-sided valvular lesions, and Eisenmenger syndrome). If necessary to control postpartum hemorrhage, oxytocics should be given in small incremental doses or in a diluted solution. Ergometrin and prostaglandin F analogues are contraindicated because of the risk of pulmonary vasoconstriction and hypertension.

General issues for obstetric/anesthetic management

Regional anesthesia in the patient with cardiac disease is strongly advised; this limits maternal sensation of pain as well as the reflexive urge to push, with their respective resultant hemodynamic changes. Slow dosing of epidural agents will prevent maternal hypotension, which, in addition to fetal heart rate abnormalities necessitating emergency uncontrolled delivery, could have disastrous consequences for poorly compensated maternal lesions or for those who are preload dependent [20]. Placement should be early in the labor course but timed appropriately, with administration or withholding of anticoagulation. Intravenous patient-controlled analgesia with opioids is a suboptimal form of pain control compared with regional anesthesia because of potential respiratory side effects. The decision for general anesthesia for cesarean section will depend on many factors and needs to be individualized based on the preferences of the anesthesiologist, obstetrician, and patient. The likelihood of cardiovascular or surgical complications, the patient's desire to view her neonate or refusal of general anesthesia, and airway compromise must all be considered. It is recommended that if general anesthesia is required opioids prior to delivery are administered, with remifentanil being the logical first choice [18].

Specific lesions

Valvular lesions

Mitral stenosis

Mitral stenosis accounts for most of the morbidity and mortality of rheumatic disease during pregnancy and is mostly encountered in the developing world. Moderate or severe mitral stenosis (valve area < 1.5 cm^2) is poorly tolerated during pregnancy because the pressure gradient over the stenotic valve may rise during pregnancy as a result of the physiological rise in heart rate and stroke volume. These changes put these patients at risk for pulmonary edema and atrial arrhythmias [21]. Prepregnancy evaluation with ergometry or treadmill allows the physician to better assess the risks and may unmask symptoms. Special attention must be paid to the immigrant population when they present with cardiac symptoms during pregnancy.

Even in previously asymptomatic women with moderate mitral stenosis, there exists a considerable risk for heart failure particularly during the second and third trimester, as the increased intravascular volume and pregnancy-induced tachycardia superimpose on the already elevated transmitral gradient. Cardiac complications are reported in more than one third of

significant rheumatic disease, mainly pulmonary edema, worsening of functional class, and arrhythmias. If atrial fibrillation develops, these patients are particularly prone to further hemodynamic deterioration and worsening of pulmonary hypertension; in atrial fibrillation or severely dilated atria, an additional risk for thromboembolic complications should be evaluated. Mortality risk is estimated between 0 and 3%. In mild mitral stenosis, symptoms can arise during pregnancy but they are usually not severe and well tolerated [17,22]. Box 23.1 outlines the management of mitral stenosis.

Aortic stenosis

If aortic stenosis in young women is found, this is most frequently related to a bicuspid aortic valve. Symptoms vary a lot and even with severe aortic stenosis, patients can still be asymptomatic. Progression rate is also considerably lower when compared with degenerative aortic stenosis in older patients [22]. Special attention should be paid to aortic root dimensions as aortic dilatation of the distal part of the ascending aorta is seen in 50% of patients with a bicuspid aortic valve stenosis. If diameters exceed 50 mm (27 mm/m^2 body surface area), surgery is recommended prior to pregnancy [23,24]. Mortality

---

Box 23.1. Management of mitral stenosis

- Prepregnancy intervention in moderate to severe mitral stenosis should be performed, preferably by percutaneous interventions if appropriate anatomical features are present
- Clinical and echocardiographic follow-up during pregnancy, at least once per trimester or bimonthly for more severe conditions is advised
- In onset of symptoms or evolution towards significant pulmonary hypertension (estimated systolic pulmonary artery pressure >50 mmHg on echocardiography): restriction of physical activities and beta-1-selective beta-blockers to prolong diastolic filling time should be implemented
- If clinical signs of congestion persist, diuretics can be used although high doses need to be avoided to minimize the risk of reducing placental flow
- Low-molecular-weight heparin is recommended in therapeutic doses in permanent or paroxysmal atrial fibrillation, left atrial thrombus, previous embolic events, or severely dilated atria (≥40 mL/m^2)
- If hemodynamic instability persists despite optimal medical treatment, percutaneous balloon mitral valvuloplasty may be considered, ideally after 20 weeks of gestation
- If percutaneous valvuloplasty fails or is not possible and the life of the mother is endangered, surgical intervention can be considered but carries a high risk of fetal loss: if gestational age is beyond 28 weeks, delivery before surgery should be considered; at 26–28 weeks of gestation, the risk balance between preterm delivery and cardiac surgery while pregnant needs to be weighed individually based on all contributing factors
- Delivery can in most cases occur vaginally; a cesarean section needs to be considered only in moderate to severe mitral stenosis and associated NYHA class III–IV without any therapeutic options predelivery

Box 23.2. Management of aortic stenosis

- Prepregnancy exercise testing helps to confirm an asymptomatic state and indicates a good prognosis if no significant strain nor pathological blood pressure drop is found
- Prepregnancy valvuloplasty or surgery should be performed in symptomatic aortic stenosis or when asymptomatic aortic stenosis is combined with impaired left ventricular function or pathological exercise test
- Prepregnancy surgery should also be considered if aortic root diameter exceeds 50 mm (i.e. 27 mm/m^2 body surface area), regardless of symptoms
- Pregnancy can be allowed even with severe aortic stenosis if asymptomatic status, preserved left ventricular function and size, no signs of severe left ventricular hypertrophy and normal exercise test can be confirmed
- Clinical and echocardiographic follow-up during pregnancy, at least once per trimester or bimonthly for more severe conditions, is advised; echocardiographic gradient across the aortic valve will rise during pregnancy because of the increased cardiac output
- If onset of symptoms or evolution towards significant pulmonary hypertension (estimated systolic pulmonary artery pressure >50 mmHg on echocardiography), restriction of physical activities and beta-1-selective beta-blockers to ameliorate coronary filling should be implemented
- If clinical signs of congestion persist, diuretics can be used although high doses need to be avoided to minimize the risk of reducing placental flow
- If hemodynamic instability persists despite optimal medical treatment, percutaneous balloon valvuloplasty may be considered, ideally after 20 weeks of gestation
- If percutaneous valvuloplasty fails or is not possible and the life of the mother is threatened, surgical intervention can be considered but carries a high risk of fetal loss: if gestational age is beyond 28 weeks, delivery before surgery should be considered; at 26–28 weeks of gestation, the risk balance between preterm delivery and cardiac surgery while pregnant needs to be weighed individually based on all contributing factors
- Delivery can in most cases occur vaginally; an abrupt decrease in peripheral vascular resistance must be avoided during regional anesthesia. A cesarean section needs to be considered only in severe aortic stenosis and disturbing symptoms without any therapeutic options predelivery
- As the anesthetic and cardiac risks in hemodynamically unstable women are worrisome, close monitoring during cesarean section, with continuous electrocardiography, pulse oximetry, and invasive arterial monitoring, is advised

is low nowadays if pregnancy is carefully supervised. Signs of heart failure are found in 10–15% of patients with severe aortic stenosis. Box 23.2 outlines the management of aortic stenosis.

Regurgitant lesions

Aortic and mitral insufficiency found in pregnant women can be of congenital, rheumatic, or degenerative origin. Left-sided regurgitant lesions, even when severe, are well tolerated during pregnancy because the decrease in systemic vascular resistance neutralizes the extra volume load. However, these women are at high risk for heart failure if severe regurgitation is associated with left ventricular impairment or if there is acute severe regurgitation. Clinical and echocardiographic follow-up is advised at least every trimester; if symptoms of congestion develop, diuretics and beta-blockers should be started and restriction of physical activities should be advised. Rarely, surgery is unavoidable when facing acute severe regurgitation

and therapy-resistant heart failure symptoms. Vaginal delivery is preferred, with epidural anesthesia and assisted second stage, in symptomatic patients and asymptomatic patients with severe left-sided regurgitant lesions.

Prosthetic valves and anticoagulation

If valvuloplasty is not an option or fails, young women and their treating physicians find themselves confronted with a difficult choice. Mechanical valves offer a superior hemodynamic profile and good long-term durability but have an increased risk of valve thrombosis, which is increased further during pregnancy because it is an hypercoagulable state. Older types of mechanical valves and single-leaflet valves are more vulnerable for thrombosis. Bioprostheses are less thrombogenic but have the risk of structural degeneration, necessitating further surgery within 10 years of implantation in almost 50% of women younger than 30 years. With normal functioning

253

bioprosthesis and good left ventricular function, pregnancy is usually well tolerated. Regular cardiac check-up with echocardiography in each trimester is advisable. The same management options apply as for patients with native valve disease.

It is, however, the need for anticoagulation with mechanical valves that is of major concern during pregnancy. Two large reviews have confirmed that oral anticoagulation with warfarin still is the safest option for the mother with a low risk of valve thrombosis (ranging from 2.4 to 3.9%), which is still higher than outside pregnancy [25,26]. Maternal mortality is generally low and almost always related to valve thrombosis. Warfarin, however, crosses the placenta and is teratogenic; its use in the first trimester can induce fetal embryopathy (1–10%) including nasal hypoplasia, stippled epiphyses, and limb hypoplasia, although the risk seems to be low (less than 3%) if the daily dose is less than 5 mg. Unfractionated heparin (UFH) and low-molecular-weight heparin (LMWH) do not cross the placenta but carry a greater risk for thromboembolic complications [27,28]. In the review by Chan et al. [25], the risk for valve thrombosis was 9.2% when UFH was used in the first trimester instead of warfarin; the risk almost tripled to 25% when UFH was used throughout pregnancy even in an adjusted dose (activated partial thromboplastin time $\geq2\times$ control). When analysing these data, one has to bear in mind that this review spans a long period, starting in 1966, and that most of the valves analysed were cage and ball or single-tilting disc types; less than 12% were less thrombogenic and bileaflet types.

The use of LMWH subcutaneously to prevent valve thrombosis during pregnancy is still controversial because of the lack of evidence. Recent literature with small retrospective series indicate, however, that the risk of valve thrombosis is lower (9–12%) with the use of LMWH in dose-adjusted manner according to anti-factor Xa levels (target 0.8–1.2 U/mL at 4–6 hours after injection). More recent reports, however, emphasize the importance of monitoring baseline levels of anti-factor Xa activity [28].

The American College of Chest Physicians (ACCP) guidelines advocate the use of daily low-dose aspirin (75–100 mg) added to UFH or LMWH in women with prosthetic valves at high risk of valve thrombosis [29]; this is not a recommendation included in the recently published European guidelines.

Whatever the regimen chosen, fetal and obstetric morbidity remains rather high because of an increased risk for spontaneous abortions, prematurity, stillbirth, and hemorraghic complications both antenatally and postnatally. A cesarean section is indicated if the mother is still taking oral anticoagulation when labor starts to avoid fetal intracranial bleeding [10], with fresh frozen plasma administered in the event of urgent delivery to achieve a target international normalized ratio of ≤2. Oral vitamin K requires 4–6 hours to influence the clotting time as measured by the international normalized ratio. The newborn of a mother on oral anticoagulants at delivery should receive vitamin K with or without fresh frozen plasma. Box 23.3 outlines the management of mechanical prosthetic valves during and at the end of pregnancy.

Congenital heart disease

There is a broad spectrum of congenital abnormalities and therefore a wide range of risk associated with pregnancy, from a risk similar to the normal population (e.g. mild pulmonary stenosis) up to very high-risk conditions such as the Eisenmenger syndrome.

Prepregnancy counseling is, therefore, strongly recommended in order to keep patients informed and minimize risks [10,23].

Shunt lesions

In general, pregnancy is well tolerated in patients with a previously closed atrial or ventricular septal defect as well as in small unrepaired atrial septal defects and restrictive perimembranous or muscular ventricular septal defects, in the absence of ventricular dilatation or dysfunction and signs of pulmonary hypertension (Figure 23.1). There is a small increased risk for atrial arrythmias in unrepaired atrial septal defect in women with long-standing volume overload and pregnancy at an older age (>30 years). Because of the risk of paradoxical embolism, preventive measures for venous pooling (compression stockings) and prophylactic use of LMWH are recommended for patients with an unrepaired atrial septal defect if they need prolonged bed rest or hospitalization.

The same approach applies for corrected atrioventricular septal defect but risks here depend mostly on residual left atrioventricular valve insuffiency and/or persisting ventricular dysfunction. If the course is uncomplicated, cardiac follow-up once per trimester is sufficient and in most cases spontaneous vaginal delivery is, from a cardiac point of view, appropriate.

Box 23.3. Management of mechanical prosthetic valves

During pregnancy
- Prepregnancy assessment of valve type and position, valvular and ventricular performance, history of valve-related complications, therapeutic compliance
- Discuss with patient and partner the problems for both mother and fetus related to the use of anticoagulation during pregnancy and make a detailed plan of the treatment chosen during pregnancy
- Choice of anticoagulation regimen has to be tailored on an individual basis after informed consent from the patient
- The ACCP guidelines advise twice-daily LMWH or UFH throughout pregnancy, or either of these until the 13th week with warfarin substitution but restarting LMWH or UFH close to delivery; for patients at very high risk of thromboembolism (older-generation prosthesis in the mitral position or history of thromboembolism), warfarin is recommended throughout pregnancy, with replacement by UFH or LMWH close to delivery, after a thorough discussion of the potential risks and benefits of this approach. In recommending this, ACCP points out that they value avoiding maternal thromboembolic complications as equal to avoiding fetal risks
- European guidelines are somewhat different and indicate that warfarin should be considered during the first trimester if the daily dose required for therapeutic levels is < 5 mg; they also state that LMWH should be replaced by UFH at least 36 hours before planned delivery
- Effectiveness of anticoagulation should be assessed weekly
- Clinical follow-up should be frequent, with a low threshold for repetitive echocardiographic examination for symptoms of dyspnea or suspicion of an embolic event

At end of pregnancy
- Switch oral anticoagulation to dose-adjusted UFH or LMWH at 36 weeks of gestation or earlier in women with prior preterm delivery; the purpose of this conversion is to avoid the risk of spinal or epidural hematoma with regional anesthesia; an alternative is to stop therapeutic anticoagulation and induce within 24 hours if clinically appropriate [30]
- The American Society of Regional Anesthesia and Pain Medicine guidelines recommend withholding neuraxial blockade for 10–12 hours after the last prophylactic dose of LMWH or 24 hours after the last therapeutic dose of LMWH; these guidelines support the use of neuraxial anesthesia in patients receiving dosages of 5000 U of UFH twice daily, but the safety in patients receiving ≥10 000 U twice daily is unknown, and in such cases, assessment on an individual basis is recommended [31]
- If preterm labor occurs and cannot be stopped while the mother is taking oral anticoagulation, cesarean delivery is preferred to prevent fetal intracranial hemorrhage in a fully anticoagulated fetus; fresh frozen plasma should be given prior to cesarean section to have an international normalized ratio of ≤2.0. Vitamin K antagonists can also be considered, although it takes 4 to 6 hours to have an effect on the clotting time [10,16]

At delivery
- Planned vaginal delivery at a tertiary center is preferable [10,16,31]
- If high risk of valve thrombosis, planned cesarean section can be an alternative [30]
- Initiate UFH at latest 36 hours before planned delivery, stop 4–6 hours before planned delivery or at onset of labor, and restart 4–6 hours after delivery
- To minimize risk of hemorrhage postpartum, a reasonable approach to resumption of full anticoagulation for women with hypercoagulable conditions is to restart UFH or LMWH no sooner than 4–6 hours after vaginal delivery or 6–12 hours after cesarean delivery
- Restart oral anticoagulation 24 hours after delivery if there are no bleeding complications
- If urgent delivery is needed while the mother is still taking oral anticoagulation, the fetus may be given fresh frozen plasma and vitamin K
- Current recommendations by American Society of Regional Anesthesia and Pain Medicine are for resumption of prophylactic LMWH no sooner than 2 hours after epidural removal; because the optimal interval for resumption of therapeutic anticoagulation after epidural removal is unclear, 12 hours may be a reasonable approach

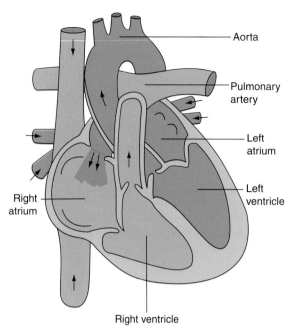

Figure 23.1. Atrial septal defect. In atrial septal defect type secundum, a left to right shunt through the defect causes a volume overload of the right heart and can lead to pulmonary hypertension.

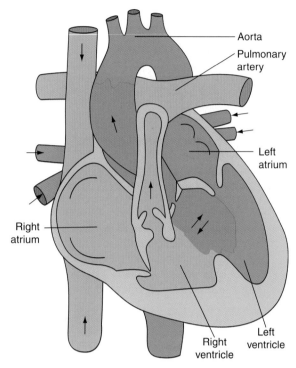

Figure 23.2. Tetralogy of Fallot. This is a combination of four heart defects including right ventricular outflow tract obstruction (infundibular stenosis), a large ventricular septal defect, an "overriding aorta," and right ventricular hypertrophy. The basic pathology is the underdevelopment of the right ventricular infundibulum. This leads to an anterior-leftward malalignment of the infundibular septum. This malalignment determines the degree of right ventricular outflow tract obstruction.

Pulmonary valve stenosis

Low and moderate pulmonary valve stenosis can be classified as low-risk conditions. Severe pulmonary stenosis (peak instantaneous gradient >60 mmHg) should be treated preferably by balloon valvuloplasty before pregnancy is undertaken. A check-up each trimester is sufficient except for severe pulmonary valve stenosis, which demands more frequent follow-up in order to detect right ventricular dysfunction and/or right heart failure in time. Vaginal delivery can be allowed for most patients; a cesarean section should, however, be considered for patients with severe symptomatic pulmonary valve stenosis in NYHA class III or IV that is refractory to medical treatment or after failure of percutaneous balloon dilatation.

Tetralogy of Fallot

Pregnancy is usually well tolerated with repaired tetralogy of Fallot if there are no severe residual sequelae and if right ventricular function is preserved (Figure 23.2). Severe pulmonary regurgitation and/or right ventricular dysfunction are, however, independent predictors of maternal complications, mostly presenting as arrhythmias or heart failure. Prepregnancy evaluation with echocardiography and/or MRI is advised to evaluate the hemodynamic status, and pre-

pregnancy valve replacement in the right ventricular outflow tract using a competent homograft is advocated if there is severe symptomatic pulmonary regurgitation or signs of severe right ventricular volume overload. Occasionally, diuretics and restriction of physical activities or bed rest may be needed during pregnancy with early delivery after induction; if not, a regular check-up during each trimester is sufficient and spontaneous vaginal delivery is preferred.

Ebstein anomaly

The variety of symptoms and complications in patients with Ebstein anomaly depend largely on the severity of tricuspid regurgitation, the right ventricular function, and the absence or presence of cyanosis caused by an associated atrial septal defect or patent foramen ovale (Figure 23.3). If there is symptomatic tricuspid insufficiency and/or clinically disabling cyanosis, repair or percutaneous closure of the atrial septal defect/patent foramen ovale is advised before

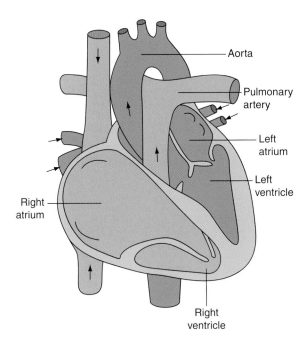

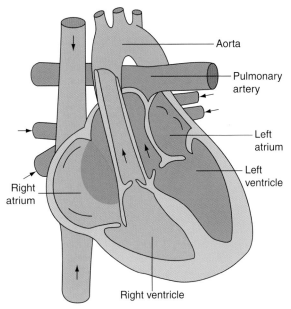

Figure 23.3. Ebstein malformation of tricuspid valve. Note the distal displacement of the septal and posterior leaflets of the tricuspid valve into the right ventricle. This lesion can be associated with stenosis and/or regurgitation of the tricuspid valve. The functional right ventricle is reduced in size because of the atrialization of part of the right ventricular cavity. A patent foramen ovale or atrial septal defect is frequently associated.

Figure 23.4. Transposition of the great arteries. The cardinal feature is ventriculo-arterial discordance. The aorta arises from the morphological right ventricle and the pulmonary artery arises from the morphological left ventricle; here, the aorta is shown displaced anteriorly and to the right of the pulmonary artery.

conception. Wolff–Parkinson–White syndrome is frequently associated with Ebstein anomaly and may become symptomatic during pregnancy. If neither cyanosis nor signs of heart failure are present, pregnancy will mostly have an uncomplicated course and vaginal delivery is preferable. Diuretics and bed rest may be needed if heart failure develops. If there is an interatrial communication, there is an increased risk of paradoxical embolism, and initiation of prophylactic LMWH may be indicated if bed rest is foreseen.

Aortic coarctation

Women with corrected aortic coarctation usually tolerate pregnancy well; however, residual hypertension, recoarctation, or aneurysmatic deformation should be excluded or treated before pregnancy starts. These women are more prone to hypertensive disorders and miscarriage, so frequent monitoring of blood pressure and a cardiac check-up during each trimester is advised. Hypertensive patients should be treated with restriction of physical activities, beta-1-selective beta-blockers or even combined pharmacological therapy, but aggressive correction should be avoided

in patients with native or recurrent coarctation because of the risk of placental hypoperfusion. Aortic dissection or rupture of a cerebral aneurysm is most feared in pregnant women with a history of corrected or uncorrected coarctation, but overall mortality is reported as rather low (0–0.8%) [32]. Spontaneous vaginal delivery with use of epidural anesthesia (to avoid hypertensive episodes) is appropriate for most women; a preterm planned elective cesarean section at 35–36 weeks is advised, however, in patients with native, unrepaired coarctation or progressive aneurysmatic deformation at the former coarctectomy site.

Transposition of the great arteries

In the 1980s, transposition of the great arteries was "repaired" by an atrial switch procedure, the so-called Mustard or Senning repair with the use of Dacron material or pericardial tissue to construct baffles to drain the systemic and pulmonary venous blood flows towards the left and right atria, respectively (Figures 23.4 and 23.5). Following this procedure, the right ventricle keeps on supporting the systemic circulation and has to adapt to an increased pressure load. Because of the increased volume load of pregnancy in addition to this, these patients are at risk for

257

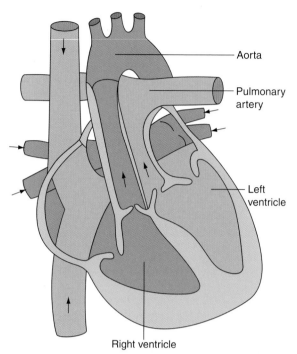

Figure 23.5. Senning repair for transposition of the great arteries. A baffle is created within the atria that redirects the deoxygenated caval blood to the mitral valve and the oxygenated pulmonary venous blood to the tricuspid valve. As a consequence, the anatomical left ventricle continues to act as the pulmonary pump and the anatomical right ventricle keeps on supporting the systemic circulation.

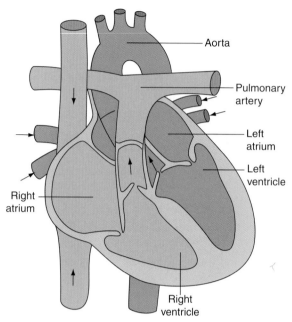

Figure 23.6. Arterial switch for transposition of the great arteries. An arterial switch is considered as the ideal operation for repair of transposition of the great arteries. It represents an anatomical repair and restores ventriculo-arterial concordance. Rarely, however, when coronary artery anatomy is abnormal (e.g. intramural coronary artery), coronary artery translocation may not be feasible and an arterial switch is not recommended.

developing or worsening of heart failure and atrial arrhythmias; an irreversible decline in right ventricular systemic function has been reported in 10% after pregnancy [33]. However, if no obstruction of the baffles can be found pre-pregnancy, and in the absence of more than moderate right ventricular dysfunction and/or severe tricuspid regurgitation, pregnancy is usually well tolerated in patients in NYHA class I–II. Patients in NYHA class III–IV or with unfavorable echocardiographic findings should be discouraged from pregnancy. Bimonthly follow-up with echocardiography is advised, and vaginal delivery is appropriate if no signs of heart failure develop. Patients being treated with angiotensin-converting enzyme inhibitors need to stop these before conception. Beta-blockers have to be used cautiously because of increased susceptibility for sinus node dysfunction as a result of extensive atrial surgery. Repair of transposition of the great arteries has moved to a more "physiological" approach by an arterial switch procedure (Figure 23.6). There are only limited data yet available on the outcome of pregnancy in

these patients; maternal and fetal outcome seems favorable if a good clinical condition exists pre-pregnancy.

Congenitally corrected transposition of the great arteries (double discordance)

The risk of pregnancy depends greatly on the functional status, ventricular function, associated valvular lesions, and antecedents of arrhythmic disturbances (Figure 23.7). However, these patients are at risk for developing or worsening of heart failure and atrial arrhythmias. Therefore, if patients are in NYHA class III–IV or are diagnosed with unfavorable echocardiographic findings (systemic ejection fraction 40% or severe tricuspid insufficiency), they should be counseled against pregnancy. Follow-up every 2 months with echocardiography is advised, and vaginal delivery is appropriate if no signs of heart failure develop. If there are signs of heart failure, cesarean section should be planned at 34–36 weeks of gestation; if there is hemodynamic instability despite optimal treatment, urgent delivery by cesarean section irrespective of gestation duration is advised.

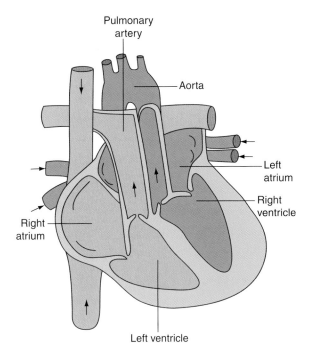

Figure 23.7. Congenitally corrected transposition of the great arteries. This is a rare condition, also called a double discordance, which describes better the nature of this defect. The anatomical left atrium (pulmonary venous atrium) is connected via a tricuspid valve with the anatomical right ventricle, from which originates the aorta. The anatomical right atrium (systemic venous atrium) is connected via a mitral valve with the anatomical left ventricle, from which originates the pulmonary artery. Consequently, two discordant connections, atrioventricular and ventriculo-arterial (double discordance), occur in sequence in the right and left side of the heart. In this condition, the right ventricle has to act as a systemic pump.

Fontan circulation

A Fontan operation is a definitive palliative procedure for a wide spectrum of complex cyanotic congenital heart defects with a univentricular physiology in which biventricular repair was not possible. Different techniques have been developed but the main issue is that systemic venous return is diverted directly to the pulmonary circulation without passing through the morphologic right ventricle. The central venous pressure and respiratory changes in intrathoracic pressures then become the driving force for preserving adequate pulmonary blood flow. However, in the long term, complications are inevitable and these patients are vulnerable to atrial arrhythmias; thromboembolic complications in a non-pulsatile, prothrombotic circuit; myocardial and hepatic dysfunction; and protein-losing enteropathy. Also, the ability to increase cardiac output is very limited. From this point of view, it is easy

to understand that pregnancy in patients who have had the Fontan operation is a high-risk condition [34]. In carefully selected patients, pregnancy is possible after extensive information if they are NYHA class I or II, have neither signs of ventricular dysfunction nor moderate to severe atrioventricular valve insufficiency, and if oxygen saturation at rest is 90% or more.

Tight surveillance with frequent echocardiography in a tertiary care center during pregnancy and after delivery is strongly recommended.

Anticoagulation is an issue, but clear guidelines even outside pregnancy do not exist. However, threshold for therapeutic anticoagulation with LMWH should be low as the thrombotic risk is more pronounced during pregnancy. If there are antecedents of atrial arrhythmias or thromboembolic complications prior to pregnancy, most of these women are already taking anticoagulation and they will be switched to fractionated heparin or LMWH during pregnancy at least in the first and third trimester (predelivery 34–36 weeks). If not, it seems prudent to consider prophylactic anticoagulation with LMWH in ongoing pregnancies [23].

Patients should be informed that fetal morbidity even in optimal settings remains high and includes prematurity, stillbirth, and low birth weight in up to 50%; neonatal outcome depends largely on the degree of prematurity. Generally, vaginal delivery is preferred but in a worsening clinical condition and/or signs of heart failure, early cesarean delivery in highly specialized centers has to be planned.

Eisenmenger syndrome

Since the recognition of Eisenmenger syndrome, a pathophysiological condition of pulmonary hypertension resulting from a reversed or bidirectional shunt in varying congenital heart defects, pregnancy has always been known as one of major causes directly related to accelerated or sudden death in these patients, particularly during delivery and early afterwards (first 2 weeks). The decrease in systemic vascular resistance resulting from hormonally mediated vasodilatation aggravates the right-to-left shunt, with further decrease in pulmonary blood flow and worsening of cyanosis. Over the last decades, maternal mortality has remained unchanged and still fluctuates around 30–50%, with poor fetal outcome and likelihood of a live birth being less than 15% if oxygen saturation at rest is < 85%. In this setting, patients should be counseled against pregnancy and if pregnancy occurs, elective abortion should be offered. However, when the patient declines termination of pregnancy, care in a specialized center and hospital admission early in the third trimester for bed rest and treatment of right heart failure may be necessary; diuretics should be used meticulously to avoid hemoconcentration and intravascular volume depletion. There is no consensus regarding use of anticoagulation, but iron deficiency should be carefully corrected to prevent microcytosis and negative disturbed rheology. Other options may be oxygen administration, inhaled nitric oxide, and intravenous prostacyclin, although it is not clear whether this reduces mortality. Experience with sildenafil is only reported in few case reports. Bosentan is contraindicated during pregnancy as animal studies have shown a possible teratogenic effect.

The mode of delivery is still a matter of debate but if there is maternal hemodynamic instability or fetal distress, an urgent cesarean section may be necessary. Most patients with Eisenmenger syndrome are referred for elective cesarean section at 30–34 weeks of pregnancy when the fetus is viable and before a hemodynamic catastrophe endangers the mother [35]. Given the risk of anesthesia, close monitoring with low-dose sequential combined spinal–epidural or incremental spinal anesthesia early in labor may reduce the effects on the peripheral circulation and improve maternal outcome [10,36].

Care for the mother with congenital heart disease

Various acronymic organizations worldwide exist for advocacy of the adult with congenital heart disease including GUCH (Grown-Up Congenital Heart Disease) in the UK, Europe, and Japan; CACH (Canadian Adult Congenital Hearts) in Canada; ACHA (Adult Congenital Heart Disease Association) in the USA; and WATCH (Working Group for Adults and Teenagers with Congenital Heart Disease) in Switzerland. In the UK, an integrated national service with four to six specialist units proximate to university centers is proposed to "concentrate" care for patients with complex conditions [37]. The International Society for Adult Congenital Heart Disease website offers a directory of GUCH centers searchable, among other criteria, by number of yearly patient visits; The Massachusetts General Hospital Heart Center ACHD Program in Boston is the largest such center in the USA, with over 2300 patient visits per year. Analysis of the Nationwide Inpatient Sample

showed that nearly 42% of GUCH parturients deliver at rural or non-teaching hospitals, and while maternal mortality and cardiac and obstetric complications were independent of hospital type, GUCH patients have increased risk of mortality and peripartum complications [38]. Multidisciplinary planning, therefore, is imperative [23].

Aortopathies

Marfan syndrome

Marfan syndrome is an autosomal dominant disorder of connective tissue caused by mutations in the gene encoding fibrillin-1 and has cardiac involvement in 80% of patients. Aortic dissection is the most feared complication, particularly in the last trimester or early postpartum. Women with Marfan syndrome and a normal sized aortic root have a risk less than 1% for aortic dissection. However, if the diameter of the aortic root exceeds 40 mm, the risk is increased up to 10%. Outside pregnancy, aortic root repair is advised when the diameter exceeds 50 mm or even at smaller diameters (45–50 mm) if there are signs of rapid growth or familial antecedents of premature dissection < 50 mm. Data on pregnancy outcome of Marfan patients with an aortic root >45 mm are lacking, but most guidelines discourage pregnancy in Marfan patients with an aortic root >45 mm and for those with a root between 40 and 45 mm if there are unfavorable familial characteristics [39]. The risk for dissection is reported to be lower after elective aortic root replacement, but patients remain at risk for dissection in the residual aorta. This means that prophylactic surgery may be considered earlier in Marfan patients if they wish to become pregnant and have an aortic root >45 mm.

Women should be informed not only on their own risks but also on the risk for their offspring. Referral for genetic counseling should be advised and beta-blockers should be continued during pregnancy. Regular monitoring by echocardiography should be provided every 3 months or more frequently if indicated. If the dimensions of the aortic root remain 40–45 mm, vaginal delivery with shortened second stage and regional anesthesia is possible. If the aortic diameter is ≥45 mm, elective cesarean section at 35–36 weeks of gestation is advised. Epidural anesthesia may be difficult in the presence of severe scoliosis or dural ectasia. If the aortic diameter index exceeds 27 mm/m^2 or 50 mm during pregnancy, aortic repair with the fetus in utero is recommended before 28–30 weeks of gestation. However, after 28–30 weeks of gestation, cesarean section followed by cardiac surgery is preferred. Aortic dissection during pregnancy is a surgical emergency necessitating rapid delivery of the fetus, if viable, through urgent cesarean section in the cardiac operating room and immediate repair of the dissection. If the fetus is not viable, all attempts should be made to save the mother's life with delivery of the fetus after repair of the dissection.

Ehlers–Danlos syndrome

Ehlers–Danlos syndrome is an autosomal inherited disorder of connective tissues with heterogeneous presentation; type IV (vascular) is associated with aortic involvement. Aortic dissection may occur without dilatation. Because of the frailty of large vessels and risk of uterine rupture, type IV Ehlers–Danlos syndrome by itself is a contraindication for pregnancy; case series have detailed a mortality rate between 11.5 and 38.5% [40]. Given the risk of poor wound healing and tissue frailty, there is no consensus regarding prophylactic aortic surgery, but generally the same criteria as for Marfan patients are used. If pregnancy occurs, close monitoring and continued treatment with beta-blockers is needed. Cervical insufficiency and preterm premature rupture of membranes are increased in the gravid patient with vascular Ehlers–Danlos syndrome; while early cesarean section at 32–36 weeks may prevent perineal trauma and intrapartum uterine rupture, perioperative complications of planned cesarean include hemorrhage and wound dehiscence, and delivery planning may be best achieved on an individual basis.

Familial thoracic aorta aneurysms

Patients with a familial occurrence of aortic dissection in the absence of an overt Marfan syndrome have been reported. This is often histopathologically related to cystic media necrosis of the aortic wall. Some of these patients can be diagnosed as having Loeys–Dietz syndrome.

Management is the same as for Marfan patients.

Turner syndrome

Almost 25–50% of patients with Turner syndrome present with cardiovascular abnormalities, mostly bicuspid aortic valve with or without stenosis, aortic coarctation, aortic dilatation, and hypertensive disorders. These patients are at increased risk for aortic dissection, particularly in the presence of aortic root dilatation and other predisposing factors such as left-sided obstructive lesions or hypertension. Hypertension should be treated aggressively, even during pregnancy. Concerning prophylactic surgery of the aortic root, the same criteria apply as for Marfan patients but the dimensions of the aortic root need to be indexed according to the body surface area of these patients (27 mm/m^2).

Coronary artery disease

Acute coronary syndromes during pregnancy are rare events with an estimated prevalence of 3–6 per 100 000 deliveries. Its occurrence is strongly related to classical coronary disease risk factors. Also maternal age (older than 35 years) and pre-eclampsia contribute to the risk for acute myocardial infarction during pregnancy. The etiology, however, is quite different to that of acute myocardial infarction occurring outside pregnancy; a review by Roth and Elkayam [41] found that less than half of the pregnancy-related myocardial infarctions could be attributed to atherosclerosis. Up to 20% and more were caused by coronary emboli in otherwise normal coronary arteries. Spontaneous coronary dissection is more frequently found among pregnant patients (16%) and is responsible for about 50% of the myocardial infarctions occurring around delivery or in the early period after birth. As a result of increased awareness and more aggressive strategies, maternal mortality has improved from 21–37% in earlier series to 5–10% in more recent reports. However according to the 2003–2005 Confidential Enquiries into Maternal Deaths and Child Health [42], maternal death during pregnancy in the UK is mainly from ischemic heart disease, which is worrisome and demands improvement in preventive strategies for high-risk patients.

In patients with ST elevation acute myocardial infarction, or non-ST elevation acute coronary syndrome, urgent percutaneous coronary intervention is the treatment of choice, particularly for the diagnosis and treatment of coronary dissection. The use of bare metal stents is preferred over drug-eluting stents because of the lack of evidence about safety. Aspirin should be continued throughout pregnancy, delivery, and lifelong. While clopidogrel is not known to be teratogenic, the safety of thienopyridines in pregnant women is not known, and their use should be restricted to the shortest duration and for strict indications. Angiotensin-converting enzyme inhibitors are teratogenic and should be withdrawn during pregnancy. Beta-blockers can be safely used. Statins are labeled as category X by the US Food and Drug Administration. While in a small prospective observational cohort study no increased risk of teratogenicity could be found, animal data on statins are conflicting. If there is no access to percutaneous coronary intervention, thrombolytic therapy is an option in case of life-threatening. acute coronary syndrome.

Hypertrophic cardiomyopathy

Hypertrophic cardiomyopathy is one of the most frequent genetic cardiac disorders encountered in adult life and may be first diagnosed during pregnancy. Symptoms may arise from diastolic dysfunction, severe left ventricular outflow tract obstruction, and arrhythmias. Asymptomatic women with known diagnosis of hypertrophic cardiomyopathy prior to pregnancy usually have an uncomplicated pregnancy course because the extra volume load of pregnancy has a beneficial effect on hemodynamics. However, patients who are symptomatic before pregnancy as a result of either severe restrictive physiology or a high outflow tract gradient are at risk for developing heart failure during pregnancy. The maternal mortality risk is negligible; fatalities are rarely reported and recent literature reports

no evidence suggesting an increased mortality risk related to pregnancy [43]. Patients should also be informed on the 50% inheritance pattern and referral for genetic counseling should be offered. Box 23.4 outlines the management of hypertrophic cardiomyopathy during pregnancy and at delivery.

Dilated cardiomyopathy

In dilated cardiomyopathy, there is dilatation of the left ventricle with systolic dysfunction of unknown etiology. Differentiation with peripartum cardiomyopathy is based on the time period of manifestation of the disease but there may be a considerable overlap. If known before conception and if left ventricular ejection fraction is 40%, women should be thoroughly informed about the high risk related to pregnancy (mortality risk 5–15%). Termination of pregnancy should be offered if ejection fraction is 20%. Management of these patients is according to guidelines for heart failure and will be discussed in the separate chapter about peripartum cardiomyopathy.

General issues for intensive care management

Box 23.5 covers the general issues for intensive care management of a pregnant woman with cardiovascular disease.

Box 23.4. Management of hypertrophic cardiomyopathy during pregnancy and at delivery

- Beta-blockers should be prescribed in case of moderate or more severe left ventricular outflow tract obstruction and/or significant hypertrophy (>15 mm wall thickness) to prevent congestion during emotional stress, physical activities and delivery
- Beta-blockers are the first choice for rate control and prevention of recurrence in atrial fibrillation, but electrical cardioversion is advised for reconversion of new-onset persistent atrial fibrillation; anticoagulation with LMWH is necessary
- Beta-blockers are the first choice for new-onset ventricular tachycardia if non-sustained and for prevention of recurrence; in sustained ventricular tachycardia with hemodynamic instability, immediate electrical cardioversion is recommended. If ventricular tachycardia is symptomatic, addition of amiodarone to the beta-blockers may be an option despite the risk of fetal hypothyroidism. An implantable cardioverter defibrillator may be considered in therapy-refractory ventricular tachycardia in high-risk patients
- If pulmonary edema or congestion develops, then admission of the patient to hospital for bed rest, close monitoring, and treatment with diuretics is advised; planned delivery preterm should be discussed if the fetus is viable
- Spontaneous labor and vaginal delivery is suitable for asymptomatic patients
- Care should be taken for potential deleterious hemodynamic effects of systemic vasodilation and hypotension with epidural anesthesia; this should be countered by careful fluid substitution in order to avoid volume overload and pulmonary congestion

Box 23.5. Intensive care management of a pregnant woman with cardiovascular disease

Before delivery
- Low threshold for admission to hospital
- Close clinical follow-up of fluid balance and signs of congestion to titrate diuretics; in severe heart failure or cardiogenic shock, start advanced therapy according to guidelines for treating acute heart failure (ACC/AHA/ESC)
- Continuous nasal oxygen to improve symptoms and arterial oxygen saturation
- Pulse oximetry, continuous electrocardiography, and invasive arterial monitoring are advised in hemodynamically unstable or critically ill patients
- Daily fetal and tocographic monitoring
- Close communication between obstetricians, cardiologists, anesthesists, intensivists, cardiac surgeons, neonatologists, and midwives to have a detailed peripartum plan and to make correct decisions in different scenarios of elective and emergency deliveries
- Prophylaxis against thromboembolic complications is advised if bed rest is prescribed
- Weekly echocardiography of the mother
- Central intravenous lines can be helpful in high-risk situations but are not generally advised; Swan–Ganz monitoring is very seldom indicated or advised, as placement of such catheters in pregnant women with complex anatomical features or cardiac conditions can be difficult or harmful and is associated with a higher risk of pulmonary artery rupture than outside pregnancy

After delivery
- Close monitoring for 24 to 72 hours postpartum in ICU as the hemodynamic changes from autotransfusion and aortocaval decompression, as well as possible (iatrogenic) fluid overload, can elicit signs of heart failure in the puerperium
- Close clinical follow-up of fluid balance and signs of congestion to titrate diuretics; in severe heart failure or cardiogenic shock start advanced therapy according to guidelines for treating acute heart failure (ACC/AHA/ESC)
- Continuous nasal oxygen to improve symptoms and arterial oxygen saturation
- Pulse oximetry, continuous electrocardiography, and invasive arterial monitoring are advised in hemodynamically unstable or critically ill patients
- Prophylaxis against thromboembolic complications is advised if bed rest is prescribed
- Weekly echocardiography of the mother
- Central intravenous lines can be helpful in high-risk situations but are not generally advised
- For very high-risk conditions such as Eisenmenger syndrome or severe pulmonary hypertension, a longer postpartum observation period (up to 2 weeks) is advised

ACC/AHA/ESC, American College of Cardiology/American Heart Association Task Force on Practice Guidelines and the European Society of Cardiology Committee for Practice Guidelines.

Key points
- Up to 4% of all pregnancies in the Western world are complicated by cardiovascular disease.
- Cardiac disease has become the major cause of non-obstetric maternal death, in particular ischemic heart disease.
- Risk in pregnancy depends on functional status but also on lesion-specific features, which have an effect on morbidity and mortality related to pregnancy.
- For most women with pre-existing cardiac disease, pregnancy will be possible.
- Cyanotic disorders and obstructive left-sided lesions are associated with significant maternal and fetal morbidity.
- Pregnancy is contraindicated in patients with Eisenmenger syndrome, severe left-sided obstructive lesions, severe left ventricular dysfunction, and aortic root >45 mm in Marfan syndrome and >50 mm in bicuspid aortic valve-associated aortic disease.

- Pre-pregnancy counseling and high suspicion for cardiac symptoms in high-risk patients, even without pre-existing heart disease, are necessary to improve outcome for more vulnerable patients. In women with high-risk cardiac conditions *no* unplanned pregnancies should occur.
- Regular clinical and echocardiographic follow-up each trimester is advised for most conditions; for more severe lesions bimonthly or even monthly follow up is recommended.
- Hospitalization for close supervision in the beginning of the third trimester may be necessary in high-risk conditions.
- For most patients, vaginal delivery with good analgesia is preferred; prolonged second stage should be avoided and instrumental delivery available.
- There are few cardiac indications for delivery by cesarean section: patients with Marfan syndrome with aortic root dilatation, aortic dissection, and refractory heart failure.
- Urgent delivery by cesarean section may be necessary in hemodynamic instability in order to improve maternal outcome and prevent fetal distress.
- For high-risk patients, delivery should be planned in an experienced center and in the presence of adequate monitoring and supervision by senior staff members.
- If cardiac surgery is unavoidable during pregnancy, gestational age and access to neonatal intensive care are important to consider in choosing the time of surgery and deciding between in utero repair or surgery after delivery of a viable fetus via urgent cesarean section. If surgery is required during the first trimester, the patient should be informed about the high risk of fetal loss (20–30%); the option to interrupt pregnancy can be discussed in these conditions.
- Women should labor in left lateral decubitus position to increase venous return, with supplemental oxygen if necessary.
- Adequate analgesia during labor and delivery is crucial to minimize the effect of possible deleterious hemodynamic changes.
- Neuraxial blocks are considered as the anesthetic of choice during labor or cesarean section. For labor analgesia, slow induction with diluted anesthetic solutions of bupivicaine or ropivacaine mixed with a small dose of an opioid followed by a continuous epidural infusion or patient-controlled epidural analgesia provide good hemodynamic stability.
- For cesarean delivery, anesthetic options are a slowly induced epidural, a low dose combined spinal–epidural, or continuous spinal anesthesia.
- Strategies to minimize the possible hypotension and tachycardia induced by anesthesia include the use of intravenous fluids or vasopressors (phenylephrine). If properly carried out by experienced anesthesiologists, analgesia can be provided with only minimal changes in maternal hemodynamics.
- General anesthesia is sometimes required in selected cases; opioids prior to delivery are administered with remifentanil being the logical first choice. Close maternal monitoring and awareness of possible neonatal respiratory depression are needed.
- Oxytocics should be used cautiously especially in patients with fixed output states in the setting of severe left-sided obstructive lesions and/or Eisenmenger syndrome.
- Close monitoring during peripartum and postpartum is warranted for high-risk patients as important changes in circulating volume and fluid shifts predispose these women for development of heart failure; additional treatment with diuretics may be necessary. In high-risk patients, a low threshold for arterial monitoring throughout labor, delivery and the postpartum is advised.

References

1. Merz WM, Keyver-Paik MD, Baumgarten G, Lewalter T, Gembruch U. Spectrum of cardiovascular findings during pregnancy and parturition at a tertiary referral center. *J Perinat Med* 2011;**39**:251–256.

2. Malhotra S, Yentis SM. Reports on Confidential Enquiries into Maternal Deaths: management strategies based on trends in maternal cardiac deaths over 30 years. *Int J Obstet Anesth* 2006;**15**:223–226.

3. Small MJ, James AH, Kershaw T, *et al.* Near-miss maternal mortality: cardiac dysfunction as the principal cause of obstetric intensive care unit admissions. *Obstet Gynecol* 2012;**119**:250–255.

4. Berg CJ, Callaghan WM, Syverson C, Henderson Z. Pregnancy-related mortality in the United States, 1998 to 2005. *Obstet Gynecol* 2010;**116**:1302–1309.

5. Siu SC, Sermer M, Colman JM, *et al.* Prospective multicenter study of pregnancy outcomes in women with heart disease. *Circulation* 2001;**104**:515–521.

6. Drenthen W, Boersma E, Balci A, *et al.* Predictors of pregnancy complications in women with congenital heart disease. *Eur Heart J* 2010;**31**:2124–2132.

7. Khairy P, Ouyang DW, Fernandes SM, *et al.* Pregnancy outcomes in women with congenital heart disease. *Circulation* 2006;**113**:517–524.

8. Criteria Committee for the New York Heart Association. *Nomenclature and Criteria for Diagnosis of Diseases of the Heart and Great Vessels*, 9th edn. New York: Little Brown, 1994, pp. 253–255.

9. World Health Organization. *International Classification of Diseases and Related Health Problems*. Geneva: World Health Organization, 1994.

10. Regitz-Zagrosek V, Blomstrom Lundqvist C, Borghi C, *et al.* ESC guidelines on the management of cardiovascular diseases during pregnancy: the Task Force on the Management of Cardiovascular Diseases during Pregnancy of the European Society of Cardiology (ESC). *Eur Heart J* 2011;**32**:3147–3197.

11. Thorne S, MacGregor A, Nelson-Piercy C. Risks of contraception and pregnancy in heart disease. *Heart* 2006;**92**:1520–1525.

12. van Mook WN, Peeters L. Severe cardiac disease in pregnancy, part I: hemodynamic changes and complaints during pregnancy, and general management of cardiac disease in pregnancy. *Curr Opin Crit Care* 2005;**11**:430–434.

13. Bowater SE, Thorne SA. Management of pregnancy in women with acquired and congenital heart disease. *Postgrad Med J* 2010;**86**:100–105.

14. Siu SC, Colman JM, Sorensen S, *et al.* Adverse neonatal and cardiac outcomes are more common in pregnant women with cardiac disease. *Circulation* 2002;**105**:2179–2184.

15. James PR. Drugs in pregnancy. Cardiovascular disease. *Best Pract Res Clin Obstet Gynaecol* 2001;**15**:903–911.

16. Elkayam U, Bitar F. Valvular heart disease and pregnancy. Part II: Prosthetic valves. *J Am Coll Cardiol* 2005;**46**:403–410.

17. Elkayam U, Bitar F. Valvular heart disease and pregnancy. Part I: Native valves. *J Am Coll Cardiol* 2005;**46**:223–230.

18. Dob DP, Yentis SM. Practical management of the parturient with congenital heart disease. *Int J Obstet Anesth* 2006;**15**:137–144.

19. Langesaeter E, Rosseland LA, Stubhaug A. Hemodynamic effects of oxytocin during cesarean delivery. *Int J Gynaecol Obstet* 2006;**95**:46–47.

20. Langesaeter E, Rosseland LA, Stubhaug A. Continuous invasive blood pressure and cardiac output monitoring during cesarean delivery: a randomized, double-blind comparison of low-dose versus high-dose spinal anesthesia with intravenous phenylephrine or placebo infusion. *Anesthesiology* 2008;**109**:856–863.

21. Bonow RO, Carabello BA, Chatterjee K, *et al.* ACC/AHA 2006 guidelines for the management of patients with valvular heart disease: a report of the American College of Cardiology/American Heart Association Task Force on Practice Guidelines (writing Committee to Revise the 1998 guidelines for the management of patients with valvular heart disease) developed in collaboration with the Society of Cardiovascular Anesthesiologists endorsed by the Society for Cardiovascular Angiography and Interventions and the Society of Thoracic Surgeons. *J Am Coll Cardiol* 2006;**48**:e1–e148.

22. Hameed A, Karaalp IS, Tummala PP, *et al.* The effect of valvular heart disease on maternal and fetal outcome of pregnancy. *J Am Coll Cardiol* 2001;**37**:893–899.

23. Warnes CA, Williams RG, Bashore TM, *et al.* ACC/AHA 2008 guidelines for the management of adults with congenital heart disease: a report of the American College of Cardiology/American Heart Association Task Force on Practice Guidelines (Writing Committee to Develop Guidelines on the Management of Adults With Congenital Heart Disease). Developed in Collaboration With the American Society of Echocardiography, Heart Rhythm Society, International Society for Adult Congenital Heart Disease, Society for Cardiovascular Angiography and Interventions, and Society of Thoracic Surgeons. *J Am Coll Cardiol* 2008;**52**:e143–e263.

24. Immer FF, Bansi AG, Immer-Bansi AS, *et al.* Aortic dissection in pregnancy: analysis of risk factors and outcome. *Ann Thorac Surg* 2003;**76**:309–314.

25. Chan WS, Anand S, Ginsberg JS. Anticoagulation of pregnant women with mechanical heart valves: a systematic review of the literature. *Arch Intern Med* 2000;**160**:191–196.

26. Sillesen M, Hjortdal V, Vejlstrup N, Sorensen K. Pregnancy with prosthetic heart valves: 30 years' nationwide experience in Denmark. *Eur J Cardiothorac Surg* 2011;**40**:448–454.

27. Abildgaard U, Sandset PM, Hammerstrom J, Gjestvang FT, Tveit A. Management of pregnant women with mechanical heart valve prosthesis: thromboprophylaxis

265

with low molecular weight heparin. *Thromb Res* 2009;**124**:262–267.

28. McLintock C, McCowan LM, North RA. Maternal complications and pregnancy outcome in women with mechanical prosthetic heart valves treated with enoxaparin. *BJOG* 2009;**116**:1585–1592.

29. Bates SM, Greer IA, Pabinger I, Sofaer S, Hirsh J. Venous thromboembolism, thrombophilia, antithrombotic therapy, and pregnancy (American College of Chest Physicians Evidence-Based Clinical Practice Guidelines, 8th edn). *Chest* 2008;**133** (Suppl):844S–886S.

30. James A. Practice Bulletin 123: thromboembolism in pregnancy. *Obstet Gynecol* 2011;**118**:718–729.

31. Horlocker TT, Wedel DJ, Rowlingson JC, Enneking FK. Executive summary: regional anesthesia in the patient receiving antithrombotic or thrombolytic therapy (American Society of Regional Anesthesia and Pain Medicine Evidence-Based Guidelines, 3rd edn). *Reg Anesth Pain Med* 2010;**35**:102–105.

32. Vriend JW, Drenthen W, Pieper PG, *et al.* Outcome of pregnancy in patients after repair of aortic coarctation. *Eur Heart J* 2005;**26**:2173–2178.

33. Guedes A, Mercier LA, Leduc L, *et al.* Impact of pregnancy on the systemic right ventricle after a Mustard operation for transposition of the great arteries. *J Am Coll Cardiol* 2004;**44**:433–437.

34. Canobbio MM, Mair DD, van der Velde M, Koos BJ. Pregnancy outcomes after the Fontan repair. *J Am Coll Cardiol* 1996;**28**:763–767.

35. Naguib MA, Dob DP, Gatzoulis MA. A functional understanding of moderate to complex congenital heart disease and the impact of pregnancy. Part II: tetralogy of Fallot, Eisenmenger's syndrome and the Fontan operation. *Int J Obstet Anesth* 2010;**19**:306–312.

36. Wang H, Zhang W, Liu T. Experience of managing pregnant women with Eisenmenger's syndrome: maternal and fetal outcome in 13 cases. *J Obstet Gynaecol Res* 2011;**37**:64–70.

37. British Cardiac Society Working Party. Grown-up congenital heart (GUCH) disease: current needs and provision of service for adolescents and adults with congenital heart disease in the UK. *Heart* 2002;**88** (Suppl 1):i1–i14.

38. Karamlou T, Diggs BS, McCrindle BW, Welke KF. A growing problem: maternal death and peripartum complications are higher in women with grown-up congenital heart disease. *Ann Thorac Surg* 2011;**92**:2193–2198; discussion 2198–2199.

39. Meijboom LJ, Vos FE, Timmermans J, *et al.* Pregnancy and aortic root growth in the Marfan syndrome: a prospective study. *Eur Heart J* 2005;**26**:914–920.

40. Hammond R, Oligbo N. Ehlers–Danlos syndrome type IV and pregnancy. *Arch Gynecol Obstet* 2012;**285**:51–54.

41. Roth A, Elkayam U. Acute myocardial infarction associated with pregnancy. *J Am Coll Cardiol* 2008;**52**:171–180.

42. Lewis G (ed.) *Saving Mothers' Lives: Reviewing Maternal Deaths to Make Motherhood Safer, 2003–2005. The Seventh Report on Confidential Enquiries into Maternal Deaths in the United Kingdom*. London: CEMACH, 2007.

43. Autore C, Conte MR, Piccininno M, *et al.* Risk associated with pregnancy in hypertrophic cardiomyopathy. *J Am Coll Cardiol* 2002;**40**:1864–1869.

Chapter

24

Respiratory disease

Stephen E. Lapinsky, Laura C. Price, and Catherine Nelson-Piercy

Introduction

The pregnant patient with pre-existing pulmonary disease is at risk of deteriorating during pregnancy. In addition, a number of respiratory conditions specific to pregnancy may produce respiratory compromise in previously healthy women. Respiratory failure carries significant risks for both mother and fetus, and many management interventions in this situation may carry risks for the fetus.

Physiological respiratory changes in pregnancy

Various physiological changes occur as a result of the pregnant state, affecting patients with pre-existing lung disease and affecting the assessment and management of the patient with respiratory failure. Estrogens produce capillary congestion and hyperplasia of mucus glands, affecting the upper respiratory tract and cause airway hyperemia and edema. Because of this mucosal edema and friability, nasal tube insertion should be avoided and endotracheal intubation may be more difficult.

Changes to the thorax occur from both the enlarging uterus and hormonal effects that produce ligamentous laxity. The diaphragm is displaced cephalad by up to 4 cm, and the potential loss of lung volume is largely offset by widening of the anteroposterior and transverse diameters. These changes in the thoracic cage produce a progressive decrease in functional residual capacity, these effects being measurable at 16 to 24 weeks of gestation and progressing to 10–25% by term [1]. Vital capacity remains unchanged, and total lung capacity decreases only minimally. Measurements of airflow and lung compliance are not altered, but chest wall and total respiratory compliance are reduced in the third trimester [2]. Transfer factor for carbon monoxide has been shown to fall from the second trimester of pregnancy, even when corrected for anemia and low alveolar volumes, and then rises to normal levels postpartum [3]. Minute ventilation increases during pregnancy, beginning in the first trimester and reaching 20–40% above baseline at term, resulting from an increase in tidal volume of approximately 30–35% [4]. These effects are mediated by the increase in respiratory drive caused by elevated serum progesterone levels. Blood gas measurements, therefore, demonstrate a respiratory alkalosis with compensatory renal excretion of bicarbonate, with arterial carbon dioxide partial pressure (Pa_{CO_2}) falling to 3.8–4.3 kPa (28–32 mmHg) and plasma bicarbonate falling to 18–21 mEq/L [5].

The difference between alveolar oxygen partial pressure (PA_{O_2}) and arterial partial pressure ($PA_{O_2} - Pa_{O_2}$) is usually unchanged by pregnancy, and mean Pa_{O_2} usually exceeds 13 kPa (100 mmHg) at sea level throughout pregnancy. As functional residual capacity diminishes towards term, mild hypoxemia and an increased $PA_{O_2} - Pa_{O_2}$ may develop in the supine position. Oxygen consumption increases because of fetal and maternal demands, reaching 20–33% above baseline by the third trimester. The reduced functional residual capacity combined with an increased oxygen consumption decreases oxygen reserve, making the pregnant patient susceptible to the rapid development of hypoxia in response to hypoventilation or apnea [6]. Alkalosis (respiratory or metabolic) adversely affects fetal oxygenation by reducing uterine blood flow [7]. Adequate pain relief with narcotics or epidural analgesia blunts the ventilatory response and can correct the gas exchange abnormalities associated with active labor.

Maternal Critical Care: A Multidisciplinary Approach, ed. Marc Van de Velde, Helen Scholefield, and Lauren A. Plante.
Published by Cambridge University Press. © Cambridge University Press 2013.

Conditions not specific to pregnancy

Asthma

Asthma affects 4–8% of the general population and may, therefore, be the most common pulmonary disorder in pregnancy. Approximately a third of women with asthma remain unchanged during pregnancy, while similar proportions either deteriorate or improve [8]. Acute asthma in labor is rare and status asthmaticus occurs in about 0.2% of pregnancies [9]. Asthma may have a number of adverse effects on both mother and fetus, including an increased incidence of preterm labor, low neonatal birth weight, increased perinatal mortality, as well as having an association with pre-eclampsia, chronic hypertension, and complicated labor [10].

Therapy of asthma in pregnancy does not differ from that for the non-pregnant patient and should be individualized according to objective measurement of lung volumes and flow. Systemic steroids may be necessary for the management of an acute attack and should be used in the same way as in the non-pregnant patient. Extensive practice algorithms are available for the management of asthma during pregnancy [11–13].

Women with asthma who become pregnant may be inclined to discontinue their treatment because of concerns regarding the effects of drugs on the fetus. A significant body of literature regarding the lack of teratogenic effects of asthma therapy now exists. In many situations, maternal (and fetal) benefit clearly outweighs fetal risk of drug exposure. The traditionally used US Food and Drug Administration pregnancy risk categories are not very useful from a clinical perspective and are being replaced by a narrative description of known drug effects with a risk summary [14,15]. Animal and human studies of selective short-acting beta-2-adrenergic agonists have demonstrated an acceptable safety profile for the fetus [16]. However, non-selective beta-adrenergic agonists (such as epinephrine) carry a risk of uterine vasoconstriction and are probably best avoided. With regard to long-acting beta-agonists, evidence from prescription event monitoring suggests that salmeterol is safe in pregnancy [17]. There are some safety data, although with small numbers, for formoterol [18]. There have been no associated obstetric complications or congenital malformations with a significant number of pregnancies where long-acting beta-agonists have been used [19]. These drugs are recommended in patients with poor asthma control on a combination of inhaled corticosteroids and short-acting beta-adrenergic agonists [11–13]. There are also encouraging early safety data on the use of some combination inhalers in pregnancy (e.g. fluticasone/salmeterol) [20]. Animal studies show an increased incidence of cleft palate with use of corticosteroids during pregnancy, but no human data support this association. Systemic corticosteroids may also cause intrauterine growth restriction but of a relatively modest degree. Halogenated corticosteroids (e.g. prednisolone, prednisone) do not cross the placenta to any significant degree, so fetal and neonatal adrenal suppression is not a major concern with these drugs. Among the inhaled steroids, beclomethasone and budesonide are preferred because of their long history of use in pregnancy and the absence of any demonstrated toxicity to the fetus in large studies [15].

Labor and delivery may carry increased risk for women with asthma, in part because of the drugs commonly administered. Narcotics other than fentanyl may release histamine, which can worsen bronchospasm. Oxytocin is commonly used as a labor induction agent and for postpartum hemorrhage and has little effect on asthma, but alternative drugs such as 15-methylprostaglandin-$F_{2\alpha}$, methylergonovine, and ergonovine may cause bronchospasm and should be avoided in women with asthma if possible.

Acute severe asthma in pregnancy may be treated as in the non-pregnant patient with intravenous beta-2-adrenergic agonists, intravenous theophylline, intravenous magnesium sulfate and steroids [11–13]. Patients with acute severe asthma require close monitoring, preferably in an intensive care unit (ICU). In addition to the asthma therapy described above, attention should be given to oxygenation, fluid hydration, and nutrition. Although intubation and mechanical ventilation may be required, these interventions carry significant risk. Application of positive pressure ventilation may induce dynamic hyperinflation ("auto-PEEP"), which causes hypotension, particularly in the volume-depleted patient. Pulseless electrical activity cardiac arrest may occur. Ventilation may be inadequate because of the small tidal volumes, necessitating a permissive hypercapnia approach until the asthma attack subsides.

Pulmonary infections

As a result of alterations in cell-mediated immunity in pregnancy, which allow tolerance to paternal fetal antigens, the pregnant woman is at risk of increased susceptibility or increased severity of certain infections.

Pneumonia is an important cause of maternal and fetal morbidity and mortality [21,22] with a reported incidence varying widely, from 1 in 367 to 1 in 2388 deliveries [21,22]. This is likely not higher than that in the general population. An increasing incidence of pneumonia in pregnancy may be occurring, with HIV and chronic disease being the major risk factors [21]. Pregnancy does appear to increase the risk for major complications of pneumonia, including respiratory failure, empyema, pneumothorax, and pericardial tamponade. Pregnancy complications may occur as a result of pneumonia, including preterm labor, small-for-gestational age, and intrauterine and neonatal death [21,22].

Bacterial pneumonia

Pneumonia in pregnancy is most commonly bacterial in origin, with the microbiological spectrum being no different to the usual organisms found in community-acquired pneumonia. The diagnosis of pneumonia is often delayed because of a reluctance to obtain a chest radiograph based on the unnecessary concern about radiation exposure. If a chest radiograph is required, this should not be witheld for this reason as the risk to the fetus is negligible (see Chapter 22). Antibacterial therapy is similar to treatment in the non-pregnant patient (Table 24.1), but some drugs such as tetracyclines and quinolones should be avoided if possible [23]. The patient with septic shock as a result of pneumonia requires aggressive fluid resuscitation and early administration of appropriate antibiotics [24].

Viral pneumonia

Viral pneumonitis is a serious concern in pregnancy with reported increased mortality rates compared with the general population, likely related to the alterations in cell-mediated immunity. Data from influenza pandemics demonstrate the maternal mortality rate to be higher than the general population: in the influenza pandemic of 1918–1919, the maternal mortality rate was as high as 27%, and in the epidemic of 1957, 50% of fatalities among women of childbearing age occurred in pregnant women [25]. The 2009 swine influenza A (H1N1) pandemic was associated with a high incidence of severe disease and respiratory failure in pregnant women, with significant mortality [26]. Early institution of antiviral therapy (within 48 hours of symptoms) is associated with an improved outcome. Amantadine has been used in pregnancy as treatment and as prophylaxis, but the 2009 pandemic strain was resistant. Oseltamivir was used quite extensively in pregnancy during the 2009 pandemic with good results [27], and zanamivir, given by inhalation, is also a treatment option. A low uptake of vaccination was common in pregnant patients developing severe respiratory failure [28], stressing the importance of H1N1 influenza vaccination in pregnancy.

Varicella pneumonia has also been associated with adverse outcomes in pregnancy. In one review, a 35% mortality rate was reported in pregnancy compared with 11% in other adults [29]. Not all studies have confirmed this increased incidence or mortality in pregnancy. This may, however, be because of early treatment with acyclovir, which reduces mortality in gravid patients [30].

Fungal pneumonia

Fungal pneumonia is uncommon, but it appears that coccidioidomycosis is more likely to disseminate in pregnancy particularly in the third trimester. This has been attributed to the impairment of cell-mediated immunity as well as to a stimulatory effect of progesterone and 17β-estradiols on fungal proliferation [31]. Amphotericin is the accepted therapy for disseminated coccidioidomycosis.

Tuberculosis

Tuberculosis is not more common nor more severe in pregnancy. Standard drug therapy, namely with isoniazid, rifampin, and ethambutol has an acceptable safety profile in pregnancy and is recommended for pregnant women by the US Centers for Disease Control and Prevention and the American Thoracic Society [32]. There is less experience with pyrazinamide, but this drug is recommended for use in pregnancy by the World Health Organization [32].

Table 24.1. Respiratory infections and treatment in pregnancy

Infection	Therapy
Bacterial pneumonia	Similar to non-pregnant patient, e.g. ceftriaxone for hospitalized patient, ceftriaxone and azithromycin in intensive care; avoid tetracyclines and quinolones if possible
Fungal pneumonia	Amphotericin B; limited data in pregnancy for newer drugs
Viral pneumonia	Oseltamivir for influenza; acyclovir for varicella
Tuberculosis	Isoniazid, rifampin, ethambutol; pyrazinamide recommended by some authorities; avoid streptomycin

Streptomycin may produce congenital deafness and is contraindicated during pregnancy (Table 24.1).

Acute respiratory distress syndrome and acute lung injury

The pregnant patient is at risk of developing pulmonary edema and acute lung injury from pregnancy-associated complications or other conditions (Table 24.2) [33]. Acute respiratory distress syndrome (ARDS) occurs fairly frequently in pregnancy and is a leading cause of maternal death [34]. The pregnant state may predispose to the development of pulmonary edema by a number of mechanisms, such as the increased circulating blood volume, reduced serum albumin [33], a possible upregulation of components of the acute inflammatory response, and increased capillary leak.

Table 24.2. Causes of acute respiratory failure in the obstetric patient

Type	Examples
Pregnancy specific	Pre-eclampsia with pulmonary edema
	Amniotic fluid embolism
	Tocolytic associated pulmonary edema
	ARDS in chorioamnionitis
	ARDS related to placental abruption
	Trophoblastic embolism
	Peripartum cardiomyopathy
Risk increased by pregnancy	Gastric acid aspiration
	Venous thromboembolism
	Asthma
	ARDS in sepsis, particularly pyelonephritis
	Transfusion-related acute lung injury
	Air embolism
	Pneumonia (e.g. varicella, fungal)
	Stenotic valvular heart disease, pulmonary hypertension
Non-specific	Trauma
	Drugs/toxins
	Pancreatitis

ARDS, acute respiratory distress syndrome.

There are few differences in the management of the pregnant patient who has ARDS compared with the non-pregnant person. The management of ARDS requires mechanical ventilation and ICU supportive care. Pressure-limited ventilation, utilizing a tidal volume of 6 mL/kg ideal body weight and limiting plateau pressure to <30 cmH$_2$O, is associated with an improved outcome [35]. Pregnant patients were not included in this study and higher plateau pressures may be needed to achieve this tidal volume because of the pregnant patient's reduced chest wall compliance. Adequate maternal oxygen saturation is essential for fetal well-being. Survival appears to be as good as, or better than, that in the general population, possibly because of these patient's young age, lack of comorbidity, and the reversibility of many of the predisposing conditions, with an anticipated 40–75% survival rate [36].

Gastric acid aspiration is an important cause of maternal acute lung injury. Contributing factors include the increased intra-abdominal pressure caused by the enlarged uterus, the effect of progesterone lowering the tone of the esophageal sphincter, and use of the supine position for delivery. About two thirds of cases of aspiration occur in the delivery suite. Aspiration of gastric contents with pH ≤2.5 causes chemical pneumonitis and permeability edema. All pregnant patients should be considered to have a full stomach, and it should be remembered that endotracheal intubation of the pregnant patient is more difficult than in the non-pregnant population [37].

Transfusion-related acute lung injury is an important complication of blood component therapy in pregnancy [38]. The clinical presentation is of sudden onset of dyspnea and tachypnea occurring during, or within 6 hours, of transfusion of plasma-containing blood products. The clinical picture is indistinguishable from ARDS and the differential diagnosis includes circulatory fluid overload. Management is supportive and most patients improve within a few days, although deaths may occur.

Pulmonary thromboembolic disease

Pulmonary embolism is a leading cause of maternal mortality, accounting for about 7–10% of pregnancy-related deaths in the USA and UK, and it is an important consideration in the evaluation of the patient with respiratory disease. This topic is covered in detail in Chapter 25.

Pulmonary arterial hypertension

Pulmonary arterial hypertension is an uncommon condition that can affect women of childbearing age, with a significant mortality rate in pregnancy (reported as 25–50%) [39,40]. Hemodynamic compromise occurs because of the inability of the right ventricle to tolerate the increases in cardiac output that occur in pregnancy and the postpartum period [39]. Although clinical trials in pregnancy are lacking, specific treatments are now available and mortality appears to be reducing, although it remains extremely high [40]. Treatment with vasodilators such as intravenous or inhaled prostacyclin or inhaled nitric oxide, as well as phosphodiesterase-5 inhibitors such as sildenafil, has been used successfully in pregnancy [41–43]. Endothelin receptor antagonists (e.g. bosentan) are teratogenic in rats. Anticoagulation is recommended for patients with pulmonary arterial hypertension , with the usual precautions during pregnancy. These patients should be managed in a center with expertise and experience in this condition, and patients should be closely followed through the peripartum period [44]. This condition is covered in more detail in Chapter 25.

Restrictive lung disease

Interstitial lung diseases are characterized by inflammation and fibrosis affecting the pulmonary parenchyma. The pathophysiology involves decreased lung volumes, loss of gas exchange units, and a diffusion abnormality. Fortunately, these conditions are not common in woman in their childbearing years, as most diseases affect an older demographic. There are conditions that may occur in this group and some, including lymphangioleiomyomatosis and systemic lupus erythematosus, may worsen in pregnancy. A concern in the woman with interstitial lung disease in pregnancy is hypoxemia and difficulty in meeting the increased oxygen consumption requirements. This requirement results in an increased cardiac output (and, therefore, shortened alveolar capillary transit time) in the face of a diffusion defect. The presence of associated pulmonary hypertension increases maternal risk significantly. Few data exist on the management and outcome in these patients, but restrictive lung disease appears reasonably well tolerated in pregnancy [45]. Oxygen supplementation may be required, particularly during exercise. Patients with a vital capacity of <1 L and those with pulmonary hypertension should consider avoiding pregnancy [46].

Patients with neuromuscular disease and respiratory compromise (e.g. severe kyphoscoliosis, muscular dystrophy) are at risk of respiratory failure as the uterus enlarges. Because there is no parenchymal disease, oxygenation problems may be less of a concern. Case reports and small case series have described successful pregnancy outcomes in women with vital capacities 40% of predicted [45,47]. Successful pregnancy in such patients requires an experienced, multidisciplinary team approach, and pregnancy should not be embarked on without significant counseling in these patients. Non-invasive ventilation has been used to support respiratory function through the latter part of pregnancy and during labor [47].

In all these patient groups, additional intercurrent illness such as pneumonia or influenza could result in significant respiratory compromise. Immunization against *Streptococcus pneumoniae*, *Haemophilus influenzae*, and viral influenza should be considered.

Other respiratory conditions

Survival of patients with cystic fibrosis is now well into the childbearing age, and 4% of women with cystic fibrosis between the ages of 17 and 37 were pregnant in 1990 [48]. This occurs despite the associated infertility of women with this condition. Pregnancy in women with cystic fibrosis may be associated with adverse fetal and maternal outcomes [49]. A somewhat dated review of 217 pregnancies, reported between 1960 and 1991 [50], showed that although more than 80% progressed to at least 20 weeks of gestation, one quarter delivered preterm and the perinatal death rate was 14%. In this series, there were three maternal deaths, and 14% of mothers had died by 2 years after delivery [50]. Pregnancy has little effect on patients with stable cystic fibrosis, although poor outcomes have been seen in those with severe disease [49,50]. Women with severe cystic fibrosis require pre-pregnancy counseling, to limit excessive maternal and fetal risk. A forced expiratory volume in 1 second (FEV1) <50% of predicted and the presence of pulmonary hypertension are poor prognostic factors for both mother and infant [49,50]. In a recent Australian series reporting 20 pregnancies from 1995 to 2009, most women tolerated pregnancy well despite most having a pre-pregnancy FEV1 <60% predicted. In addition to pre-pregnancy lung function, body mass index <20 kg/m^2 was an important predictor of worse fetal outcomes [51].

There have even been successful pregnancies in patients following lung transplantation for cystic fibrosis lung disease as well as for other end-stage lung diseases. There are few data on long-term outcomes of this high-risk group, although a stable interval of at least 3 years post-transplant is associated with a more favorable outcome [52]. Additional considerations include the potential adverse fetal effects of maternal immunosuppressive agents, and the marked reduction in life expectancy of the mother.

Pregnancy may be complicated by obstructive sleep apnea, potentially having adverse effects on both mother and fetus [53]. Hypopnea should be uncommon in pregnancy because of the respiratory stimulatory effect of progesterone. Obstructive sleep apnea may, however, occur in obese patients being precipitated by the upper airway mucosal edema and vascular congestion that accompany pregnancy. Although nocturnal hypoxemia may be associated with poor fetal growth, snoring alone does not increase fetal risk [54]. Treatment with nasal continuous positive airway pressure is safe and effective.

Venous air embolism has been reported during pregnancy, resulting from air entry through the subplacental venous sinuses [55]. This disorder has been documented during labor and delivery, during cesarean section, during abortions, in patients with placenta previa, and related to blowing air into the vagina during orogenital sex during pregnancy.

Pulmonary arteriovenous malformations may expand during pregnancy because of the general vascular distensibility and the increase in blood volume. The likelihood of bleeding is, therefore, increased. Embolization and surgical management have been utilized successfully during pregnancy [56].

Pregnancy-specific conditions

Amniotic fluid embolism

Amniotic fluid embolism is an important cause of sudden respiratory failure in pregnancy and is covered in detail in Chapter 40. Survivors of the initial event may go on to develop ARDS, requiring ventilatory support. Treatment is predominantly supportive, although there may be a role for steroid therapy.

Pulmonary edema secondary to pre-eclampsia

Pre-eclampsia is a pregnancy-induced condition (see Chapter 36). Acute respiratory failure with bilateral pulmonary infiltrates occurs in a small proportion of

patients (approximately 3%) and is more common in obese, chronically hypertensive women [57]. The mechanism is likely multifactorial in origin, with a component being hydrostatic edema related to the increased afterload and diastolic dysfunction, aggravated by the lowered serum oncotic pressure. Pre-eclampsia can progress to ARDS. The pathophysiology of pre-eclampsia involves activation of an inflammatory process [58], which may initiate a lung injury process. Acute respiratory failure in the pre-eclamptic patient occurs most commonly in the early postpartum period, often associated with intrapartum fluid administration and return of blood to the central circulation as the uterus contracts. Treatment of respiratory failure is supportive, with recovery time varying depending on the underlying pathological mechanism.

Tocolytic pulmonary edema

Uterine contractions in preterm labor may be inhibited with beta-adrenergic agonists, as well as several other drugs such as calcium antagonists, indomethacin, atosiban and magnesium sulfate. Use of beta-adrenergic agonists has become less common because of the associated risk of pulmonary edema [59]. The frequency of tocolytic-induced pulmonary edema varies from 0.3% to 9%. Possible mechanisms include prolonged exposure to catecholamines causing myocardial dysfunction, increased capillary permeability, large volumes of intravenous fluid administration (often in response to drug-induced maternal tachycardia), and reduced osmotic pressure. Glucocorticoids administered to enhance fetal lung maturity in preterm labor may compound fluid retention.

The clinical presentation is with respiratory distress and clinical features of pulmonary edema, during or immediately following intravenous infusion of the tocolytic drug. Treatment involves discontinuing the drug and supportive measures such as oxygen and diuresis [33,59]. Early recognition and management reduces the need for mechanical ventilation. Failure of the pulmonary edema to resolve in 12–24 hours should prompt a search for an alternative diagnosis [33].

Gestational trophoblastic disease

Pulmonary hypertension and pulmonary edema may rarely occur in the setting of benign hydatidiform mole, as a result of trophoblastic pulmonary embolism. This is an uncommon event, and other pulmonary complications such as fluid overload, ventricular dysfunction, and systemic inflammatory response with associated thyrotoxicosis may produce a similar clinical picture. Pulmonary complications as a result of trophoblastic embolism most commonly occur during evacuation of the uterus, with a higher incidence of pulmonary complications occurring in woman later in pregnancy. Treatment is supportive, and resolution usually occurs within 48–72 hours [60]. Molar pregnancy may also be associated with choriocarcinoma, which can produce multiple, discrete pulmonary metastases.

Management of respiratory failure in pregnancy

Some of the respiratory conditions discussed in this chapter may be complicated by the development of respiratory failure. Intubation and mechanical ventilation in the pregnant patient are covered in detail elsewhere in this book (see Chapters 17 and 18). Endotracheal intubation in the pregnant patient carries significant risks, and the pregnant patient will experience much more rapid oxygen desaturation during apnea than the non-pregnant patient [6]. Intubation should be performed by the most skilled operator available. Marked sedation of the mother, producing apnea, should be avoided in the absence of a skilled intubator. Non-invasive ventilation using an oronasal mask avoids the potential complications of endotracheal intubation and is well suited to the short-term ventilatory support that may be needed in obstetric respiratory complications that reverse rapidly. The major concern with mask ventilation in pregnancy is the risk of aspiration, and, therefore, non-invasive ventilation should be reserved for the patient who is alert, protecting her airway, and where there is an expectation of a relatively brief requirement for ventilatory support. Furthermore, non-invasive ventilation may carry significant risks in the setting of severe acute lung injury during pregnancy, such as in influenza H1N1 pneumonitis [61].

No prospective studies exist to guide the prolonged mechanical ventilation of pregnant patients in the ICU. Several approaches to respiratory support, including conventional mechanical ventilation, airway pressure release ventilation, high-frequency oscillation, and extracorporeal membrane oxygenation, have been used successfully in pregnancy. It is essential that oxygenation be optimized to ensure adequate fetal oxygen delivery. Respiratory alkalosis should be avoided because of its adverse effects on placental circulation. It is unclear whether carbon dioxide targets should mirror the slightly reduced levels found in the spontaneously breathing pregnant patient, or whether permissive hypercapnia is tolerated in pregnancy. Limited clinical reports suggest that mild hypercapnia may be tolerated [62]. Maternal respiratory acidosis may produce fetal acidemia, but these changes do not have the same ominous implications as fetal acidosis occurring through lactic acidosis resulting from fetal hypoxia [63]. However, the right shift of the hemoglobin–oxygen dissociation curve caused by acidosis may negate the beneficial oxygen-carrying characteristics of fetal hemoglobin.

Because of the respiratory physiological changes of late pregnancy, it may be considered that delivery of the pregnant patient with respiratory failure will result in improvement in the mother's condition [64]. However, limited case series addressing this issue have not always found a significant benefit to the mother, and delivery carries a risk of harm [65,66]. Some degree of improvement in oxygenation has been noted, but without improvement in respiratory system compliance or level of positive end-expiratory pressure ventilation needed [64]. Delivery should, therefore, not be performed purely in the hope of improving "maternal condition." However, if the fetus is viable but is at risk because of intractable maternal hypoxia, consultation with a neonatologist may identify a benefit to the fetus in being delivered. Obstetric indications should determine the mode of delivery; while cesarean section allows more rapid delivery in the critically ill patient, the increased physiological stress of operative delivery is associated with higher mortality in these patients.

References

1. Elkus R, Popovich J. Respiratory physiology in pregnancy. *Clin Chest Med* 1992;**13**:555–565.

2. Marx GF, Murthy PK, Orkin LR. Static compliance before and after vaginal delivery. *Br J Anaesth* 1970;**42**:1100–1104.

3. Milne JA, Mills RJ, Coutts JR, *et al*. The effect of human pregnancy on the pulmonary transfer factor for carbon monoxide as measured by the single-breath method. *Clin Sci Mol Med* 1977;**53**:271–276.

4. Rees GB, Pipkin FB, Symonds EM, Patrick JM. A longitudinal study of respiratory changes in normal human pregnancy with cross-sectional data on subjects with pregnancy-induced hypertension. *Am J Obstet Gynecol* 1990;**162**:826–830.

5. Lucius H, Gahlenbeck HO, Kleine O, *et al*. Respiratory functions, buffer system, and electrolyte concentrations of blood during human pregnancy. *Respir Physiol* 1970;**9**:311–317.

6. Archer GW, Marx GF. Arterial oxygen tension during apnoea in parturient women. *Br J Anaesth* 1974;**46**:358–360.

7. Buss DD, Bisgard GE, Rawlings CA, Rankin JHG. Uteroplacental blood flow during alkalosis in the sheep. *Am J Physiol* 1975;**228**:1497–1500.

8. Stenius-Aarniala B, Piirilä P, Teramo K. Asthma and pregnancy: a prospective study of 198 pregnancies. *Thorax* 1988;**43**:12–18.

9. Mabie WC, Barton JR, Wasserstrum N, *et al*. Clinical observations on asthma in pregnancy. *J Matern Fetal Med* 1992;**1**:45–50.

10. Nelson-Piercy C. Asthma in pregnancy. *Thorax* 2001;**56**:325–328.

11. Scottish Intercollegiate Guidelines Network and the British Thoracic Society. *British Guideline on the Management of Asthma*. Edinburgh: Scottish Intercollegiate Guidelines Network, 2011 (http://www.sign.ac.uk/guidelines/fulltext/101/index.html, accessed 7 December 2012).

12. National Asthma Council Australia. *Asthma Management Handbook 2006*. Melbourne: National Asthma Council Australia, 2006 (http://www.nationalasthma.org.au/uploads/handbook/370-amh2006_web_5.pdf, accessed 7 December 2012).

13. NAEPP Working Group. *Report on Managing Asthma During Pregnancy Managing Asthma During Pregnancy: Recommendations for Pharmacologic Treatment*. Bethesda, MD: National Heart, Lung, and Blood Institute, 2004 (http://www.nhlbi.nih.gov/health/prof/lung/asthma/astpreg/astpreg_qr.pdf, accessed 7 December 2012).

14. Law R, Bozzo P, Koren G. FDA pregnancy risk categories and the CPS: do they help or are they a hindrance? *Can Fam Physician* 2010;**56**:239–241.

15. Schatz M. The efficacy and safety of asthma medications during pregnancy. *Semin Perinatol* 2001;**25**:145–152.

16. Schatz M, Zeiger RS, Harden K, *et al*. The safety of asthma and allergy medications during pregnancy. *J Allergy Clin Immunol* 1997;**100**:301–306.

17. Mann RD, Kubota K, Pearce G, Wilton L. Salmeterol: a study by prescription-event monitoring in a UK cohort of 15,407 patients. *J Clin Epidemiol* 1996;**49**:247–250.

18. Wilton LV, Shakir SA. A post-marketing surveillance study of formoterol (Foradil): its use in general practice in England. *Drug Saf* 2002;**25**:213–223.

19. Tata LJ, Lewis SA, McKeever TM, *et al*. Effect of maternal asthma, exacerbations and asthma medication use on congenital malformations in offspring: a UK population-based study. *Thorax* 2008;**63**:981–987.

20. Perrio MJ, Wilton LV, Shakir SA. A modified prescription-event monitoring study to assess the introduction of Seretide Evohaler in England: an example of studying risk monitoring in pharmacovigilance. *Drug Saf* 2007;**30**:681–695.

21. Berkowitz K, LaSala A. Risk factors associated with the increasing prevalence of pneumonia during pregnancy. *Am J Obstet Gynecol* 1990;**163**:981–985.

22. Richey SD, Roberts SW, Ramin KD, *et al*. Pneumonia complicating pregnancy. *Obstet Gynecol* 1994;**84**:525–528.

23. Lim WS, Macfarlane JT, Colthorpe CL. Pneumonia and pregnancy. *Thorax* 2001;**56**:398–405.

24. Dellinger RP, Levy MM, Carlet JM, *et al*. Surviving Sepsis Campaign: international guidelines for management of severe sepsis and septic shock: 2008. *Crit Care Med* 2008;**36**:296–327.

25. McKinney P, Volkert P, Kaufman J. Fatal swine influenza pneumonia occurring during late pregnancy. *Arch Intern Med* 1990;**150**:213–215.

26. Jamieson DJ, Honein MA, Rasmussen SA, *et al*. H1N1.2009 influenza virus infection during pregnancy in the USA. *Lancet* 2009;**374**:451–458.

27. Tanaka T, Nakajima K, Murashima A, *et al*. Safety of neuraminidase inhibitors against novel influenza A (H1N1) in pregnant and breastfeeding women. *CMAJ* 2009;**181**:55–58.

28. Pierce M, Kurinczuk JJ, Spark P, Brocklehurst P, Knight M; UKOSS. Perinatal outcomes after maternal 2009/H1N1 infection: national cohort study. *BMJ* 2011;**342**:d3214.

29. Haake DA, Zakowski PC, Haake DL, Bryson YJ. Early treatment with acyclovir for varicella pneumonia in otherwise healthy adults: retrospective controlled study and review. *Rev Infect Dis* 1990;**12**:788–798.

30. Broussard RC, Payne DK, George RB. Treatment with acyclovir of varicella pneumonia in pregnancy. *Chest* 1991;**99**:1045–1047.

31. Catanzaro A. Pulmonary mycosis in pregnant women. *Chest* 1984;**86**:14S–18S.

32. Blumberg HM, Burman WJ, Chaisson RE, *et al*. American Thoracic Society/Centers for Disease Control and Prevention/Infection Diseases Society of America: treatment of tuberculosis. *Am J Resp Crit Care Med* 2003;**167**:603–662.

33. Bandi VD, Munnur U, Matthay MA. Acute lung injury and acute respiratory distress syndrome in pregnancy. *Crit Care Clin* 2004;**20**:577–607.

34. Perry KG, Martin RW, Blake PG, *et al*. Maternal mortality associated with the adult respiratory distress syndrome. *South Med J* 1998;**91**:441–444.

35. Acute Respiratory Distress Syndrome Network. Ventilation with lower tidal volumes as compared with traditional tidal volumes for acute lung injury and the acute respiratory distress syndrome. *N Engl J Med* 2000;**342**:1301–1308.

36. Cole DE, Taylor TL, McCullough DM, Shoff CT, Derdak S. Acute respiratory distress syndrome in pregnancy. *Crit Care Med* 2005;**33**(Suppl): S269–S278.

37. Rasmussen GE, Malinow AM. Toward reducing maternal mortality: the problem airway in obstetrics. *Int Anesthesiol Clin* 1994;**32**:83–101.

38. Cantwell R, Clutton-Brock T, Cooper G, *et al*. Saving Mothers' Lives: Reviewing Maternal Deaths to make Motherhood Safer 2006–2008. The Eighth Report of the Confidential Enquiries into Maternal Deaths in the United Kingdom. *BJOG* 2011;**118** (Suppl 1):1–203.

39. Weiss BM, Zemp L, Seifert B, Hess OM. Outcome of pulmonary vascular disease in pregnancy: a systematic overview from 1978 through 1996. *J Am Coll Cardiol* 1998;**31**:1650–1657.

40. Bédard E, Dimopoulos K, Gatzoulis MA. Has there been any progress made on pregnancy outcomes among women with pulmonary arterial hypertension? *Eur Heart J* 2009;**30**:256–265.

41. Ray P, Murphy GJ, Shutt LE. Recognition and management of maternal cardiac disease in pregnancy. *Br J Anaesth* 2004;**93**:428–439.

42. Easterling TR, Ralph DD, Schmucker BC. Pulmonary hypertension in pregnancy: treatment with pulmonary vasodilators. *Obstet Gynecol* 1999;**93**:494–498.

43. Higton AM, Whale C, Musk M, Gabbay E. Pulmonary hypertension in pregnancy: two cases and review of the literature. *Intern Med J* 2009;**39**:766–770.

44. Kiely DG, Condliffe R, Webster V, *et al*. Improved survival in pregnancy and pulmonary hypertension using a multiprofessional approach. *BJOG* 2010;**117**:565–574.

45. Boggess KA, Easterling TR, Raghu G. Management and outcome of pregnant women with interstitial and restrictive lung disease. *Am J Obstet Gynecol* 1995;**173**:1007–1014.

46. King TE. Restrictive lung disease in pregnancy. *Clin Chest Med* 1992;**13**:607–622.

47. Bach JR. Successful pregnancies for ventilator users. *Am J Phys Med Rehabil* 2003;**82**:226–229.

48. Kotloff RM, FitzSimmons SC, Fiel SB. Fertility and pregnancy in patients with cystic fibrosis. *Clin Chest Med* 1992;**13**:623–635.

49. Edenborough FP, Mackenzie WE, Stableforth DE. The outcome of 72 pregnancies in 55 women with cystic fibrosis in the United Kingdom 1977–1996. *BJOG* 2000;**107**:254–261.

50. Kent NE, Farquharson DF. Cystic fibrosis in pregnancy. *CMAJ* 1993;**149**:809–813.

51. Lau EM, Barnes DJ, Moriarty C, *et al*. Pregnancy outcomes in the current era of cystic fibrosis care: a 15-year experience. *Aust N Z J Obstet Gynaecol* 2011;**51**:220–224.

52. Gyi KM, Hodson ME, Yacoub MY. Pregnancy in cystic fibrosis lung transplant recipients: case series and review. *J Cyst Fibrosis* 2006;**5**:171–175.

53. Edwards N, Middleton PG, Blyton DM, Sullivan CE. Sleep disordered breathing and pregnancy. *Thorax* 2002;**57**:555–558.

54. Littner MR, Brock BJ. Snoring in pregnancy. Disease or not? *Chest* 1996;**109**:859–860.

55. Gottlieb JD, Ericsson JA, Sweet RB. Venous air embolism. *Anesth Analg* 1965;**44**:773–779.

56. Esplin MS, Varner MW. Progression of pulmonary arteriovenous malformation during pregnancy: case report and review of the literature. *Obstet Gynecol Surv* 1997;**52**:248–253.

57. Sibai BM, Mabie BC, Harvey CJ, *et al*. Pulmonary edema in severe preeclampsia-eclampsia: Analysis of thirty-seven consecutive cases. *Am J Obstet Gynecol* 1987;**156**:1174–1179.

58. Kronborg CS, Gjedsted J, Vittinghus E, *et al*. Longitudinal measurement of cytokines in pre-eclamptic and normotensive pregnancies. *Acta Obstet Gynecol Scand* 2011;**90**:791–796.

59. Pisani RJ, Rosenow EC III. Pulmonary edema associated with tocolytic therapy. *Ann Intern Med* 1989;**110**:714–718.

60. Twiggs LB, Morrow CP, Schlaerth JB. Acute pulmonary complications of molar pregnancy. *Am J Obstet Gynecol* 1979;**135**:189–194.

61. Cabrini L, Silvani P, Landoni G, *et al*. Noninvasive ventilation in H1N1-correlated severe ARDS in a pregnant woman: please, be cautious! *Intensive Care Med* 2010;**36**:1782.

62. Ivankovic AD, Elam JO, Huffman J. Effect of maternal hypercarbia on the newborn infant. *Am J Obstet Gynecol* 1970;**107**:939–946.

63. Low JA, Panagiotopoulos C, Derrick EJ. Newborn complications after intrapartum asphyxia with metabolic acidosis in the term fetus. *Am J Obstet Gynecol* 1994;**170**:1081–1087.

64. Daily WH, Katz AR, Tonnesen A, Allen SJ. Beneficial effect of delivery in a patient with adult respiratory distress syndrome. *Anesthesiology* 1990;**72**:383–386.

65. Tomlinson MW, Caruthers TJ, Whitty JE, Gonik B. Does delivery improve maternal condition in the respiratory-compromised gravida? *Obstet Gynecol* 1998;**91**:108–111.

66. Mabie WC, Barton JR, Sibai BM. Adult respiratory distress syndrome in pregnancy. *Am J Obstet Gynecol* 1992;**167**:950–957.

Chapter 25

Thromboembolism

Andra H. James and Ian A. Greer

Introduction

The thrombotic risk of pregnancy is a consequence of the hypercoagulability resulting from suppressed fibrinolysis and increased levels of procoagulant factors, venous stasis, and, reflecting the likely inevitable trauma to pelvic vessels at delivery, endothelial damage [1]. Therefore, all three factors in Virchow's triad occur in the course of pregnancy and delivery. Unsurprisingly, the risk is greatest immediately postpartum.

The coagulation changes in pregnancy include:

- coagulation factors increased: factors VII, VIII, andX; von Willebrand factor; fibrinogen
- suppressed endogenous anticoagulant activity
- reduced protein S
- acquired activated protein C resistance
- suppressed fibrinolysis
- increased plasminogen activator inhibitor types 1 and 2 (type 2 is produced by the placenta).

The hypercoagulable state of pregnancy has likely evolved to meet the hemostatic challenge of hemorrhage at the time of miscarriage or childbirth. Indeed, in the developing world, the leading cause of maternal death remains obstetric hemorrhage, but in Western Europe and the USA, where hemorrhage is more likely to be successfully prevented or treated, a leading cause of maternal death is thromboembolic disease, with recent reports from the UK suggesting a decline that is temporally associated with the introduction of greater thrombotic risk assessment and prophylaxis guidelines [2].

During pregnancy, the risk of venous thromboembolism is increased four- to five-fold; postpartum, the risk of venous thromboembolism is even higher (20-fold) and does not approach baseline until 6 weeks after delivery [3,4]. Despite the high relative risk, the absolute risk remains low, with the overall incidence of thromboembolic events during pregnancy approximately 2 per 1000 deliveries [4].

Approximately 80% of venous thromboembolic events during pregnancy and the postpartum period present as deep vein thrombosis (DVT), the other 20% as pulmonary emboli [4]; one third of pregnancy-related DVT and half of pregnancy-related pulmonary emboli occurring after delivery [5]. In contrast to DVT outside of pregnancy, the majority of DVT during pregnancy are proximal, massive, and in the left lower extremity [1,5]. This left-sided predominance, accounting for 80% of all pregnancy-related lower extremity DVT, may reflect a relative stenosis of the left common iliac vein where it lies between the lumbar vertebral body and the right common iliac artery. Pelvic vein thrombosis, which is rare outside of pregnancy or pelvic surgery, accounts for approximately 10% of DVT during pregnancy and the postpartum period.

Risk factors for thrombosis in pregnancy

Risk factors for thrombosis are largely those that enhance each of the components of Virchow's triad. However, since the risk of thrombosis is as high during the first trimester of pregnancy as during the remainder of gestation [6], while venous flow reaches its lowest point in the third trimester, this suggests that, overall, the most important reason for the increased risk during pregnancy is hypercoagulability induced by the hormonal changes of pregnancy.

The most important risk factor for thrombosis in pregnancy is a history of thrombosis. Recurrent events

Maternal Critical Care: A Multidisciplinary Approach, ed. Marc Van de Velde, Helen Scholefield, and Lauren A. Plante. Published by Cambridge University Press. © Cambridge University Press 2013.

Table 25.1. Risk of venous thromboembolism conferred by type of thrombophilia

Thrombophilia	Odds ratio (95% confidence interval)
Factor V Leiden, homozygosity	34.40 (9.86–120.05)
Factor V Leiden, heterozygosity	8.32 (5.44–12.70)
Prothrombin gene mutation, homozygosity	26.36 (1.24–59.29)
Prothrombin gene mutation, heterozygosity	6.80 (2.46–18.77)
Protein C deficiency	4.76 (2.15–10.57)
Protein S deficiency	2.19 (1.48–6.00)
Antithrombin deficiency	4.76 (2.15–10.57)
Methylenetetrahydrofolate reductase C677T homozygosity	0.74 (0.22–2.48)

Source: adapted from Robertson *et al.*, 2006 [13].

Table 25.2. Medical conditions and complications of pregnancy and delivery associated with an increased risk of venous thromboembolism in pregnancy

Risk factor	Odds ratio (95% confidence interval)
Medical conditions	
Heart disease	7.1 (6.2–8.3)
Sickle cell disease	6.7 (4.4–10.1)
Lupus	8.7 (5.8–13.0)
Obesity	4.4 (3.4–5.7)
Anemia	2.6 (2.2–2.9)
Diabetes	2.0 (1.4–2.7)
Hypertension	1.8 (1.4–2.3)
Smoking	1.7 (1.4–2.1)
Complications of pregnancy and delivery	
Multiple gestation	1.6 (1.2–2.1)
Hyperemesis	2.5 (2.0–3.2)
Fluid and electrolyte imbalance	4.9 (4.1–5.9)
Antepartum hemorrhage	2.3 (1.8–2.8)
Cesarean delivery	2.1 (1.8–2.4)
Postpartum infection	4.1 (2.9–5.7)
Postpartum hemorrhage	1.3 (1.1–1.6)
Transfusion	7.6 (6.2–9.4)

Source: adapted from Pabinger *et al.*, 2002 [7].

account for 15–25% of all thromboembolic events in pregnancy. Among pregnant women with a history of venous thromboembolism (VTE), the risk of recurrent VTE is increased three- to four-fold (relative risk, 3.5; 95% confidence interval (CI), 1.6–7.8) [7]. In current practice, many of these women now receive prophylactic antithrombotic therapy. However, the rate of recurrent VTE in women who did not receive prophylactic anticoagulation has been reported to range from 2.4% to 12.2% [8–10], whereas in those who did receive anticoagulation, it is reported as 0.0–5.5% [8,11,12]. Thrombophilia is also an important risk factor [13] and is a positive finding in 20–50% of women who experience VTE during pregnancy and the postpartum period (Table 25.1). Risk factors are summarized in Table 25.2 [4].

Treatment of patients with thrombotic problems in pregnancy

Because coumarins, the preferred agents for long-term anticoagulation outside of pregnancy, have harmful maternal and fetal effects in terms of bleeding, warfarin embryopathy, and adverse neurodevelopmental issues, the preferred agents for anticoagulation in pregnancy are heparins [1,14]. Neither unfractionated heparin (UFH) nor low-molecular-weight heparin (LMWH) crosses the placenta, and both are considered safe in pregnancy [1,14]. The main issues with UFH are heparin-induced osteoporosis, allergy and heparin-induced thrombocytopenia for the mother. In women treated exclusively with LMWH, heparin-induced thrombocytopenia is not a significant issue; platelet count monitoring is not considered necessary in these women [14]. Heparin-induced osteoporosis has been reported, but is much less common than with UFH and may be associated with comorbid conditions or other treatments when it does occur in women on LMWH [11]. Unique aspects of anticoagulation in pregnancy include an increase in maternal blood volume of 40–50% and an increase in the volume of distribution. An increase in glomerular filtration results in increased renal excretion of heparin compounds, which are eliminated by this route. Additionally, there is an increase in protein binding of heparin. During pregnancy, both UFH and LMWH have shorter half-lives and lower peak plasma concentrations, hence a rationale for higher doses and more frequent administration.

Diagnosis of acute venous thromboembolism in pregnancy

There are no large clinical trials to support the management of suspected VTE in pregnancy; therefore, guidelines are based on extrapolation from studies performed in the non-pregnant state and from expert opinion and consensus. Clinical diagnosis of VTE is unreliable and is particularly unreliable during pregnancy because the key symptoms and signs of VTE (leg swelling, chest pain, and dyspnea) are commonly encountered, with a further reduction in reliability of clinical diagnosis. Objective diagnosis is, therefore, critical in women with suspected VTE. If objective testing is unavailable, then the woman with suspected VTE should be commenced on anticoagulant therapy until imaging studies are available, unless there are contraindications to anticoagulant therapy. Diagnosis of thromboembolism in pregnancy is similar to that in individuals who are not pregnant. Fear of fetal radiation exposure should not deprive women of a timely and proper diagnostic evaluation.

In pregnancy, compression Duplex ultrasound of the entire proximal venous system is the first-line diagnostic test for DVT [15]. As the most gestational DVTs are ileofemoral, and the ileofemoral veins are usually easily visualized, the diagnosis of proximal DVT is confirmed. Anticoagulant treatment should then be commenced or continued. However, an initial negative ultrasound examination does not completely exclude a distal (calf) DVT. Therefore, with a high level of clinical suspicion and a negative ultrasound examination, the patient should remain on anticoagulation and the ultrasound repeated 1 week later (or an alternative diagnostic test employed). If repeated testing is negative, it is appropriate to discontinue treatment. When pelvic vein thrombosis in the iliac veins is suspected, often because of symptoms of back pain and swelling of the entire limb, pulsed Doppler, MR venography, or, if required, conventional contrast venography should be considered.

With suspected pulmonary thromboembolism (PE) in a hemodynamically stable pregnant patient, chest radiography should be performed, as this may diagnose other pulmonary disease such as pneumonia or pneumothorax. Often (in >50% of cases), the chest radiograph is normal even with objectively proven PE, but abnormal chest radiography findings associated with PE include atelectasis, effusion, focal opacities, and regional oligemia. The radiation dose to the fetus from chest radiography performed at any stage of pregnancy is negligible and there is no reason to withhold this test in pregnancy on fetal concerns. If the radiograph is abnormal with a high clinical suspicion of PE, CT pulmonary angiography (CTPA) should be performed because isotope ventilation–perfusion (V/Q) scanning is unreliable. However, if leg symptoms are also present, then Doppler ultrasound of the legs is useful as a diagnosis of DVT indirectly confirms PE as the etiology of chest symptoms, and the anticoagulant management is the same for both DVT and PE. Thus further pulmonary imaging can be avoided.

In the UK, the British Thoracic Society recommends CTPA as first-line investigation for non-massive PE in non-pregnant patients (often the non-pregnant patient will have comorbid chest pathology, limiting the value of V/Q scans, but this is not the case in most young pregnant women). There are also several advantages of CTPA over V/Q scans: better sensitivity and specificity and the ability to identify other possible diagnoses such as aortic dissection. There is disagreement as to whether CPTA delivers a lower fetal radiation dose than a V/Q scan, but measured doses are low for both modalities. Measured fetal radiation doses for V/Q scans versus CPTA were recently and systematically reviewed by the American Thoracic Society and Society of Thoracic Radiology for a clinical practice guideline on the evaluation of suspected pulmonary embolism in pregnancy. The fetal radiation dose was 0.32–0.74 mGy for a V/Q scan and 0.03–0.66 mGy for CPTA. The wide range of values reflects heterogeneity in protocols and equipment, as well as the size and gestational age of the fetus at the time of the exposure[15], but it does not account for the increasing radiation exposure from current equipment. Disadvantages of CTPA include a high radiation dose to the maternal breasts (overall maternal radiation dose is 4–18 mSv with CPTA compared with 1–2.5 mSv with a V/Q scan), which is associated with an increased lifetime risk of developing breast cancer (note that only around 1 in 20 of such investigations will have a positive result in pregnancy). Despite these potential advantages of CTPA, many authorities in the UK still recommend V/Q scanning, where available, as a first-line investigation in pregnancy because of the high negative predictive value, its substantially lower radiation dose to pregnant breast tissue, and because most pregnant women will not have comorbid pulmonary pathology [16]. The American Thoracic Society, Society of Thoracic

Radiology, and American College of Obstetricians and Gynecologists also recommend V/Q scanning as the first-line investigation [15]. The choice of technique for definitive diagnosis (V/Q scan or CTPA) will, therefore, be influenced by local availability and guidelines. Note that with a V/Q scan in pregnancy, the perfusion component may be all that is required if the chest radiograph is normal.

In non-pregnant patients, plasma D-dimer levels are useful in assessing the likelihood of VTE. However, D-dimer levels increase physiologically throughout gestation and fall outside the "normal" range in most normal pregnancies. Levels also increase with conditions such as pre-eclampsia and placental abruption. Therefore a "positive" D-dimer test in pregnancy is not necessarily consistent with VTE. The European Society of Cardiology [17] recommends that D-dimer levels should be measured even though the probability of a negative result is lower than in other patients with suspected VTE, in order to avoid unnecessary exposure of the fetus to radiation. However, false negative D-dimer results have been reported in cases of VTE in pregnancy. The American Thoracic Society, Society of Thoracic Radiology, and American College of Obstetricians and Gynecologists recommend that D-dimer levels should *not* be used to exclude PTE in pregnancy [15].

Maternal and fetal radiation issues

The risk of fatal cancer to the age of 15 years after in utero exposure to CTPA is 1 in 1 000 000 and with V/Q scan is 1 in 280 000 [12].

Use of CTPA is associated with relatively high radiation dose (20 mGy) to the mother's chest and breasts; 10 mGy of radiation to a woman's breast is estimated to increase her lifetime risk of developing breast cancer by around 14%.

Management of venous thromboembolism in pregnancy

Prior to commencing anticoagulation, it is usual to perform a full blood count, coagulation screen, urea, electrolytes, and liver function tests (the last to exclude renal or hepatic dysfunction, which are cautions for anticoagulant therapy). It is not useful to perform a thrombophilia screen as this will not alter the immediate management. Further, results of protein S tests are unreliable in pregnancy as around 40% of pregnant women develop acquired activated protein C resistance,

and levels of antithrombin may be low in the presence of thrombosis.

In both Europe and North America, LMWH has largely replaced UFH for the immediate management of VTE in pregnancy. As noted above, since there are no sufficiently powered trials within pregnancy, evidence is extrapolated from the non-pregnant situation and supported by observational studies in pregnancy. Outside of pregnancy, LMWH is more effective, with lower mortality and a lower risk of hemorrhagic complications than UFH in the initial treatment of DVT. There is also similar efficacy in the initial treatment of PE. These findings are confirmed in a large systematic review of LMWH in pregnancy [11]; further, compared with UFH, LMWH is associated with a substantially lower risk of heparin-induced thrombocytopenia, hemorrhage, and heparin-induced osteoporosis.

In non-pregnant patients, LMWH is usually administered in a once-daily dose, but because of alterations in the pharmacokinetics of LMWH during pregnancy, a twice-daily dosage regimen has often been recommended for treatment of VTE in pregnancy (e.g. enoxaparin 1 mg/kg twice daily; dalteparin 100 U/kg twice daily) [14,16–19]. There are no data using ideal body weight; actual body weights are used for calculations. The rationale for twice-daily dosing is based on the pharmacokinetics of these agents in pregnancy [20–23]. In actual clinical practice, a retrospective study of once-daily versus twice-daily dosing of LMWH for VTE in pregnancy found no recurrent VTE in 125 women, 83 (66%) of whom received once-daily LMWH [24]. Another study comparing once-daily versus twice-daily tinzaparin for the treatment of VTE in pregnancy did find that a higher than recommended dosage was required in women who took tinzaparin only once a day [21]. Another retrospective study of the once-daily tinzaparin regimen found two unusual thrombotic complications among 37 pregnancies [25]. However, there is increasing experience to suggest once-daily dosing may be satisfactory [26]. In the initial management of DVT, leg elevation and application of a graduated elastic compression stocking to reduce pain and swelling are useful, and the patient can be encouraged to mobilize (early mobilization and use of a graduated elastic compression stocking do not increase the risk of PE). Once a woman is able to self-administer LMWH by subcutaneous injection, outpatient management until delivery is appropriate. Continued use of graduated elastic compression stockings may reduce the likelihood of post-thrombotic syndrome. In the rare event that major occlusive DVT risks leg viability, surgical embolectomy or thrombolysis should be considered.

Satisfactory anti-factor Xa levels (peak anti-factor Xa activity, 3–4 hours after injection, of 500–1200 U/L) are usually achieved using a weight-based dose. In addition, there are concerns over the accuracy and consistency of anti-factor Xa monitoring, thus monitoring of anti-factor Xa is not routinely advocated. The need for monitoring is, perhaps, more appropriate at extremes of body weight (50 kg and ≥90 kg), with suspected non-compliance, or with comorbid conditions such as renal disease and recurrent VTE. Recently published guidelines from the American College of Chest Physicians acknowledge that, on the basis of small studies that demonstrated a need to escalate doses to maintain a therapeutic concentration of anti-factor Xa, some authorities do recommend measuring anti-factor Xa every 1–3 months to maintain concentrations in the therapeutic range; however, the authors of the guidelines concluded that with the current lack of data about the benefits of monitoring anti-factor Xa, the costs were difficult to justify [14].

The activated partial thromboplastin time (aPTT) is used to monitor UFH. When UFH is used, or if the woman is receiving LMWH after first receiving UFH or with previous exposure to UFH, the platelet count should ideally be monitored every 2–3 days from day 4 to day 14, or until heparin is stopped.

LMWH (or UFH) is recommended for the remainder of the pregnancy, with treatment continued for a minimum of 3 months and until 6 weeks after delivery. Outside pregnancy, the initial dose of LMWH may be reduced to an intermediate dose after several weeks of therapeutic anticoagulation. In pregnancy data are limited, but reducing to an intermediate dose after several months (or earlier in pregnant women at increased risk of bleeding or osteoporosis) can be considered.

To avoid delivery while a woman is taking therapeutic anticoagulation, a planned delivery, either through induction of labor or elective cesarean section, facilitates anticoagulant management. A pragmatic approach is to reduce LMWH to a once-daily thromboprophylactic dose on the day before induction of labor or cesarean section such that when delivery occurs in 24 hours or more from the previous LMWH injection, its effect on hemostasis will be absent or minimal. In North America, it is more common than in Europe to convert women who are being treated with LMWH to intravenous or subcutaneous UFH when delivery is imminent or anticipated. Disadvantages of UFH include difficulties in control, as the aPTT is unreliable, particularly in pregnancy, and the patient also incurs the risk of problems such as heparin-induced thrombocytopenia, which would be avoided by exclusive use of LMWH. When women present in labor while on therapeutic LMWH, the main issue is regional anesthesia techniques, as these should not normally be employed for at least 24 hours after the last dose of LMWH. In addition, LMWH should be avoided for at least 4 hours after epidural catheter removal. The catheter should not be removed within 12 hours of the most recent injection. When delivery is by scheduled cesarean section, *therapeutic doses of LMWH should be omitted for 24 hours prior to surgery.* However, a *thromboprophylactic* dose of LMWH (e.g. enoxaparin 40 mg, dalteparin 5000 IU, tinzaparin 75 IU/kg) can be given as early as 3 hours postoperatively (>4 hours after removal of the epidural catheter, if appropriate), and the treatment dose recommended later that day.

Both UFH and LMWH increase the risk of wound hematoma following cesarean section, with an incidence around 2%. Surgical drains should, therefore, be considered at operation. Closure of the skin incision should ideally be with staples or interrupted sutures to allow easy drainage of any hematoma that might develop.

A particular problem that obstetricians may face is thrombosis presenting close to delivery. In this event, UFH should be considered (since it can be reversed using protamine sulfate and has a short duration of action) or the timing of LMWH administration adjusted. When labor occurs in a woman on therapeutic UFH, the aPTT is used to assess the anticoagulant effect. In general, subcutaneous UFH should be discontinued 12 hours before, and intravenous UFH 6 hours before, induction of labor/regional anesthesia. It should be noted that the aPTT is less reliable in pregnancy because of the increased levels of factor VIII and heparin-binding proteins, which, in turn, may lead to an apparent heparin resistance.

Although both heparin and warfarin are satisfactory for use postpartum, including in women who are breastfeeding, many women prefer to use LMWH (with once-daily dosing postpartum) because they have become accustomed to its administration and because they can avoid the monitoring associated with coumarin therapy.

Massive or life-threatening pulmonary embolism

Massive or life-threatening PE is indicated if

- systolic blood pressure is 90 mmHg, *or*
- there is a fall in systolic blood pressure of >40 mmHg from baseline, not otherwise explained by hypovolemia, sepsis, or new arrhythmia, *or*
- there is evidence of cardiogenic shock, manifested by tissue hyperperfusion (altered level of consciousness; oliguria; or cool, clammy extremities) and hypoxia.

With massive life-threatening PE, the pregnant woman needs emergency assessment by a multidisciplinary team of obstetricians, surgeons, and radiologists, who should decide rapidly on appropriate treatment ranging from intravenous UFH to systemic thrombolysis, catheter thrombolysis or embolectomy, or surgical embolectomy. In contrast to thrombolytic therapy, anticoagulant therapy will not reduce the obstruction of the pulmonary circulation. When used in pregnancy, thrombolytic therapy is associated with a maternal hemorrrhagic complication (including genital tract bleeding) rate of approximately 6%, similar to non-pregnant patients [27,28]. The great danger in pregnancy is that appropriate treatment will be delayed out of fear of genital tract bleeding or of the fetal consequences of intervention, but hemodynamically unstable PE, defined as PE with arterial hypotension or cardiogenic shock at presentation, is otherwise associated with a poor short-term prognosis [29] and pregnant patients are no exception.

As soon as massive PE is suspected, therapeutic intravenous UFH should be initiated. In massive PE, most patients should receive a bolus of at least 80 U/kg UFH followed by a minimum of 18 U/kg per hour to maintain a target aPTT of at least 80 seconds [30]. The rationale for aggressive dosing of UFH is the empirical observation that patients with massive PE require more than standard doses of UFH and that subtherapeutic doses can be fatal [30]. If signs and symptoms of massive PE persist despite intravenous UFH, and there is no contraindication to fibrinolysis, new evidence-based guidelines from the American Heart Association for the management of massive PE recommend proceeding to thrombolysis with the recombinant tissue plasminogen activator altepase 100 mg intravenous over 2 hours [31]. Patients who remain unstable despite thrombolysis may be candidates for catheter thrombolysis or embolectomy, or for surgical embolectomy. These procedures should be performed in institutions experienced in them and, consequently, patients may need to be transferred [31]. Embolectomy requires cardiopulmonary bypass and experienced thoracic surgeons.

Data specific to the management of massive PE in pregnant women are limited. A recent review reported on 13 women who were managed with thrombolysis [32] and five other women have been reported subsequently. In these five women, all of the patients carried their pregnancies to term without bleeding complications. In the review of the 13 women, the rate of complications was higher than among other series of patients receiving thrombolysis, perhaps reflecting the severe morbidity of the patients at the time of therapy. The rate of major bleeding was 30.8% (95% CI, 9.1–61.4]), of fetal death 15.4% (95% CI, 1.9–45.5), and of preterm delivery 38.5% (95% CI, 13.9–68.4). There were no maternal deaths [32]. The same authors reported on eight women who had surgical embolectomy. There were three fetal deaths (37.5%; 95% CI, 8.5–75.5) and four preterm deliveries (50%; 95% CI, 15.7–84.3). There were no maternal deaths. The same authors also reported on four women who received catheter thrombolysis or embolectomy. One fetal death (25%; 95% CI, 0.63–80.6) and one preterm delivery (25%; 95% CI, 0.63–80.6) occurred.

In unstable situations where reversal of anticoagulation may be required, such as when surgery or other invasive procedure is required, intravenous UFH may be employed. Vena caval filters can be used, but these are rarely required and are generally considered only when there is recurrent VTE despite adequate anticoagulation [16] or new-onset VTE within the previous 2–4 weeks. Filters can be associated with tears in the vena cava and serious hemorrhage; filter fracture and movement can also occur. If the filter is not removed, the woman will require lifelong anticoagulation with coumarins.

In the exceptionally rare, but possible, scenario where the patient with recent PE and persistent right heart strain requires emergency surgery with general anesthesia, the highest risk period for hemodynamic collapse is during induction of anesthesia and initiation of positive pressure ventilation. Monitoring should be performed with transesophageal echocardiography. The need for cardiopulmonary bypass and surgical embolectomy must be anticipated. The patient should be in the appropriate operating room suite and the cardiac surgical team should be immediately available [33].

Thromboprophylaxis

Women with significant risk factors should be considered for prophylactic low-dose LMWH (e.g. enoxaparin 40 mg/day or dalteparin 5000 IU/day). For the pregnant woman with previous VTE, postpartum prophylaxis for 6 weeks is usually advocated. Where the risk of antenatal recurrence is considered higher because of a previous unprovoked VTE, or a previous pregnancy- or estrogen-associated event or more than one previous VTE (where she is not receiving long-term anticoagulation), prophylactic low-dose or intermediate-dose LMWH is usually employed antenatally starting from the diagnosis of pregnancy. For those women with a single previous VTE associated with a transient risk factor unrelated to pregnancy or use of estrogen, it is not routine to use prophylaxis antenatally: experts recommend only postpartum prophylaxis. Where a woman has multiple other risk factors, prophylaxis should also be considered both antenatally and postpartum, particularly after cesarean section. When a woman is on long-term coumarin therapy, it is usual to switch to LMWH (adjusted or intermediate dose) prior to 6 weeks of gestation (to avoid the risk of embryopathy) with resumption of long-term anticoagulants postpartum [14,28].

Pregnant and postpartum patients in the ICU who have not experienced a thromboembolic event remain at high risk of experiencing one. In addition to their hypercoagulable state, they are frequently postoperative from cesarean delivery or hysterectomy and have one or more of the medical conditions or complications of pregnancy and delivery listed in Table 25.2, all compounding the risk of thrombosis. Thromboprophylaxis based on usual ICU protocols is essential.

Conclusions

Women are at an increased risk of VTE during pregnancy. Additional risk factors include a history of thrombosis, thrombophilia, certain medical conditions, and some complications of pregnancy and childbirth. Despite the increased risk of thrombosis during pregnancy and in the postpartum period, most women do not require anticoagulation. Exceptions are women at high risk of thrombosis. Unique aspects of anticoagulation in pregnancy include both maternal and fetal issues. For fetal reasons, the preferred agents for anticoagulation in pregnancy are heparin compounds. In anticipation of delivery, surgery, or other invasive procedures, anticoagulation should be manipulated to reduce the risk of bleeding complications while minimizing the risk of thrombosis.

References

1. Greer IA. Thrombosis in pregnancy: maternal and fetal issues. *Lancet* 1999;**353**:1258–1256.
2. Cantwell R, Clutton-Brock T, Cooper G, *et al.* Saving Mothers' Lives: Reviewing Maternal Deaths to make Motherhood Safer 2006–2008. The Eighth Report of the Confidential Enquiries into Maternal Deaths in the United Kingdom. *BJOG* 2011;**118**(Suppl 1):1–203.
3. Heit JA, Kobbervig CE, James AH, *et al.* Trends in the incidence of venous thromboembolism during pregnancy or postpartum: a 30-year population-based study. *Ann Intern Med* 2005;**143**:697–706.
4. James AH, Jamison MG, Brancazio LR, Myers ER. Venous thromboembolism during pregnancy and the postpartum period: incidence, risk factors, and mortality. *Am J Obstet Gynecol* 2006;**194**:1311–1315.
5. Ray JG, Chan WS. Deep vein thrombosis during pregnancy and the puerperium: a meta-analysis of the period of risk and the leg of presentation. *Obstet Gynecol Surv* 1999;**54**:265–271.
6. Jacobsen AF, Skjeldestad FE, Sandset PM. Incidence and risk patterns of venous thromboembolism in pregnancy and puerperium: a register-based case–control study. *Am J Obstet Gynecol* 2008; **198**:233 e1–e7.
7. Pabinger I, Grafenhofer H, Kyrle PA, *et al.* Temporary increase in the risk for recurrence during pregnancy in women with a history of venous thromboembolism. *Blood* 2002; **100**: 1060–1062.
8. Brill-Edwards P, Ginsberg JS, Gent M, *et al.* Safety of withholding heparin in pregnant women with a history of venous thromboembolism. Recurrence of clot in this pregnancy study group. *N Engl J Med* 2000; **343**: 1439–1444.
9. Pabinger I, Grafenhofer H, Kaider A, *et al.* Risk of pregnancy-associated recurrent venous thromboembolism in women with a history of venous thrombosis. *J Thromb Haemost* 2005; **3**: 949–954.
10. De Stefano V, Simioni P, Rossi E, *et al.* The risk of recurrent venous thromboembolism in patients with inherited deficiency of natural anticoagulants antithrombin, protein C and protein S. *Haematologica* 2006; **91**: 695–698.
11. Greer IA, Nelson-Piercy C. Low-molecular-weight heparins for thromboprophylaxis and treatment of venous thromboembolism in pregnancy: a systematic review of safety and efficacy. *Blood* 2005; **106**: 401–407.

12. Roeters van Lennep JE, Meijer E, *et al.* Prophylaxis with low-dose low-molecular-weight heparin during pregnancy and postpartum: is it effective? *J Thromb Haemost* 2011. **9**: 473–480.

13. Robertson L, Wu O, Langhorne P, *et al.* Thrombophilia in pregnancy: a systematic review. *Br J Haematol* 2006;**132**:171–196.

14. Bates SM, Greer IA, Middeldorp S, *et al.* VTE, thrombophilia, antithrombotic therapy, and pregnancy: Antithrombotic Therapy and Prevention of Thrombosis, 9th edn: American College of Chest Physicians Evidence-Based Clinical Practice Guidelines. *Chest* 2012;**141**(Suppl):e691S–736S.

15. Leung AN, Bull TM, Jaeschke R, *et al.* An official American Thoracic Society/Society of Thoracic Radiology clinical practice guideline: evaluation of suspected pulmonary embolism in pregnancy. *Am J Resp Crit Care Med* 2011;**184**:1200–1208.

16. Thompson AJ, Greer I. *Thromboembolic Disease in Pregnancy and the Puerperium: Acute Management (Green-top Guideline 28)*. London: Royal College of Obstetricians and Gynaecologists, 2007.

17. Torbicki A, Perrier A, Konstantinides S, *et al.* Guidelines on the diagnosis and management of acute pulmonary embolism: the Task Force for the Diagnosis and Management of Acute Pulmonary Embolism of the European Society of Cardiology (ESC). *Eur Heart J* 2008;**29**:2276–2315.

18. James A. Practice Bulletin No. 123: thromboembolism in pregnancy. *Obstet Gynecol* 2011;**118**:718–729.

19. Casele HL, Laifer SA, Woelkers DA, Venkataramanan R. Changes in the pharmacokinetics of the low-molecular-weight heparin enoxaparin sodium during pregnancy. *Am J Obstet Gynecol* 1999;**181**:1113–1117.

20. Barbour LA, Oja JL, Schultz LK. A prospective trial that demonstrates that dalteparin requirements increase in pregnancy to maintain therapeutic levels of anticoagulation. *Am J Obstet Gynecol* 2004;**191**:1024–1029.

21. Lykke JA, Gronlykke T, Langhoff-Roos J. Treatment of deep venous thrombosis in pregnant women. *Acta Obstet Gynecol Scand* 2008;**87**:1248–1251.

22. Norris LA, Bonnar J, Smith MP, Steer PJ, Savidge G. Low molecular weight heparin (tinzaparin) therapy for moderate risk thromboprophylaxis during pregnancy. A pharmacokinetic study. *Thromb Haemost* 2004;**92**:791–796.

23. Lebaudy C, Hulot JS, Amoura Z, *et al.* Changes in enoxaparin pharmacokinetics during pregnancy and implications for antithrombotic therapeutic strategy. *Clin Pharmacol Ther* 2008;**84**:370–377.

24. Voke J, Keidan J, Pavord S, Spencer NH, Hunt BJ. The management of antenatal venous thromboembolism in the UK and Ireland: a prospective multicentre observational survey. *Br J Haematol* 2007;**139**:545–558.

25. Ni Ainle F, Wong A, Appleby N, *et al.* Efficacy and safety of once daily low molecular weight heparin (tinzaparin sodium) in high risk pregnancy. *Blood Coagul Fibrinolysis* 2008;**19**:689–692.

26. Nelson-Piercy C, Powrie R, Borg JY, *et al.* Tinzaparin use in pregnancy: an international, retrospective study of the safety and efficacy profile. *Eur J Obstet Gynecol Reprod Biol* 2011;**159**:293–299.

27. Ahearn GS, Hadjiliadis D, Govert JA, Tapson VF. Massive pulmonary embolism during pregnancy successfully treated with recombinant tissue plasminogen activator: a case report and review of treatment options. *Arch Intern Med* 2002;**162**:1221–1227.

28. Leonhardt G, Gaul C, Nietsch HH, Buerke M, Schleussner E. Thrombolytic therapy in pregnancy. *J Thromb Thrombolysis* 2006;**21**:271–276.

29. Imberti D, Ageno W, Manfredini R, *et al.* Interventional treatment of venous thromboembolism: A review. *Thromb Res* 2012;**129**:418–425.

30. Kucher N, Goldhaber SZ. Management of massive pulmonary embolism. *Circulation* 2005;**112**:e28–e32.

31. Jaff MR, McMurtry MS, Archer SL, *et al.* Management of massive and submassive pulmonary embolism, iliofemoral deep vein thrombosis, and chronic thromboembolic pulmonary hypertension: a scientific statement from the American Heart Association. *Circulation* 2011;**123**:1788–1830.

32. te Raa GD, Ribbert LS, Snijder RJ, Biesma DH. Treatment options in massive pulmonary embolism during pregnancy; a case-report and review of literature. *Thromb Res* 2009;**124**:1–5.

33. Rosenberger P, Shernan SK, Shekar PS, *et al.* Acute hemodynamic collapse after induction of general anesthesia for emergent pulmonary embolectomy. *Anesth Analg* 2006;**102**:1311–1315.

Chapter 26

Neurological disease and neurological catastrophes

Cynthia A. Wong and Roland Devlieger

Introduction

Pregnant women may have chronic neurological disease or may develop neurological disease during pregnancy and the postpartum period. Some neurological conditions are more likely to occur or be exacerbated during pregnancy, including posterior spinal encephalopathy syndrome (PRES), cortical vein thrombosis, and hemorrhagic or thrombotic stroke. Other neurological conditions may occur during pregnancy by chance, for example Guillain-Barré syndrome. Obstetric disease such as eclampsia may present with neurological symptoms. Finally, rare complications of neuraxial procedures administered during childbirth, including spinal/epidural hematoma or abscess, meningitis, or subdural hematoma, may occur in the postpartum period. The initial signs and symptoms of these life-threatening neurological conditions may overlap with more common and benign pregnancy-associated conditions. Therefore, both obstetricians and anesthesiologists/intensivists caring for obstetric patients must be well versed in the neurological diseases and complications associated with, or exacerbated by, pregnancy and anesthesia.

Epilepsy

Epidemiology

Approximately 3 to 5 births per 1000 occur to women with epilepsy [1]. The International Registry of Antiepileptic Drugs and Pregnancy (EURAP registry) summarized data from 1956 pregnancies between 1999 and 2004 [2]; 1095 (58%) women remained seizure free throughout pregnancy. Seizures occurred during delivery in 3.5% of women and status epilepticus occurred in 1.8%.

In 2009, the American Academy of Neurology and the American Epilepsy Society published Practice Parameters Updates for the management of pregnant women with epilepsy. The review concluded that there is insufficient evidence to determine whether there is a consistent change in seizure frequency during pregnancy in women with epilepsy [1]. Switching seizure medications during pregnancy is not recommended, as this increases the likelihood of seizures. Approximately 90% of women who have been seizure-free at least 9 months prior to conception are likely to remain seizure-free during pregnancy. Changes in blood volume, hepatic metabolism, and protein binding during pregnancy generally result in decreased serum anticonvulsant concentrations; inadequate drug levels may explain recurrent seizures.

Diagnosis, clinical features, and investigations

New-onset seizures during pregnancy may represent epilepsy, but other acute etiologies of seizure must be excluded and the underlying disease process treated appropriately (Box 26.1). Eclamptic seizures are the most common cause of seizures during pregnancy and may present without hypertension, proteinuria, and edema. A careful history, including information from witnesses and family members, and physical examination are essential. The setting, onset, duration, and characteristics of the seizure should be elicited, including the presence of an aura, loss of consciousness, incontinence, and whether the seizure was associated with a secondary injury. Knowledge of inciting factors, such as prior history of chronic disease, acute illness, drug non-compliance, and history of recent trauma are critical to making the correct diagnosis. A thorough physical examination includes vital signs, a complete neurological examination, and a search for associated trauma. Laboratory screening should include serum

Box 26.1. Differential diagnosis of new-onset seizures during pregnancy

- Eclampsia
- Posterior reversible encephalopathy syndrome
- Cerebral vein thrombosis
- Intracranial hemorrhage
- Subarachnoid hemorrhage
- Ischemic stroke
- Brain tumor
- Metabolic causes
    - hyperemesis gravidarum
    - acute hepatitis (fatty liver of pregnancy)
    - acute intermittent porphyria
    - electrolyte imbalances
- Infections
- Toxins
    - drug withdrawal
    - drug overdose
- Epilepsy: gestational epilepsy
- Pseudoseizures

glucose, electrolyte levels, and liver function tests. A toxicology screen may be indicated, and serum levels of antiepileptic drugs should be measured in patients taking these medications. Hypoglycemia is the most common cause of metabolic seizures.

A lumbar puncture is indicated if meningitis is suspected, although seizure activity causes hyperthermia, leukocytosis, and cerebrospinal fluid (CSF) pleocytosis, thus confusing the diagnosis. Neuroimaging (usually CT) may be considered for a suspected acute intracranial event, particularly intracranial hemorrhage. Magnetic resonance imaging without gadolinium may be preferable to exclude other intracranial pathology.

Management

Treatment of seizure during pregnancy mimics standard seizure treatment in adults. Although drugs used to treat seizures cross the placenta, this is of secondary importance when treating pregnant patients. It is more important to both the mother and fetus to prevent the direct adverse physiological effects of seizure, including hypoxemia, acidosis, and hyperthermia. Modifications of standard treatment during pregnancy include positioning the patient in the left lateral decubitus position after the 20th week of gestation to prevent aortocaval compression, and fetal heart rate monitoring after the age of viability. Additionally, pregnant women are at increased risk of gastroesophageal reflux; therefore, prompt control of the airway to prevent pulmonary aspiration of gastric contents is indicated in unconscious patients. In case of (suspicion) of eclamptic seizure, magnesium sulfate should be initiated promptly.

Status epilepticus

The definition of status epilepticus is evolving, but many experts define status epilepticus as continuous seizure activity for 5 minutes or more. Several population-based studies estimate the risk of status epilepticus during pregnancy as being between 0 and 1.3% [1]. The American Academy of Neurology and the American Epilepsy Society have concluded that there is insufficient evidence to support or refute an increased risk of status epilepticus during pregnancy [1].

Historically, status epilepticus has been associated with a high risk of maternal morbidity and mortality, as well as fetal mortality; however, more recent data suggest that poor outcomes are not inevitable. [2]. Given the historically poor outcomes, experts agree that immediate and effective treatment of status epilepticus is necessary. Maternal morbidity and mortality are related to the etiology of the seizure disorder, as well as duration and systemic consequences of the inciting event and seizure. The European Society of Neurological Societies published guidelines for the management of status epilepticus in adults in 2010 (Box 26.2) [3]. Modifications suggested for pregnant women include positioning the patient in the left lateral decubitus position and fetal heart rate monitoring in women in whom the fetus has reached the age of viability.

Stroke

Epidemiology and etiology

Cardiovascular accidents are responsible for 10–14% of all maternal deaths, and a significant proportion of those who survive are left with permanent disability. The risk of stroke is increased by as much as 12- to 13-fold in pregnant compared with non-pregnant women [4]. A review of the world's literature published in 2006 found that the incidence of pregnancy-related stroke ranged from 8.9 to 67.1 per 100 000 deliveries [5].

Cardiovascular accidents are usually classified as hemorrhagic or ischemic. Conditions highly associated

Box 26.2. Initial treatment of generalized convulsive and complex partial seizure status epilepticus

Position patient in left lateral decubitus position

Assessment and control of the airway, oxygenation, and ventilation:

- oxygen administration
- arterial blood gas measurement

Assessment and monitoring of circulation:

- electrocardiogram
- blood pressure

Establish intravenous access
Treat seizures

- lorazepam 0.1 mg/kg IV (may be administered out of hospital)
- if lorazepam not available, diazepam 10 mg intravenous followed by phenytoin 18 mg/kg (50 mg/min infusion)

Laboratory measurements

- glucose, electrolytes, magnesium, calcium
- hematological screen
- hepatic and renal function
- thiamine
- antiepileptic drug levels

Fetal heart rate assessment (if fetus is viable)

Assess for and treat cause of status epilepticus (e.g. glucose, thiamine)

Refractory generalized convulsive status epilepticus
Intensive care unit

Anesthetic agents (chose one):

- midazolam (titrated to seizure suppression): initial dose 0.2 mg/kg followed by infusion 0.05 –0.4 mg/kg per hour
- propofol (titrated to electroencephalograph burst suppression): initial dose 2–3 mg/kg, further boluses of 1–2 mg/kg until seizure control, followed by infusion 4–10 mg/kg per hour
- thiopental (titrated to electroencephalograph burst suppression): initial dose 3–5 mg/kg, further boluses of 1–2 mg/kg, followed by infusion 3–7 mg/kg per hour

Refractory complex partial status epilepticus
Trial of further non-anesthetizing anticonvulsants:

- phenobarbital (avoid if possible during pregnancy)
- valproic acid (avoid if possible during pregnancy)
- levetiracetam

Source: Modified from Meierkord *et al.*, 2010 [3].

with stroke during pregnancy include advanced maternal age, migraine headache with aura, thrombophilia, thrombocytopenia, systemic lupus erythematosus, sickle cell disease, heart disease, hemorrhage, and pregnancy-related hypertensive conditions [4]. An estimated 25–45% of pregnancy-related strokes are associated with pre-eclampsia or eclampsia, and stroke is the most common cause of death in women with pre-eclampsia [5]. Several studies have found cesarean delivery and multiple gestation to be risk factors [5]. In the USA, African-Americans were found to be at increased risk compared with Caucasian Americans [4]. The results of several studies suggest that the greatest incidence of stroke occurs in the postpartum period [4,5].

Care of pregnant patients with stroke should be centralized to facilities with multidisciplinary teams of obstetricians, neurologists, intensivists, and rehabilitation specialists. In general, pregnancy should not alter the diagnosis and management of cerebrovascular accidents. As with all stroke patients, quickly differentiating between hemorrhagic and ischemic etiologies is of utmost importance for determining therapy. A thorough history and physical examination, as well as imaging of the head are required. Although CT scanning involves exposure to ionizing radiation, the fetus is exposed to <0.1 mGy per test; therefore, indications for single scans should not be altered by pregnancy. Triiodinated contrast agents are probably safe for use during pregnancy; they are not detectable in the fetus and amniotic fluid. In contrast, gadolinium, used in MRI, crosses the placenta and appears rapidly in the fetal bladder and amniotic fluid. Its half-life and safety in the fetus are unknown and its use should be avoided if possible.

Cerebral vein thrombosis

Pregnancy is a "hypercoagulable" state, and the risk of thrombotic events, including cerebral thrombosis, is increased compared with the non-pregnant state. Approximately 2% of pregnancy-associated strokes are caused by cerebral vein thrombosis (CVT) and up to 73% of CVT events in women occur during pregnancy or the postpartum period [6]. Associated factors include hypovolemia, operative delivery, hypertension, and infections.

Diagnosis and clinical features

The onset of symptoms is usually insidious. Progressive, diffuse headache over several days is common. In the postpartum period, the headache from CVT has been misdiagnosed as postdural puncture headache in patients who had an intrapartum neuraxial procedure with dural puncture. (Intracranial hypotension from a CSF leak may increase the risk of CVT.) Isolated headache without other symptoms occurs in up to 25% of patients. Other symptoms include progressive focal neurological deficits, visual changes, psychosis, and seizures (up to 40%). Symptoms may be bilateral. Seizures can be misdiagnosed as eclamptic seizures. Cerebral vein thrombosis may also masquerade as intracranial hemorrhage or idiopathic intracranial hypertension, and clinicians should have a high index of suspicion. For example, up to 50% of patients may present with an isolated headache or headache with papilledema or sixth cranial nerve palsy, suggestive of idiopathic intracranial hypertension [6]. Finally, a small proportion of patients will present with isolated mental status changes without focal neurological symptoms.

The most common sites of thrombosis in pregnancy are the sagittal sinus with extension into the cortical veins, or primary thrombosis of the cortical veins. Clinical features depend on the location of the thrombus and relate to obstruction of venous return and impaired CSF absorption (causing increased intracranial pressure (ICP)), and/or ischemia, infarction, cytotoxic or vasogenic edema, and bleeding [6].

Workup for suspected CVT should include routine blood studies (including prothrombin time and activated partial thromboplastin time) and thrombophilia screening. While normal D-dimer levels have been shown to identify a subset of patients with low probability for CVT, the test is unlikely to be helpful in pregnancy because D-dimer levels are normally elevated. The most sensitive imaging technique for diagnosing CVT is MRI with gadolinium, particularly in combination with MR venography. Conventional CT scanning may be normal as often as 70% of the time. As always, the risk of gadolinium to the fetus must be weighed against the risk of missing the diagnosis in the mother.

Treatment of cerebral vein thrombosis

Guidelines from several professional organizations have recently been published to guide treatment of CVT [6,7]. Figure 26.1 shows the management algorithm proposed by the American Heart Association/American Stroke Association (AHA/ASA). Full anticoagulation with intravenous unfractionated heparin (titrated to activated partial thromboplastin time 2× normal), or weight-adjusted subcutaneous low-molecular-weight heparin (LMWH) remains the mainstay of therapy. Anticoagulation should be

continued for a total duration of 6 months and for at least 6 weeks after delivery. Oral anticoagulation may be substituted after delivery (international normalized. ratio goal of 2.0–3.0). There is currently limited evidence for fibrinolytic or endovascular therapy.

Early complications of CVT include seizures, intracranial hypertension, and hydrocephalus. Initiation of anticonvulsant therapy is reasonable in patients who have had a seizure, although the optimal duration of therapy is not known. In the absence of seizures, therapy is not recommended [6]. Acetazolamide may be initiated for patients with increased ICP. If increased ICP is associated with progressive visual loss, other therapies (lumbar puncture, optic nerve compression, shunts) should be considered. Decompressive hemicraniotomy may be considered in patients with neurological deterioration who are unresponsive to other therapies. Steroid therapy is not recommended.

Obstetric and anesthetic management

Fetal surveillance is indicated for pregnant women hospitalized for CVT. Plans for delivery and anesthetic care are based on obstetric indications and will need to account for the patient's anticoagulation status. Anticoagulant therapy is suspended intrapartum, and then restarted within 12 to 24 hours following delivery. A history of CVT during pregnancy is not a contraindication for future pregnancies [6]. Prophylaxis with LMWH is a reasonable plan for future pregnancies.

Hemorrhagic stroke

Hemorrhagic strokes can be categorized as intracerebral or subarachnoid. Intracerebral or intraparenchymal hemorrhage involves bleeding from small arteries or arterioles directly into brain matter. Intracranial hemorrhage during pregnancy is usually associated with severe hypertension secondary to pre-eclampsia/eclampsia but may also be secondary to drug abuse (cocaine or methamphetamines), trauma, or tumors. Subarachnoid hemorrhage (SAH) is bleeding into the subarachnoid space between the arachnoid and pia mater. It is most commonly secondary to spontaneous leaking, to rupture of an aneurysm, or rupture of an arteriovenous malformation (AVM) but may also be secondary to trauma, hypertension-induced rupture of pial vessels, or intracranial thrombosis.

Indirect evidence suggests pregnancy may play a role in SAH, although data are inconsistent. The ratio of AVM to aneurysm incidence is significantly higher in pregnant than in non-pregnant patients, and aneurysm

Proposed Algorithm for the Management of CVT

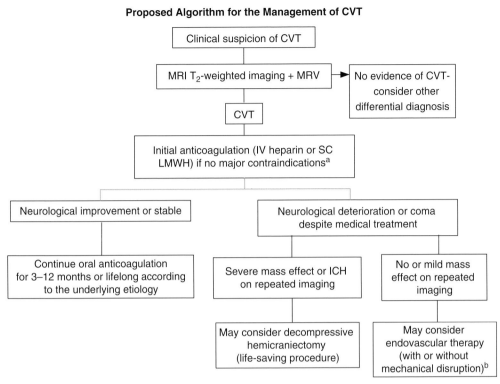

Figure 26.1. Proposed management algorithm for cerebral vein thrombosis (CVT). The algorithm is not comprehensive and may not be applicable to all clinical scenarios; patient management must be individualized. CTV, CT venography; CVST, cerebral venous and sinus thrombosis; ICH, intracranial hemorrhage; IV, intravenous; LMWH, low-molecular-weight heparin; MRV, magnetic resonance venography; SC, subcutaneous; Tx, therapy.
[a]Intracranial hemorrhage that occurred as a consequence of CVST is not a contraindication for anticoagulation.
[b]Endovascular therapy may be considered in patients with absolute contraindications for anticoagulation therapy or failure of initial therapeutic doses of anticoagulant therapy. (Modified from the American Heart Association/American Stroke Association [6].)

rupture is clustered in the peri- and postpartum periods, suggesting pregnancy may contributed to rupture and bleeding from both aneurysms and AVMs [8]. It is hypothesized that the increases in blood volume and cardiac output, and hormone-induced changes to the arterial wall, may contribute to rupture. Mortality rates from SAH are as high as 50%, and survivors often have severe functional deficits [9]. Mortality rates in pregnant women are lower than overall mortality rates, likely secondary to a higher rate of non-aneurysmal hemorrhage during pregnancy. In an analysis of data from the US Nationwide Inpatient Sample from 1995 to 2008, the overall SAH rate was 5.8 per 100 000 deliveries, and SAH was responsible for 4.1% of all pregnancy-related in-patient deaths [8].

Aneurysmal subarachnoid hemorrhage

Diagnosis and clinical features

The most common presentation of SAH is a sudden, diffuse, severe headache ("worst headache of my life").

Other symptoms include nausea and vomiting, meningismus, decreased level of consciousness, speech and visual deficits, hemiparesis, cranial third nerve palsy, and seizure. Urgent evaluation of suspected SAH is recommended as there is a least a 3–4% risk of rebleeding of untreated, ruptured aneurysms in the first 24 hours after the initial ictus [10]. Non-contrast CT is the screening imaging technique currently recommended by the AHA/ASA management guidelines [10]. Sensitivity in the first 24 hours approaches 100% but decreases over time. If SAH is suspected, but the CT scan is negative, a lumbar puncture should be performed, looking for elevated opening pressure and an increase in CSF red blood cell count and/or xanthochromia. If SAH is diagnosed, further imaging studies, such as selective cerebral angiography or MR angiography, are indicated to further characterize the source of hemorrhage.

The Hunt and Hess or World Federation of Neurosurgeons grading scales are utilized to describe the patient's condition, propose treatment, and assess

Table 26.1. Hess and Hunt severity scale for subarachnoid hemorrhage

Grade	Description
0	Unruptured aneurysm
1	Asymptomatic or mild headache
2	Moderate to severe headache, nuchal rigidity, and no neurological deficit other than possible cranial nerve palsy
3	Mild alteration in mental status (confusion, lethargy), mild focal neurological deficit
4	Stupor and/or hemiparesis
5	Comatose and/or decerebrate rigidity

Table 26.2. World Federation of Neurological Surgeons scale

Grade	Glasgow Coma Scale score	Motor deficit
I	15	Absent
II	13–14	Absent
III	13–14	Present
IV	7–12	Present/absent
V	3–6	Present/absent

Table 26.3. Modified Fisher scale[a]

Grade	CT scan appearance
1	Focal or diffuse thin SAH, no intraventricular hemorrhage
2	Focal or diffuse thin SAH, with intraventricular hemorrhage present
3	Thick SAH present, no intraventricular hemorrhage
4	Thick SAH present, with intraventricular hemorrhage present

SAH, subarachnoid hemorrhage.
[a] Describes amount and location of blood on CT scan: useful for predicting likelihood of vasospasm.

prognosis (Tables 26.1 and 26.2). The modified Fisher scale describes the amount of blood observed on CT imaging (Table 26.3). Combining the clinical scale with the imaging scale improves ability to predict outcome [9]. Clinical outcome is primarily dependent on the severity of the initial bleed. Other factors include age, gender, medical comorbidities, size and location of the aneurysm, and services available in the facility where the patient is first evaluated.

Management of subarachnoid hemorrhage

Early support therapy is summarized in Box 26.3. Management of SAH is complicated by a number of neurological and medical complications. Rebleeding is most likely to occur in the first 24 hours after ictus; the risk gradually decreases after 1–6 months to 3% per year. Systolic blood pressure >160 mmHg is an independent risk factor for rebleeding; however, it is not known whether treatment of hypertension decreases the risk. Blood pressure should be monitored (usually

invasively) and controlled, taking into account the risk of rebleeding, stroke, and maintenance of cerebral perfusion pressure [10]. Hypotension may contribute to cerebral ischemia. Higher blood pressures may be tolerated once the aneurysm is secured. Agents used to treat hypertension should be easily titratable with minimal effects on cerebral blood flow. Nicardipine and labetalol are commonly used.

The AHA/ASA guidelines recommend stabilization of the aneurysm to decrease the risk of (re)bleeding, either with surgical clipping of the aneurysm or endovascular coiling. The International Subarachnoid Aneurysm Trial was a large randomized controlled trial that compared clipping with endovascular coiling [11]. Mortality was lower at 1 year in the endovascular coiling group than in the clipping group. The risk of rebleeding was small in both groups, but slightly higher in the endovascular coiling group. There were no differences in the proportion of survivors who were functionally independent at 5 years. Therefore, in this population of patients (low-grade aneurysms), both therapies appear to have equivalent outcomes.

The risk of rebleeding is reduced with the use of the antifibrinolytics, tranexamic acid and aminocaproic acid. However, long-term use is associated with an increased risk of cerebral ischemia. The AHA/ASA guidelines state that a short-term course of antifibrinolytic therapy of up to 72 hours may be reasonable [10].

Other neurological complications of aneurysmal SAH include acute and chronic hydrocephalus, seizure, vasospasm, and delayed ischemic neurological deficits. Obstruction of CSF drainage by the intraventricular clot results in increased ICP. Aggressive treatment of ICP greater than 20 to 25 mmHg is warranted, as high ICP is associated with secondary brain ischemia.

The incidence of seizures is low (6–18%); however, seizures can cause hypertension and increased ICP. Prophylactic use of anticonvulsants has been associated with poor functional and cognitive outcome and does

Box 26.3. Management of subarachnoid hemorrhage

Intervention/treatment
- Initial care
- Intravenous fluids (isotonic or hypertonic) to achieve euvolemia
- Support circulation
- Support airway, ventilation, oxygenation

Prevention of rebleeding
- Maintain systolic blood pressure <160 mmHg until aneurysm is secured: intravenous nicardipine infusion 2.5–5 mg/h titrated up to 15 mg/h; labetalol bolus 10–20 mg every 5 minutes or continuous infusion 0.5 mg/min titrated up to 2 mg/min
- Tranexamic acid (1 g every 6 hours for 72 hours or until aneurysm is secured) or epsilon-aminocaproic acid (4 g over 1 hour, then 1 g/h for 72 hours or until 4 hours prior to angiography)
- Early clipping or coiling
- Stool softener
- Pain management
- Sedation

Seizure prophylaxis
- Consider short term in immediate posthemorrhage or postoperative period
- Consider long term if risk factors are present (prior history of seizures, parenchymal hematoma, cerebral infarct, middle cerebral artery aneurysm)

Hydrocephalus
- External ventricular drain

Prevention of delayed ischemic neurological deficits
- Maintenance of normothermia
- Maintenance of euglycemia
- Maintenance of euvolemia
- Nimodipine 60 mg orally every 4 hours for 21 days starting within 96 hours of ictus

Prevention of medical complications
- Mucosal damage prophylaxis (histamine H_2 blockers or proton pump inhibitors)
- Venous embolism prophylaxis: mechanical or unfractionated heparin 5000 U subcutaneous every 8 hours or low-molecular-weight heparin (enoxaparin) 30 mg subcutaneous every 12 hours
- Glycemic control (serum glucose 80–140 mg/dL)

Management of medical complications
- Hyponatremia
- Hypovolemia
- Dysrhythmias (ventricular, torsades de pointes): ST segment, T waves changes, and prolongation of QT interval are common
- Cardiomyopathy (neurogenic stunned myocardium)
- Pulmonary edema
- Fever
- Anemia (target hemoglobin value not known)

Manage vasospasm
- Triple-H therapy: treating hypervolemia, hemodilution, and induced hypertension; although target values are not well studied, central venous pressure is usually maintained between 8 and 12 mmHg, hematocrit between 30% and 35%, and systolic blood pressure between 180 and 200 mmHg (see text for discussion)
- Consider cerebral angioplasty and/or selective intra-arterial vasodilator therapy

Management of increased intracranial pressure
- Ventriculostomy
- Acute hyperventilation (target arterial partial pressure carbon dioxide of 30–35 mmHg)
- Sedation
- Osmotherapy (mannitol)
- Metabolic suppression

Source: adapted from Rhoney *et al.*, 2010 [9] and Bederson *et al.*, 2009 [10].

not reduce the incidence of seizures [9]. The AHA/ASA guidelines state that short-term prophylactic anticonvulsants may be considered in the immediate posthemorrhage period [9].

The presence of blood in the subarachnoid space causes dysregulation of vasoconstriction and vasodilatation, free radical formation, and an inflammatory response [9]. Breakdown of erythrocytes and release of oxyhemoglobin results in cerebral vasoconstriction, usually of the large capacitance arteries at the base of the brain. Vasospasm occurs in 30–70% of patients with SAH; onset is typically 3 to 5 days after the hemorrhage and maximal narrowing occurs at 5 to 14 days, with gradual resolution over 2 to 4 weeks. Vasospasm is a leading cause of death after SAH. Delayed ischemic neurological deficits were traditionally thought to result from decreased cerebral perfusion from vasospasm; however, newer evidence suggests that other mechanisms of brain tissue injury may also play a role.

Management of vasospasm centers on both prevention and treatment. Unfortunately, randomized controlled trials are lacking and no single therapy has been shown to prevent or treat vasospasm effectively. The most common therapy for prevention of vasospasm is nimodipine. Meta-analysis of clinical trials has demonstrated that nimodipine decreases vasospasm-induced morbidity and mortality compared with placebo, although the incidence of vasospasm did not differ. Therefore, oral nimodipine is currently recommended in the AHA/ASA guidelines for prevention of vasospasm; therapy should be initiated within 96 hours of ictus [10]. Hypovolemia is associated with an increased risk of vasospasm; however, prophylactic, so-called triple-H therapy (hypervolemia, hemodilution, induced hypertension) has not been shown to be effective for prevention of vasospasm. Use of hydroxymethylglutaryl coenzyme A reductase inhibitors (statins) and magnesium is currently being investigated.

Diagnosis of vasospasm, particularly in comatose patients, is difficult. The literature regarding the use of serial transcranial Doppler technology is inconclusive [10]. The gold standard diagnostic technique for vasospasm is cerebral catheter angiography. This is an invasive procedure with significant risks for mother and fetus, but an advantage is that it can be combined with selected intra-arterial vasodilator therapy.

Historically, triple-H therapy has been the standard treatment of vasospasm following SAH. The level of evidence for triple-H therapy is moderate, at best. It is not clear which components of triple-H therapy are important, alone or in combination. Recent physiological studies suggest that normovolemic hypertension may increase cerebral blood flow, whereas hypervolemia hemodilution may be associated with increased complications [12]. The AHA/ASA guidelines consider triple-H therapy to be a reasonable approach. Cerebral angioplasty and/or selective intra-arterial vasodilator therapy may be reasonable therapies with, after, or instead of triple-H therapy, depending on the clinical scenario [10].

In the future, intraparenchymal brain monitoring may play an increasingly important role in neurocritical care. Probes are now available that can provide measurement of cerebral blood flow and brain oxygen. Microdialysis probes allow measurement of interstitial glucose, glutamate, lactate, pyruvate, and pH. Outcome research is currently lacking.

Obstetric and anesthetic management of subarachnoid hemorrhage

The fetus may be indirectly compromised in women with SAH by maternal hypo- or hypertension, hypo- or hyperventilation, hypoxemia, acid–base changes, or indeed any perturbations that compromise uteroplacental perfusion or fetal gas exchange. Direct effects include adverse effects of drugs administered to the mother. If neurosurgical or interventional neuroradiology therapy occurs before fetal viability (24 weeks of gestation), care should focus on the mother. If the fetus is viable at the time of surgery, a decision must be made whether delivery is appropriate. There is no evidence that one mode of delivery results in better outcomes compared with others. Options include performing neurosurgery with the plan to maintain the pregnancy and deliver at a later date, or cesarean delivery followed by immediate neurosurgery. Cesarean delivery of a viable fetus may be considered in patients with poor neurological status (Hunt and Hess grade 4 or 5), if labor begins during the period that the patient is at risk for rebleeding or vasospasm, or if the rupture occurs during labor. If vaginal delivery is chosen in a patient with a history of SAH, neuraxial analgesia is recommended in order to mitigate the urge to bear down. A shortened second stage is indicated.

Arteriovenous malformation

Diagnosis and clinical features

Rupture of AVM accounts for approximately 2% of all strokes. The most common presentations of AVM is SAH (most common) or intracranial hemorrhage, usually between 20 and 40 years of age [13]. Other presenting signs include seizures, mass effect, and ischemic steal, as well as headaches in the absence of bleeding. The overall risk of hemorrhage is estimated at 2–4% per year. Hemorrhage is associated with a 5–10% chance of death and a 30–50% chance of permanent neurological deficits. The risk of rebleeding is slightly increased during the first year. Whether pregnancy affects these risks is not clear. The most important risk factor for bleeding is hypertension. Cerebral angiography is the gold standard imaging modality by which to evaluate the architecture of the AVM. Three-dimensional MR angiography may provide details regarding surrounding cerebral structures.

Management of arteriovenous malformation

Management decisions must weigh the risk of leaving the AVM untreated, risking (re)bleeding, against risks of the intervention. Which patients should be treated and the best time and therapy remain uncertain [13]. Procedures are usually scheduled electively. The Spetzler–Martin grading scale (Table 26.4) has been validated for operative risk assessment and outcome. Patients with Spetzler-Martin grade I and II lesions are usually considered candidates for surgical resection; the risk is low and outcome is good. Patients with grade III lesions may be offered surgery after embolization. Grades IV and V lesions are associated with poor outcomes after surgical resection [13]. Another option, particularly if the lesion is located in an eloquent area, is radiosurgery. A disadvantage is that there is a lag period of 1–3 years before obliteration is complete. During this time the patient is still at risk for bleeding. Additionally, the cure rate for lesions

Table 26.4. Spetzler–Martin grading scale for arteriovenous malformation

Characteristic	Classification	Points[a]
Eloquent brain area[b]	No	0
	Yes	1
Venous drainage	Superficial only	0
	Deep	1
Size	Small (3 cm)	1
	Medium (3–6 cm)	2
	Large (>6 cm)	3

[a] Points are added up; the possible grades are I–V based on 1–5 points.
[b] Sensorimotor, language, or visual cortex; hypothalamus or thalamus; internal capsule; brainstem; cerebellar peduncles; or cerebellar nuclei.

<3 cm is only 81–90%, and lower yet for larger lesions. Embolization using endovascular catheters to deposit occlusive material into the AVM feeding arteries and nidus is another treatment option. It results in complete cure for only very small lesions. Aneurysms are found in up to 58% of patients with AVM and may complicate management.

Obstetric and anesthesia management of arteriovenous malformation

Some data suggest that pregnant women who present with hemorrhage from AVM are at high risk for rebleeding, implying that consideration should be given for definitive AVM therapy during pregnancy; however, the data are inconsistent [13,14]. A proposed algorithm for the management of pregnant patients with AVM is presented in Figure 26.2 [14]. The decision to proceed with definitive treatment during pregnancy must also consider potential risks to the fetus. Women with a known AVM who are considering pregnancy should consider definitive therapy before conception [15].

There are no data to suggest that one mode of delivery is safer than another [14]. Options include a cesarean delivery or an instrumental vaginal delivery with neuraxial analgesia, although there is evidence that increased venous pressure during a Valsalva maneuver is not directly transmitted to AVM draining veins [15].

Posterior reversible encephalopathy syndrome

Epidemiology and etiology

The term posterior reversible encephalopathy syndrome (PRES) was first coined in 1996 to describe a

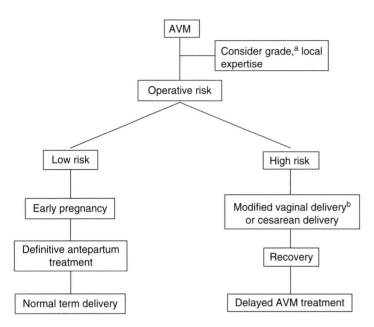

Figure 26.2. Algorithm for management of the pregnant patient with an arteriovenous malformation (AVM).
[a]Spetzler–Martin grade;
[b]see text. (Modified from Trivedi and Kirkpatrick, 2003 [14].)

syndrome consisting of headache, vomiting, confusion, seizures, and visual abnormalities in combination with a pathognomonic MRI pattern of bilateral white matter abnormalities in the posterior cerebral hemispheres. It is likely a form of hypertensive encephalopathy. Theories as to the etiology of PRES include breakdown in cerebral autoregulation leading to disruption in the blood–brain barrier or endothelial dysfunction caused by circulating toxins, or a combination of these two mechanisms [16]. Failure of the blood–brain barrier, which may result from severe hypertension, toxins, or systemic illness, causes endothelial injury or dysfunction. The relative contribution of these mechanisms may vary by disease state, but the clinical syndrome is similar. Secondary effects of cerebral edema include focal cerebral vasospasm and microvascular thrombosis [16].

An association of PRES with several diseases has been noted, including pre-eclampsia/eclampsia. Both hypertension-induced breakdown in the blood–brain barrier, as well as toxin-induced endothelial dysfunction, are thought to play a role in pre-eclampsia-associated PRES. Other entities associated with PRES include abrupt hypertension, impaired renal function, autoimmune diseases, infection, and immunosuppressive drug therapy. The nature of the inciting event is not well understood. Animal and human data support both a hypoperfusion/ischemia mechanism and a hyperperfusion/edema mechanism.

Diagnosis and clinical features

Signs and symptoms of PRES are described in Table 26.5. Seizure occurs in most patients, usually accompanied by other symptoms. Papilledema is uncommon. The absolute degree of hypertension is highly variable [16]. The change in blood pressure, rather than the absolute blood pressure value, may be the more important contributing factor in PRES. Symptoms usually develop quickly over several hours, peak in severity between 12 and 48 hours, and resolve over 7 days. Although the presentation of PRES is often severe, recovery generally occurs. However, the differential diagnosis includes life-threatening disorders that must be excluded (Table 26.6) [17]. In women with pre-eclampsia/eclampsia, PRES may present in the antepartum, intrapartum, and postpartum periods.

The gold standard imaging technique is MRI; CT shows lesions in only about 50% of patients with PRES. The MRI lesions can be confluent or patchy, and are bright on T_2-weighted and fluid-attenuated inversion recovery imaging. The lesions represent areas of vasogenic edema. About one third of patients have lesions in atypical places, but almost all patients have involvement of the parietal–occipital area. Although PRES is a leukoencephalopathy, the cortex is also frequently involved. Hemorrhage may also be present. Patients with widespread lesions tend to have poor outcomes.

Table 26.5. Signs and symptoms of posterior reversible encephalopathy syndrome

Symptoms/sign	Characteristics
Seizures	Generalized tonic–clonic, may start focally; status epilepticus may occur
Vision abnormalities	Cortical blindness, homonymous hemianopia, blurred vision, vision neglect, visual hallucinations
Altered mental status	Confusion, lethargy, slowed motor responses, stuporous
Headache	Bilateral, dull
Other neurologic	Nausea, vomiting, occasional hemiparesis, Babinski's sign, brainstem features
Blood pressure	Hypertension

Table 26.6. Differential diagnosis of posterior reversible encephalopathy syndrome

Differential diagnosis	Characteristics
Posterior circulation stroke	No seizures, cytotoxic edema[a]
Reversible cerebral vasoconstriction syndrome	Thunderclap headache, MRI-identified lesions of PRES usually not observed
Primary central nervous system vasculitis	Insidious onset of symptoms; abnormal CSF; MRI may show multiple infarcts
Migraine headache	Aura may cause occipital symptoms
Encephalitis	Confusion, seizures, aphasia; systemic signs and symptoms of inflammation (fever, leukocytosis)
Status epilepticus	MRI lesions usually cortical and unilateral

CSF, cerebral spinal fluid; PRES, posterior reversible encephalopathy syndrome.
[a] MRI imaging, particularly diffusion-weighted imaging, shows hyperintensity with low signal on the apparent diffusion map, whereas PRES shows the opposite pattern.

Management

Clinical trials of PRES treatment are lacking. Intensive care is usually indicated, with continuous blood pressure monitoring, treatment of hypertension, and if possible, removal of the underlying cause. In pre-eclampsia/eclampsia, delivery and magnesium sulfate therapy are indicated. The goal of antihypertensive therapy is to reduce blood pressure below the threshold for vasoregulatory breakthrough without causing a precipitous drop, which might decrease cerebral perfusion [16]. The ideal agent is not known but should be easily titratable. Patients are often hypovolemic and may, therefore, require fluid replacement.

Guillain–Barré syndrome

Epidemiology and etiology

Guillain–Barré syndrome occurs rarely during pregnancy. Retrospective data suggest that the incidence is no different in pregnancy than in the general population, although the risk may be increased immediately postpartum [18]. Guillain–Barré syndrome is thought to result from abnormal immune responses to peripheral nerves. About two thirds of cases follow an infectious event. *Campylobacter jejuni* and cytomegalovirus are two common associated infections.

Diagnosis and clinical features

Initial signs and symptoms, as well as laboratory data, are non-specific and vague; consequently, diagnosis is often delayed [19]. Symptoms include weakness, neck and back pain, paresthesia, cranial nerve palsies (most commonly facial nerve), and autonomic dysfunction. Progressive muscle weakness may include limbs and respiratory, facial, and bulbar muscles. Total areflexia usually evolves over several days. By definition, the progression of symptoms from normal to the nadir occurs in under 4 weeks. The differential diagnosis of Guillain–Barré syndrome includes infection (e.g. Lyme disease, diphtheria); inflammatory, paraneoplastic, malignant (from nerve infiltration), vasculitic, and metabolic (e.g. beri-beri) diseases. Diagnostic criteria are shown in Box 26.4.

Tests should be conducted primarily to exclude other diseases. Nerve conduction studies demonstrate an evolving multifocal demyelinating polyneuropathy. Lumber puncture should be performed to rule out alternative diagnoses. Typically in Guillain–Barré syndrome, CSF protein is elevated. The presence of antiganglioside antibodies is suggestive of Guillain–Barré syndrome, although their absence does not exclude the diagnosis.

Management

Randomized controlled trials support treatment with intravenous immunoglobulin or plasmapheresis. The safety of both treatments in pregnancy has been demonstrated with other disease states. Among 30 pregnant

Box 26.4. Diagnostic criteria for Guillain–Barré syndrome

Required criteria
- Absent reflexes
- Progressive weakness of more than one limb
- Absence of other causes for neuropathy

Supportive criteria
- Symmetrical
- Mild sensory signs
- Cranial nerves affected
- Autonomic dysfunction
- No fever
- Cerebral spinal fluid protein increased
- Cerebral spinal fluid cell count <100/μL
- Slowed nerve conduction
- Progression in under 4 weeks

women with Guillain–Barré syndrome between 1986 and 2002, there were no reports of adverse effects with either therapy [18]. The current first-line treatment is usually intravenous immunoglobulin because it is easier to administer. Treatment should be started as soon as possible. There is no evidence that steroid therapy is helpful. Support of ventilation may be life saving. Patients who present with progressive disease should be monitored with hourly vital capacity measurements, and cardiac rhythm and oxygen saturation monitoring. Other measures include a chest radiograph, swallowing assessment, and thrombosis prophylaxis. Pregnancy and the gravid uterus may exacerbate circulatory instability and the need for ventilatory support.

A multidisciplinary approach to the care of the pregnant patient with Guillain–Barré syndrome is essential. Important components of care include prevention and treatment of infectious complications, prevention of venous thromboembolism, and pain management.

Obstetric management
Several reviews of Guillain–Barré syndrome in pregnancy suggest that termination of pregnancy does not hasten recovery of the disease nor improve maternal outcome, nor is there evidence that the disease itself alters pregnancy outcome [18]. There is no evidence that uterine contractile activity is adversely affected and, therefore, vaginal delivery is possible. Cesarean delivery should be reserved for patients with obstetric indications.

Anesthetic management
Both neuraxial (including both spinal and epidural anesthesia/analgesia) and general anesthesia have been described for delivery of patients with Guillain–Barré syndrome. Autonomic instability predisposes patients to hemodynamic instability during both types of anesthesia.

Succinylcholine should be avoided in these patients because of the risk of hyperkalemia due to postsynaptic receptor proliferation. Patients also have increased sensitivity to non-depolarizing neuromuscular-blocking agents, and well as to respiratory depressants. Bulbar weakness may increase the risk of pulmonary aspiration.

There is no evidence that neuraxial anesthesia/analgesia worsens the outcome of Guillain–Barré syndrome [18]. Patients may have increased sensitivity to neuraxial local anesthetic agents; therefore, doses should be carefully titrated. Direct-acting vasopressors should be used to treat hypotension. High sensory–motor blockade may exacerbate respiratory compromise.

Acute spinal cord injury
Spinal cord injury (SCI) affects thousands of people each year, and many are women in their reproductive years.

Management
As with other neurological trauma during pregnancy, ensuring stabilization of the mother is the best therapy for the fetus. Early acute management in adults with SCI has been summarized in a clinical practice guideline by the Consortium for Spinal Cord Medicine [20]. Highlights of the recommendations are summarized in Table 26.7.

High thoracic or cervical spinal cord lesions are associated with neurogenic shock because of blockade of autonomic function at the level of the SCI. Parasympathetic effects predominate; the patient may be hypotensive and have profound bradycardia and decreased cardiac output. Hypothermia results from peripheral vasodilatation. Neurogenic shock must be differentiated from hypovolemia caused by trauma and hemorrhage. The backboard to which the pregnant patient is initially secured can be tilted to the left, or the uterus can be moved to the left, in order to relieve aortocaval compression without rotating the spine.

The use of high-dose steroids in the setting of acute SCI remains controversial. Their use is associated with significant side effects, such as severe sepsis, pneumonia, hyperglycemia, and wound disruption. Pregnant

Table 26.7. Initial management of acute spinal cord injury

Action	Description
Triage protocols and systems of care	Prehospital triage, transportation to trauma centers and spinal cord injury centers
Spinal stabilization and immobilization	Immobilize spine of all patients with potential spinal cord injury (risk factors: altered mental status, intoxication, extremity fracture of distracting injury, spinal pain) until definitive diagnosis/treatment
ABCs and resuscitation	Airway, ventilation, circulatory support
Neuroprotection	Currently no evidence to definitely recommend any pharmacological agent
Diagnosis	Baseline and serial neurological assessment; MRI
Associated conditions and injuries	Survey for other injuries (brain, limb, chest, abdomen, artery, penetrating)
Surgical procedures	Early open or closed reduction of bilateral cervical facet dislocation; consider early surgical spinal canal decompression
Anesthetic concerns	Airway, circulation support (hypotension, bradycardia) Avoid succinylcholine after the first 48 hours after injury Maintain normothermia Consider intraoperative spinal cord function monitoring
Analgesia and sedation	Treat pain; thoughtful patient handling
Secondary prevention	Prevent skin breakdown Thromboembolism prophylaxis Respiratory management (baseline and serial parameters, early tracheostomy for ventilator-dependent patients, pulmonary hygiene, protocol to prevent ventilator-associated pneumonia) Genitourinary tract (urinary catheter) Gastrointestinal (stress ulcer prophylaxis, assess swallowing function) Bowel care (initiate bowel protocol) Nutrition (enteral) Glycemic control
Rehabilitation	Rehabilitation specialists; psychosocial family issues; health-promotion behaviors; mental health

Source: adapted from Steering Committee for the Consortium for Spinal Cord Medicine, 2008 [20].

women may be at increased risk for some of these adverse effects. There is no proven benefit to initiating steroids beyond 8 hours after the injury.

Obstetric and anesthetic management

The uterus functions as an end-organ. Therefore, onset of fetal heart rate abnormalities is a sign of maternal circulatory or metabolic derangement. In trauma, fetal–maternal transfusion should be quantified in all patients and anti-D administered to rhesus D-negative women. Additionally, placental abruption must be ruled out.

It is almost always proper to focus initial resuscitative measures on the mother. However, providers should consider immediate delivery in two circumstances: a viable fetus in a dying or arrested mother, or a dying fetus in a stable mother. Perimortem cesarean delivery should be initiated after 4 minutes of unsuccessful cardiopulmonary resuscitation with the intent to deliver the fetus by 5 minutes [21]. Delivery may improve the chances for maternal survival because it relieves aortocaval compression and is followed by autotransfusion secondary to the contracted uterine vascular bed.

Fetal surveillance should be a part of the primary survey performed immediately after admission of a pregnant patient to the trauma unit. If the mother is stable, but fetal status is not, emergency cesarean delivery can be considered. Most women will require anesthesia despite a high SCI. If the initial fetal surveillance is reassuring, continuous fetal heart rate monitoring is appropriate.

Progression of pregnancy with its accompanying decrease in functional residual capacity and encroachment of the gravid uterus on the diaphragm, as well as increase in oxygen consumption, may compromise ventilation and oxygenation in women with SCIs. Therefore, respiratory surveillance is indicated.

Labor may be painless and fast; therefore, regular tocometry is indicated. In general, cesarean delivery is indicated for obstetric reasons. Pelvic fractures may hamper vaginal delivery. Patients, particularly those with SCIs above T5–T6, are at risk of autonomic hyper-reflexia after the neurogenic shock resolves. Labor is a frequent trigger of autonomic hyper-reflexia. Optimal management includes early initiation of epidural analgesia. An instrumental vaginal delivery will shorten the second stage and assist with deliver of the fetus past the perineum. Neuraxial anesthesia is possible for women undergoing cesarean delivery; however, consideration must be given to the compromised respiratory musculature in the parturient with an SCI.

Neurologic complications of neuraxial anesthesia

Local anesthetic toxicity

Clinical features

Although a rare event, local anesthetic systemic toxicity is a feared complication of regional anesthetic procedures. Subtoxic concentrations of local anesthetics cause complaints of tongue numbness, lightheadedness, and muscle twitching. Higher levels cause convulsions and coma, followed by respiratory arrest. Very high levels lead to cardiac dysrhythmias, profound myocardial depression, and vasodilatation. Studies assessing whether pregnancy lowers the threshold for local anesthetic systemic toxicity are inconsistent. Anecdotally, it appears much more difficult to resuscitate a pregnant patient with local anesthetic systemic toxicity.

Management

New resuscitation guidelines from professional organizations include the use of lipid emulsion for treatment (Box 26.5). While the exact mechanism is unknown, it is hypothesized that the lipid emulsion acts as a "lipid sink," sequestering the local anesthetic and reducing the tissue concentration. Alternatively, lipid emulsion may impede local anesthetic inhibition of acylcarnitine, thus improving mitochondrial metabolism, or it may increase intracellular calcium concentration, thus improving contractility [22].

Neuraxial infections

Meningitis and spinal epidural abscess are rare complications of neuraxial anesthesia. Neuraxial infections occur less commonly in obstetric patients than in general surgical patients.

Spinal epidural abscess

The most common causative organism of epidural abscess is *Staphylococcus aureus*, most likely as a result of skin contamination. Updated antisepsis guidelines from multiple professional organizations state that chlorhexidine in alcohol is the preferred antiseptic

Box 26.5. Management of severe local anesthetic toxicity

1. Stop injecting local anesthetic
2. Call for help
3. Maintain/secure airway, ventilate with 100% oxygen, consider hyperventilation
4. Confirm/establish intravenous access
5. Control seizures (benzodiazepines, propofol)
6. Assess/treat hemodynamic instability

In cardiac arrest
- Start standard cardiopulmonary resuscitation
- Consider cardiopulmonary bypass
- Give lipid emulsion[a]

Without cardiac arrest
- Support circulation
- Consider lipid emulsion[a]

[a] Lipid emulsion dose: 20% lipid emulsion, initial intravenous dose of 1.5 mL/kg over 1 minute. Start an intravenous infusion of 15 mL/kg per hour. After 5 minutes, repeat dose if hemodynamic stability has not returned or adequate circulation deteriorates. Give a maximum of three boluses. The infusion rate may be doubled if hemodynamic stability is not been restored or deteriorates. The maximum cumulative dose is 12 mL/kg.

Source: modified from Association of Anaesthetists of Great Britain and Ireland, 2010 [23].

solution for decontaminating the back prior to initiation of neuraxial procedures.

Diagnosis, clinical features, and management

Onset of symptoms of epidural abscess is usually 4 to 10 days after epidural catheterization. The most common symptoms are severe backache and localized tenderness. Other signs and symptoms include fever, neck stiffness and headache, and elevated white blood cell count and erythrocyte sedimentation rate. Late-onset symptoms include radicular pain, lower limb and sacral numbness, loss of muscle stretch reflexes, and bladder dysfunction. The catheter entry site may be inflamed and there may be a fluid leak. Gadolinium MRI is the gold standard for diagnosis. Early diagnosis and treatment are essential to a good outcome; delayed decompression is associated with permanent neurological sequelae. Surgical decompression and drainage is the norm, although occasionally, antibiotic therapy alone suffices.

Meningitis

Meningitis is a rare, but potentially deadly complication of neuraxial anesthesia. It occurs more commonly after neuraxial procedures involving dural puncture and more commonly in women following labor and vaginal delivery than with scheduled cesarean delivery [24].

Diagnosis, clinical features, and management

In contrast to community-acquired meningitis, post-dural puncture meningitis is most commonly caused by viridans type streptococci. Viridans streptococci colonize the upper respiratory tract, the female genital tract, and the gastrointestinal tract. Although not normally virulent, they thrive in watery media such as CSF. Reports of iatrogenic meningitis tend to occur in clusters, suggesting contamination occurs because of a breakdown in sterile technique during the neuraxial procedure. Contamination by organisms residing in the nasopharynx of medical personnel during dural puncture has been identified as a source of infection in the anesthesiology, radiology, and neurology literature, suggesting that droplet contamination plays a role in transmission. Updated professional organization guidelines recommend that practitioners wear a clean mask while performing neuraxial procedures [25].

Symptom onset, including fever, headache, photophobia, nausea, vomiting, and neck stiffness, is typically 12 hours to several days after dural puncture. Other signs and symptoms include confusion, drowsiness, and a positive Kernig sign. Diagnostic lumbar puncture reveals an elevated CSF protein level and white blood cell count, and a CSF glucose level that is lower than the plasma glucose concentration. Because viridans streptococci are the most likely pathogens, bacteria should be cultured in broth. Treatment with the appropriate antibiotics should not await culture results.

Spinal/epidural hematoma

Epidemiology and etiology

Spinal/epidural hematoma is a rare complication of neuraxial procedures in the obstetric population. Pregnant patients are hypercoagulable and this may confer some degree of protection. A "bloody tap" in a healthy parturient does not increase the risk for spinal/epidural hematoma. Because pulmonary embolism is a major cause of maternal mortality, many more patients are presenting with pharmacological anticoagulation. Professional society guidelines are available to guide anticoagulation

management relative to initiation of neuraxial anesthesia/analgesia. Low-dose aspirin is not a contraindication to neuraxial procedures. Spontaneous epidural hematomas during pregnancy have been described.

Diagnosis, clinical features, and management

Signs and symptoms of a spinal/epidural hematoma include acute onset of back and radicular leg pain, lower extremity weakness and numbness, and bladder and bowel dysfunction. These complaints should generate prompt evaluation, including neurosurgical evaluation and MRI if indicated. Adverse neurological outcome is directly related to the duration of symptoms. For best recovery of neurological function, the hematoma should be decompressed within 6 to 8 hours of the onset of symptoms.

Cranial subdural hematoma

Epidemiology and etiology

Subdural hematoma is a rare complication of dural puncture. Reduced CSF pressure may cause traction and tearing of the bridging veins. It has been reported after dural puncture with small-gauge spinal needles, as well as unintentional dural puncture with large-gauge epidural needles.

Diagnosis, clinical features, and management

Subdural hematoma should be suspected if a headache persists after epidural blood patch, particularly if the nature of the headache changes or it is accompanied by altered mental status, seizures, or other focal neurological findings. An urgent MRI is warranted, with neurosurgical depression if indicated.

References

1. Harden CL, Hopp J, Ting TY, *et al.* Practice parameter update: management issues for women with epilepsy: focus on pregnancy (an evidence-based review). Obstetrical complications and change in seizure frequency: report of the Quality Standards Subcommittee and Therapeutics and Technology Assessment Subcommittee of the American Academy of Neurology and American Epilepsy Society. *Neurology* 2009;**73**:126–132.

2. EURAP Study Group. Seizure control and treatment in pregnancy: observations from the EURAP epilepsy pregnancy registry. *Neurology* 2006;**66**:354–360.

3. Meierkord H, Boon P, Engelsen B, *et al.* EFNS guideline on the management of status epilepticus in adults. *Eur J Neurol* 2010;**17**:348–355.

4. James AH, Bushnell CD, Jamison MG, Myers ER. Incidence and risk factors for stroke in pregnancy and the puerperium. *Obstet Gynecol* 2005;**106**:509–516.

5. Tang SC, Jeng JS. Management of stroke in pregnancy and the puerperium. *Expert Rev Neurother* 2010;**10**:205–215.

6. Saposnik G, Barinagarrementeria F, Brown RD Jr., *et al.* Diagnosis and management of cerebral venous thrombosis: a statement for healthcare professionals from the American Heart Association/American Stroke Association. *Stroke* 2011;**42**:1158–1192.

7. Einhäupl K, Stam J, Bousser MG, *et al.* EFNS guideline on the treatment of cerebral venous and sinus thrombosis in adult patients. *Eur J Neurol* 2010;**17**:1229–1235.

8. Bateman BT, Olbrecht VA, Berman MF, *et al.* Peripartum subarachnoid hemorrhage: nationwide data and institutional experience. *Anesthesiology* 2012;**116**:1–10.

9. Rhoney DH, McAllen K, Liu-DeRyke X. Current and future treatment considerations in the management of aneurysmal subarachnoid hemorrhage. *J Pharm Pract* 2010;**23**:408–424.

10. Bederson JB, Connolly ES Jr., Batjer HH, *et al.* Guidelines for the management of aneurysmal subarachnoid hemorrhage: a statement for healthcare professionals from a special writing group of the Stroke Council, American Heart Association. *Stroke* 2009;**40**:994–1025.

11. Molyneux AJ, Kerr RS, Birks J, *et al.* Risk of recurrent subarachnoid haemorrhage, death, or dependence and standardised mortality ratios after clipping or coiling of an intracranial aneurysm in the International Subarachnoid Aneurysm Trial (ISAT): long-term follow-up. *Lancet Neurol* 2009;**8**:427–433.

12. Chittiboina P, Conrad S, McCarthy P, Nanda A, Guthikonda B. The evolving role of hemodilution in treatment of cerebral vasospasm: a historical perspective. *World Neurosurg* 2011;**75**:660–664.

13. Friedlander RM. Clinical practice. Arteriovenous malformations of the brain. *N Engl J Med* 2007;**356**:2704–2712.

14. Trivedi RA, Kirkpatrick PJ. Arteriovenous malformations of the cerebral circulation that rupture in pregnancy. *J Obstet Gynaecol* 2003;**23**:484–489.

15. Ogilvy CS, Stieg PE, Awad I, *et al.* AHA Scientific Statement: recommendations for the management of intracranial arteriovenous malformations: a statement for healthcare professionals from a special writing group of the Stroke Council, American Stroke Association. *Stroke* 2001;**32**:1458–1471.

16. Feske SK. Posterior reversible encephalopathy syndrome: a review. *Semin Neurol* 2011;**31**:202–215.

17. Roth C, Ferbert A. The posterior reversible encephalopathy syndrome: what's certain, what's new? *Pract Neurol* 2011;**11**:136–144.

18. Chan LY, Tsui MH, Leung TN. Guillain–Barré syndrome in pregnancy. *Acta Obstet Gynecol Scand* 2004;**83**:319–325.

19. Pritchard J. Guillain–Barré syndrome. *Clin Med* 2010;**10**:399–401.

20. Steering Committee for the Consortium for Spinal Cord Medicine. Early acute management in adults with spinal cord injury: a clinical practice guideline for health-care professionals. *J Spinal Cord Med* 2008;**31**:403–479.

21. Vanden Hoek TL, Morrison LJ, Shuster M, *et al.* Part 12: Cardiac arrest in special situations. 2010 American Heart Association Guidelines for Cardiopulmonary Resuscitation and Emergency Cardiovascular Care. *Circulation* 2010;**122**: S829–S861.

22. Toledo P. The role of lipid emulsion during advanced cardiac life support for local anesthetic toxicity. *Int J Obstet Anesth* 2011;**20**:60–63.

23. Association of Anaesthetists of Great Britain and Ireland. *Safety Guideline: Management of Severe Local Anesthetic Toxicity.* London: Association of Anaesthetists of Great Britain and Ireland, 2010 (http://www.aagbi.org/sites/default/files/la_toxicity_2010_0.pdf, accessed 7 December 2012).

24. Reynolds F. Neurological infections after neuraxial anesthesia. *Anesthesiol Clin* 2008;**26**:23–52.

25. American Society of Anesthesiologists Task Force on Infectious Complications Associated with Neuraxial Techniques. Practice advisory for the prevention, diagnosis, and management of infectious complications associated with neuraxial techniques. *Anesthesiology* 2010;**112**:530–545.

Chapter 27

Acute kidney injury in pregnancy and critical care emergencies

Michelle Hladunewich and John Davison

Introduction

The approach to and the assessment of acute kidney injury (AKI) in pregnancy should not differ from the non-pregnant population with awareness of potential prerenal, renal, and postrenal etiologies. There are, however, conditions that can impair kidney function that are either unique to pregnancy or potentially worsened by the pregnant state and these require heightened clinical acumen to ensure the proper diagnosis is made in the face of the sometimes confusing gestational physiological changes. Furthermore, the management of these conditions, which might include immunosuppressive therapy, plasmapheresis, and/or dialysis, must take into account the potential impact on both the mother and unborn fetus.

Renal physiological changes associated with pregnancy

Renal anatomy and physiology are significantly affected by pregnancy, with changes to kidney size as well as glomerular and tubular function. These physiological changes are critical for an optimal pregnancy outcome and awareness of this healthy accommodation is necessary to assist with the diagnosis of kidney problems in the context of pregnancy (Table 27.1).

Healthy women accommodate to pregnancy via the upregulation of vasodilatory and the downregulation of vasoconstricting hormones, resulting in a decrease in the systemic vascular resistance and mean arterial pressure despite an increase in cardiac output. At the level of the kidney, these hormonal alterations result in dilatation of the collecting system with a small increase in renal size as well as vasodilatation with increased renal plasma flow and glomerular filtration rate (GFR). Although precise mechanisms are not completely understood, the enhanced GFR that accompanies healthy pregnancy along with altered tubular reabsorption may be responsible for increased urinary levels of glucose, amino acids, uric acid, and protein. The decreased renal tubular threshold for bicarbonate reabsorption results in a net decrease in serum bicarbonate by 4–5 mmol/L, despite progesterone-governed stimulation of the respiratory center. Finally, an intricate balance of natriuretic, anti-natriuretic, and osmoregulatory factors governs gestational changes in serum electrolytes, resulting in mild hyponatremia and hypokalemia as well as a lowered plasma osmolality. Table 27.1 summarizes these key anatomical and physiological alterations associated with the pregnant state.

Prerenal etiologies

In the critically ill pregnant or postpartum woman, the most common cause of acute renal insufficiency lies along the continuum from prerenal hemodynamic compromise through acute tubular damage to the final irreversible state of cortical necrosis. Prolonged renal hypoperfusion, the result of insufficient cardiac output, extreme hypovolemia, and/or vasodilatation, often coupled with other nephrotoxic insults, is the most common cause of prerenal insufficiency, which can progress to more sustained tubular damage as ischemia produces a cascade of damaging inflammatory mediators as well as reactive oxygen species. Acute cortical necrosis would be the result of an overwhelming hypotensive and toxic insult wherein the complete absence of cellular ATP results in cell swelling, loss of membrane integrity, and disruption of active transport with the subsequent release of proteolytic enzymes. This can result in rapid cellular demise and death. Fortunately, this final progression to acute cortical necrosis with non-recoverable renal function is rare, but it has been documented in critically ill pregnant women who develop disseminated

Maternal Critical Care: A Multidisciplinary Approach, ed. Marc Van de Velde, Helen Scholefield, and Lauren A. Plante. Published by Cambridge University Press. © Cambridge University Press 2013.

Table 27.1. Pregnancy-associated anatomical and physiological renal changes

Physiological change	Clinical implication
Increase in kidney size (1 cm) Dilatation of the collecting system (right more than left)	Complicate diagnosis of true obstruction
Increase in renal plasma flow and hence glomerular filtration rate Altered tubular reabsorption of protein, glucose, amino acids, uric acid, and bicarbonate	Decreased serum creatinine Slight increase in urine protein excretion, with abnormal proteinuria defined as >300 mg daily Glycosuria and aminoaciduria in some women Decreased uric acid in first and second trimesters, thereafter increasing towards term as a result of the fetal and placental mass Decreased serum bicarbonate by 4–5 mmol/L
Increase in total body sodium by 3–4 mEq/day (net balance of 900–1000 mEq) and total body potassium up to 320 mEq Decrease in set point for thirst and antidiuretic hormone release Expansion of plasma volume	Decreased plasma osmolality Decreased serum sodium and potassium levels

Table 27.2. Pregnancy-specific etiologies of prerenal insufficiency and acute tubular injury

Mechanism	Etiology
Volume contraction/hypotension	Massive hemorrhage Hyperemesis gravidarum Adrenocortical failure (usually through failure to augment steroids to cover delivery in patients on long-term therapy)
Volume contraction/hypotension and coagulopathy	Coagulopathy secondary to massive hemorrhage Aamniotic fluid embolus Acute fatty liver of pregnancy
Volume contraction/hypotension, coagulopathy, and infection	Septic abortion Chorioamnionitis Pyelonephritis Puerperal sepsis

intravascular coagulation [1]. Acute cortical necrosis is primarily noted in developing countries but recently decrements in the prevalence were reported by investigators in India citing improvements in medical management of obstetrical complications including septic abortion and haemorrhage from placental abruption [2].

Table 27.2 summarizes potential pregnancy-specific causes of prerenal insufficiency with the potential to progress to acute tubular injury and cortical necrosis. The diagnosis is typically based on a thorough search for hemodynamic and nephrotoxic insults. On physical examination, particular attention must be paid to the patient's volume status as adequate fluid resuscitation may arrest prerenal insufficiency, whereas fluid overload is an indication for urgent diuresis and/or dialysis.

The urine sediment may reveal the presence of heme-granular casts, pathognomonic of tubular injury, whereas abrupt anuria accompanied by hematuria and flank pain, particularly in the context of disseminated intravascular coagulation, is suggestive of cortical necrosis.

Renal interstitial, vascular, and glomerular etiologies

Any potential interstitial, vascular, or glomerular cause of renal insufficiency and/or proteinuria can present or worsen during pregnancy. A careful nephrological assessment must include examination of the urine sediment and quantification of urine protein, as well as the appropriate laboratory and serological assessments as guided by the clinical presentation (Table 27.3). Further, a renal biopsy might be considered to assist in the diagnosis and to guide treatment if the clinical presentation includes nephrotic syndrome or deterioration in renal function in early pregnancy without an established diagnosis. Data are limited with respect to the safety of kidney biopsy in pregnancy, with the only sizable series from 1987 reporting a low complication rate of 4.5% based on 111 renal biopsies in 104 women over 20 years [3]. This was confirmed by a smaller subsequent series in women before 30 weeks of gestation [4]. Expert opinion, therefore, recommends a cut-off for renal biopsy of approximately 30–32 weeks of gestation, as the further along in gestation, the more likely that pre-eclampsia could hamper the safety of the procedure through evolving hypertension and abnormal coagulation indices.

Table 27.3. Recommended assessment and interpretation of urine and blood samples in pregnant women with acute deterioration in kidney function with or without proteinuria

Assessment	Findings
Urinalysis and urine microscopy	RBCs and RBC casts (vasculitis, lupus nephritis, and other inflammatory causes of acute glomerulonephritis) WBCs and WBC casts (pyelonephritis, acute interstitial nephritis secondary to allergic reactions to medications, lupus nephritis) Oval fat bodies (severe nephrotic syndrome of any cause)
Quantification of urine protein	Urine dipstick too dependent on urine concentration Protein–creatinine or albumin–creatinine ratio can screen 24 hour collections remains the gold standard
Common laboratory assessments: complete blood counts, liver function tests, uric acid, peripheral smear, lactate dehydrogenase, haptoglobin	Increased uric acid, aspartate transaminase, and alanine transaminase with decreased platelet count: pre-eclampsia/HELLP syndrome Peripheral smear for schistocytes and RBC fragments, decreased haptoglobin, and increased lactate dehydrogenase with low platelets: thrombotic thrombocytopenic purpura/hemolytic uremic syndrome
Serological assessment: complement, specific autoantibodies, lupus anticoagulant and/or anti-cardiolipin antibodies	Decreased complement levels (C3, C4), positive anti-nuclear antibodies, anti-double-stranded DNA and/or extractable nuclear antigens (anti-Ro/SSA, anti-La/SSB): lupus nephritis Positive lupus anticoagulant and/or anti-cardiolipin antibodies: antiphospholipid antibody syndrome Positive extractable nuclear antigens: lupus, mixed connective tissue disease, or scleroderma Positive anti-Ro, anti-La: lupus with the potential for fetal heart block Positive anti-neutrophil cytoplasmic antibody or anti-glomerular basement membrane antibodies: pulmonary renal syndrome Other serology may also be indicated depending on associated morbidities and clinical presentation (e.g. for HIV, hepatitis viruses)

RBC, red blood cell; WBC, white blood cell; HELLP, hemolysis, elevated liver enzymes, low platelets.

Although a thorough assessment is necessary in each presenting woman, there are a number of important conditions that are either exacerbated specifically by pregnancy (acute pyelonephritis, lupus nephritis, thrombotic thrombocytopenic purpura/hemolytic uremic syndrome (TTP/HUS)) or are unique to pregnancy (acute fatty liver of pregnancy, pre-eclampsia/HELLP syndrome (hemolysis, elevated liver enzymes, and low platelets)). Finally, special consideration to the etiology of renal compromise must be given to women with established chronic kidney disease (CKD) or a renal allograft, as it is often difficult to distinguish pregnancy-associated conditions from deterioration in native kidney or graft function.

Pyelonephritis

Urinary tract infection is among the most common complication noted in pregnancy and *Escherichia coli* is the most frequently cultured bacterial organism [5]. Because of the pregnancy-associated dilatation of the urinary tract, asymptomatic bacteriuria can progress to cystitis and/or pyelonephritis, along with more severe maternal complications such as septicemia and renal insufficiency, if not promptly treated.

Screening for bacteriuria using urine dipstick followed by urine culture when positive is, therefore, recommended [6]. Subsequent initiation of antibiotic therapy based on culture sensitivity will reduce progression to cystitis and more importantly to pyelonephritis [7]. In women presenting with symptoms of cystitis, empiric therapy may be recommended [8], including trimethoprim–sulfamethoxazole, nitrofurantoin, and cephalexin. Current guidelines support the use of therapy for 3 days in healthy women or for 7 days to increase the likelihood of definitive cure in women with comorbidities [6]. Acquisition of a negative follow-up urine culture after completion of the antibiotic regimen is required, along with periodic screening throughout the remainder of the pregnancy [6].

Vigilance for pyelonephritis is necessary at all stages of pregnancy along with aggressive management with prompt empiric treatment until culture and sensitivity results are available. Recent data from 440 inpatients with antepartum pyelonephritis noted respiratory insufficiency in 10% and septicemia in 20%, based on blood culture results [5]. However, a decrease in the prevalence of renal dysfunction was noted (20% to 2%), a finding that the authors attributed to early, aggressive treatment [5].

Lupus nephritis and other connective tissue diseases

Autoimmune diseases are covered in more depth in Chapter 35, but those with the potential to cause renal involvement include lupus, anti-neutrophil cytoplasmic antibody-associated vasculitis, Goodpasture syndrome, and scleroderma renal disease. Lupus nephritis can present or flare during any trimester or the early postpartum period, and active nephritis predicts a particularly poor pregnancy outcome [9]. The literature notes a number of cases of anti-neutrophil cytoplasmic antibody-associated vasculitis, either presenting in pregnancy or relapsing during pregnancy, sufficient to suggest the possibility that, as in lupus, pregnancy might result in disease activation [10]. Despite an approximate 75% live birth rate, there are numerous complications, with pre-eclampsia complicating approximately 25% and preterm delivery occurring is just over 40% of reported cases [10]. Goodpasture syndrome is a rare disease where anti-glomerular basement membrane antibodies result in pulmonary hemorrhage and crescentic renal disease. The handful of cases in the literature suggest overall poor maternal and fetal outcomes [11]. Fortunately, scleroderma is also rare, and women whose disease is limited to the skin do reasonably except for increased rates of pre-eclampsia (22.9%) and intrauterine growth retardation (5.3%) [12]. Those women with underlying vascular involvement can have devastating outcomes in terms of maternal morbidity and mortality through accelerated hypertension, renal failure, and pulmonary hypertension.

Thrombotic microangiopathies

The renal thrombotic microangiopathies include TTP and HUS, disorders characterized by disseminated occlusion of arterioles and capillaries with agglutinated platelets, resulting in ischemia (see Chapter 25). With recent insights into pathophysiology, TTP is becoming better understood in the context of pregnancy, and, more recently, the pregnancy outcomes in atypical HUS-associated complement gene mutations have been described [13]. This heightened understanding is critical to the differentiation of these potentially treatable conditions (where plasmapheresis is the standard of care and even eculizumab may prove to have a role in pregnancy [14]) from other pregnancy-related conditions, including pre-eclampsia, the HELLP syndrome, and acute fatty liver of pregnancy (where delivery may be imminently necessary) (Table 27.4).

Acute fatty liver of pregnancy

In acute fatty liver of pregnancy (see Chapter 37), the mechanism of renal failure is unclear. A single series of four patients where renal pathology was documented included tubular damage secondary to lipid accumulation along with mesangial cell interposition and subendothelial electron-dense deposits not unlike the findings noted in pre-eclampsia [15]. Therefore, both acute fatty liver of pregnancy and pre-eclampsia/HELLP syndrome are similar with respect to the reported presence of hypertension and proteinuria [16].

Pre-eclampsia/HELLP syndrome

Pre-eclampsia, the most common cause of the constellation of renal insufficiency, hypertension, and proteinuria (see Chapter 36), is essentially a disease of the placenta, wherein the release of anti-angiogenic factors (soluble fms-like tyrosine kinase 1 and soluble endoglin) from an abnormal, ischemic placenta causes injury to the maternal endothelium. Consequently, on renal biopsy, glomerular endotheliosis is the hallmark finding [17]. In the future, assays for anti-angiogenic factors might prove useful in discriminating between pre-eclampsia and other etiologies of renal injury and deterioration that contribute to the often complex clinical diagnostic dilemmas. To date these assays have proven useful in a variety of clinical scenarios, including presumed glomerulonephritis [18], lupus [19], and in patients on hemodialysis [20], but they are not as yet widely commercially available.

Chronic kidney disease

Women who enter pregnancy with established CKD are a challenging, high-risk population because their

Table 27.4. Differential diagnosis of pre-eclampsia, acute fatty liver of pregnancy, thrombotic thrombocytopenic purpura, and hemolytic uremic syndrome

	Pre-eclampsia	AFLP	TTP	HUS
Symptoms				
Onset	>20 weeks	>28 weeks	Anytime	Peripartum
Nausea/vomiting	− or +	+++	− or +	− or +
Abdominal pain	+ to +++	++	0 to +	0′ to +
Signs				
Hypertension	+ to +++	−/+	+ to +++	+ to +++
Fever	−	−/+	+	−/+
Abnormal mentation	− to +++	− to +++	− to +++	−/+
Liver function tests				
Bilirubin	N to 5×N	S to 30×N	↑ Indirect	↑ Indirect
Aalanine transaminase	S to 100×N	S to 20×N	N to S	N to S
Glucose	N (rarely ↓)	N or ↓	N	N
Ammonia	N	↑	N	N
Hematology				
White blood cell count	N to ↑	↑↑	N or ↑	N or ↑
Schistocytes	+/++	+/++	+++	+++
Normoblasts	−	+/++	+++	+++
Platelets (× 10^9/L)	30 to N	20–150	5–100	5–100
Prothrombin time/partial thromboplastin time	N or S↑	N to ↑↑↑	N	N
Fibrinogen	N or S↓	N or ↓	N	N or S↓
Fibrin degradation products	N or S↑	N or ↑	N	N or S↑
Antithrombin III	↓	↓	N	N
ADAMST13	N	N	↓	N
C3/C4	N	N	N	↓
Renal				
Creatinine	N to 5×N	N to 10×N	N to 5×N	Rapid ↑
Proteinuria	+ to ++++	0 to ++++	+ to ++++	+ to ++++
Uric acid	↑	N or ↑	N or ↑	N or ↑

AFLP, acute fatty liver of pregnancy; TPP, thrombotic thrombocytopenic purpura; HUS, hemolytic uremic syndrome; N, normal; S, slightly raised.

renal disease can flare, their renal dysfunction proteinuria can worsen, and/or their hypertension may accelerate and prove more difficult to manage. Further, they are at considerable risk for untoward maternal and fetal outcomes, including fetal growth restriction, fetal demise, pre-eclampsia, and preterm delivery. Indeed, the presence of pre-pregnancy renal insufficiency, proteinuria, and hypertension are all factors that contribute to poor pregnancy outcomes in an additive manner.

Early studies tended to utilize the serum creatinine to stratify pregnancy risk. A typical classification defined mild renal insufficiency as a serum creatinine 123 μmol/L (1.4 mg/dL), moderate renal insufficiency as 124–220 μmol/L (1.4–2.4 mg/dL), and severe renal insufficiency as a creatinine ≥221 μmol/L (2.5 mg/dL). In a classic paper by Jones and Hayslett published over two decades ago, pregnancy-related loss of kidney function was noted in a staggering 43% of pregnancies with moderate to severe disease, of which 10% rapidly progressed to end-stage renal disease [21]. Serum creatinine, however, is likely too imprecise to be utilized to stratify all women prior to pregnancy as it does not take into account patient size and muscle mass, and in young women serum creatinine often inadequately reflects the actual degree of histological renal damage. Tubulointerstital changes involving >20% of the cortical area, glomerulosclerosis, and severe arteriolar hyalinosis have all been deemed important with respect to pregnancy outcome [22,23].

More recently, therefore, studies have prognosticated pregnancy outcome on the basis of an estimated GFR, which has served to increase the reported prevalence of CKD in pregnancy significantly from 1 to 3% as women with more subtle renal insufficiency are identified [24]. Two formulas frequently applied to calculate the estimated GFR include the Cockcroft–Gault formula, which estimates GFR from gender, age, and weight, and the Modified Diet in Renal Disease (MDRD) formula, which was developed in a multiethnic population of men and women with moderate renal impairment. The latter has the advantage of not requiring patient weight to calculate the estimated GFR. Importantly, neither formula can be used during pregnancy to estimate renal function as the Cockcroft–Gault formula can substantially overestimate or underestimate true GFR [25], while the MDRD equation consistently underestimates true GFR as measured by inulin clearance [25]. However when used to stratify risk pre-pregnancy, studies have noted adverse outcomes even at earlier stages of CKD when associated with proteinuria and hypertension [26]. A recent systematic review summarizing 13 studies concluded adverse pregnancy outcomes to be at least twice as common in women with CKD than in women without CKD [27]. Therefore, women with identified CKD of various histological types, along with varying degrees of renal insufficiency, proteinuria, and hypertension, require preconception planning to improve pregnancy outcomes and increase awareness of potential risks and complications so that informed decision making can occur.

Renal allograft dysfunction

Similar to native kidneys, allografts adapt to pregnancy with increased kidney volume [28], increased GFR, and hence enhanced creatinine clearance (34% on average; range 10–60%), with better pre-pregnancy function predicting more robust pregnancy adaptation [29]. Therefore, a decrease in serum creatinine is to be expected in women with renal allografts. When allograft function worsens during pregnancy, there must be the same meticulous assessment as in women with native kidneys, including urinalysis, quantification of urine protein, and scrutiny for laboratory clues that might indicate de novo renal disease or a superimposed pregnancy-related condition such as pre-eclampsia. Pre-pregnancy graft dysfunction and hypertension, shorter mean intervals between transplantation and pregnancy, as well as previous rejection episodes have been noted to be risk factors for untoward pregnancy outcomes, including pre-eclampsia 27% (95% confidence interval (CI), 25–29) and preterm delivery 46% (95% CI, 44–48) [30].

Unique to a renal allograft is the potential for acute rejection, which may present with increased creatinine, fever, and graft tenderness. Pregnancy per se is not a risk factor, but gestational alterations in drug metabolism can precipitate rejection. For example, cyclosporine metabolism tends to increase and, therefore, higher doses may be required, whereas tacrolimus metabolism may decrease by inhibition of hepatic cytochrome P450 enzymes, with the potential for exacerbating hypertension and causing nephrotoxicity.

The mandated immunosuppressed state also places these women at increased risk of infections. Ongoing close surveillance for bacterial infections, including regular urine cultures, and prompt treatment is necessary. A number of potential infectious complications can also result in serious neonatal compromise, the most common and significant being primary or reactivated cytomegalovirus infection during pregnancy [31]. Primary maternal infection has a 30–40% risk of intrauterine transmission and a 20–25% risk for the development of fetal sequelae, including microcephaly, hearing loss, visual impairment, mental retardation, and also more subtle learning disabilities [32]. The transmission rate to the fetus is significantly lower in reactivated cytomegalovirus disease.

The diagnosis of primary maternal cytomegalovirus infection is based on the de novo appearance of virus-specific immunoglobulin (Ig) M or G if the woman was previously known to be IgG seronegative. Prenatal diagnosis of fetal infection should be based on presence of the virus in amniotic fluid. The diagnosis of secondary infection is based on a significant rise in IgG antibody titer; the risk–benefit ratio of amniocentesis in secondary infection must then be carefully considered given the lower rate of transmission. The incidence of primary or reactivated infections in transplant recipients, however, is largely unknown, with very few cases reported [33].

Postrenal aetiologies

Obstructive causes of renal insufficiency, such as nephrolithiasis, should be less likely as pregnancy progresses. Dilatation of the right kidney usually exceeds that of the left kidney, and begins in the 6th week of gestation, with maximal dilatation progressing at a rate of 0.5 mm/week until week 24–26, thereafter slowing to 0.3 mm/week until term [34]. Although over 50% of pregnant women demonstrate some degree of dilatation, there is significant variability between patients, and even serial variability within the same patient, making the diagnosis of true obstruction challenging [35]. A baseline scan in women at risk along with serial radiological evaluations may be necessary to determine if worsening renal function has an obstructive cause. Further, documented nephrolithiasis needs prompt urological assessment as stones large enough to cause obstruction in pregnancy have also been associated with higher rates of urinary tract infection and pyelonephritis [36], with preterm delivery nearly doubling in one study involving over 2000 women admitted for nephrolithiasis (adjusted odds ratio 1.8; 95% CI, 1.5–2.1) [37]. Recent developments in endoscopic equipment may allow for more definitive treatments, including ureteroscopy and even yttrium–aluminum–garnet lithotripsy, as opposed to temporary ureteral stenting procedures and nephrostomy tubes, both of which postpone definitive management until after delivery and further heighten the risk for potential infectious complications [38–41]. Surgical trauma is another rare cause of postobstructive renal failure and can include damage to the ureters during cesarean section or with repair of cervical and/or vaginal lacerations, as well as from significant pelvic or broad ligament hematomas.

General principles of hypertension management

Hypertension is a common complication of CKD and renal disease and a well-established risk factor for the development of pre-eclampsia. The principles of hypertension management do not differ from pregnant women without CKD (see Chapter 36), but blood pressure targets are typically more stringent, with most obstetric societies recommending targeting a blood pressure consistently < 140/90 mmHg. Commonly used, safe, intravenous and oral options for the treatment of hypertension in women with and without CKD include, but are not limited to, methyldopa, labetalol, hydralazine, and nifedipine (Table 27.5). Although it may have a blood pressure-lowering effect, magnesium sulfate should not be used specifically for that purpose particularly in women with advanced CKD as it undergoes renal clearance and can readily cause toxicity.

Table 27.5. Commonly used drugs for the treatment of hypertension that are considered pregnancy safe options[a]

Drug	Dosing	Onset of action	Duration of action
Methyldopa	*Initial*: 250 mg oral twice a day *Maximum*: 3 g oral daily	3–6 hours	12–24 hours
Labetalol	*Acute option*: 10 mg intravenous; can be repeated at 10 minute intervals to a maximum of 300 mg	5–10 minutes	Dose dependent (2–18 hours)
	Initial: 100 mg oral twice a day *Maximum*: 2.4 g oral daily	1–4 hours	8–12 hours
Hydralazine	*Acute option*: 2.5–10 mg intravenous; can be repeated at 10–20 minute intervals	5–20 minutes	1–4 hours
	Initial: 10 mg oral four times a day *Maximum*: 300 mg oral daily	20–30 minutes	8–12 hours
Nifedipine	*Acute option*: 10 mg oral	≈20 minutes	2–5 hours
Nifedipine XL	*Initial*: 30–60 mg oral once or twice a day *Maximum*: 90–120 mg daily	1–4 hours	8–24 hours

[a] This is not a comprehensive list; other drugs might also be useful and might be used if the benefits outweigh the risks.

Many young women with CKD may be taking renin–angiotensin system blockers, which are absolutely contraindicated in pregnancy. Teratogenicity in the second and third trimester secondary to use of angiotensin-converting enzyme inhibitors is well described and includes oligohydramnios, neonatal anuria and renal failure, limb contractures, craniofacial abnormalities, pulmonary hypoplasia, and patent ductus arteriosus [42]. Angiotensin receptor blockers may be more teratogenic, with case reports of significant malformations emerging after first trimester exposure [43]. As yet, there are no case reports of teratogenicity after exposure to the newer direct renin inhibitors, but there is no reason to expect that they will not be equally or even more teratogenic; consequently, these must be used with caution in young women with reproductive potential. That being said, unintentional trimester exposure does not require termination, but careful assessment by fetal imaging is mandatory [44].

Immunosuppressive therapies

Although there are no immunosuppressive medications adequately tested in pregnancy to be designated by the US Food and Drug Administration as pregnancy category A, there are a number of medications where the risk–benefit ratio is appropriate for use in pregnancy. These include prednisone, azathioprine, calcineurin inhibitors, and possibly rituximab, but not mycophenolate mofetil or cyclophosphamide.

Only a fraction of the oral dose of prednisone reaches the fetus. Therefore, prednisone is considered a safe option at low doses. Higher doses, however, may not be completely without risk, as first trimester exposure maybe associated with an increased risk of cleft palate (approximately 3/1000 compared with 1/1000 in the general population) and exposure later in pregnancy can be associated with increased potential for the development of gestational diabetes and exacerbation of hypertension. Azathioprine requires inosine triphosphate pyrophosphorylase for conversion to its active metabolite, an enzyme lacking in fetal liver. Both cyclosporine and tacrolimus can be safely used in pregnant women. Although smaller babies have been reported in conjunction with use of these medications, it is not clear if this is a direct drug effect or secondary to the underlying disease that necessitated their use. The calcineurin inhibitors do have the potential to exacerbate hypertension and can be nephrotoxic. At present, there are some reassuring data on the use of rituximab primarily from the oncology literature. To date, no fetal malformations have been noted, but CD19 B-cells were either undetectable or severely decreased in exposed neonates, returning to normal levels by 3–6 months later without documented serious infections [45].

Mycophenolate mofetil is a human teratogen with an identifiable pattern of malformations: craniofacial (microtia or anotia, absent auditory canal, cleft palate, hypertelorism) and limb anomalies [46]. Cyclophosphamide is contraindicated at least in the first trimester where it has been noted to cause spontaneous pregnancy loss, growth deficiency, developmental delay, craniosynostosis, blepharophimosis, flat nasal bridge, abnormal ears, and distal limb defects, including hypoplastic thumbs and oligodactyly [47].

Dialysis, plasmapheresis, and extracorporeal removal of antiangiogenic factors

Acute kindney injury, if severe enough, may require renal replacement therapy irrespective of the etiology. Indications for dialysis are no different in pregnancy and include imbalances in electrolytes and volume status that cannot be managed medically. Dialysis may, however, be considered at an earlier stage or at a higher intensity during pregnancy in an attempt to decrease fetal risks such as stillbirth and to manage polyhydramnios. Fetal mortality and polyhydramnios have been noted to be directly related to level of blood urea nitrogen (BUN), with no successful documented pregnancies once that exceeds 21.4 µmol/L (60 mg/dL) [48]. More recently, in a series of 28 pregnant women receiving hemodialysis with 18 surviving infants, a significant negative relationship was noted between BUN and birth weight and gestational age [49]. A birth weight of at least 1500 g was achieved at a BUN of 17.9 µmol/L (49 mg/dL) and a gestational age of at least 32 weeks was achieved at a BUN of 17.1 µmol/L (48 mg/dL). Although this level of BUN is the accepted target in many centers, the best pregnancy outcomes have been noted in patients receiving daily nocturnal hemodialysis [50]. Ultrafiltration goals must be determined carefully to avoid hypotension during dialysis, which could impair placental and fetal perfusion. Drugs typically given to dialysis patients, including erythropoietin-stimulating agents and heparin, are safe.

The delivery of plasmapheresis does not differ in pregnancy, but the same precautions apply as with hemodialysis – avoid hypotension. Recently, a small pilot study in three women with severe early-onset pre-eclampsia utilized dextran sulfate cellulose apheresis treatments to reduce circulating soluble fms-like tyrosine kinase 1 levels in a dose-dependent fashion [51]. Proteinuria was reduced and blood pressure stabilized without apparent adverse effects to mother or fetus. The future potential for this therapy remains to be determined.

Anaesthetic considerations

With reference to renal patients, specific issues include early recognition and treatment of sepsis, regular frequent blood pressure monitoring in severe hypertension, avoidance and/or treatment of fluid overload, awareness of unpredictable responses to vasoactive medications, and assessment of the impact of blood loss at the time of delivery on the overall renal situation. The use of general anesthetic and regional anesthetic techniques in relation to delivery has been discussed in Section 3 and the basic principles enunciated there apply equally to renal patients. Unique to renal patients, uremia may result in platelet dysfunction with increased bleeding potential, and non-steroidal anti-inflammatory drugs, often an integral component of postpartum pain management, should be employed with extreme caution in women who already have hypertension and/or renal compromise.

Considerations for future pregnancies

Reassessment of women with hypertension and/or renal compromise following a complicated pregnancy is critical to improve her long-term health as well as to safely plan future pregnancies. Pregnancy can be the first time many young women are assessed by a medical team. Indeed, the diagnosis of chronic hypertension or renal disease may not be made until this time, and as both are strong predictors of pregnancy complications, early onset of severe placental disease should have made their consideration as possible risk factors obvious. In a study where women who presented with severe pre-eclampsia had a postpartum renal biopsy, unrecognized kidney pathology, most commonly IgA nephropathy, was diagnosed in 22% and a strong relationship between pre-eclampsia severity (delivered prior to 30 weeks of gestation) and the presence of undiagnosed renal disease was

noted [52]. Consequently, all women with kidney disease should consult with a nephrologist and obstetrician to discuss the potential impact of their renal pathology – the degree of renal insufficiency, the amount of proteinuria, and presence of hypertension – on their future obstetric outcomes.

Further, women with renal disease with the potential to flare during pregnancy also need careful counseling and optimization. In women with lupus nephritis, 6 months of sustained disease quiescence prior to considering a pregnancy, and converting a young woman to pregnancy-safe treatment, has been recommended based on studies that show the disease flared in 7% of patients with inactive disease compared with 61% of patients with active disease at the time of conception [53]. In women with pregnancy-associated TTP, the overall risk of recurrent TTP is reported to be rare (14%) [54]. The risk of recurrence in congenital TTP, however, is reported to be 100% [55]. Therefore the detection of severe deficiency of ADAMTS13 or of congenital defects in the alternative complement pathway (atypical HUS) may assist with future pregnancy planning.

Although it was previously thought that the consequences of maternal placental disease resolved quickly and completely after delivery of the placenta, it is now apparent that placental disease is a marker of future adverse maternal vascular health. This relationship between pre-eclampsia and cardiovascular disease was first noted in a study that utilized the Norwegian Medical Birth Registry [56], demonstrating an almost three-fold increased risk of death and an eight-fold increased risk of cardiovascular death in women who delivered prior to 37 weeks of gestation, interpreted as a surrogate marker for more severe disease because there was no increased risk of death among women with pre-eclampsia who delivered at term. In addition to an increased risk of cardiovascular disease, an increased risk of cerebrovascular disease, peripheral vascular disease, and end-stage renal disease was also noted [57,58]. The impact of increased vascular risk is, however, best demonstrated by the Child Health and Development cohort, with data from over 14 000 women with, on average, 30 years of follow-up. This indicated that the median age for cardiovascular events was 56 years, with a cumulative survival of 85.9% for early-onset pre-eclampsia compared with 98.3% for late-onset pre-eclampsia and 99.3% for healthy pregnancies [59]. Therefore, the immediate postpartum period becomes a crucial time for health education with respect to cardiovascular risk reduction and long-term health maintenance strategies, including exercise, healthy eating habits, salt reduction, blood pressure monitoring, and medications as appropriate.

References

1. Matlin RA, Gary NE. Acute cortical necrosis. Case report and review of the literature. *Am J Med* 1974;**56**:110–118.

2. Prakash J, Vohra R, Wani IA, *et al*. Decreasing incidence of renal cortical necrosis in patients with acute renal failure in developing countries: a single-centre experience of 22 years from Eastern India. *Nephrol Dial Transplant* 2007;**22**:1213–1217.

3. Packham D, Fairley KF. Renal biopsy: indications and complications in pregnancy. *Br J Obstet Gynaecol* 1987;**94**:935–939.

4. Chen HH, Lin HC, Yeh JC, Chen CP. Renal biopsy in pregnancies complicated by undetermined renal disease. *Acta Obstet Gynecol Scand* 2001;**80**:888–893.

5. Hill JB, Sheffield JS, McIntire DD, Wendel GD Jr. Acute pyelonephritis in pregnancy. *Obstet Gynecol* 2005;**105**:18–23.

6. American College of Obstetricians and Gynecologists. Educational Bulletin 245: antimicrobial therapy for obstetric patients. *Int J Gynaecol Obstet* 1998;**61**:299–308.

7. Smaill F, Vazquez JC. Antibiotics for asymptomatic bacteriuria in pregnancy. *Cochrane Database Syst Rev* 2007:CD000490.

8. Vazquez JC, Abalos E. Treatments for symptomatic urinary tract infections during pregnancy. *Cochrane Database Syst Rev* 2011:CD002256.

9. Smyth A, Oliveira GH, Lahr BD, *et al*. A systematic review and meta-analysis of pregnancy outcomes in patients with systemic lupus erythematosus and lupus nephritis. *Clin J Am Soc Nephrol* 2010;**5**:2060–2068.

10. Koukoura O, Mantas N, Linardakis H, Hajiioannou J, Sifakis S. Successful term pregnancy in a patient with Wegener's granulomatosis: case report and literature review. *Fertil Steril* 2008;**89**:457 e1–5.

11. Hatfield T, Steiger R, Wing DA. Goodpasture's disease in pregnancy: case report and review of the literature. *Am J Perinatol* 2007;**24**:619–621.

12. Chakravarty EF, Khanna D, Chung L. Pregnancy outcomes in systemic sclerosis, primary pulmonary hypertension, and sickle cell disease. *Obstet Gynecol* 2008;**111**:927–934.

13. Fakhouri F, Roumenina L, Provot F, *et al*. Pregnancy-associated hemolytic uremic syndrome revisited in the era of complement gene mutations. *J Am Soc Nephrol* 2010;**21**:859–867.

14. Kose O, Zimmerhackl LB, Jungraithmayr T, Mache C, Nurnberger J. New treatment options for atypical hemolytic uremic syndrome with the complement inhibitor eculizumab. *Semin Thromb Hemost* 2010;**36**:669–672.

15. Slater DN, Hague WM. Renal morphological changes in idiopathic acute fatty liver of pregnancy. *Histopathology* 1984;**8**:567–581.

16. Vigil-De Gracia P. Acute fatty liver and HELLP syndrome: two distinct pregnancy disorders. *Int J Gynaecol Obstet* 2001;**73**:215–220.

17. Lafayette RA, Druzin M, Sibley R, *et al*. Nature of glomerular dysfunction in pre-eclampsia. *Kidney Int* 1998;**54**:1240–1249.

18. Hladunewich MA, Steinberg G, Karumanchi SA, *et al*. Angiogenic factor abnormalities and fetal demise in a twin pregnancy. *Nat Rev Nephrol* 2009;**5**:658–662.

19. Williams WW, Ecker JL, Thadhani RI, Rahemtullah A. Case 38-2005. *N Engl J Med* 2005;**353**: 2590–2600.

20. Shan HY, Rana S, Epstein FH, *et al*. Use of circulating antiangiogenic factors to differentiate other hypertensive disorders from preeclampsia in a pregnant woman on dialysis. *Am J Kidney Dis* 2008;**51**:1029–1032.

21. Jones DC, Hayslett JP. Outcome of pregnancy in women with moderate or severe renal insufficiency. *N Engl J Med* 1996;**335**:226–232.

22. Abe S, Amagasaki Y, Konishi K, *et al*. The influence of antecedent renal disease on pregnancy. *Am J Obstet Gynecol* 1985;**153**:508–514.

23. Packham DK, North RA, Fairley KF, *et al*. Primary glomerulonephritis and pregnancy. *Q J Med* 1989;**71**:537–553.

24. Piccoli GB, Attini R, Vasario E, *et al*. Pregnancy and chronic kidney disease: a challenge in all CKD stages. *Clin J Am Soc Nephrol* 2010;**5**:844–855.

25. Koetje PM, Spaan JJ, Kooman JP, Spaanderman ME, Peeters LL. Pregnancy reduces the accuracy of the estimated glomerular filtration rate based on Cockroft–Gault and MDRD formulas. *Reprod Sci* 2011;**18**:456–462.

26. Piccoli GB, Conijn A, Attini R, *et al*. Pregnancy in chronic kidney disease: need for a common language. *J Nephrol* 2011;**24**:282–299.

27. Nevis IF, Reitsma A, Dominic A, *et al*. Pregnancy outcomes in women with chronic kidney disease: a systematic review. *Clin J Am Soc Nephrol* 2011;**6**:2587–2598.

28. Absy M, Metreweli C, Matthews C, Al Khader A. Changes in transplanted kidney volume measured by ultrasound. *Br J Radiol* 1987;**60**:525–529.

29. Davison JM. The effect of pregnancy on kidney function in renal allograft recipients. *Kidney Int* 1985;**27**:74–79.

30. Deshpande NA, James NT, Kucirka LM, *et al.* Pregnancy outcomes in kidney transplant recipients: a systematic review and meta-analysis. *Am J Transplant* 2011;**11**:2388–2404.

31. Yinon Y, Farine D, Yudin MH. Screening, diagnosis, and management of cytomegalovirus infection in pregnancy. *Obstet Gynecol Surv* 2010;**65**:736–743.

32. McCarthy FP, Giles ML, Rowlands S, Purcell KJ, Jones CA. Antenatal interventions for preventing the transmission of cytomegalovirus (CMV) from the mother to fetus during pregnancy and adverse outcomes in the congenitally infected infant. *Cochrane Database Syst Rev* 2011;(3):CD008371.

33. Coscia LA, Constantinescu S, Moritz MJ, *et al.* Report from the National Transplantation Pregnancy Registry (NTPR): outcomes of pregnancy after transplantation. *Clin Transpl* 2009: 103–122.

34. Faundes A, Bricola-Filho M, Pinto e Silva JL. Dilatation of the urinary tract during pregnancy: proposal of a curve of maximal caliceal diameter by gestational age. *Am J Obstet Gynecol* 1998;**178**:1082–1086.

35. Fried AM, Woodring JH, Thompson DJ. Hydronephrosis of pregnancy: a prospective sequential study of the course of dilatation. *J Ultrasound Med* 1983;**2**:255–259.

36. Rosenberg E, Sergienko R, Abu-Ghanem S, *et al.* Nephrolithiasis during pregnancy: characteristics, complications, and pregnancy outcome. *World J Urol* 2011;**29**:743–747.

37. Swartz MA, Lydon-Rochelle MT, Simon D, Wright JL, Porter MP. Admission for nephrolithiasis in pregnancy and risk of adverse birth outcomes. *Obstet Gynecol* 2007;**109**:1099–1104.

38. Lifshitz DA, Lingeman JE. Ureteroscopy as a first-line intervention for ureteral calculi in pregnancy. *J Endocrinol* 2002;**16**:19–22.

39. Watterson JD, Girvan AR, Beiko DT, *et al.* Ureteroscopy and holmium:YAG laser lithotripsy: an emerging definitive management strategy for symptomatic ureteral calculi in pregnancy. *Urology* 2002;**60**:383–387.

40. Isen K, Hatipoglu NK, Dedeoglu S, *et al.* Experience with the diagnosis and management of symptomatic ureteric stones during pregnancy. *Urology* 2012;**79**:508–512.

41. Khoo L, Anson K, Patel U. Success and short-term complication rates of percutaneous nephrostomy during pregnancy. *J Vasc & Intervasc Radiol: JVIR* 2004;**15**:1469–1473.

42. How HY, Sibai BM. Use of angiotensin-converting enzyme inhibitors in patients with diabetic nephropathy. *J Matern Fetal Neonatal Med* 2002;**12**:402–407.

43. Enzensberger C, Eskef K, Schwarze A, Faas D, Axt-Fliedner R. Course and outcome of pregnancy after maternal exposure to angiotensin-II-receptor blockers: case report and review of the literature. *Ultraschall Med* 2012;**33**:493–461.

44. Diav-Citrin O, Shechtman S, Halberstadt Y, *et al.* Pregnancy outcome after in utero exposure to angiotensin converting enzyme inhibitors or angiotensin receptor blockers. *Reprod Toxicol* 2011;**31**:540–545.

45. Azim HA Jr., Azim H, Peccatori FA. Treatment of cancer during pregnancy with monoclonal antibodies: a real challenge. *Expert Rev Clin Immunol* 2010;**6**:821–826.

46. Anderka MT, Lin AE, Abuelo DN, Mitchell AA, Rasmussen SA. Reviewing the evidence for mycophenolate mofetil as a new teratogen: case report and review of the literature. *Am J Med Genet* 2009;**149A**:1241–1248.

47. Enns GM, Roeder E, Chan RT, *et al.* Apparent cyclophosphamide (cytoxan) embryopathy: a distinct phenotype? *Am J Med Genet* 1999;**86**:237–241.

48. Mackay EV. Pregnancy and Renal Disease A Ten-Year Survey. *Aust N Z J Obstet Gynaecol* 1963;**3**:21–34.

49. Asamiya Y, Otsubo S, Matsuda Y, *et al.* The importance of low blood urea nitrogen levels in pregnant patients undergoing hemodialysis to optimize birth weight and gestational age. *Kidney Int* 2009;**75**:1217–1222.

50. Barua M, Hladunewich M, Keunen J, *et al.* Successful pregnancies on nocturnal home hemodialysis. *Clin J Am Soc Nephrol* 2008;**3**:392–396.

51. Thadhani R, Kisner T, Hagmann H, *et al.* Pilot study of extracorporeal removal of soluble fms-like tyrosine kinase 1 in preeclampsia/clinical perspective. *Circulation* 2011;**124**:940–950. doi: 10.1161/circulationaha.111.034793.

52. Murakami S, Saitoh M, Kubo T, Koyama T, Kobayashi M. Renal disease in women with severe preeclampsia or gestational proteinuria. *Obstet Gynecol* 2000;**96**:945–949.

53. Bobrie G, Liote F, Houillier P, Grunfeld JP, Jungers P. Pregnancy in lupus nephritis and related disorders. *Am J Kidney Dis* 1987;**9**:339–343.

54. George JN. The thrombotic thrombocytopenic purpura and hemolytic uremic syndromes: overview of pathogenesis (Experience of the Oklahoma TTP-HUS Registry, 1989–2007). *Kidney Int Suppl* 2009;**112**: S8–S10.

55. Vesely SK, Li X, McMinn JR, Terrell DR, George JN. Pregnancy outcomes after recovery from thrombotic thrombocytopenic purpura-hemolytic uremic syndrome. *Transfusion* 2004;**44**:1149–1158.

56. Irgens HU, Reisaeter L, Irgens LM, Lie RT. Long term mortality of mothers and fathers after pre-eclampsia: population based cohort study. *BMJ* 2001;**323**:1213–1217.

57. Ray JG, Vermeulen MJ, Schull MJ, Redelmeier DA. Cardiovascular health after maternal placental syndromes (CHAMPS): population-based

retrospective cohort study. *Lancet* 2005;**366**:1797–1803.

58. Vikse BE, Hallan S, Bostad L, Leivestad T, Iversen BM. Previous preeclampsia and risk for progression of biopsy-verified kidney disease to end-stage renal disease. *Nephrol Dial Transplant* 2010;**25**:3289–3296.

59. Mongraw-Chaffin ML, Cirillo PM, Cohn BA. Preeclampsia and cardiovascular disease death: prospective evidence from the child health and development studies cohort. *Hypertension* 2010;**56**:166–171.

Chapter 28

Cancer

Kristel Van Calsteren and Frederic Amant

Introduction

Cancer is the second leading cause of death in women during the reproductive years and complicates 1 in 1500 pregnancies. This means that every year 3300 and 4000 women are diagnosed with cancer during pregnancy in Europe and the USA, respectively. This number may increase as women in developed societies delay childbearing, as the incidence of most malignancies rises with increasing age. The cancers most frequently diagnosed in pregnancy reflect the most common cancer types in women between the ages of 20 and 40 years, including breast cancer, malignant melanoma, cervical cancer, lymphoma, leukemia, and thyroid cancer [1,2].

The diagnosis and treatment of cancer in pregnant women is a clinical and ethical challenge for medical care workers. The risk–benefit balance of diagnostic and therapeutic options should be carefully weighed in an effort to achieve optimal benefit to the mother and minimal harm to the fetus.

Diagnosis of cancer during pregnancy

Tiredness, constipation, changes in breast constitution, (postcoital) blood loss, and abdominal inconvenience are often seen in pregnancy simply from the physiological changes. With a low index of suspicion and a tendency to ignore many symptoms as being pregnancy related, a malignancy may easily be missed. Therefore, when history and physical examination are suspicious, a low threshold for requesting additional examinations is advised. In general, fine needle aspiration and excisional or incisional biopsies of lumps can be performed safely. Endoscopy, including laparoscopy, lumbar puncture, and bone marrow aspiration/biopsy are quite safe and should be performed when clinically indicated.

With regard to imaging studies, the radiation dose should be kept as low as reasonably achievable; however, a missed diagnosis or delayed treatment often poses a greater risk to the patient and her pregnancy than the hazard associated with ionizing radiation. Therefore, if a radiography scan is medically indicated for the benefit of the mother, it should be performed as long as a safety limit of a maximum fetal radiation exposure of 100 mGy is respected (see Chapter 22). This threshold dose was determined based on extrapolations of studies on the damaging effect of ionizing radiation in the Japanese atomic bombing disasters, assuming a linear dose–response relationship.

Table 28.1 shows the estimated fetal doses from common radiological diagnostic procedures, which are all below the threshold dose of 100 mGy [3]. In addition a 50–75% dose reduction from leaked radiation shielding and scatter can be achieved by adequate shielding. Nevertheless, it is generally advised, whenever possible, to replace a radiograph examination in pregnancy with ultrasonography or nuclear medicine [4].

Iodinated contrast media and gadolinium are known to cross the placenta and have a potentially toxic effect on thyroid and renal function, respectively. However, clinical sequelae from brief exposures have not been reported.

In cases where the result obtained with a nuclear medicine examination (positron emission tomography, ventilation/perfusion scan, bone scan) can change therapeutic management, these examinations are also allowed during pregnancy. Most such examinations during pregnancy have been performed with technetium-99m; iodine-131 is avoided during pregnancy.

For most radioisotopes, the main fraction of fetal exposure derives from proximity to radionuclides excreted into the maternal bladder. Maternal

Table 28.1. Approximate fetal doses from common radiological and nuclear diagnostic procedures

Procedure	Mean (mGy)	Maximum (mGy)
Conventional X ray examination		
Abdomen	1.4	4.2
Chest	<0.01	<0.01
Intravenous urogram	1.7	10
Lumbar spine	1.7	10
Pelvis	1.1	4
Skull	<0.01	<0.01
Thoracic spine	<0.01	<0.01
Fluoroscopic examination		
Barium meal (upper gastrointestinal tract)	1.1	5.8
Barium enema	6.8	24
Computed tomography		
Abdomen	8.0	49
Chest	0.06	0.96
Head	<0.005	<0.005
Lumbar spine	2.4	8.6
Pelvis	25	79
Nuclear examinations		
Positron emission tomography	5–6	
Pulmonary ventilation/perfusion scan (to 80 MBq ^{99}Tc)	0.4	
Bone scan (~740 MBq ^{99}Tc-medronic acid)	2.0	
Sentinel node mapping (no blue dye)		
Breast (40 MBq ^{99}Tc–nanocolloid fetal	0.05	
Vulvar cancer (60–80 MBq ^{99}Tc)	0.1	

^{99}Tc, technetium-99m.
Source: International Atomic Energy Agency, 2009 [3].

hydration and an indwelling catheter to prevent retention of radioactive agents in the bladder can reduce this exposure [3].

Management of cancer during pregnancy

The therapeutic strategy will be determined by the stage of disease, gestational period at diagnosis, and the patient's wishes concerning the pregnancy. The complex medical, ethical, psychological, and religious issues arising in pregnant women with cancer demand care from a multidisciplinary team with obstetricians, oncologists, radiation oncologists, surgeons, pediatricians, geneticists, and psychologists. The patient and her family should be actively involved in the decision-making process.

While curing the mother should be the priority, fetal health may be taken into consideration, and modifications may, therefore, be made in the mother's treatment, but unnecessary delay in diagnosis or treatment must be avoided. Standard cancer treatment includes surgery, systemic treatment (chemotherapy and targeted treatment), and radiotherapy, or a combination of these.

Surgery

Surgery can be performed safely during pregnancy. The use of most anesthetic agents is considered safe for the developing fetus, but hypoxia, hypercapnia, hypotension, hypoglycemia, fever, pain, infections, or thrombosis can have serious adverse effects on fetal development and so should be prevented. Very important is the left lateral tilt position to avoid vena cava compression [5].

Whether or not to monitor the fetus during surgery should be discussed with the obstetrician. Since no data are available supporting the benefit of systematic use of tocolytic drugs, this should only be considered if there are uterine contractions.

Adequate postoperative analgesia should be prescribed. Moreover, since pregnancy includes an additional risk for thrombosis – apart from the malignant disease – surgical intervention in these patients is an indication for thromboprophylaxis with low-molecular-weight heparin.

The sentinel lymph node procedure with technetium-99m can be relatively safely performed during pregnancy. Studies in breast cancer show that after injection of 18.5 MBq technetium-99m, the fetal dosage approximately ranges between 0.0 and 0.05 mGy, which is far below the deterministic threshold dosage [6,7]. This is mainly because of the low dosages that are administered and the fact that technetium-99m is captured in the lymph nodes for a period, during which radioactivity decreases considerably. It should be noted that some radiopharmaceuticals, such as iodine isotopes, do cross the placenta and concentrate in a specific organ or tissue and can, therefore, pose substantial fetal risk [8]. Blue dye should not be used during pregnancy as it includes a potential risk of an allergic or anaphylactic maternal reaction, which can be harmful to the fetus [5–7].

Chemotherapy

The placenta seems to fulfill its barrier role for most of the chemotherapeutic drugs and reduces fetal exposure to chemotherapy. Transplacental transfer mainly occurs by passive diffusion and is, therefore, determined by the concentration gradient and the physicochemical drug characteristics of the agents, where unbound, uncharged, lipid-soluble molecules with a low molecular weight (<300 Da) will easily cross the placenta [9]. Furthermore, there is also active transport by placental protein pumps as P-glycoprotein, multidrug resistance proteins, and breast cancer resistance protein. These pumps work as protective mechanisms for the fetus against potential toxic agents and have been shown to have a regulating role in the transfer of certain chemotherapeutic agents such as vinblastine, doxorubicin, epirubicin, and paclitaxel [9]. Preclinical research in a mouse and a baboon model showed a wide variation in transplacental transfer of different chemotherapeutic agents. While for carboplatin and cytarabine, significant drug concentrations were detected in fetal plasma samples (57–100% and 40% of maternal plasma, respectively), fetal plasma levels of anthracyclines, taxanes, vinblastine, cytarabine, and 4-hydroxycyclophosphamide

were substantially lower than the maternal drug concentrations (0–25% of maternal) [10–12].

The potential risk of fetal damage induced by cytotoxic treatment depends on the gestational age at exposure and the type and dosage of the applied agent(s). An overview is given in Table 28.2 [8,13,14]. Congenital malformations are reported in 7–17% after single-agent chemotherapy; after combination therapy, the risk rises to 25%. Excluding the folic acid antagonists, a risk of 6% is reported [15].

To prevent malformations, the use of cytotoxic agents is considered contraindicated until 8 weeks after conception (10 weeks after the last menstrual period). Mostly, a "safety period" of 2–4 weeks is added, allowing chemotherapy to start from a gestational age of 12–14 weeks (10–12 weeks postconception). Following chemotherapy in the second and third trimesters, short-term outcomes in the offspring are reassuring overall [1,16]. There is no increased incidence of congenital anomalies. Concerns for fetal growth restriction and preterm labor appear to be limited to certain subgroups of patients (hematological malignancies and high-dose chemotherapy). Neonatal hematopoietic suppression has been described in patients who deliver within 3 weeks of chemotherapy administration, so delivery within this time frame should be avoided if possible.

The fact that the central nervous system continues to develop throughout gestation raises concerns regarding the long-term neurodevelopmental outcome. Aviles and Neri [17] examined 84 children exposed to

Table 28.2. Overview of the potential fetal damage induced by cytotoxic treatment depending on the gestational age at exposure

	Gestational period		
	0–10 days after conception	10 days to 8 weeks after conception	>9 weeks after conception (gestational age of >11 weeks)
Embryological phase	Implantation phase	Organogenesis	Fetal developmental phase (fetal growth and maturation; organogenesis is completed with the exception of eyes, gonads, and central nervous system)
Effect expected of cytotoxic exposure (chemotherapy, targeted therapy, fetal radiation exposure of >100 mGy)	"All-or-nothing" phenomenon; when sufficient cells remain the embryo will develop normally, otherwise a miscarriage occurs	Congenital malformations[a]	No congenital malformations *Described effects*: growth restriction, prematurity, intrauterine and neonatal death, hematopoietic suppression *Potential effects*: neurodevelopmental delay, fertility problems, carcinogenesis, genetic defects

[a] The type of malformation depends on the timing of exposure in the embryological development; the most frequently described malformations are skeletal problems (face, limbs).

chemotherapy in utero and reported that all the children's learning and educational performances were normal and they were without congenital, neurological, psychological, cardiac, and cytogenetic abnormalities, or malignancies. Hahn et al. [18] surveyed parents/guardians by mail or telephone regarding outcomes of 40 children exposed in utero to chemotherapy for breast cancer (age, 2–157 months). Medical problems that were reported at that time included allergy, eczema, asthma, and upper respiratory interactions; 2 of the 18 children who went to school needed special attention [18]. More recently Amant et al. [19] presented a prospective study on 70 children with a median follow-up period of 22.3 months (range, 16.8–211.6). Children's behavior, general health, hearing, and growth were reported to be as in the general population. However, a severe neurodevelopmental delay was seen in both members of a twin pair (3%).

A high incidence of preterm, mostly induced, deliveries were noticeable in the study of Amant et al. [19]. The median gestational age at birth was 35.7 weeks (range, 28.3–41.0); 16 children were born before 34 weeks of gestation, 31 at 34–37 weeks, and 23 at term. Birth weight was below the 10th percentile for gestational age and gender in 14 of the 70 children (20·6%). The mothers of these children were treated for leukemia (four), lymphoma (four), breast cancer (two), colon cancer (one), and ovarian cancer (three) [19]. Echocardiographic follow-up data suggest normal cardiac function in children following in utero exposure to cytotoxic drugs, including anthracyclines [19–21].

As of writing, only one case of a secondary malignancy (thyroid and neuroblastoma) after prenatal exposure to chemotherapy (cyclophosphamide) has been reported; this was in a dizygotic twin boy, but his twin sister was healthy [22].

It can be concluded that, while the long-term outcome of children exposed in utero to chemotherapy is poorly documented, the available, though limited, evidence is reassuring with regard to outcome, and chemotherapy should not be withheld for fetal reasons in the second and third trimester.

Radiation therapy

Radiation doses used in cancer therapy are in the range 30–70 Gy. The fetal exposure depends on the size of the radiation field, the distance to the fetus, the target dose, the shielding measures, the specific radiation machine, and leakage. External beam radiotherapy has been used for the treatment of breast cancer, supradiaphragmatic

Hodgkin disease, head and neck cancer, and brain tumors in pregnant women [8,23–25].

In a review of 109 women who were treated with radiation for different malignancies during pregnancy [26], there were 13 adverse outcomes: two spontaneous abortions, five perinatal deaths, one stillbirth; one child born with hypospadias; one child reported as a slow learner and with scoliosis; one child with sensory hearing loss from an inner ear defect after mantle irradiation for Hodgkin disease starting at 3 weeks of gestation; one child diagnosed with intrauterine growth restriction where the mother was treated for non-Hodgkin lymphoma; and one mother ruptured membranes spontaneously and developed chorioamnionitis at 38 weeks of gestation. Labor was induced with pitocin in this last patient, but the fetal heart rate tracing showed moderate variable decelerations and a fetal scalp pH was 7.21. A primary transverse lower segment cesarean section was performed through a Pfannenstiel incision. The baby was a viable female weighing 2015 g, with Apgar scores of 8 at 1 minute and 9 at 5 minutes. At 6 years, she remains below the 5th percentile for height and weight, has expressive problems, attention deficit disorder, and delayed co-ordination and motor development.

One child whose mother had axillary irradiation for melanoma (starting at 24 weeks) was diagnosed at birth with an undescended left testicle and an uncomplicated, restricted, perimembranous ventricular septal defect. From these case reports with adverse outcomes, estimated fetal dosages were available in four patients and all had received <100 mGy [26].

Targeted therapy

Biological agents have the potential to affect the fetus and should be used with caution during pregnancy. However, in circumstances where better alternative treatments do not exist, or where failure to use targeted treatments would result in suboptimum patient care or survival, the risk–benefit analysis might favor the use of potentially effective molecular treatment during pregnancy [27,28]. Most frequently used agents in the treatment of breast cancer and hematological tumors are selective estrogen receptor modulators and aromatase inhibitors, trastuzumab, rituximab, imatinib, and interferon-alpha.

The use of hormonal agents, such as the selective estrogen receptor modulators and aromatase inhibitors, interferes with the hormonal environment of a normal pregnancy and should be avoided. These drugs are associated with vaginal bleeding, spontaneous abortion, birth defects including craniofacial malformations and ambiguous genitalia, and fetal death [29].

Trastuzumab is a humanized recombinant monoclonal antibody (IgG) that blocks the human epidermal growth factor receptor-2 (HER2) and has been shown to inhibit expression of angiogenic factors such as vascular endothelial growth factor. Trastuzumab is used in the treatment of HER2-positive breast cancers. In 15 fetuses exposed to trastuzumab, three had renal failure and four died. In eight women, the volume of amniotic fluid was reduced [28]. This phenomenon is explained by the fact that *HER2* is stongly expressed in the fetal renal epithelium, and IgG molecules cross the placenta. Based on these data, trastuzumab is contraindicated during pregnancy.

Rituximab, used in B-cell lymphoma and leukemia, is also a monoclonal antibody of the IgG isotype, so crosses the placental barrier and interacts with fetal B-cells. One case report compared maternal and fetal rituximab concentrations and B-cells. Although at birth rituximab concentrations were similar in mother and child, the fetal B-cells were severely diminished (1% of normal); the B-cells recovered after 6 weeks, to reach a normal level at 12 weeks. No further adverse events or malformations were seen during 16 months of follow-up [30]. For this reason, rituximab, seems to be safe and without significant consequences for the fetus [30].

Administration of imatinib mesylate, a tyrosine kinase inhibitor used in the treatment of chronic myelogenous leukemia, during the first trimester is associated with a considerable risk of congenital anomalies and spontaneous abortions, while late exposure seems to have less impact [31]. In a series of 125 patients, 63 (50%) delivered normal infants; 35 (28%) had elected termination (three for known malformations of the fetus), and 12 newborns were born with abnormalities. The authors concluded that, although the majority of patients had normal outcomes, there is a significant risk for serious fetal malformations after exposure to imatinib [32]. Very few data are available about the safety of second-generation oral tyrosine kinase inhibitors during pregnancy and it is recommended that patients on these drugs should avoid pregnancy [33].

Interferon-alpha, an immune modulator, does not cross the placenta to a great extent because of its high molecular weight (19 kDa) and does not inhibit DNA synthesis. Interferon use in pregnancy for a variety of hematological malignancies has been published for 40 women (eight during first trimester). No fetal malformations were reported when interferon was administered as monotherapy. Given the available preclinical and clinical data, interferon can be safely administered throughout pregnancy and it is the treatment of choice for patients diagnosed with chronic myeloid leukaemia in pregnancy [34].

Supportive treatment

Supportive treatment for pregnant women is possible, similar to non-pregnant women. Granulocyte colony-stimulating factor and erythropoetin have been used safely in pregnant patients, and their use should follow current guidelines for growth factor support during chemotherapy [35]. First choice pain relief consists of acetaminophen and tramadol. Non-steroidal anti-inflammatory drugs are associated with congenital anomalies after first trimester exposure, and with preterm closure of the fetal ductus arteriosus after exposure after 30 weeks of gestation. Consequently, it is preferred to avoid these in pregnancy. The use of steroids deserves attention since repeated antenatal exposure is associated with increased incidence of attention problem and higher rates of cerebral palsy [36]. In contrast to dexamethasone and betamethasone, methylprednisolone and hydrocortisone are extensively metabolized in the placenta and are, therefore, the preferred steroids to use during pregnancy, except when being used to achieve fetal lung maturation.

Obstetrical care

Pregnancies complicated by a maternal cancer diagnosis are at high risk. At diagnosis it is important to evaluate fetal growth and development to date by ultrasound and to exclude pre-existing malformations. For patients treated during pregnancy, fetal well-being should be assessed before and after each major intervention. Special attention is required for fetal growth, preterm contractions, and potential fetal anemia or cardiotoxicity after (anthracycline-based) chemotherapy [1]. The timing of delivery should be determined based on the oncological treatment schedule and the maturation of the fetus. As in non-cancer patients, term delivery (≥37 weeks) should be the aim [1]. Early induction results in prematurity and low birth weight, which have been identified as contributing factors in the cognitive and emotional development of children. When preterm delivery is indicated, antenatal steroids should be administered to improve fetal lung maturation, according to local policy.

The mode of delivery should be determined following general obstetric guidelines. When continuation of chemotherapy is required postpartum, an interval of a few days after a vaginal delivery is advised; after an uncomplicated cesarean section, an interval of 1 week is necessary. To allow bone marrow to recover and to minimize the risk of maternal and fetal neutropenia, delivery should be planned 3 weeks after the last dose of chemotherapy [7]. Neonates, particularly preterm babies, have limited capacity to metabolize and eliminate drugs because of their immature liver and kidneys. Delaying delivery after chemotherapy will allow fetal drug excretion via the placenta. For the same reason, chemotherapy should not be administered after 35 weeks of gestation since spontaneous labor becomes more likely. Although placental metastases are rare, the placenta should always be analysed histopathologically after delivery [37]. Documented reports of maternal malignant metastases in the placenta are rare. Since the first description in 1866, fewer than 80 cases have been described. Proven maternal metastasis to the fetus is exceptional, with only 11 cases reported so far. Malignancies that can spread to the products of conception are melanoma (32%), leukemia and lymphomas (15%), breast cancer (13%), lung cancer (11%), sarcoma (8%), gastric cancer (3%), and gynecological cancers (3%), reflecting malignancies with a high incidence in women of reproductive age [38–40]. Despite this, each placenta should be thoroughly examined for metastasis, which, if present, should alert the clinician to monitor the infant for development of malignant disease.

In the absence of safety data, breastfeeding during or shortly after chemotherapy is contraindicated.

Critical illness in pregnant women with cancer

Cancer is life threatening, but in most cases in a chronic way. Nevertheless, cancer and its treatment are associated with a high rate of complications that can result in acute life-threatening situations.

In our experience, hematopoietic suppression or insufficiency related to chemotherapy or leukemia is most frequently seen. Neutropenia with the risk of overwhelming infections and sepsis and thrombocytopenia with the risk of major hemorrhages (spontaneous, peripartum, after intramuscular or epidural puncture) can clearly lead to significant maternal and fetal morbitidy and mortality. Therefore, it is important to treat these complications in the same manner as in non-pregnant patients.

Furthermore, there is an increased risk of deep venous thrombosis with both the malignancy and the pregnancy. While there is a theoretical base for administration of low-molecular-weight heparin to all pregnant patients with cancer, in clinical practice this is only prescribed after surgery or long-term immobilization.

The relative immunosuppression of pregnancy increases the mortality risk of infectious diseases such as influenza, and this risk will increase even more in women with hematopoietic suppression after chemotherapy. In addition, pyelonephritis is seen more frequently, and associated with sepsis, in pregnant women.

Depending on the location, solid tumors can also cause a mass effect on blood vessels, urinary tract, or gastrointestinal tract, leading to organ failure.

Less frequent dangerous side effects of cancer therapy are, for example, cardiotoxicity associated with anthracycline exposure and nefrotoxicity with platinum exposure. In patients with disseminated malignancy or specific chemotherapeutic treatment, such as gemcitabine, cyclophosphamide, cisplatin and bevacizumab, there is an increased risk of thrombotic thrombocytopenic purpura/hemolytic uremic syndrome.

It is important to screen for these complications in order to treat them adequately.

Psychosocial and ethical concerns of cancer diagnosis during pregnancy

Pregnant women diagnosed with cancer experience high emotional distress and even long-term emotional sequelae. Cancer diagnosis brings fear of death, worry about continuation of the pregnancy, anxiety about the impact of cancer treatment on the fetus, fear for not being able to raise the child into adulthood, and anxiety about future fertility. Emotional and psychological support is imperative. The partner, or other family member, runs a risk of raising the child alone and should be involved. It is advisable to engage the expertise of other members of the healthcare team, such as psychologists and social workers, especially during the time that treatment decisions are being made. Ongoing psychological support during treatment and delivery should be available for the parents.

Termination of pregnancy

Termination of pregnancy does not seem to improve survival. Most data are available on breast cancer during pregnancy. These studies showed a worsening trend for survival in patients choosing termination, but no statistically significant difference in 5-year survival when these groups were compared by several authors [41–43]. However, not all studies matched patients for stage of disease or provided explanations affecting patient choices. Therefore, it is difficult to determine whether women with advanced stage disease, or a worse prognosis at diagnosis, were encouraged to terminate their pregnancy, whereas women with earlier stage disease or a better prognosis at diagnosis were not.

Nowadays, termination of pregnancy is recommended if the required treatment is associated with unacceptable risks for the health of mother and fetus; when it is morally unacceptable to continue the pregnancy in the presence of incurable maternal cancer; or when the pregnancy itself makes the target of local treatment unreachable (abdominal/pelvic tumors with a need for immediate local treatment). It should be stressed that most case series did not show induced abortion to be associated with improved outcome of pregnant women with cancer when appropriate antineoplastic therapy was implemented.

Prognosis of cancer during pregnancy

Literature on cancer during pregnancy is mainly composed of small retrospective studies and case reports. When interpreting the results obtained in the reported cases, a positive publication bias should be kept in mind.

Recent data suggest that the maternal prognosis is probably similar to non-pregnant women when women are matched by age and cancer stage, provided that the same treatment strategies are applied and unnecessary delay in treatment is avoided [2].

Stensheim et al. [2] reported on the cause-specific survival for women with cancer during pregnancy or lactation in a Scandinavian population. They concluded that the cause-specific death for most cancer types was not increased when diagnosed during pregnancy or lactation. However, in the subgroups of lactating women with breast or ovarian cancer, the hazard ratios were doubled, even when adjusted for age. Pregnant women diagnosed with malignant melanoma had a slightly elevated risk of cause-specific death [2].

The poorer outcome of breast cancer diagnosed postpartum is probably related to more advanced stages of disease diagnosed among these patients, as changes or lumps in the breast during pregnancy or lactation may be regarded as normal, leading to delay.

However, the disease-free and overall survivals were not adversely affected by pregnancy in women who became pregnant after successfully treated cancer; these women seemed to have a better prognosis, the so-called "healthy mother effect" [2,44]. Nevertheless, it is recommended that pregnancy is delayed until 2 to 3 years after completion of treatment, particularly if axillary nodes were positive for tumor. During this period, the tumor biology will become clear, since aggressive tumors often relapse within these first years. In this way, the delay of 2–3 years is used to defer childbearing until after the period of greatest risk of recurrence.

Conclusions

Pregnancy complicated by maternal cancer is a rare and challenging problem requiring a multidisciplinary approach. Diagnostic and staging examinations can be performed safely during pregnancy and are required to determine an optimal treatment strategy. A delay in diagnosis leads to more advanced stages of the disease at presentation and should be avoided by all means. Treatment should adhere to standard treatment for non-pregnant cancer patients. Considering the gestational period, surgery, chemotherapy (not in the first trimester), and radiotherapy (not in the third trimester) can safely be applied in pregnancy. Hormonal therapy and trastuzumab should be deferred until after birth.

Acute critical illness in these patients is mostly related to hematopoietic insufficiency caused either by the malignancy or chemotherapy, with complications of sepsis and hemorrhage. It is important to screen for these complications and treat them adequately.

References

1. Van Calsteren K, Heyns L, De Smet F, et al. Cancer during pregnancy: an analysis of 215 patients emphasizing the obstetrical and the neonatal outcomes. *J Clin Oncol* 2010;**28**:683–689.

2. Stensheim H, Moller B, van Dijk T, Fossa SD. Cause-specific survival for women diagnosed with cancer during pregnancy or lactation: a registry-based cohort study. *J Clin Oncol* 2009;**27**:45–51.

3. International Atomic Energy Agency. *Pregnancy and Radiation Protection of Patients: Pregnant Women*. Vienna: International Atomic Energy Agency, 2009

(http://rpop.iaea.org/RPOP/RPoP/Content/
SpecialGroups/1_PregnantWomen/index.htm,
accessed 7 December 2012).

4. Rajaraman P, Simpson J, Neta G, *et al.* Early life
exposure to diagnostic radiation and ultrasound scans
and risk of childhood cancer: case–control study. *BMJ*
2011;**342**:d472.

5. Kizer NT, Powell MA. Surgery in the pregnant patient.
Clin Obstet Gynecol 2011;**54**:633–641.

6. Khera SY, Kiluk JV, Hasson DM, *et al.*
Pregnancy-associated breast cancer patients can
safely undergo lymphatic mapping. *Breast J*
2008;**14**:250–254.

7. Amant F, Deckers S, Van Calsteren K, *et al.* Breast
cancer in pregnancy: recommendations of an
international consensus meeting. *Eur J Cancer*
2010;**46**:3158–3168.

8. Kal HB, Struikmans H. Radiotherapy during
pregnancy: fact and fiction. *Lancet Oncol*
2005;**6**:328–333.

9. Syme MR, Paxton JW, Keelan JA. Drug transfer and
metabolism by the human placenta. *Clin
Pharmacokinet* 2004;**43**:487–514.

10. Van Calsteren K, Verbesselt R, Devlieger R, *et al.*
Transplacental transfer of paclitaxel, docetaxel,
carboplatin, and trastuzumab in a baboon model. *Int J
Gynecol Cancer* 2010;**20**:1456–1464.

11. Van Calsteren K, Verbesselt R, Beijnen J, *et al.*
Transplacental transfer of anthracyclines, vinblastine,
and 4-hydroxy-cyclophosphamide in a baboon model.
Gynecol Oncol 2010;**119**:594–600.

12. Van Calsteren K, Verbesselt R, Van Bree R, *et al.*
Substantial variation in transplacental transfer of
chemotherapeutic agents in a mouse model. *Reprod Sci*
2011;**18**:57–63.

13. Cardonick E, Iacobucci A. Use of chemotherapy during
human pregnancy. *Lancet Oncol* 2004;**5**:283–291.

14. De Santis M, Di Gianantonio E, Straface G, *et al.*
Ionizing radiations in pregnancy and teratogenesis: a
review of literature. *Reprod Toxicol* 2005;**20**:323–329.

15. Ebert U, Loffler H, Kirch W. Cytotoxic therapy and
pregnancy. *Pharmacol Ther* 1997;**74**:207–220.

16. Cardonick E, Usmani A, Ghaffar S. Perinatal
outcomes of a pregnancy complicated by cancer,
including neonatal follow-up after in utero
exposure to chemotherapy: results of an
international registry. *Am J Clin Oncol*
2010;**33**:221–228.

17. Aviles A, Neri N. Hematological malignancies and
pregnancy: a final report of 84 children who received
chemotherapy in utero. *Clin Lymphoma*
2001;**2**:173–177.

18. Hahn KM, Johnson PH, Gordon N, *et al.* Treatment of
pregnant breast cancer patients and outcomes of
children exposed to chemotherapy in utero. *Cancer*
2006;**107**:1219–1226.

19. Amant F, Van CK, Halaska MJ, *et al.* Long-term
cognitive and cardiac outcomes after prenatal
exposure to chemotherapy in children aged 18
months or older: an observational study. *Lancet
Oncol* 2012;**13**:256–264.

20. Meyer-Wittkopf M, Barth H, Emons G, Schmidt S.
Fetal cardiac effects of doxorubicin therapy for
carcinoma of the breast during pregnancy: case report
and review of the literature. *Ultrasound Obstet Gynecol*
2001;**18**:62–6.

21. Aviles A, Neri N, Nambo MJ. Long-term evaluation of
cardiac function in children who received
anthracyclines during pregnancy. *Ann Oncol*
2006;**17**:286–288.

22. Zemlickis D, Lishner M, Erlich R, Koren G.
Teratogenicity and carcinogenicity in a twin exposed in
utero to cyclophosphamide. *Teratog Carcinog Mutagen*
1993;**13**:139–143.

23. Mazonakis M, Damilakis J, Theoharopoulos N,
Varveris H, Gourtsoyiannis N. Brain radiotherapy
during pregnancy: an analysis of conceptus dose using
anthropomorphic phantoms. *Br J Radiol*
1999;**72**:274–278.

24. Mazonakis M, Varveris H, Fasoulaki M, Damilakis J.
Radiotherapy of Hodgkin's disease in early pregnancy:
embryo dose measurements. *Radiother Oncol*
2003;**66**:333–339.

25. Mazonakis M, Varveris H, Damilakis J,
Theoharopoulos N, Gourtsoyiannis N. Radiation dose
to conceptus resulting from tangential breast
irradiation. *Int J Radiat Oncol Biol Phys*
2003;**55**:386–391.

26. Luis SA, Christie DR, Kaminski A, Kenny L, Peres MH.
Pregnancy and radiotherapy: management options for
minimising risk, case series and comprehensive
literature review. *J Med Imaging Radiat Oncol*
2009;**53**:559–568.

27. Robinson AA, Watson WJ, Leslie KK. Targeted
treatment using monoclonal antibodies and
tyrosine-kinase inhibitors in pregnancy. *Lancet Oncol*
2007;**8**:738–743.

28. Azim HA Jr., Azim H, Peccatori FA. Treatment of
cancer during pregnancy with monoclonal antibodies:
a real challenge. *Expert Rev Clin Immunol*
2010;**6**:821–826.

29. Isaacs RJ, Hunter W, Clark K. Tamoxifen as systemic
treatment of advanced breast cancer during pregnancy:
case report and literature review. *Gynecol Oncol*
2001;**80**:405–408.

30. Decker M, Rothermundt C, Hollander G, Tichelli A, Rochlitz C. Rituximab plus CHOP for treatment of diffuse large B-cell lymphoma during second trimester of pregnancy. *Lancet Oncol* 2006;7:693–694.

31. Pye SM, Cortes J, Ault P, *et al.* The effects of imatinib on pregnancy outcome. *Blood* 2008;**111**:5505–5508.

32. Shapira T, Pereg D, Lishner M. How I treat acute and chronic leukemia in pregnancy. *Blood Rev* 2008;**22**:247–259.

33. Conchon M, Sanabani SS, Serpa M, *et al.* Successful pregnancy and delivery in a patient with chronic myeloid leukemia while on dasatinib therapy. *Adv Hematol* 2010;**2010**:136–152.

34. Rizack T, Mega A, Legare R, Castillo J. Management of hematological malignancies during pregnancy. *Am J Hematol* 2009;**84**:830–841.

35. Dale DC, Cottle TE, Fier CJ, *et al.* Severe chronic neutropenia: treatment and follow-up of patients in the Severe Chronic Neutropenia International Registry. *Am J Hematol* 2003;**72**:82–93.

36. Wapner RJ, Sorokin Y, Mele L, *et al.* Long-term outcomes after repeat doses of antenatal corticosteroids. *N Engl J Med* 2007;**357**:1190–1198.

37. Pavlidis N, Pentheroudakis G. Metastatic involvement of placenta and foetus in pregnant women with cancer. *Recent Results Cancer Res* 2008;**178**:183–194.

38. Jackisch C, Louwen F, Schwenkhagen A, *et al.* Lung cancer during pregnancy involving the products of conception and a review of the literature. *Arch Gynecol Obstet* 2003;**268**:69–77.

39. Alexander A, Samlowski WE, Grossman D, *et al.* Metastatic melanoma in pregnancy: risk of transplacental metastases in the infant. *J Clin Oncol* 2003;**21**:2179–2186.

40. Miller K, Zawislak A, Gannon C, Millar D, Loughrey M. Maternal gastric adenocarcinoma with placental metastases: what is the fetal risk? *Pediatr Dev Pathol* 2012;**15**:237–239.

41. Cardonick E, Dougherty R, Grana G, *et al.* Breast cancer during pregnancy: maternal and fetal outcomes. *Cancer J* 2010;**16**:76–82.

42. Zemlickis D, Lishner M, Degendorfer P, *et al.* Maternal and fetal outcome after breast cancer in pregnancy. *Am J Obstet Gynecol* 1992;**166**:781–787.

43. Pavlidis N, Pentheroudakis G. The pregnant mother with breast cancer: diagnostic and therapeutic management. *Cancer Treat Rev* 2005;**31**:439–447.

44. Sankila R, Heinavaara S, Hakulinen T. Survival of breast cancer patients after subsequent term pregnancy: "healthy mother effect." *Am J Obstet Gynecol* 1994;**170**:818–823.

Chapter 29

Endocrine disorders

Patricia Peticca, Erin Keely, and Tracey Johnston

Introduction

Endocrine disorders are common in women of reproductive age, but fortunately endocrine emergencies are rare. There is little evidence base for pregnancy-specific management of endocrine crises, and in the majority of cases the underlying condition should be treated as it would be outside of pregnancy, with no need for immediate delivery. If delivery is indicated or labor coincides, mode of delivery will depend on maternal and fetal clinical conditions and how easily vaginal birth can be achieved, taking into account parity and cervical status. If anesthesia is required, the most appropriate mode will depend on the maternal condition. Close liaison and early involvement of an experienced obstetric anesthesiologist is essential. In most cases, there is no contra-indication to epidural or combined spinal–epidural anesthesia with appropriate monitoring and hemo-dynamic support.

Thyroid emergencies

Thyroid dysfunction occurs in 2.5% of all pregnancies in overt and subclinical forms [1]. Critical illness in the pregnant patient can result from two extremes of thyroid dysfunction: thyroid storm and myxedema coma.

Thyroid storm

Clinical presentation

Thyroid storm, also known as thyrotoxic crisis, is an endocrinological emergency caused by exaggeration of the signs/symptoms of thyrotoxicosis (Table 29.1). Clinical presentation is characterized by thermoregulatory dysfunction, altered mental status, and multiorgan failure. Though rare, it is associated with a mortality of 20–30% if untreated [2,3]. Thyroid storm can be precipitated by surgery, trauma, parturition, stroke, myocardial infarction, severe infection, diabetic ketoacidosis, withdrawal of antithyroid medications, radioactive iodine therapy, and administration of iodinated radiocontrast dyes [3,4]. The severity is related to the hypermetabolic and hyperadrenergic effects of thyroxinemia on the cardiovascular and central nervous systems.

Diagnosis

Thyroid storm is a clinical diagnosis based on severity of clinical features (Table 29.2). The scoring system devised by Burch and Wartofsky [5] has been used to differentiate severe thyrotoxicosis from thyroid storm. A cumulative score of ≥ 45 is highly suggestive of thyroid storm [4]; however, this scoring system has not been validated in pregnancy. Levels of thyroid-stimulating hormone (TSH) will be suppressed and free thyroid hormones (thyroxine (T_4) and triiodothyronine (T_3)) elevated. There is no arbitrary serum T_4 or T_3 cut-off that discriminates severe thyrotoxicosis from thyroid storm. Since critical illness can impair peripheral conversion of T_4 to T_3, a mildly elevated free T_3 or "normal" T_3 should be considered inappropriate in the setting of severe systemic illness [3,4]. Other laboratory findings may include mild hyperglycemia (from catecholamine-mediated inhibition of insulin release), mild hypercalcemia, elevated liver enzymes (hepatic dysfunction), and a leukocytosis with a left shift or, conversely, leukopenia [4]. Adrenocortical function may also be impaired because of acceleration of cortisol production and degradation, leading to a state of relative adrenal insufficiency [6].

Maternal Critical Care: A Multidisciplinary Approach, ed. Marc Van de Velde, Helen Scholefield, and Lauren A. Plante.
Published by Cambridge University Press. © Cambridge University Press 2013.

Table 29.1 Signs and symptoms of severe thyrotoxicosis

Organ system	Clinical manifestations
Cardiovascular	Tachycardia, high-output heart failure, arrhythmia (e.g. atrial fibrillation), systolic hypertension, wide pulse pressure
Skin and soft tissue	Lid lag, proptosis (Graves disease), warm moist skin, hyperhydrosis
Neurological	Hyperthermia, lethargy, altered mental status, psychosis, seizures, hyperkinesis, hyper-reflexia
Gastrointestinal	Abdominal pain, vomiting, diarrhea, nausea
Respiratory	Tachypnea, dyspnea

Source: adapted from Goldberg and Inzucchi, 2003 [3].

Table 29.2. The predictive clinical scale for thyroid storm

Parameter	Points[a]
Thermoregulatory dysfunction (oral temperature°C [°F])	
37.2–37.7 (99–99.9)	5
37.8–38.3 (100–100.9)	10
38.3–38.8 (101–101.9)	15
38.9–39.4 (102–102.9)	20
39.4–39.9 (103–103.9)	25
>40 (>104)	30
Central nervous system effects	
Absent	0
Mild (agitation)	10
Moderate (delirium, psychosis, extreme lethargy)	20
Severe (seizures, coma)	30
Gastrointestinal–hepatic dysfunction	
Absent	0
Moderate (diarrhea, nausea/vomiting, abdominal pain)	10
Severe (unexplained jaundice)	20
Tachycardia (beats/min)	
99–109	5
110–119	10
120–129	15
130–139	20
>140	25
Congestive cardiac failure	
Absent	0
Mild (pedal edema)	≥5
Moderate (bibasal rales)	10
Severe (pulmonary edema)	15
Atrial fibrillation	
Absent	0
Present	10
Precipitating event	
Absent	0
Present	10

[a] A cumulative score ≥45 is highly suggestive of thyroid storm, 25–44 is suggestive of "impending" storm, and 25 is unlikely to represent thyroid storm.
Source: with permission from Burch and Wartofsky, 1993 [5].

Maternal and fetal/neonatal risks

Adverse maternal outcomes, including cardiovascular collapse, heart failure, metabolic derangements, acid–base disorders, coma, and death, are directly related to the elevated T_4 and T_3. Thyroid storm is also associated with placental abruption, and increased rates of cesarean section. Women with uncontrolled hyperthyroidism have a five-fold increased risk of developing severe pre-eclampsia and should be monitored closely for this.

Adverse perinatal outcomes include premature birth, intrauterine death, and low birth weight [1,6]. Beginning at 10–12 weeks of gestation, thyroid-stimulating antibodies can cross the placenta, resulting in neonatal Graves disease [2]. The risk of thyrotoxicosis in the fetus and newborn is greatest when the mothers have positive antibody titers [2,7]. There are different commercial assays that have different normal values. In one study, a thyroid receptor antibody titer >5 IU (normal ≤1.3 IU) had a 100% specificity and 76% sensitivity for predicting fetal Graves disease [8].

Fetal hyperthyroidism should be strongly suspected with evidence of a fetal goiter on sonography (earliest sign), impaired growth, accelerated bone maturation, and/or fetal tachycardia [7]. Cordocentesis can be performed to obtain a sample of blood to directly assess fetal thyroid function. However, in the vast majority of cases, direct fetal blood sampling is not required as fetal thyroid function can be determined with using serial sonographic assessments [9].

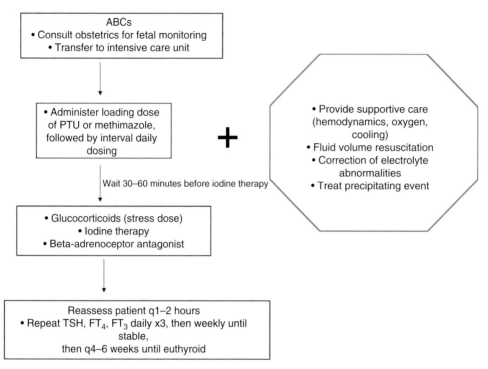

Figure 29.1. Management of thyroid storm in the pregnant patient. ABC, airway, breathing and circulation; FT$_3$, free triiodothyronine; FT$_4$, free throxine; PTU, propylthiouracil; TSH, thyroid-stimulating hormone.

Management

Thyroid storm necessitates immediate recognition and aggressive management in an intensive care setting. Goals of management should be directed at inhibiting further production and release of T$_4$, reducing conversion of T$_4$ to T$_3$ in peripheral tissues, ameliorating systemic effects of severe uncontrolled hyperthyroidism (e.g. hyperthermia), and treatment of the precipitating event. A stepwise approach to treatment of the pregnant patient in thyroid storm is provided in Figure 29.1. The order of therapy in treating thyroid storm is crucial and should begin with administration of thionamides in order to prevent synthesis of new T$_4$/T$_3$ [1]. Medical therapies are reviewed in Box 29.1 [10].

Thionamides, namely propylthiouracil and methimazole, are first-line agents in the treatment of severe thyrotoxicosis. These compounds interfere with the coupling process by which iodotyrosine residues are combined to form T$_4$ and T$_3$. Propylthiouracil offers the added benefit of blocking peripheral conversion of T$_4$ to T$_3$. Thionamides may also have immunosuppressive effects, reducing antithyrotropin receptor antibodies titers over time. Both propylthiouracil

and methimazole can be administered by oral and/or rectal route [10]. The more serious adverse reactions are agranulocytosis (0.1–0.4%), hepatotoxicity (0.1–0.2%), and systemic vasculitis [1,10]. Reports to the US Food and Drug Administration suggest that there is an increased risk of hepatotoxicity with propylthiouracil compared with methimazole; however, propylthiouracil remains the preferred agent in pregnancy.

Following administration of antithyroid medications, iodine should be given. Iodine therapy (Lugol's solution or saturated solution of potassium iodide) decreases release of stored T$_4$ and, in high doses, inhibits new hormone production [4,10]. It is imperative that iodine administration does not precede administration of thionamides as this will fuel increased synthesis and release of T$_4$ [2]. Radiographic contrast agents (sodium ipodate or iopanoic acid) inhibit release of T$_4$ from the thyroid gland and block peripheral conversion T$_4$ to T$_3$ as well as blocking binding of T$_3$ to its receptors.

Beta-blockers play a pivotal role in the treatment of thyroid storm, ameliorating the severe cardiovascular consequences. The excess adrenergic stimulation results from the increased adrenergic receptor density,

Box 29.1. Medical therapies for management of thyroid storm in pregnancy

Inhibition of new thyroid hormone production
- Propylthiouracil, 200–400 mg orally every 6–8 hours (also decreases conversion of thyroxine to triiodothyronine)
- Methimazole, 20–25 mg orally every 6–12 hours

Inhibition of thyroid hormone release from the gland
- Potassium iodide, 5 drops orally every 6 hours
- Lugol's solution, 4–8 drops orally every 6–8 hours
- Sodium ipodate (308 mg iodine per 500 mg tablet), 1–3 g orally daily (also inhibits conversion of thyroxine to triiodothyronine)
- Iopanoic acid, 1 g orally every 8 hours for 24 hours, then 500 mg orally every 12 hours (also inhibits conversion of thyroxine to triiodothyronine)

Beta-adrenergic antagonism
- Propranolol, 60–80 mg orally every 4 hours or 80–120 mg every 6 hours
- Metoprolol, 100–200 mg orally daily

Supportive treatment
- Acetaminophen, 325–650 mg oral/rectal every 4–6 hours as needed: treatment of hyperthermia
- Hydrocortisone 100 mg intravenous every 8 hours: decreases conversion of thyroxine to triiodothyronine, improves vasomotor stability

Alternative therapies
- Colestyramine (oral 4 g four times a day): decreases reabsorption of thyroid hormone from enterohepatic circulation (NB no human studies in pregnancy have been conducted so use with caution)

Source: adapted from Nayak and Burman, 2006 [10].

which translates into a requirement for much higher doses of beta-blocker to control hemodynamic sequelae adequately [4]. Propranolol is often the preferred drug of choice because of its added benefit of reducing conversion of T_4 to T_3. Relative contraindications are the presence of reactive airway disease and a history of moderate to severe congestive heart failure.

Glucocorticoids are usually given to inhibit the peripheral conversion of T_4 to T_3. Stress doses should be used as excess thyroid hormone can cause adrenal insufficiency [10] by increasing cortisol metabolism and clearance.

Antithyroid medications and iodides cross the placenta and can effectively treat fetal hyperthyroidism. The effect on the fetus, however, is not easily predicted, and caution is required to not overtreat as this will result in fetal hypothyroidism and goiter [7,10,11]. Radioactive iodine is contraindicated in pregnancy [11]. The dose of antithyroid medications to control fetal hyperthyroidism occasionally requires the mother to receive concurrent T_4 (levothyroxine) to prevent maternal hypothyroidism. Fetal hyperthyroidism will

persist to birth and may last for several months until maternal antibodies are cleared from the neonatal circulation [9].

Supportive care is needed in combination with thyroid-targeted pharmacological therapies, including acetaminophen for treatment of pyrexia, external cooling methods, correction of fluid losses, and dextrose supplementation to replenish glycogen stores. Nutritional deficiencies may coexist. Administering thiamine before glucose prevents the potential development of Wernicke's encephalopathy [10]. Salicylates should be avoided as they decrease thyroid-binding globulin, thereby increasing free T_4 in circulation [10].

Labor and delivery considerations

At or near term, delivery should be considered in the case of impending thyroid storm once the maternal condition is stabilized. Close maternal observation for deterioration is essential, as both labor and cesarean section can precipitate thyroid storm.

It is important to assess for fetal goiter prior to delivery, as this can cause hyperextension of the neck and malposition/malpresentation, which may necessitate delivery by cesarean section. In severe goiter where the airway is potentially compromised, cesarean section and a fetal EXIT (ex utero intrapartum treatment) procedure must be considered [12].

Fetal tachycardia is often found alongside maternal tachycardia and can cause problems with interpretation of electronic fetal monitoring. Close liaison with the neonatologist to ensure appropriate postnatal investigation and monitoring is essential.

During thyroid storm, it is essential to stabilize the maternal condition before embarking upon elective delivery [1,13]. Once the storm is under control, it is likely that pregnancy can continue if preterm.

Thyroid storm is associated with an increased risk of preterm labor [14], and staff in the critical care setting should be aware of this, along with the signs and symptoms of labor. Beta-blockers have been used effectively during labor to control maternal tachycardia.

Mxyedema coma

Clinical presentation

Myxedema coma is a life-threatening condition that results from decompensated hypothyroidism. Though rare, myxedema coma is a challenge to diagnose because of its insidious onset and lack of classic signs and symptoms (Table 29.3). Mortality in the non-pregnant population is estimated at 20–25% [15]. Patients present with profound slowing and impairment of metabolic and thermoregulatory functions, accompanied by central nervous system and hemodynamic instability; there is often an inciting event such as infection, cold exposure, lung disease, stroke, heart failure, gastrointestinal bleeding, acute trauma, poor compliance with thyroid hormone replacement, or drugs (e.g. sedatives, tranquilizers, narcotics, amiodarone) [16].

Diagnosis

The diagnosis of myxedema coma is confirmed by elevated serum TSH accompanied by low or undetectable free T_4 and free T_3. Critical illness can also provoke a non-thyroidal illness – which may lower TSH levels into the low–normal range [16]. Arterial blood gas analysis can show hypercapnia, hypoxia, and respiratory acidosis [15]. Additional laboratory findings include hypoglycemia, hyponatremia, elevated creatine kinase, elevated creatinine, hypercholesterolemia, elevated lactate dehydrogenase, and normocytic anemia [15].

Table 29.3. Signs and symptoms of myxedema coma

Organ system	Clinical manifestations
Central nervous system	Hypothermia (≤32.2°C), lethargy, slow mentation, frank psychosis, focal or generalized seizure (25% prevalence), delayed or absent deep tendon reflexes, poor memory
Cardiovascular	Bradycardia, hypotension, shock, pericardial effusion, heart failure (from cardiac enlargement, depressed cardiac contractility)
Respiratory	Pleural effusion, marked hypoxia and hypercapnia (from alveolar hypoventilation), macroglossia and submucosal edema of upper airways, respiratory muscle weakness (from hypothyroid myopathy)
Renal	Hyponatremia (increased antidiuretic hormone secretion), decreased glomerular filtration rate
Gastrointestinal	Paralytic ileus, megacolon (from gastric atony or dysmotility), neurogenic oropharyngeal dysphagia
Dermatological	Dry, coarse skin, sparse hair, edema of periorbital tissues/hand/feet

Maternal and fetal/neonatal risks

Maternal neurological, respiratory, and cardiovascular dysfunction can lead to death if treatment is not initiated promptly. The metabolic consequences of severe thyroid deficiency, largely hyponatremia and decreased serum osmolality, contribute to progressive deterioration [15]. Other adverse outcomes include placental abruption, preterm birth, and low birth weight [6,17]. Poor prognostic indicators include persistent hypothermia below 33.9°C (93°F) after 3 days of thyroid hormone replacement, advanced age, bradycardia, hypotension, and cardiac complications (e.g. heart failure, myocardial infarction) [6].

Management

Similar to thyroid storm, the management of the pregnant patient with mxyedema coma requires continuous monitoring in an intensive care unit. A standardized approach to thyroid hormone replacement has not been developed, and the use of levothyroxine (T_4) monotherapy versus combination therapy with levothyroxine and liothyronine (T_3) continues to be a topic of debate [16]. Current recommended dosing regimens for treatment of severe hypothyroidism is based on clinical opinion rather than scientific evidence. Monotherapy with levothyroxine is often preferred because it provides a steady, gradual onset of action without increased risk of metabolic effects. Conversely, monotherapy with liothyronine may provide better clinical response in the setting of superimposed non-thyroidal illness, given the impairment in T_4 to T_3 conversion. Liothyronine therapy may expedite neurological recovery as studies in baboons have shown that T_3 crosses the blood–brain barrier more readily than T_4 [15,16]. However, these potential benefits do not overshadow the risk of tachyarrhythmias and acute coronary events associated with liothyronine administration [16].

Combination therapy (T_4/T_3) has been cited in several review articles. A loading dose of levothyroxine (200–400 µg) for the initial 24–48 hours [15] is followed by a physiological dose of 50–100 µg daily. Liothyronine can be added at a dose of 10–20 µg intravenously every 4 hours on the first day, followed by gradual tapering and discontinuation by day 4 (Figure 29.2) [15]. Treatment of the pregnant patient may require higher or more frequent dosing given changes in body mass and circulating binding globulins. Glucocorticoids in stress doses (50–100 mg every 6 or 8 hours) should also be administered intravenously because of the risk of relative adrenal insufficiency that can accompany severe thyroid disease [3,15,16]. Finally, management should also include treatment of any precipitating factor, such as infection.

Labor and delivery considerations

Close liaison with neonatologists to ensure appropriate postnatal investigation and monitoring is essential.

Severe hypothyroidism can slow metabolism of anesthetic agents and increase the risk of hypothyroidism and bradycardia.

Adrenal crisis

Adrenal crisis refers to an acute state of glucocorticoid deficiency either as a de-novo presentation or in someone known to have adrenal insufficiency. Precipitating

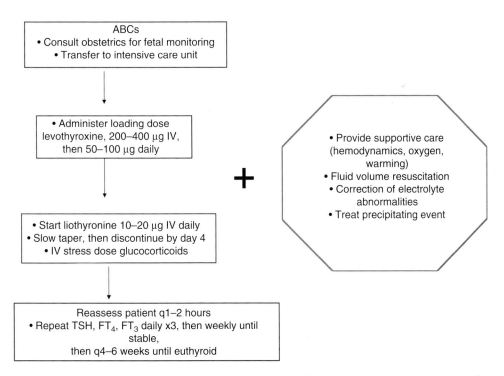

Figure 29.2. Management of myxedema coma in the pregnant patient. ABC, airway, breathing, and circulation; FT_3, free triiodothyronine; FT_4, free throxine; IV, intravenous.

Table 29.4. Etiology of adrenal insufficiency

Primary (adrenal gland)	Secondary (hypothalamic–pituitary)
Autoimmune	Abrupt withdrawal of exogenous
Bilateral adrenalectomy	Exogenous corticosteroid therapy
Trauma, hemorrhage	Lymphocytic hypophysitis
Drugs (ketoconazole, mitotane, metyrapone, aminoglutethamide)	Tumor (hypothalamic or pituitary tumor, craniopharyngioma, meningioma, glioma, chordoma, metastases)
Infection (tuberculosis, HIV, fungal)	Infections (meningitis, encephalitis, tuberculoma)
Genetic (hyperplasia, familial glucocorticoid deficiency)	Trauma, hemorrhage, infarction (Sheehan syndrome, eclampsia, apoplexy)
Neoplasia (lung, breast, gastric, malignant melanoma, lymphoma)	Infiltrative (sarcoidosis, amyloidosis, hemochromatosis, histiocytosis)

events include infection, sepsis, pregnancy, labor and delivery, surgery, pre-eclampsia, heat, fever, and illness that requires intensive care [18]. The causes of adrenal insufficiency are listed in Table 29.4 [18].

Clinical presentation

The pregnant patient with acute adrenocortical failure will present with rapid onset of hemodynamic instability, fever, and altered level of consciousness. Other clinical manifestations include bradycardia, hypothermia, refractory hypoglycemia, malaise, non-specific abdominal pain, nausea and vomiting, anorexia, weight loss, and slow respirations [18]. Loss of mineralocorticoid function (from aldosterone deficiency) results in hyperkalemia, hyponatremia, and intravascular volume depletion. Primary adrenal insufficiency is also associated with excess melanocyte-stimulating hormone (cleavage product of the adrenocorticotropic hormone (ACTH) precursor), resulting in hyperpigmentation [18].

Diagnosis

Women with mild adrenal insufficiency may only present at the onset of labor, in the early postpartum period, or with intercurrent illness in pregnancy. If clinically suspected, serum cortisol and ACTH should be immediately measured and then treatment with intravenous glucocorticoids can be started while awaiting results. Baseline cortisol levels can be higher than expected in the non-pregnant state because of the physiological changes of pregnancy [19]. A definitive diagnosis requires dynamic testing with an ACTH (cosyntropin) stimulation test (Figure 29.3) [18]. Serum cortisol levels are expected to at least double from baseline within 30 minutes of ACTH administration [19]. Serum ACTH levels distinguish primary (adrenal) from secondary (hypothalamic–pituitary) causes of adrenal insufficiency. Dexamethasone does not interfere with dynamic testing and can be safely administered while waiting to conduct the ACTH stimulation test [19].

Maternal and fetal/neonatal risks

Acute adrenal crisis in the pregnant patient, if left untreated, is associated with high risk of maternal and fetal mortality. Maternal adrenal insufficiency is also reported to confer risk of intrauterine growth restriction, neonatal hypoglycemia, and low birth weight [19].

Management

In general, the patient should receive 150–300 mg hydrocortisone intravenously over 24 hours either with a continuous infusion or as dosing every 6–8 hours. A gradual tapering in dose and conversion to the oral route occurs with clinical improvement (Box 29.2) [19,20]. Any precipitating stressors (i.e. infection) should be treated. Mineralocorticoid replacement is unnecessary in the acute phase, as hydrocortisone doses of 50 mg or more per day are equivalent to $\geq$0.1 mg fludrocortisone [20]. Once the acute situation resolves, chronic glucocorticoid (hydrocortisone or prednisone) and aldosterone (i.e. fludrocortisone) replacement should continue [19]. Prior to discharge, patients should be educated on the signs and symptoms of emerging adrenal crisis, including dose adjustments during acute physical stress and illness.

Labor and delivery considerations

If labor coincides with adrenal crisis, or delivery is indicated, steroid administration and correction of electrolyte imbalances are essential.

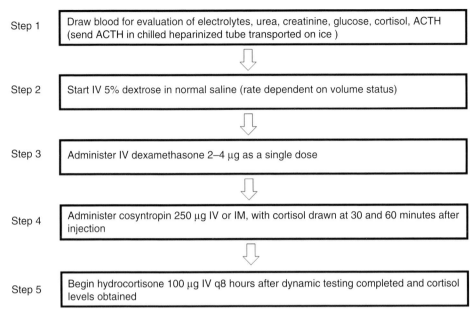

Step 1 — Draw blood for evaluation of electrolytes, urea, creatinine, glucose, cortisol, ACTH (send ACTH in chilled heparinized tube transported on ice)

Step 2 — Start IV 5% dextrose in normal saline (rate dependent on volume status)

Step 3 — Administer IV dexamethasone 2–4 μg as a single dose

Step 4 — Administer cosyntropin 250 μg IV or IM, with cortisol drawn at 30 and 60 minutes after injection

Step 5 — Begin hydrocortisone 100 μg IV q8 hours after dynamic testing completed and cortisol levels obtained

Figure 29.3. Diagnosis of adrenal insufficiency with concomitant treatment. ACTH, adrenocorticotropic hormone; IM, intramuscular; IV, intravenous.

Box 29.2. Glucocorticoid therapy for adrenal crisis in the pregnant patient in labor, surgery, or other severe stress

1. Airway, circulation, and breathing check, supportive care (i.e. vasopressors, fluid, correction of electrolyte abnormalities)
2. Consult obstetrics
3. Hydrocortisone 150 mg intravenous continuously for first 24 hours, or hydrocortisone 100 mg intramuscular or intravenous every 6 or 8 hours
4. Hydrocortisone 100 mg intramuscular or intravenous on call to operating room or at onset of labor, and for duration of event
5. Postpartum day 1: taper hydrocortisone to 50 mg intramuscular or intravenous every 8 hours
6. Postpartum day 2: taper hydrocortisone to 25–50 mg orally or intravenous every 8 hours; resume higher doses of hydrocortisone for major procedures or if patient becomes unstable and reinstate a slower tapering regimen
7. Postpartum day 3: hydrocortisone 25 mg orally or intravenous every 8–12 hours and start fludrocortisone 0.1 mg orally daily
8. Discharge regimen: hydrocortisone 15 mg orally in the morning and 10 mg in the evening plus fludrocortisone 0.1 mg orally daily (range, 0.05–0.2 mg daily)
9. Referral to endocrinology or internal medicine for outpatient management

Source: Malcolm and Keely, 2008 [19].

Pituitary apoplex

Pituitary tumor apoplexy is a life-threatening condition of acute pituitary insufficiency, often secondary to, but not exclusive to, infarction or hemorrhage of an existing pituitary adenoma. Hyperplasia of the lactotroph cells results in an increase in pituitary gland size by 70% by the third trimester, which increases the risk of apoplexy for pregnant women [21], with tumors >1.0 cm associated with the greatest risk [19]. This differs from Sheehan syndrome, which is postpartum hypopituitarism that results from pituitary necrosis caused by severe hypotension or shock secondary to massive bleeding during or shortly after delivery [17].

Clinical presentation

The presentation of apoplexy depends on the effects of the space-occupying mass and loss of pituitary function. Classic symptoms include severe headache (often frontal or retro-orbital), nausea, vomiting, vision loss, and cranial nerve (III, IV, V, VI) palsies [3,25]. In rare cases, the internal carotid artery can be compressed or have vasospasm, causing syncope, hemiplegia, or seizure. Superior extension will compress the optic apparatus, causing decreased visual acuity and visual field deficits. Signs of meningismus (e.g. fever, meningismus, altered level of consciousness, nausea, and vomiting) may also be present [3]. Inferior expansion can be associated with epistaxis or cerebral spinal fluid rhinorrhea.

Diagnosis

Prompt recognition and diagnosis can reduce maternal morbidity, including vision loss, progressive cranial nerve palsies, and consequences of untreated hypopituitarism.

Biochemical testing should include serum electrolytes, glucose, creatinine, serum osmolality, random cortisol, ACTH, TSH, free T_4, prolactin, growth hormone, insulin-growth factor 1, and urine electrolytes and osmolality. Interpretation must take into account normal pregnancy changes. Magnetic resonance imaging is most specific. If not available, CT with abdominal shielding may be done [22].

Maternal and fetal/neonatal risks

The impact of apoplexy on maternal and fetal well-being is dependent on the degree of pituitary gland dysfunction. Deficits in ACTH result in glucocorticoid insufficiency, manifesting as maternal hypotension, fetal distress from placental hypoperfusion, and hyponatremia [22,23]. Serum potassium is unaffected because of stimulation of aldosterone by the renin–angiotensin system. Central hypothyroidism, caused by TSH deficiency, may carry the same risks as discussed above. Growth hormone is reported to play an important role in placental function and fetal growth, particularly preconception and in early pregnancy [23]. Acute deficiency may predispose to placental dysfunction and poor fetal growth. If the posterior pituitary function is compromised, insufficient

antidiuretic hormone (diabetes insipidus) can cause severe intravascular volume depletion, hypernatremia, and death.

Management

The patient should be managed in an intensive care setting, with close monitoring of neurological and vital signs and surveillance for development of deficits. The most clinically relevant and life-threatening risk to both mother and fetus is ACTH deficiency. If possible, serum for baseline biochemistry and pituitary hormone function should be collected before administration of stress-dose glucocorticoids [19]. Dosing of glucocorticoids and tapering regimen is the same as discussed above for adrenal crisis. Thyroid hormone replacement is not required in the acute setting of pituitary apoplexy because of the long half-life of T_4, but should be evaluated again by measuring free T_4 4–6 weeks after apoplexy, or earlier if the patient develops symptoms of hypothyroidism. Once stable, the patient should undergo urgent imaging of the sella and suprasellar regions.

Trans-sphenoidal decompression should be considered if there is coma, visual loss, or a rapidly deteriorating clinical course [3,21]. Conversely, a conservative approach (non-surgical) has been recommended in patients with unilateral ophthalmoplegia and/or partial visual field deficits, and stable mental status, as most will resolve with expectant management (watchful waiting with close monitoring). This is particularly applicable in patients with prolactin-secreting adenomas, as dopamine agonist therapy is highly effective and recommended as first-line therapy [19,23]. Several published case series have found similar rates of improvement in visual field deficits or acuity with conservative treatment and surgical decompression (mean improvement 70% and 75%, respectively).

Labor and delivery considerations

If labor coincides with pituitary apoplexy, or delivery is indicated, steroid administration and correction of electrolyte imbalances are essential. If there is hemorrhage or a rapidly expanding tumor, neurosurgical input is required to assess whether the Valsalva maneuver in the second stage is safe or not. If deemed unsafe, delivery by cesarean section, or elective forceps delivery, would be indicated.

Regional anesthetic techniques may not be appropriate in patients with a rapidly expanding

Table 29.5. Symptoms of severe hypercalcemia

Symptoms	Causes
Dehydration	Electrolyte disturbances (e.g. hyper- or hyponatremia)
Renal	Nephrolithiasis, nephrocalcinosis, renal failure, hyperchloremic metabolic acidosis
Cardiac	Hypertension (pre-eclampsia), arrhythmias
Gastrointestinal	Peptic ulcer, pancreatitis, constipation, anorexia, nausea, vomiting
Neurologic	Weakness, depression, impaired memory, hyporeflexia, psychosis, stupor, coma

large pituitary tumor, and close liaison with the neurosurgeon and early involvement of an experienced obstetric anesthesiologist is essential in these cases.

Management of hypercalcemia in pregnancy

Calcium homeostasis is altered in pregnancy and must adapt to the increased demands of the fetus and placenta. Levels of calcitriol (1,25-dihydroxyvitamin D), parathyroid hormone (PTH)-related peptide, and urinary calcium excretion are increased. Total serum calcium is slightly decreased [24]; however, ionized calcium levels remain unchanged. Serum PTH levels initially decline, reaching a nadir between 16 and 20 weeks of gestation, followed by a gradual increase thereafter [25]. Several pregnancy tissues produce PTH-related peptide, including placenta, amnion, decidua, mammary tissue, and fetal parathyroid glands [26].

Hypercalcemic crisis. Fewer than 200 cases of hyperparathyroidism in pregnancy have been reported, with hypercalcemic crisis occurring in only 8% [26]. Benign parathyroid adenomas account for 89% of cases diagnosed during pregnancy or after delivery [27].

Hypocalcemia crisis. This is rare and most often exclusive to patients with previous thyroid or parathyroid surgery, when replacement doses of calcium and vitamin D may be inadequate.

Because of the rarity of hypocalcemia crisis, this section will focus on hypercalcemic crisis (Table 29.5).

Clinical presentation

Severe hypercalcemia is life threatening to both mother and fetus, with profound dehydration and neuromuscular complications that quickly develop without proper management. Hyperchloremic metabolic acidosis develops under the influence of PTH from decreased bicarbonate reabsorption in the proximal renal tubule [25]. The symptoms of severe hypercalcemic crisis are listed in Table 29.5.

Diagnosis

The classic findings of serum PTH at the upper limit of normal or higher, elevated ionized calcium levels, and low–normal or decreased serum phosphorus (phosphates) confirm the diagnosis of primary hyperparathyroidism [28]. If PTH is suppressed, other causes, in particular malignancy-associated hypercalcemia, sarcoidosis, and ingestions, should be pursued.

Localization of a parathyroid adenoma or glandular hyperplasia in pregnancy can be more challenging as parathyroid scintigraphy (e.g. Sestamibi scan) requires ionizing radiation and should not be used [29]. Ultrasound can be safely used; however, the sensitivity in localizing a parathyroid adenoma is suboptimal at 50–60% [29].

Maternal and fetal/neonatal risks

Hyperparathyroidism can result in considerable morbidity for the mother and fetus. Maternal risks include pancreatitis, nephrolithiasis, changes in mental status, nausea, vomiting, seizures, and pre-eclampsia.

Neonatal tetany is the most frequent complication associated with untreated maternal hyperparathyroidism, occurring in 15% of affected pregnancies [24]. Chronic maternal hypercalcemia creates high levels of serum calcium in the fetus and suppresses the fetal parathyroid glands. Neonatal hypocalcemia and hypoparathyroidism are often transient and typically resolve within 3 to 5 months. Severe maternal hypercalcemia also increases stillbirth and miscarriage rates [24,26]. Perinatal mortality of 25% has been reported [29].

Management

A multidisciplinary team including a maternal–fetal medicine specialist, an endocrinologist, and an experienced parathyroid surgeon should guide treatment. Vigorous intravenous fluid therapy is essential to replace volume losses caused by increased diuresis. Surgical treatment of primary hyperparathyroidism should be considered for all pregnant women with symptomatic and/or severe hypercalcemia. Ideally, surgery should be performed during the middle of the second trimester, following completion of embryogenesis and before the gestational age of viability [25]. This period is thought to reduce risk of premature labor and anesthesia exposure to the fetus. However, parathyroid surgery has also been safely performed in the third trimester [30]. No satisfactory medical therapy exists as an alternative and superior management option. Bisphosphonates are contraindicated because of their effects on fetal skeletal development [24,29]. Calcitonin does not cross the placenta and has been used safely in pregnancy [30]. High-dose magnesium has also been proposed, because of its activation of the calcium-sensing receptor, which leads to a reduction in serum PTH and calcium, although its true effectiveness remains unclear [31]. In extremely resistant hyperparathyroidism, unstable patients, or poor surgical candidates, dialysis may be used [28].

Labor and delivery considerations

At or near term, medical management and maternal stabilization, using dialysis if necessary, followed by delivery (vaginally unless there are other contraindications) should occur prior to surgery. In the preterm situation, definitive maternal treatment should allow the pregnancy to continue. If delivery occurs at the time of a hypercalcemic crisis, close attention to fluid balance and renal function are essential.

Close liaison with the neonatologists to ensure appropriate postnatal investigation and monitoring for neonatal tetany is essential.

Diabetes emergencies

In pregnancy, diabetic ketoacidosis (DKA) and the hyperosmolar hyperglycemic state (HHS) typically occur in the second and third trimesters, affecting an estimated 1–2% of pregnancies [32]. Traditionally, DKA has been associated with the insulin deficiency that occurs in type 1 diabetes; however, it is now recognized to occur in some subgroups of type 2 diabetes that are relatively insulin insufficient and ketosis prone. There are rare reports in gestational diabetes [33,34].

Causes of DKA in pregnancy include interruption of insulin treatment, previously undiagnosed type 1 diabetes, infection, emesis, glucocorticoid administration for fetal lung maturation, and beta-mimetic tocolytics [32–36]. Several changes that occur in pregnancy

predispose to DKA, including an accelerated starvation state with enhanced lipolysis, lower buffering capacity (i.e. from lower serum bicarbonate to compensate for a baseline primary respiratory alkalosis), and relative insulin resistance [32].

Clinical presentation

The onset of DKA is typically rapid, developing within 24 hours, although the symptoms may be present for several days:

- malaise
- dehydration
- polydipsia
- polyuria
- acetone breath
- cardiovascular: hypotension, tachycardia
- gastrointestinal: nausea, vomiting, abdominal pain, ileus
- respiratory: tachypnea, Kussmaul respiration
- neurologic: drowsiness, mental status change, lethargy, coma, shock.

In contrast, HHS develops over days to weeks. Clinical signs and symptoms often overlap for both conditions and include profound volume contraction, nausea, vomiting, abdominal pain, altered mental status (worse with HHS caused by elevated serum osmolality), acetone-odoured breath and Kussmaul breathing (DKA only), polyuria, polydipsia, and hypothermia [32]. Depletion of the effective circulating volume should not be underestimated; average water loss is 100 mL/kg in DKA and 100–200 mL/kg in HHS [37].

Diagnosis

The classic biochemical findings are arterial pH ≤ 7.3, plasma glucose ≥ 14 mmol/L, positive serum and/or urine ketones, elevated anion gap >12, and serum bicarbonate ≤ 15 mmol/L [37]. In HHS, there is more profound hyperglycemia (plasma glucose ≥ 34 mmol/L) and volume contraction, with minimal acid–base disturbance [37]. Hyperglycemia and profound water losses result in elevation of plasma osmolality. In DKA, plasma osmolality is generally ≤ 320 mmol/kg, while HHS results in an increase to ≥ 320 mmol/kg.

The pregnant patient will develop more rapid changes in pH because of the physiological respiratory alkalosis, lower bicarbonate levels, and associated reduced buffering capacity. Glucose levels will be lower compared with the severity of the acidosis than normally seen in the non-pregnant state. In one cohort study comparing pregnant and non-pregnant women with DKA, the initial glucose was 16.3 and 27.5 mmol/ L, respectively [38]. Plasma sodium is appropriately lower in the setting of hyperglycemia [32].

Maternal and fetal/neonatal risks

The impact of hyperglycemic emergencies affects both mother and fetus simultaneously. Estimates for rates of fetal loss range from 9 to 35%, but this can be greatly reduced by prompt recognition and treatment [32]. The passage of ketone bodies across the placenta predisposes to fetal acidosis and blood flow redistribution, which is reversible with medical management of the mother [32].

Management

Patients with DKA and HHS require close monitoring in an intensive care unit and frequent biochemical reassessments (every 1–2 hours) until the patient is stabilized and metabolic derangements corrected. Goals of management include restoration of the effective circulating volume and tissue perfusion, correction of electrolyte imbalance and hyperglycemia, and cessation of ketoacid production via administration of insulin [37]. Starvation ketosis often plays a significant role in ketoacid production in the pregnant patient, so administration of dextrose with insulin is essential to meet the needs of the fetal–placental unit until the patient is eating normally [36,39]. Given that fetal condition improves with maternal stabilization, immediate delivery of the fetus is not recommended. Fetal assessment should be undertaken at regular intervals, under the direction of an obstetrician.

We caution against rapid re-expansion of extracellular fluid volume because of the risk of cerebral edema. Plasma osmolality should be lowered no faster than 3 mmol/kg per hour [37]. Short-acting insulin dosed at 0.1 U/kg per hour should be administered intravenously for both DKA and HHS [37]. Use of intravenous sodium bicarbonate is reserved for patients in shock or with arterial pH ≤7.0 to avoid the potential risks of hypokalemia and induction of metabolic alkalosis [37]. Potassium chloride should be added to intravenous fluid therapy as soon as its serum level is 5.0 mmol/L [37]. If potassium levels are low on initial investigations, there is a severe potassium

deficiency and it must be replaced urgently to avoid further falls when intravenous insulin is initiated.

Labor and delivery considerations

Abnormal fetal monitoring often seen during DKA (e.g. reduced baseline variability and recurrent late decelerations) reverses with maternal treatment and resolution of DKA [40,41] and is not an indication for immediate delivery, as this may compromise the mother further with no evidence of benefit for the baby [32,36]. If labor coincides with DKA, close maternal and fetal monitoring are indicated with aggressive maternal treatment. Mode of delivery is dictated by obstetric indications.

References

1. Rashid M, Rashid MH. Obstetric management of thyroid disease. *Obstet Gynecol Surv* 2007;**62**:680–688.

2. Waltman PA, Brewer JM, Lobert S. thyroid storm during pregnancy: a medical emergency. *Crit Care Nurse* 2004;**24**:74–79.

3. Goldberg PA, Inzucchi SE. Critical issues in endocrinology. *Clin Chest Med* 2003;**24**:583–606.

4. Sarlis NJ, Gourgiotis L. Thyroid emergencies. *Rev Endocrinol Metab Dis* 2003;**4**:129–136.

5. Burch HB, Wartofsky L. Life-threatening thyrotoxicosis. Thyroid storm. *Endocrinol Metab Clin North Am* 1993;**22**:263–277.

6. Keely E, Barbour LA. Thyroid disorders. In Rosene-Montella K, Keely E, Barbour LA, Lee RL (eds.) *Medical Care of the Pregnant Patient*, 2nd edn. Philadelphia, PA: ACP Press, 2008, pp. 253–270.

7. Polak M, Van Vliet G. Therapeutic approach of fetal thyroid disorders. *Horm Res Paediatr* 2010;**74**:1–5.

8. Peleg D, Cada S, Peleg A, Ben-Ami M. The relationship between maternal serum thyroid-stimulating immunoglobulin and fetal and neonatal thyrotoxicosis. *Obstet Gynecol* 2002;**99**:1040–1043.

9. Laurberg P, Bournaud C, Karmisholt J, Orgiazzi J. Management of Graves' hyperthyroidism in pregnancy: focus on both maternal and foetal thyroid function, and caution against surgical thryoidectomy in pregnancy. *Eur J Endocrinol* 2009;**160**:1–8.

10. Nayak B, Burman K. Thyrotoxicosis and thyroid storm. *Endocrinol Metab Clin N Am* 2006;**35**:663–686.

11. Endocrine Society. Management of thyroid dysfunction in pregnancy and postpartum: an Endocrine Society clinical practice guideline. *J Clin Endocrinol Metab* 2007;92(Suppl), S1–S47.

12. Abraham RJ, Sau A, Maxwell D. A review of the EXIT (Ex utero intrapartum treatment) procedure. *J Obstet Gynecol* 2010;**30**:1–5.

13. American College of Obstetrics and Gynecology. Practice Bulletin 37: thyroid disease in pregnancy. *Int J Gynecol Obstet* 2002;**79**:171–180.

14. Hague WM. Pre-existing endocrine disease in relation to pregnancy: thyroid disorders. *Curr Obstet Gynecol* 1999;**9**:63–68.

15. Devdhar M, Ousman YH, Burman KD. Hypothyroidism. *Endocrinol Metab Clin N Am* 2007; **36**:595–615.

16. Wartofsky L. Myxedema coma. *Endocrinol Metab Clin N Am* 2006;**35**:687–698.

17. Molitch ME. Endocrine emergencies in pregnancy. *Ballieres Clin Endocrinol Metab* 1992;**6**:1992.

18. Aron DC, Findling JW, Tyrrell JB. Glucocorticoids and adrenal androgens. In Gardner DG, Shoback D (eds.) *Greenspan's Basic and Clinical Endocrinology*, 8th edn. New York: McGraw-Hill, 2007, pp. 346–395.

19. Malcolm J, Keely E. Pituitary and adrenal disorders. In Rosene-Montella K, Keely E, Barbour LA, Lee RL (eds.) *Medical Care of the Pregnant Patient*, 2nd edn. Philadelphia, PA: ACP Press, 2008, pp. 285–305.

20. Hahner S, Allolio B. Therapeutic management of adrenal insufficiency. *Best Pract Res Clin Endocrinol Metab* 2009;**23**:167–179.

21. De Heide LJ M, van Tol KM, Doorenbos B. Pituitary apoplexy presenting during pregnancy. *Neth J Med* 2004;**62**:393–396.

22. Nawar RN, AbdelMannan D, Selman WR, Arafah BM. Pituitary tumor apoplexy: a review. *J Intensive Care Med* 2008;**23**:75–90.

23. Karaca Z, Tanriverdi F, Unluhizarci K, Kelestimur F. Pregnancy and pituitary disorders. *Eur J Endocrinol* 2010;**162**:453–475.

24. Kovacs CS, Fuleihan GEH. Calcium and bone disorders during pregnancy and lactation. *Endocrinol Metab Clin N Am* 2006;**35**:21–51.

25. Lippes H. (2008). Parathyroid disorders and calcium metabolism. In Rosene-Montella K, Keely E, Barbour LA, Lee RL (eds.) *Medical Care of the Pregnant Patient*, 2nd edn. Philadelphia, PA: ACP Press, 2008, pp. 271–284.

26. Mestman JH. Parathyroid disorders of pregnancy. *Semin Perinatol* 1998;**22**:485–496.

27. Kelly TR. Primary hyperparathyroidism during pregnancy. *Surgery* 1991;**110**:1028–1034.

28. Shoback D, Sellmeyer D, Bikle DD. Metabolic bone disease. In Gardner DG, Shoback D (eds.) *Greenspan's Basic and Clinical Endocrinology*, 8th edn. New York: McGraw-Hill, 2007, pp. 281–345.

29. Pothiwala P, Levine SN. Parathyroid surgery in pregnancy: review of the literature and localization by aspiration for parathyroid hormone levels. *J Perinat* 2009;**29**:779–784.

30. Schnatz PF, Thaxton S. Parathyroidectomy in the third trimester of pregnancy. *Obstet Gynecol Surv* 2005;**60**:672–682.

31. Rajala B, Abbasi RA, Hutchinson HT, Taylor T. Acute pancreatitis and primary hyperparathyroidism in pregnancy: treatment of hypercalcemia with magnesium sulphate. *Obstet Gynecol* 1987;**70**:460–462.

32. Carroll MA, Yeomans ER. Diabetic ketoacidosis in pregnancy. *Crit Care Med* 2005;**33**(Suppl):S347–S353.

33. Pinto ME, Villena JE. Diabetic ketoacidosis during gestational diabetes: A case report. *Diabetes Res Clin Pract* 2011;**93**: e92–e94.

34. Maislos M, Harman-Bohem I, Weitzman S. Diabetic ketoacidosis: a rare complication of gestational diabetes. *Diabetes Care* 1992;**15**:968–970.

35. Chaisson JL, Aris-Jilwan N, Belanger R, *et al.* Diagnosis and treatment of diabetic ketoacidosis and the hyperglycaemic hyperosmolar state. *CMAJ* 2003;**168**:859–866.

36. Kamalakannan D, Baskar V, Barton DM, Abdu TA. Diabetic ketoacidosis in pregnancy. *Postgrad Med J* 2003;**79**:454–457.

37. Canadian Diabetes Association. Clinical Practice Guidelines for Prevention and Management of Diabetes in Canada. Can J Diab 2008;32:S1–S201.

38. Guo RX, Yang LZ, Li LX, Zhao XP. Diabetic ketoacidosis in pregnancy tends to occur at lower blood glucose levels: case–control study and a case report of euglycemic diabetic ketoacidosis in pregnancy. *J Obstet Gynecol Res* 2008;**34**:324–330.

39. Montoro MN, Myers VP, Mestman JH, *et al.* Outcome of pregnancy in diabetic ketoacidosis. *Am J Perinatol* 1993;**10**:17–20.

40. Lobue C, Goodlin RC. Treatment of fetal distress during diabetic ketoacidosis. *J Reprod Med* 1978;**20**:101–104.

41. Greco P, Vimercati A, Giorgino F, *et al.* Reversal of foetal hydrops and foetal tachyarrhythmia associated with maternal diabetic coma. *Eur J Obstet Gynecol Reprod Biol* 2000;**93**:33–35.

Chapter 30

Acute abdomen

Stephen Lu, Nova Szoka, Ulrich J. Spreng, and Vegard Dahl

Introduction

The term acute abdomen refers to the sudden onset of severe abdominal pain, tenderness, and muscular rigidity, which may be caused by inflammation, obstruction, perforation, infarction, or rupture of abdominal organs. In addition, medical illnesses such as diabetic ketoacidosis or a serious general viral infection such as influenza can mimic an acute abdomen. During pregnancy, the obstetrician/gynecologist and/or surgeon face the difficult task of distinguishing between obstetric and non-obstetric causes of the acute abdomen and in determining appropriate surgical and non-surgical management. Historically, there has been a general reluctance to operate on pregnant women because of concerns that surgical intervention may jeopardize the well-being of either mother or fetus. Approximately 1–2% of all pregnant women will undergo non-obstetric surgery during gestation [1].

Differential diagnosis

Figure 30.1 shows the potential causes.

Management of acute abdomen in pregnancy

Management of the pregnant woman with an acute abdomen is a typical multidisciplinary challenge. Regardless of the type of surgery and anesthesia, close cooperation and communication between surgeons, anesthesiologists, obstetricians, radiologists, the intensivist, as well as nurses and midwives, is essential. Box 30.1 recommends how to proceed with diagnosis and treatment.

In the subsequent sections of this chapter, it is important to note there is little literature on how critical illness alters the presentation of surgical disease

in the gravid patient. It is, therefore, necessary to extrapolate somewhat from how critical illness affects the presentation of non-pregnant women.

Non-obstetric causes of acute abdomen in pregnancy

Gastrointestinal causes

Appendicitis

Appendectomy is the most common non-gynecological surgery performed for pregnant women and approximately 50% present during the second trimester [2]. The incidence of appendicitis during pregnancy is 1 in 1500 [3]. Although growth of the gravid uterus pushes the appendix superiorly and posteriorly in the peritoneal cavity, the literature consistently reports right lower quadrant pain being the most common presenting symptom of appendicitis in any trimester. Additional symptoms include nausea, vomiting, anorexia, fever, and leukocytosis. Since nausea, vomiting, and leukocytosis may occur during normal pregnancy, the diagnosis of appendicitis can be challenging. Leukocytosis, which is a useful diagnostic sign in the non-pregnant population, cannot be trusted in pregnant women [3].

A critically ill patient with appendicitis may have a more severe presentation of the above symptoms, including a higher white blood cell count, criteria of the systemic inflammatory response syndrome or sepsis, or possible appendiceal perforation.

The initial workup for appendicitis should include history and physical examination and laboratory tests (electrolytes, complete blood count/differential) followed by selective use of imaging. Few data exist on the accuracy of imaging studies in the diagnosis of appendicitis in pregnancy [4]. The initial imaging

Maternal Critical Care: A Multidisciplinary Approach, ed. Marc Van de Velde, Helen Scholefield, and Lauren A. Plante. Published by Cambridge University Press. © Cambridge University Press 2013.

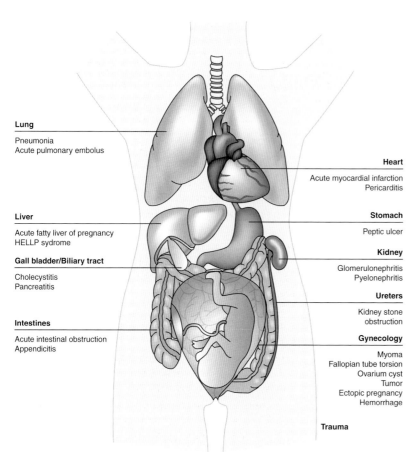

Figure 30.1. Differential diagnosis in acute abdomen in pregnancy.

Lung

Pneumonia
Acute pulmonary embolus

Heart

Acute myocardial infarction
Pericarditis

Liver

Acute fatty liver of pregnancy
HELLP sydrome

Stomach

Peptic ulcer

Gall bladder/Biliary tract

Cholecystitis
Pancreatitis

Kidney

Glomerulonephritis
Pyelonephritis

Ureters

Kidney stone
obstruction

Intestines

Acute intestinal obstruction
Appendicitis

Gynecology

Myoma
Fallopian tube torsion
Ovarium cyst
Tumor
Ectopic pregnancy
Hemorrhage

Trauma

Box 30.1. Management of acute abdomen in pregnancy

- Obtain history
- Physical examination
- Place peripheral intravenous line and begin fluid resuscitation if indicated
- Insert nasogastric tube if significant vomiting is present
- Evaluate laboratory studies: serum electrolytes, complete blood count with differential, liver function tests, lipase, partial thromboplastin time, prothrombin time/international normalized. ratio, urinalysis
- Consider radiographic studies: ultrasonography, radiography, CT, MRI
- Fetal monitoring is recommended after the 24th week of gestation
- Identify conditions that require immediate operation.

modality of choice is right lower quadrant ultrasound, which is reported to have a sensitivity of 86% and specificity of 81%. Although this test is non-invasive, rapid, inexpensive, and does not use ionizing radiation, it is operator dependent and is often difficult to interpret because of patient characteristics, such as obesity or a retrocecal appendix [4]. Additional imaging with CT or MRI can decrease the negative appendectomy rate [4,5]. One study demonstrated the negative appendectomy rate to be 54% in patients with clinical evaluation alone, 36% in patients who undergo abdominal ultrasound, and 8% in patients who have both ultrasound and CT scan. There was a significant reduction in the negative appendectomy rate in the ultrasound/CT scan group compared with the clinical evaluation group (54% versus 8%) [4]. Because of concerns about the radiation exposure incurred from CT, MRI is also being explored as a diagnostic modality for pregnant women, with one study reporting a negative appendectomy rate for MRI of 3% [5].

Once the diagnosis of appendicitis has been established, treatment is surgical, via an open or laparoscopic appendectomy. Multiple small case series since the early 2000s show that laparoscopic appendectomy is a safe procedure for pregnant women and has few complications, with low rates of maternal mortality and fetal loss. There is no difference in preterm delivery rates or fetal outcome in open versus laparoscopic appendectomy [2]. The benefit of the laparoscopic approach includes decreased postoperative pain, shorter hospital stay, and lower hospital costs. The most common complications following surgery for appendicitis include premature uterine contractions (25%) and preterm labor (13%), wound infection (8%), sepsis (2%), and miscarriage (2%) [6]. Also of concern are postoperative deep venous thrombosis and pulmonary embolism.

An area of controversy is the treatment of perforated appendicitis during pregnancy. One study reports a perforation rate of 15%, with 25% of perforations occurring in the third trimester. The rate of complications is higher in perforated appendicitis (52% versus 17%) [6]. Perforation is associated with a maternal mortality rate close to zero, an infant mortality rate of 3–8%, and a miscarriage rate of 8% [4,6]. In the non-pregnant patient, the trend has been toward non-operative management of perforated appendicitis, with drain placement and consideration of interval appendectomy. There are no studies that have evaluated drain placement and interval appendectomy for pregnant women with perforated appendicitis.

Laparoscopic appendectomy is a feasible procedure for the treatment of acute appendicitis in all trimesters of pregnancy. The current literature suggests that there is no significant difference in outcomes between the trimesters, although definitive conclusions are difficult because of the small sample sizes.

Bowel obstruction

Bowel obstruction in pregnancy is a rare condition, with a reported incidence varying widely, from 1 in 1500 to 1 in 66 000 [7]. Many of the data are decades old, representing individual case reports with low statistical power. Newer data indicate that the rate of bowel obstruction may be higher than previously estimated. Since the 1980s, maternal mortality has decreased from 12% to 6%; however, infant mortality has remained high at 20–26% [8].

This condition presents with diffuse abdominal pain, nausea/vomiting, and loss of appetite. In pregnant women, causes include adhesions (58%), volvulus (24%), intussusception (5%), as well as hernia, carcinoma, and appendicitis [7]. Small bowel obstruction is more common than large bowel obstruction. Large bowel obstruction is caused by cecal or sigmoid volvulus.

Diagnosis can be made with an upright abdominal film demonstrating air–fluid levels. The use of ultrasound has a low sensitivity, whereas MRI will achieve a correct diagnosis more often.

Treatment is an exploratory laparotomy when signs of intestinal ischemia or bowel perforation are present; otherwise conservative management with serial abdominal examinations and close monitoring can be used. Because of the high rate of maternal morbidity and fetal mortality associated with this condition, a high index of suspicion is necessary for prompt diagnosis, particularly in women presenting with a history of previous abdominal or pelvic surgery, and aggressive intervention is warranted [7,8].

The critically ill parturient is at high risk of developing non-obstructive motility disorders of both the small bowel and colon. Both ileus and acute colonic pseudo-obstruction are associated with a variety of metabolic and pharmacological conditions, ischemia, sepsis, and narcotic use. Critically ill patients are also at a risk of developing toxic megacolon, which is a serious complication of inflammatory bowel disease (IBD) or infectious colitis. Treatment is generally supportive, with source control and appropriate antibiotics for sepsis, along with restoration of vascular volume. For colonic pseudo-obstruction (Ogilvie syndrome), with impending cecal ischemia, it is important to exclude mechanical obstruction. A trial of neostigmine can then be considered. As neostigmine may cause bradyarrythmia and bronchospasm, the patient should be adequately monitored and atropine should be available. If neostigmine is not successful, colonoscopic decompression may be considered. Resection may be required in a minority of patients.

Inflammatory bowel disease

The term inflammatory bowel disease encompasses both Crohn's disease and ulcerative colitis. It affects women during their reproductive years and can, therefore, impact family planning decisions. Several studies have demonstrated that there is an increased risk of preterm birth and low birth weight among infants of women with IBD. Disease activity at conception and during pregnancy is associated with increased complications; however, pregnant women with Crohn's disease or ulcerative colitis are as likely to flare as nonpregnant women with the disease (~30% per year). There are few data published on acute abdominal complications of women with IBD. One study from 2005 described five patients who underwent subtotal colectomy for fulminant ulcerative colitis and then went on to have successful pregnancies [9]. Other sources report the ideal window for non-obstetric surgical intervention in patients with IBD is the second trimester, but that the third trimester is also low risk without significant adverse pregnancy outcomes. Data also indicate women with IBD have a higher rate of cesarean sections than the general population.

Spontaneous esophageal rupture

Nausea and vomiting affect the majority of pregnant women. Spontaneous esophageal rupture (Boerhaave syndrome) is a rare condition usually caused by intense vomiting; there are five reported cases of spontaneous esophageal rupture in pregnancy caused by vomiting. This condition requires prompt diagnosis and treatment to prevent fulminant mediastinitis and death. Presenting symptoms include vomiting, sudden chest and abdominal pain, and subcutaneous or mediastinal emphysema. Chest radiograph can aid in diagnosis. Treatment is emergency surgical repair [10].

Peptic ulcer disease and perforated gastric ulcer

Several epidemiological studies support a decreased incidence of peptic ulcer disease during pregnancy. One study of 17 032 women reported a rate of 0.26 peptic ulcers per 1000 pregnant women [11]. Another 10-year multicenter study reported six cases of peptic ulcer disease among 149 500 pregnancies [12]. Several endoscopic studies confirm that gastroesophageal reflux disease is increased while peptic ulcer disease is decreased during pregnancy. Several hypotheses exist as to why pregnant women have a decreased incidence of peptic ulcer disease, including increased gastric mucus production, protective effect of pregnancy hormones, and immunological tolerance; however, these have not been confirmed. Risk factors for pregnant women are the same as those for the general population and include smoking, use of non-steroidal anti-inflammatory drugs, alcoholism, gastritis, and *Helicobacter pylori* infection. Symptoms include burning epigastric pain, anorexia, nausea/vomiting, and abdominal distention. Initial therapy includes lifestyle and diet changes. Women are recommended to avoid stress, anxiety, night-time snacks, fatty foods, acidic drinks, caffeine, chocolate, salicylates, alcohol, and tobacco. Treatment is with histamine receptor antagonists. Failure of conservative therapy warrants invasive testing (esophagogastroduodenoscopy) or proton pump inhibitor therapy; however, the proton pump inhibitors have a less favorable safety profile in the pregnant population. Pregnant women with hemodynamically significant upper gastrointestinal bleeding should undergo esophagogastroduodenoscopy. Indications for surgery include ulcer perforation, ongoing active bleeding from an ulcer requiring transfusion of six or more units of packed erythrocytes, gastric outlet obstruction refractory to intense medical therapy, and a malignant gastric ulcer without evident metastases [13].

Biliary tree and pancreas

Cholecystitis

Acute cholecystitis is the second most common non-obstetric emergency in pregnant women. Risk factors include age, female sex, recent pregnancy, and family history. The reported incidence of gallstones varies between 1 and 12% of parturient patients, and biliary sludge is present in up to 30%. Elevated estrogen and progesterone levels are believed to predispose pregnant women to biliary sludge and gallstone formation. Estrogen increases bile lithogenicity and progesterone impairs gallbladder emptying [14]. Despite the increased tendency toward biliary sludge and gallstone formation in pregnancy, acute cholecystitis does not occur more often in pregnant women, affecting 1 in 1000.

The presentation of acute cholecystitis in pregnant women is identical to its presentation in the general population. Symptoms include postprandial right upper quadrant pain that can radiate to the epigastrium or back, with associated nausea, vomiting, and anorexia. Additional findings may include fever, tachycardia, leukocytosis, positive Murphy's sign, sepsis, or jaundice. Ultrasonography is the most accurate test for detecting gallstones. Positive findings include gallstones, gallbladder wall thickening (3–5 mm), pericholecystic fluid, a sonographic Murphy's sign, and a normal common bile duct.

Approximately a third of pregnant patients with cholelithiasis become symptomatic, and they may require surgical intervention with open or laparoscopic cholecystectomy [14]. Newer data show that women with symptomatic biliary colic treated conservatively have a recurrence rate as high as 38%. Relapse can lead to longer hospital stay, premature delivery, and labor induction.

As use of laparoscopic cholecystectomy has increased, multiple small case series show no significant differences in preterm delivery rates and fetal outcomes in patients treated with open versus laparoscopic cholecystectomy. Similar data suggest that laparoscopic cholecystectomy is safe throughout pregnancy, although published guidelines still state a preference for open surgery during the second semester.

Another complication of gallstones is choledocholithiasis, when a gallstone obstructs the common bile duct, leading to severe right upper quadrant pain associated with jaundice and fevers. The incidence is 1 in 1200 deliveries [14]. Choledocholithiasis during pregnancy, although infrequent, usually requires therapeutic intervention. Endoscopic retrograde cholangiopancreatography (ERCP) is safe during pregnancy. Indications for its use include recurrent biliary colic, abnormal liver function tests with hyperbilirubinemia, dilated common bile duct on ultrasound, and obstructive jaundice.

A procedure with ERCP followed by sphincterotomy and stone extraction is very effective and can be performed safely during all trimesters of pregnancy, with a premature delivery rate less than 5% [14]. Endoscopic ultrasonography is accurate for the detection of common bile duct stones and may be useful before ERCP in select patients.

Critically ill parturient patients with cholecystitis frequently do not present with the usual signs and symptoms, as listed above. Acute cholecystitis may occur as a complication of trauma, burn, sepsis, cardiovascular diseases, malignancy, biliary stasis, and total parenteral nutrition. About half of those with acute cholecystitis in an intensive care setting have acalculous disease. Acalculous cholecystitis is frequently seen in the critically ill patient population and is hypothesized to be related to biliary stasis, gastrointestinal hypomotility, narcotic use, and microvascular ischemia. The best initial test is ultrasonography. (We were unable to find any published guidelines regarding the use of hepatobiliary iminodiacetic acid scan in the pregnant population.) In patients too unstable to tolerate a general anesthetic, a percutaneous cholecystostomy tube is the most appropriate treatment.

Pancreatitis

Pancreatitis in pregnancy is a rare condition, with an incidence of 1 per 1000–4000 pregnancies [15]. Older literature on the subject of acute pancreatitis in pregnancy reported maternal and fetal mortality rates as high as 20% and 50%; however, contemporary data show decreased risk, with no maternal mortality and a 5% rate of fetal loss [15].

During pregnancy, gallstones are the most common cause of pancreatitis; this etiology is found in 70–90%. Symptoms include diffuse abdominal pain with elevated amylase and lipase. Workup should include liver function tests, calcium, and a right upper quadrant ultrasound. Diagnostic findings include gallstones or sludge in the gallbladder and/or biliary tree. Biliary duct dilatation and elevated bilirubin are signs of ductal involvement. Additional imaging modalities include endoscopic ultrasound, MR cholangiopancreatography, or ERCP.

Treatment of pancreatitis with a biliary etiology is with laparoscopic cholecystectomy or ERCP. Conservative management has a 50–70% recurrence rate; therefore, newer data favor intervention over watchful waiting [15]. Treatment of pancreatitis with a non-biliary etiology includes bowel rest, correcting hypovolemia with intravenous fluid resuscitation, nasogastric tube placement, analgesia, and correcting the calcium level. No antibiotics are needed.

A critically ill parturient patient with pancreatitis is likely to have the severe acute form of the disease, which is responsible for most of the morbidity and mortality associated with pancreatitis. Severe acute pancreatitis is associated with the systemic inflammatory response syndrome and end-organ dysfunction; additional complications include pancreatic necrosis with or without infection. In the critically ill patient population, 80% of deaths from acute pancreatitis are related to infectious complications. One recent retrospective review of 25 cases reported that 40% of this population had severe acute pancreatitis. Perinatal mortality rate was 8% and preterm labor rate was 32% [16].

Liver

Spontaneous hepatic rupture

Spontanous hepatic rupture during pregnancy is a rare, serious complication associated with eclampsia or pre-eclampsia and is associated with a 75% mortality [6]. Risk factors include multiparous patients with an average age of 30 years. The rupture can occur at any time from 16 weeks of pregnancy to a few days after a full-term delivery [6]. In one study of 437 women with the HELLP syndrome (hemolysis, elevated liver enzymes, and low platelets), the incidence of subcapsular liver hematoma was 0.9% [17]. Symptoms of hepatic rupture include acute onset of right upper quadrant abdominal pain and hypovolemic shock. In a stable patient, CT has been used to aid diagnosis. Treatment includes selective embolization of the hepatic artery or surgical intervention.

Two extremely rare conditions that can affect the liver during pregnancy are Budd–Chiari syndrome/portal vein thrombosis and hepatic hemangioma. As there are few data published on these, a high index of suspicion in addition to the proper imaging studies is necessary for diagnosis.

Abdominal vascular emergencies

Ruptured splenic artery aneurysm

There have been over 100 cases of reported ruptured splenic artery aneurysm in pregnancy, with only 10 cases of maternal and fetal survival; maternal and fetal mortality rates are 75% and 95%, respectively. The majority (69%) have presented during the third trimester[18]. Symptoms include sudden onset severe left upper quadrant abdominal pain. Multiparity increases the risk of rupture and, in one study, 78% of affected women were in their third pregnancy [19]. One study recommends that women of childbearing age or pregnant women with a known splenic artery aneurysm with a diameter of ≥2 cm should be treated electively because of the increased risk of rupture during pregnancy, in contrast to the low mortality rates of 0.5% and 1.3% for mother and fetus, respectively, for elective surgery [20].

Aortic aneurysm and dissection

Symptoms associated with aortic aneurysm or dissection include chest or abdominal pain radiating to the back, as well as a pulsatile abdominal mass. Diagnosis can be made with CT angiography. Treatment is not recommended for otherwise healthy pregnant patients with asymptomatic aortic aneurysms 5.5 cm in diameter. If symptoms develop or aneurysm size is ≥6 cm, referral to a vascular surgeon to discuss elective repair is recommended. Pregnant women with Marfan syndrome have an increased risk of developing an aortic dissection and should undergo appropriate screening before or during pregnancy to evaluate their thoracic and abdominal aortic anatomy. Repair is indicated if symptoms develop.

Renal tract

Nephrolithiasis

Nephrolithiasis, or kidney stones, is uncommon in pregnancy. Its incidence is 1.7 admissions per 1000 deliveries. Presenting symptoms include colicky flank pain radiating to the groin, with microscopic or gross hematuria. Confirmatory radiological tests include abdominal plain film, ultrasound, and non-contrast CT scan. The risks and benefits of using these studies on the parturient must be considered. One study demonstrated that women admitted for symptomatic nephrolithiasis had nearly double the risk of preterm delivery than the control group (10.6% versus 6.4%) [21]. In addition, pregnant women admitted for nephrolithiasis were more like to undergo induction of labor or receive tocolytic therapy and women with nephrolithiasis had a four-fold risk of pyelonephritis (7.9%) compared with non-pregnant women (1.7%). Undergoing a therapeutic procedure and the trimester of admission did not affect the risk of preterm delivery [21].

Trauma

Trauma is one of the leading coincidental causes of maternal death and morbidity [22]. Fetal death in this situation may be from severe hemorrhage and hypovolemia, placental abruption, or maternal death. An early diagnostic ultrasound is important to establish the viability of the fetus. Fetal monitoring should be continued if possible. Acute cesarean delivery may be indicated if the mother is stable and the fetus is in distress, the mother is dead and the fetus still alive, or if there is a traumatic uterine rupture. If the pregnancy itself makes emergency intra-abdominal procedures difficult, a termination of the pregnancy or an emergency cesarean section may be necessary in order to save the mother.

When receiving a pregnant patient to the trauma room, the special physiological and anatomical changes that occur in pregnant women must be borne in mind in order to stabilize the mother and fetus adequately. Treatment should include left lateral tilt position, extra oxygen supply, and maintenance of perfusion pressure.

Medical conditions mimicking the acute abdomen

Many serious medical illnesses can mimic an acute abdomen in pregnancy. These include severe sepsis of any causes, diabetic ketoacidosis, and serious viral infections such as influenza. Diabetic ketoacidosis may be associated with abdominal pain, nausea, and dehydration. Blood and urine samples (showing hyperglycemia and ketonuria) are useful diagnostic tools in the differential diagnosis.

Gynecologic and obstetrical causes of acute abdomen

The most frequent cause of an acute abdomen in early pregnancy is ectopic pregnancy. The incidence has been rising during the past decades and is now estimated to be around 2% [23]. Ultrasonography and hormonal markers such as human beta-chorionic gonadotropin are used to verify the diagnosis. Recent advances in surgical and medical therapy such as laparoscopy and methotrexate have made the treatment less invasive. Other possible causes for an acute abdomen that should be considered in early pregnancy are rupture or torsion of an ovarian cyst, torsion of a fallopian tube, or an infectious disease such as a tubo-ovarian abscess. Torsion, degeneration, or infection of uterine myomas are other possibilities that should be considered.

In late pregnancy, some of the hypertensive diseases in pregnancy such as the HELLP syndrome will often manifest by abdominal pain. Other serious complications of late pregnancy such as placental abruption can also start with acute abdominal pain. The diagnosis and treatment of these disorders are discussed in other chapters of this book.

Anesthesia for the acute abdomen in pregnancy

General considerations

Ideally, in order to avoid possible harm to the fetus, any surgery would be postponed until after delivery. However, when presented with a pregnant woman with an acute abdomen, the emergency situation and illness is by far more dangerous to both mother and fetus than anesthesia. Regardless of the type of anesthesia, close cooperation and communication between the surgeon, the anesthesiologist, and the obstetrician are essential when the pregnant patient presents with an acute abdomen and requires surgery.

Careful preoperative assessment of the woman should be made, and all preparative measures taken in order to minimize the risk and possible harm of the anesthetic procedure. Moreover, optimal perioperative care in pregnancy requires knowledge and understanding of the changes in anatomy and physiology taking place during pregnancy (Table 30.1) [24,25].

When anesthetizing a pregnant patient, it is crucial to preserve maternal hemodynamic stability and uteroplacental blood flow. Hypotension (>20% decrease from baseline or <100 mmHg) should be avoided and

Table 30.1. Anatomic and physiological changes and consequences in pregnancy, anesthesiological implications and precautions

Changes	Consequences	Precautions
Circulation		
Systemic vascular resistance ↓	Hypotension	Fluid load, use vasoconstrictor
Cardiac output ↑	Oxygen consumption ↑	Fraction of inspired oxygen ↑
Aortocaval compression (>12 weeks)	Preload ↓	Lateral decubitus position
Airway and respiration		
Venous engorgement, upper airway edema	Intubation difficulties	Equip for difficult airway management
Functional residual capacity ↓	Early desaturation	Preoxygenation
Oxygen consumption ↑		Rapid sequence induction
Hyperventilation	Respiratory alkalosis	Normoventilation
Gastrointestinal		
Gastric emptying delayed		Rapid sequence induction

its treatment is mandatory [25]. Perioperative maternal and fetal hypoxia must be avoided and normoventilation is essential [25,26].

Both general and regional anesthesia techniques can be used in pregnancy dependent on the volemic situation and the site and nature of surgery.

Most acute abdominal surgical procedures will require general anesthesia [1], and the airway should be secured with an endotracheal tube after a rapid sequence induction.

Preoperative period

Premedication to allay anxiety and pain may be beneficial since maternal stress may decrease uterine blood flow. The use of an anticholinergic agent (e.g. glycopyrrolate) decreases oral secretions and may prevent bradycardia during anesthesia [1].

Aspiration prophylaxis with an antacid, metoclopramide, and/or a histamine H_2 receptor antagonist may be beneficial, particularly during the third trimester [27].

Intraoperative period

General anesthesia in pregnancy is more often associated with intubation difficulties than in the general population [28]. Therefore, careful pre-anesthetic evaluation of the patient as well as preparedness for a difficult airway and training in airway management are mandatory [28]. Equipment for difficult airway management (e.g. gum elastic bougie, video laryngoscope, and intubation laryngeal mask such as the LMA Fasttrach) should be easily accessible.

Pregnant women desaturate faster during induction of anesthesia. Therefore, effective preoxygenation with a tight face mask is crucial. Preoxygenation should be performed either for 3 minutes with normal tidal volumes or with the eight deep breath technique. Orotracheal intubation is necessary in most patients undergoing abdominal surgery because of the increased aspiration risk in pregnancy. The use of cricoid pressure during rapid sequence induction is controversial.

Appropriate anesthetic drugs for the pregnant women undergoing abdominal surgery include hypnotics, analgesics, and muscle relaxants. The primary goals for choosing a drug for anesthesia are:

- to preserve maternal blood pressure, cardiac output, and uterine blood flow, thus avoiding hypotension

- to avoid maternal hypoxia, hypocapnia, and/or hypercapnia
- to ensure maternal hypnosis, analgesia and amnesia.

Volatile halogenated agents (e.g. sevoflurane, desflurane, or isoflurane) are frequently used for anesthesia during pregnancy. Animal studies have shown that moderate concentrations of these agents (minimum alveolar concentration, 0.5–1.0%) had little influence on maternal and fetal hemodynamics and blood gases. However, high concentrations of sevoflurane and isoflurane (miniumum alveolar concentration, 1.5–2.0%) may induce hemodynamic instability in both the mother and the fetus. Boat et al. [29] have recently shown that high MAC values of desflurane can reduce fetal cardiac function.

Nitrous oxide is frequently used for cesarean section when general anesthesia is necessary. However, the use of nitrous oxide in abdominal surgery, particularly laparoscopic, remains controversial because of the influence of this agent on bowel distention.

Opioids are used to provide analgesia during intubation and surgery. Opioids may decrease fetal heart rate variability. Moreover, opioids can induce fetal respiratory depression. This is only relevant if cesarean section is to be performed in relation to the non-pregnancy-related surgical procedure [1].

Thiopental, etomidate, and propofol can be used for induction of anesthesia. All three drugs rapidly cross the placenta and are rapidly cleared from the neonatal circulation. Experience with thiopental is greatest.

Ketamine provides both hypnosis and analgesia and is recommended in hemodynamic unstable patients.

To provide good conditions for endotracheal intubation and abdominal surgery, muscle relaxants should be used. Succinylcholine and high-dose rocuronium are the drugs of choice for rapid sequence induction. The advantage of rocuronium is that the muscle block can be reversed by sugammadex in the rare case of a "cannot intubate–cannot ventilation" situation [30].

Teratogenicity of anesthetic agents

The possible teratogenic effect of any anesthetic agent is probably minimal. Although there are animal studies supporting teratogenic effects of some anesthetic drugs, such as nitrous oxide and benzodiazepines, no such effect has ever been demonstrated in humans.

Lately, more focus has been set on the possible behavioral teratogenic effect of anesthetic drugs. The use of N-methyl-D-aspartate receptor (NMDA) antagonists (ketamine, nitrous oxide) and gamma-aminobutyric acid (GABA) receptor enhancers (benzodiazepines, intravenous induction agents and volatile agents) in a period of extensive receptogenesis has been associated with long-lasting cognitive deficits. Although these new results are disturbing, there are still substantial controversies regarding the risks of anesthetic drugs on fetuses exposed to maternal anesthesia in utero. When anesthesia is inevitable, it is probably better to avoid nitrous oxide and ketamine if possible.

Prevention and treatment of preterm labor

Non-obstetric surgery during pregnancy will increase the risk of abortion and preterm delivery. It is unclear whether it is the disease itself, the anesthesia, or the surgery that is responsible. The gravity of the disease, as well as early diagnosis and management, will influence the frequency. The use of laparoscopic techniques does not seem to reduce the numbers of preterm labors [2]. Procedures performed in the second trimester seem to have the lowest risk for preterm labor. From a theoretical point of view, the use of volatile agents, which is known to relax the uterine wall, would be advantageous. This has, however, never been proven. Evidence does not support any one anesthetic drug as better than any other; neither does the use of preoperative tocolytics appear to improve the outcome. In order to reduce the possibility of abortion or preterm labor, measures should be taken during anesthesia and surgery to maintain uteroplacental blood flow, keep the pregnant patient normoventilated and normovolemic, and perform surgery carefully with the least manipulation of the uterus as possible. The risk of preterm labor or delivery during the operation and for several days after necessitates careful observation of the pregnant woman, and treatment with tocolytic agents may be necessary. The oxytocin antagonist atosiban seems particularly useful in preventing preterm labor [31]. The prophylactic use of glucocorticoids is advised between gestation weeks 24 and 34 in order to mature the fetal lungs in case of preterm delivery. Progesterone substitution should be used in early pregnancy (until week 9) if surgery, which includes removal of the corpus luteum, is performed.

Monitoring during anesthesia

In addition to standard monitoring, fetal heart rate and uterine activity should be monitored with Doppler and a tocodynamometer before the start of anesthesia. An obstetric consultation before the start of the procedure is advised in order to document the well-being of the fetus. If possible, monitoring should be continued during induction, surgery, and emergence from anesthesia. When this is performed, loss of beat-to-beat variability is normal during anesthesia but fetal bradycardia is not, and this must initiate immediate reactions. In the postoperative period, fetal monitoring should be performed and the well-being of the fetus should be documented.

Postoperative period

Pregnant patients are at high risk for thromboembolism during the postoperative period. Early mobilization is important and prophylaxis with anticoagulants should be considered. Furthermore, postoperative pain should be treated adequately. Acetaminophen as analgetic is safe, as are opioids. Non-steroidal anti-inflammatory drugs should be avoided in late pregnancy. For major abdominal surgery, the use of epidural analgesia is safe and beneficial provided there is a stable hemodynamic situation. Careful hemodynamic monitoring and prompt treatment of hypotension is mandatory. Box 30.2 gives the key principles for anesthesia in pregnancy.

Box 30.2. Key principles for anesthesia in pregnancy

Preoperative
- Understanding of the anatomical and physiological changes in pregnancy
- Interdisciplinary communication
- Information for the mother

Intraoperative
- Difficult airway management
- Maintenance of maternal blood-pressure and uterine blood flow
- Avoidance of hypotension, hypoxia, and hyperventilation
- Use of established drugs
- Fetal monitoring (if possible)

Postoperative
- Early mobilization, prophylaxis of thromboembolism
- Treatment of postoperative pain

Key learning points

1. Surgical intervention for non-obstetric reasons will be needed in 1–2% of all pregnancies.
2. The most frequent cause of an acute abdomen in pregnancy is appendicitis, followed by acute cholecystitis and bowel obstruction.
3. Laparoscopic appendectomy is feasible in all stages of pregnancy.
4. The presentation of acute cholecystitis in pregnant women is identical to the general population.
5. Critically ill parturient patients are at a high risk of developing acalculous cholecystitis, severe acute pancreatitis, ileus, and colonic pseudo-obstruction.
6. In trauma, an early diagnostic ultrasound is important to establish the viability of the fetus.
7. The frequency of an ectopic pregnancy is rising and is now around 20 in 1000 pregnancies.
8. If a pregnant woman needs anesthesia, the most important single point is to maintain maternal hemodynamic stability in order to preserve uteroplacental blood flow.
9. General anesthesia during pregnancy is more often associated with intubation difficulties.
10. The possible teratogen effect of any anesthetic drug is probably minimal and should be disregarded. Recent studies on behavioral teratogen effect indicate that some anesthetic drugs may have more negative impact.
11. Imaging procedures in order to establish a proper diagnosis is safe, and MRI without intravenous contrast is a useful tool.

References

1. Kuczkowski KM. The safety of anaesthetics in pregnant women. *Expert Opin Drug Saf* 2006;**5**:251–264.

2. Ueberrueck T, Koch A, Meyer L, Hinkel M, Gastinger I. Ninety-four appendectomies for suspected acute appendicitis during pregnancy. *World J Surg* 2004;**28**:508–511.

3. Mourad J, Elliott JP, Erickson L, Lisboa L. Appendicitis in pregnancy: new information that contradicts long-held clinical beliefs. *Am J Obstet Gynecol* 2000;**182**:1027–1029.

4. Wallace CA, Petrov MS, Soybel DI, *et al.* Influence of imaging on the negative appendectomy rate in pregnancy. *J Gastrointest Surg* 2008;**12**:46–50.

5. Cobben L, Groot I, Kingma L, *et al.* A simple MRI protocol in patients with clinically suspected appendicitis: results in 138 patients and effect on outcome of appendectomy. *Eur Radiol* 2009;**19**:1175–1183.

6. Yilmaz HG, Akgun Y, Bac B, Celik Y. Acute appendicitis in pregnancy – risk factors associated with principal outcomes: a case control study. *Int J Surg* 2007;**5**:192–197.

7. Perdue PW, Johnson HW Jr., Stafford PW. Intestinal obstruction complicating pregnancy. *Am J Surg* 1992;**164**:384–388.

8. Connolly MM, Unti JA, Nora PF. Bowel obstruction in pregnancy. *Surg Clin North Am* 1995;**75**:101–113.

9. Dozois EJ, Wolff BG, Tremaine WJ. Maternal and fetal outcome after colectomy for fulminant ulcerative colitis during pregnancy: case series and literature review. *Dis Colon Rectum* 2006;**49**:64–73.

10. Eroğlu A, Kürkçüoğlu C, Karaoğlanoğlu N, Tekinbaş C, Cesur M. Spontaneous esophageal rupture following severe vomiting in pregnancy. *Dis Esophagus* 2002;**15**:242–243.

11. Vessey MP, Villard-Mackintosh L, Painter R. Oral contraceptives and pregnancy inrelation to peptic ulcer. *Contraception* 1992;**46**:349–357.

12. Durst JB, Klieger JA. A report of a fatal hemorrhage due to peptic ulcer in pregnancy. *Am J Obstet Gynecol* 1955;**70**:448–451.

13. Cappell M. Gastric and duodenal ulcers during pregnancy. *Gastroenterol Clin North Am* 2003;**32**:263–308.

14. Al-Hashem H, Muralidharan V, Cohen H, Jamidar PA. Biliary disease in pregnancy with an emphasis on the role of ERCP. *J Clin Gastroenterol* 2009;**43**:58–62.

15. Hernandez A, Petrov MS, Brooks DC, *et al.* Acute pancreatitis and pregnancy: a 10-year single center experience. *J Gastrointest Surg* 2007;**11**:1623–1627.

16. Li HP, Huang YJ, Chen X. Acute pancreatitis in pregnancy: a 6-year single center clinical experience. *Chin Med J* 2011;**124**:2771–2775.

17. Sibai BM, Ramadan MK, Usta I, *et al.* Maternal morbidity and mortality in 442 pregnancies with hemolysis, elevated liver enzymes, and low platelets (HELLP syndrome) *Am J Obstet Gynecol* 1993;**169**:1000–1006.

18. Herbeck M, Horbach T, Putzenlechner C, Klein P. Lang W. Ruptured splenic artery aneurysm during pregnancy: A rare case with both maternal and fetal survival *Am J Obstet Gynecol* 1999;**181**:763–764.

19. Trastek VF, Pairolero PC, Bernatz PE. Splenic artery aneurysms. *World J Surg* 1985;**9**:694–699.

20. De Perrot M, Bühler L, Deléaval J, *et al.* Management of true aneurysms of the splenic artery. *Am J Surg* 1998;**175**:466–8.

21. Swartz M, Lydon-Rochelle MT, Simon D, Wright JL, Porter MP. Admission for nephrolithiasis in pregnancy and risk of adverse birth outcomes. *Obstet Gynecol* 2007;**109**:1099–1104.

22. Cantwell R, Clutton-Brock T, Cooper G, *et al.* Saving Mothers' Lives: Reviewing Maternal Deaths to make Motherhood Safer 2006–2008. The Eighth Report of the Confidential Enquiries into Maternal Deaths in the United Kingdom. *BJOG* 2011;**118** (Suppl 1):1–203.

23. Farquhar CM. Ectopic pregnancy. *Lancet* 2005;**366**:583–591.

24. Palmer CM, D'Angelo R, Paech MJ. *Handbook of Obstetric Anesthesia*. Oxford: BIOS, 2002.

25. Goodman S. Anesthesia for nonobstetric surgery in the pregnant patient. *Semin Perinatol* 2002;**26**:136–145.

26. Littleford J. Effects on the fetus and newborn of maternal analgesia and anesthesia: a review. *Can J Anaesth* 2004;**51**:586–609.

27. American Society of Anesthesiologists Task Force on Obstetric Anesthesia. Practice guidelines for obstetric anesthesia: an updated report. *Anesthesiology* 2007;**106**:843–863.

28. Biro P. Difficult intubation in pregnancy. *Curr Opin Anaesthesiol* 2011;**24**:249–254.

29. Boat A, Mahmoud M, Michelfelder EC, *et al.* Supplementing desflurane with intravenous anesthesia reduces fetal cardiac dysfunction during open fetal surgery. *Paediatr Anaesth* 2010;**20**:748–756.

30. Williamson RM, Mallaiah S, Barclay P. Rocuronium and sugammadex for rapid sequence induction of obstetric general anaesthesia. *Acta Anaesthesiol Scand* 2011;**55**:694–699.

31. Usta IM, Khalil A, Nassar AH. Oxytocin antagonists for the management of preterm birth: a review. *Am J Perinatol* 2011;**28**:449–460.

Chapter 31

Sepsis

Luis D. Pacheco and Joost J. Zwart

Sepsis and pregnancy

Sepsis occurs as the result of a systemic maladaptive inflammatory response to an infectious insult. It is the leading cause of mortality in intensive care units (ICUs) in developed countries and the incidence is increasing worldwide [1]. Sepsis is also one of the leading causes of maternal mortality [2]. The incidence of death from severe sepsis in the obstetric population is lower than that of non-obstetric patients. The latter is likely secondary to a younger population with less coexisting medical pathologies.

Pregnancy affects both humoral and cell-mediated immunological functions. The white blood cell count rises as pregnancy progresses, and some authors have described these neutrophils as "activated," favoring severe inflammatory reactions to infectious stimuli [3]. Cellular immunity is compromised as a consequence of the decline in T-helper type 1 and natural killer cells. The decrease in cellular immunity predisposes pregnant women to infections from viruses and parasites. In contrast, antibody-mediated immunity is enhanced in pregnancy despite the fact that levels of immunoglobulins are depressed (likely from hemodilution). Pregnancy is not a state of generalized immunosuppression, instead, it is a state of immunomodulation, with compromised cellular and enhanced humoral immunity.

The literature regarding management of sepsis in the pregnant patient is extremely limited, and pregnant women have typically been excluded from landmark trials that have dictated the management of sepsis over the last decades. Most patients with severe sepsis/septic shock are managed in ICU, and most obstetricians and maternal fetal medicine specialists are unfamiliar with its management principles. This chapter will discuss key aspects of the diagnosis and treatment of severe sepsis and will comment on the likely effects/modifications of such interventions during pregnancy.

Definition of (maternal) sepsis

The following definitions are used.

> *Maternal sepsis.* Any sepsis of a woman during pregnancy, delivery, or puerperium up to the 42nd postpartum day.
>
> *Sepsis.* Infection plus systemic manifestations of infection, known as the systemic inflammatory response syndrome (SIRS).
>
> *Severe sepsis.* Sepsis with signs of at least one organ dysfunction (e.g. confusion, respiratory failure, acute kidney injury, thrombocytopenia, prolongation of clotting times, elevation of liver enzymes, hypotension).
>
> *Septic shock.* Severe sepsis with hypotension despite adequate fluid resuscitation.

A patient is considered to have SIRS if two or more of the following are present:

- temperature >38°C or <36°C
- heart rate >90 beats/min
- respiratory rate >20 breaths/min or arterial carbon dioxide partial pressure (Pa_{CO_2}) <32 mmHg
- white blood cell count $>12 \times 10^9$/L or $<4000 \times 10^9$/L or bandemia >10%.

The concept of SIRS was introduced by the American College of Chest Physicians and the Society of Critical Care Medicine in 1992 [4].

The definition of sepsis has been criticized for being too sensitive and non-specific as most patients in ICU will meet SIRS criteria [5]. Adding to the problem, *physiological* changes of pregnancy may include a heart rate >90 beats/min, a Pa_{CO_2} <32 mmHg, and a white blood cell count $>12 \times 10^9$/L. This definition is even more non-specific in the pregnant population.

Maternal Critical Care: A Multidisciplinary Approach, ed. Marc Van de Velde, Helen Scholefield, and Lauren A. Plante.
Published by Cambridge University Press. © Cambridge University Press 2013.

In 2001, extended criteria for the diagnosis of sepsis were developed to improve the diagnostic capacity of the clinical response to infection [6]. These signs and symptoms are depicted in Box 31.1 [7]. The reader should understand that this list of signs is a guide and not all patients with sepsis will have them, just as nonseptic patients may have some of them.

It is important to realize that sepsis can present atypically in pregnant women, with diarrhea, vomiting, and severe lower abdominal pain being common and important early symptoms of genital tract sepsis. The same goes for abnormal smell of vaginal discharge, vaginal bleeding, severe "after-pains" that require frequent analgesia or do not respond to the usual analgesia, and for abnormal or absent fetal heart beat with or without placental abruption.

Epidemiology of maternal sepsis

Sepsis accounts for 2% of all hospital admissions and 11–20% of all ICU admissions [5]. It is the most important cause of death among ICU patients, with reported rates of 33% for severe sepsis and 59% for septic shock. Sepsis is also among the leading causes of maternal mortality in low-income as well as high-income countries, accounting for up to 15% of maternal deaths [8]. The latest triennial report of the Confidential Enquiries into Maternal Deaths and Child Health in the UK showed – despite an overall decrease in maternal deaths – an increase in maternal mortality rate related to sepsis from 0.85 deaths per 100 000 maternities in 2003–2005 to 1.13 in 2006–2008, and sepsis is now the most common cause of direct maternal death in the UK [2].

In absolute numbers, maternal sepsis causes at least 75 000 maternal deaths annually, mostly in low-income countries. In high-income countries, 2.1% (95% confidence interval (CI), 0.0–5.9) of maternal deaths are caused by sepsis [8]. Much higher rates in low-income countries can be mainly attributed to the high incidence of septic abortion.

Nowadays, in most high-income countries, maternal mortality is too rare to be used as a sensitive marker for the quality of care, and *severe acute maternal morbidity* has been introduced as an additional marker. Two prospective population-based studies from Europe have reported incidences of 0.2 and 0.8 per 1000 deliveries [9]. Reported incidences from Canada and the USA were 0.1–0.3 per 1000 in Canada to 0.4–0.6 per 1000 the USA, based on retrospective studies using large discharge databases. In the Netherlands, 8% of all obstetric ICU admissions were for sepsis, with a case fatality rate of 7.7%.

The single most important risk factor for postpartum infection seems to be cesarean section, with average rates of endometritis for non-elective cesarean section being higher than those for elective cesarean section (28.6% versus 9.2%). Prophylactic antibiotics during the procedure substantially reduce the infection risk [10].

The main causative microorganisms of maternal sepsis are group A streptococci, responsible for 39–43% of direct maternal deaths [2] and 32% of severe obstetric morbidity from sepsis [9]. Most important sources of maternal sepsis include pyelonephritis, chorioamnionitis, postpartum endometritis, wound infection, and pneumonia. Coincidental non-pregnancy-related infections such as appendicitis and cholecystitis should also be considered and their course can be atypical [11].

Pathophysiology of sepsis

The pathophysiology of sepsis is extremely complicated and not completely understood. After exposure to a microorganism (bacteria, virus, parasite, fungi), the inflammatory cascade is activated. Massive production of inflammatory (interleukin-1β, tumor necrosis factor-alpha, interleukin-6, interleukin-8) and anti-inflammatory (interleukin-4, interleukin-10) cytokines, together with endothelial factors such as nitric oxide and other mediators such as prostaglandins, leukotrienes, and complement, lead to loss of vasomotor tone with profound vasodilation and increased vascular permeability (secondary to cytokine-induced endothelial injury) plus subsequent third spacing [1]. The profound decrease in systemic vascular resistances facilitates the so-called "increased cardiac output" seen in septic patients. However, the myocardium function in sepsis is also profoundly altered by the action of substances such as nitric oxide, interleukin-1, oxygen-derived free radicals, and tumor necrosis factor-alpha. Up to 60% of patients with sepsis have an ejection fraction < 45%. Both systolic and diastolic dysfunction may occur. Not infrequently, myocyte injury from proinflammatory cytokines may lead to leakage of troponins. Typically, patients with systolic dysfunction tend to present with biventricular dilatation. This appears to be an adaptive response since the dilation will allow for more intracavitary filling, leading to an increased stroke volume despite a decrease in ejection fraction

(preload recruitment). These cardiac changes tend to resolve spontaneously among survivors of sepsis.

Almost all patients with severe sepsis have clotting anomalies ranging from silent biochemical changes to full-blown disseminated intravascular coagulopathy (DIC) [1]. Activation of the clotting cascade in sepsis results from tissue factor expression in mococytes, neutrophils, and the endothelium as part of the inflammatory response. Once tissue factor is expressed in the surface of these cells, it binds factor VII, activating the clotting cascade through the extrinsic pathway. Development of DIC contributes to organ hypoperfusion (secondary to microvascular occlusion) and multiorgan failure.

Another important pathway is that of activated protein C. Once thrombin is generated, it interacts with an endothelial surface receptor known as thrombomodulin. This interaction leads to activation of protein C, which inhibits clotting factors V and VIII, promotes fibrinolysis, and has anti-inflammatory properties. Cytokines decrease the activity of thrombomodulin, leading to a lack of protein C activity in sepsis.

Mitochondrial dysfunction is also commonly seen in severe sepsis [1]. Even in the presence of adequate oxygen delivery, adequate oxygen consumption cannot be guaranteed if the mitochondria are dysfunctional and cannot extract oxygen and use it in oxidative respiration. This explains why patients with sepsis may have normal or above normal saturations of hemoglobin in the central or pulmonary circulations despite poor oxygen tissue utilization.

In summary, sepsis is characterized by a massive inflammatory response leading to hypotension secondary to a decrease in systemic vascular resistance, cardiac dysfunction, activation of the clotting cascade, inhibition of natural anticoagulant pathways, and mitochondrial impairment.

Management of maternal sepsis

Before discussing the management of sepsis, the importance of prevention must be emphasized, as this is probably the one intervention that most affects the incidence of sepsis and its mortality. Prevention includes hygienic measures, antibiotic prophylaxis, selective gastrointestinal decontamination, and optimizing the metabolic and nutritional condition of women.

Infections in pregnant women should never be underestimated as onset can be insidious but progression to fulminating sepsis and maternal death can develop very rapidly. The women are generally young and healthy, being able to maintain good vital signs until final stages of sepsis. Management of maternal sepsis is even more encompassing since there is a second patient to consider – the fetus. As effective maternal resuscitation is the cornerstone for optimizing fetal well-being, the focus should be on the mother.

The Surviving Sepsis Campaign

The Surviving Sepsis Campaign highlights the importance of the rapid diagnosis and management of sepsis that is critical to successful treatment. The patient with sepsis is usually already critically ill and requires immediate attention to avoid rapid deterioration; therefore, it is necessary to treat the patient at the same time as confirming the diagnosis. The management of maternal sepsis involves a wide range of clinical specialties in its diagnosis and treatment. Treatment is more likely to be effective, and severe sepsis avoided, if appropriate therapy is used early. Obstetricians may not have sufficient training to identify the symptoms to reach a timely diagnosis in this complex condition. Because of the challenges of diagnosing and treating this sepsis, approximately 10% of patients with sepsis do not receive prompt appropriate antibiotic therapy, which increases mortality by 10–15% [5].

Sepsis Bundles

Reducing mortality from severe sepsis requires an organized process that guarantees early recognition and consistent application of evidence-based practices. The "Severe Sepsis Bundles" are a series of therapies that, when implemented together, achieve better outcomes than when implemented individually. They are a distillation of the evidence-based recommendations found in the 2008 practice guidelines promulgated by the Surviving Sepsis Campaign to clearly articulate a therapeutic framework that will function as a lever for change. Making the Severe Sepsis Bundles standard practice will eliminate the piecemeal or chaotically applied of standards for sepsis care that characterize many clinical environments today.

The Sepsis Resuscitation Bundle is a combined evidence-based set of goals that must be completed within 6 hours for patients with severe sepsis, septic shock, and/or lactate >4 mmol/L (36 mg/dL) (Box 31.2).

Box 31.2. The Sepsis Resuscitation Bundle

Tasks must be completed within 6 hours for patients with severe sepsis, septic shock, and/or lactate >4 mmol/L (36 mg/dL).

1. Measure serum lactate
2. Obtain blood cultures prior to antibiotic administration
3. Administer broad-spectrum antibiotic *within 3 hours of emergency department admission and within 1 hour of ICU admission*
4. In the event of hypotension and/or a serum lactate > 4 mmol/L:
   (a) Deliver an initial minimum of 20 mL/kg of crystalloid or an equivalent
   (b) Apply vasopressors for hypotension not responding to initial fluid resuscitation to maintain mean arterial pressure >65 mmHg
5. In the event of persistent hypotension despite fluid resuscitation (septic shock) and/or lactate >4 mmol/L:
   (a) achieve a central venous pressure of >8 mmHg
   (b) achieve a central venous oxygen saturation of >70% or mixed venous oxygen saturation >65%

Source control and antibiotic therapy

Of pivotal importance in the management of sepsis is to achieve early source control and institute adequate antibiotic therapy. Any infected collections or tissues should be drained/excised as clinically indicated [12]. This includes prompt evacuation of the pregnancy after initiation of antibiotic therapy if the source is thought to be inside the womb. This means dilatation and curettage for septic abortion, delivery for chorioamnionitis, or hysterectomy or curettage for endometritis/retained products of conception in the puerperium.

Adequate empiric broad-spectrum antibiotic therapy covering Gram-negative and anaerobic organisms should start as soon as possible. Early administration of antimicrobial drugs in septic shock (within 1 hour of recognizing severe sepsis) has consistently been shown to decrease mortality. Regimens suggested by the Surviving Sepsis Campaign include

- co-amoxiclav 1.2 g plus metronidazole 500 mg every 8 hours or

- cefuroxime 1.5 g plus metronidazole 500 mg every 8 hours or
- cefotaxime 1–2 g every 6 to 12 hours plus metronidazole 500 mg every 8 hours [7].

Once culture results are obtained, the initial broad-spectrum coverage should be narrowed accordingly. In case of group A streptococcal infection, known for its rapid progress to maternal death, clindamycin is the first choice as it inhibits exotoxin production.

Apart from early initiation, efforts should be made to optimize antibiotic therapy based on the pharmacokinetic/pharmacodynamic properties of different agents. Critical illness is characterized by third spacing, with a significant increase in volume of distribution (mainly for hydrophilic antibiotics) [13]. Such increase in volume of distribution frequently leads to a decrease in plasma concentration and requires the use of higher doses of antibiotics in sepsis [13]. Tissue penetration of antimicrobial drugs in sepsis is limited by coexisting perivascular edema, with small vessel compression, hypotension leading to less perfusion pressure, and microvascular occlusion in DIC. Use of higher doses may help to overcome this problem. The pregnant patient may be particularly vulnerable as volume of distribution and glomerular filtration rate increase during normal pregnancy [14]. Needless to say, dosing should also be adjusted in the presence of liver or renal failure.

Concentration-dependent antibiotics (e.g. aminoglycosides, daptomycin) should be administered in high doses once a day since clinical success is directly proportional to the maximum concentration achieved. By comparison, time-dependent antibiotics (e.g. betalactams) require a plasma concentration above the minimal inhibitory concentration to achieve efficacy [13]. The latter has led clinicians to administer betalactam antibiotics over prolonged periods or even as continuous infusions in an attempt to maximize efficacy. Unfortunately, the evidence so far does not indicate that such practices improve outcomes [15].

Controversy surrounds the efficacy of initial combination antibiotic therapy compared with monotherapy. In the subgroup of patients with septic shock, the available evidence suggests that combination therapy may be superior.

If possible, teratogenicity and fetotoxicity of antibiotics should play a role in selecting the most appropriate antibiotic therapy. Cephalosporins, erythromycin, and penicillins are considered safe during pregnancy. Tetracyclins and sulfonamides should be avoided if possible. Nitrofuran derivates should not be used beyond 36 weeks of gestational age or when preterm delivery is anticipated because they interfere with the immature enzyme systems in red blood cells of newborns. Short courses of gentamycin at standard doses are generally considered safe. No increased incidence of congenital malformations has been found after use of metronidazol, but data are limited. Breastfeeding can be safely continued in mothers taking cephalosporins, erythromycin, gentamycin, or penicillins. Metronidazol is considered safe as a single dose, but there are insufficient data regarding safety for the neonate during multiple doses.

In summary, in the setting of sepsis, it is recommended that surgical control (if indicated) of the infectious process is completed without delay. Broad-spectrum antibiotics at the highest recommended doses should be instituted promptly. Antimicrobial therapy should be narrowed afterwards based on culture results.

Fluid therapy

The cornerstone of resuscitation in sepsis is fluid administration. Classically, hemodynamic resuscitation in severe sepsis has been directed to achieve a mean arterial blood pressure of 65 mmHg. The placenta, oxygenating the fetus, should be regarded as the one maternal end-organ that is most sensitive to hypoperfusion. For this reason, fetal heart rate decelerations on electronic fetal monitoring are often the first sign of maternal hypoperfusion.

Early aggressive fluid resuscitation improves tissue perfusion by increasing driving pressure and also modulates early inflammation by decreasing concentrations of proinflammatory cytokines. The Surviving Sepsis Campaign guidelines recommend the use of either crystalloid or colloid for the early resuscitation of sepsis [7]. We agree that, on the available evidence, either crystalloids or colloids may be used in severe sepsis and this should be no different in the pregnant population. Crystalloids (normal saline, Ringer's lactate, Plasmalyte) have an intravascular half-life of 30–60 minutes, compared with 16 hours for colloids such as albumin. Theoretically, the use of colloids leads to a more efficient resuscitation, but the largest trial available to date comparing the use of crystalloids and colloids in critically ill patients found no difference in outcomes [16]. A subgroup analysis suggested that septic patients with low serum albumin could benefit from albumin administration [17].

Some evidence suggests that hydroxyethyl starch (e.g. 6% Hespan) could increase the incidence of acute kidney injury when used in the septic patient.

One of the most challenging clinical decisions in daily critical care practice is the precise identification of adequate fluid resuscitation: it is clearly known that aggressive fluid therapy is fundamental in the initial management of sepsis, but the question is when to stop giving fluids. Premature initiation of vasopressors may be harmful as it will worsen tissue ischemia; however, excessive fluid resuscitation and positive fluid balances in the critically ill patient have consistently been associated with increased mortality. It appears that early in sepsis (first 6 hours), patients benefit from aggressive fluid therapy. Later, a conservative fluid strategy might be beneficial. Rivers et al. [18] demonstrated that early aggressive fluid resuscitation up to a central venous pressure of 8–12 mmHg coupled with the use of vasopressors, inotropes, and blood transfusions as needed leads to a decrease in mortality in septic patients from 46.5% to 30.5%. A subsequent trial in patients with acute lung injury and acute respiratory distress syndrome showed that after the initial phase of resuscitation, patients who received more fluid had a tendency to higher mortality and spent more days on a ventilator and in the ICU [19].

Traditionally, clinicians have titrated fluid therapy to static measurements such as central venous pressure or the pulmonary artery occlusion pressure. In fact, the Surviving Sepsis Campaign still recommends fluid therapy targeting a central venous pressure between 8 and 12 mmHg (12–15 mmHg if the patient is on mechanical ventilation) [7]. This recommendation likely also applies to pregnancy, as neither central venous pressure nor pulmonary artery occlusion pressure change during gestation.

Unfortunately, static measurements of preload are less than ideal for predicting fluid responsiveness, being effective in only 47% to 54% of cases. Echocardiographic-derived measurements suffer from the same limitations.

Current evidence suggests titrating fluid therapy to dynamic (rather that static) measurements of preload [20]. This topic is discussed in more detail in Chapter 27. More data are needed to validate the accuracy of pulse pressure variation and passive leg raising to predict fluid response during pregnancy.

Vasopressors, inotropes, and steroid therapy

When fluid therapy alone is unable to achieve a mean arterial blood pressure above 60–65 mmHg, vasopressors are commonly utilized. The pressor of choice in septic shock is either dopamine or norepinephrine [7]. Norepinephrine increases blood pressure mainly by increasing systemic vascular resistance, dopamine mainly by increasing stroke volume. Although most studies did not find one vasopressor to be clearly superior over others, a recent meta-analysis of randomized controlled trials and observational studies found dopamine to be associated with greater mortality and a higher incidence of arrhythmic events compared with norepinephrine [21]. The clinician may use the agent he or she is more familiar with. Concern has traditionally existed among obstetricians regarding the potential side effects of vasopressors on uterine perfusion. However, in the setting of shock, restoring maternal organ perfusion pressure is paramount, also for fetal survival. Multiple case reports attest to fetal status improvement with the use of vasopressors to improve mean arterial blood pressure.

Vasopressin is a peptide hormone synthesized in the hypothalamus and stored in the pituitary gland. A relative deficiency of vasopressin has been described during septic shock. Vasopressin causes direct vascular smooth muscle constriction via V_1 receptors and also increases cathecolamine responsiveness, probably by increasing cortisol secretion through its action on V_3 receptors in the pituitary gland. Additionally, vasopressin achieves vasoconstriction by closing ATP-dependent potassium channels. Observational studies have shown that the addition of low-dose vasopressin (0.04 U/min) can raise blood pressure in pressor-refractory septic shock. A recent large randomized clinical trial reported no improvement in mortality in patients with pressor-dependent septic shock who received vasopressin [22]. This trial did not address the use of vasopressin as a rescue therapy for septic shock that is resistant to conventional vasopressors. We believe that, in cathecolamine-resistant shock, the addition of low-dose vasopressin is indicated. No good data exist regarding the use of vasopressin during septic shock in pregnant women. Theoretically, it may activate uterine $V_{1\alpha}$ receptors, leading to uterine contractions. Extreme caution is recommended if this agent is used during pregnancy.

Contrary to popular belief, myocardial contractility is compromised in septic shock as tumor necrosis factor-alpha and interleukin-1 lead to myocardial depression. Patients may develop both systolic and diastolic dysfunctions, commonly involving both ventricles. The subgroup of patients with mainly systolic dysfunction usually will dilate the ventricles in order to accommodate more preload. This adaptive mechanism allows a transient increase in stroke volume and has been associated with improved outcomes. Patients with predominant diastolic dysfunction do not usually develop this compensatory chamber dilatation.

Septic cardiomyopathy may be "unmasked" when vasopressors are used to increase systemic vascular resistance. We recommend assessment of cardiac output (e.g. bedside transthoracic echocardiography) when vasopressors (mostly norepinephrine and vasopressin) are used without any inotropic support. If worsening cardiac output is noticed after initiating vasopressors, inotropic support (dobutamine or dopamine) is recommended.

Approximately 50–75% of patients with severe sepsis/septic shock have critical-illness-related corticosteroid insufficiency. Cytokines lead to a dysfunctional hypothalamic–pituitary–adrenal axis with a consequent decrease in cortisol secretion. Cortisol plays a pivotal role in upregulating catecholamine receptors at the vascular level (leading to increased response to endogenous and exogenous catecholamines).

The use of steroids in septic shock has been controversial for many years. In the past, large doses of steroids led to increased mortality, likely from immunosuppression. Currently, physiological doses of steroids are recommended in patients who fail to respond to catecholamines [7]. Patients who receive vasopressors and are unable to maintain a systolic blood pressure >90 mmHg are candidates for steroid therapy [7,23]. The agent of choice is hydrocortisone at doses of 50 mg intravenously every 6 hours or a continuous intravenous infusion at 10 mg/h. Such low doses of glucocorticoids are believed to be immunomodulatory, downregulating the excessive immune response that leads to shock without causing immunosuppression. Once started, treatment should be maintained for at least 4–7 days and the dose should be tapered over 1 week to avoid rebound inflammation and shock. The adrenocorticotropic hormone stimulation test should not be used to identify those patients with septic shock who should receive glucocorticoids. We recommend that the same guidelines be applied

during pregnancy to decide when steroid therapy is required. The clinician should be cognitive of the small association between steroid use and fetal facial clefting when deciding to use steroids during the first 8 weeks of pregnancy.

Anecdotal data suggest that cathecholamines may not be effective in the setting of severe acidemia. However, no data support use of sodium bicarbonate therapy during resuscitation to improve outcome. In the setting of sepsis, such therapy is not indicated if the pH is >7.15 [7]. If pH is <7.15, use of sodium bicarbonate should be individualized.

Particular care should be taken if the clinician opts to use this agent during pregnancy as bicarbonate does not cross the placenta but the carbon dioxide generated from the administration does cross to the fetal compartment, leading to potential fetal acidemia.

Resuscitation targets

Commonly, the main goal of resuscitation efforts in sepsis has been to achieve "normal" vital signs (mean arterial blood pressure >65 mmHg, urine output >0.5 mL/kg per hour, normal heart rate). Unfortunately, clinical signs and symptoms lack sensitivity to predict tissue hypoperfusion. Patients may have "normal" vital signs and still present organ hypoperfusion and anaerobic metabolism. Different strategies have been proposed to detect these patients with "occult shock." Resuscitation may be guided by serum lactate levels. Patients with persistent lactic acidosis despite apparent normal vital signs may require further resuscitation in order to increase tissue oxygen delivery.

Another option is to optimize hemodynamic support using central ($Scvo_2$) and mixed venous (Svo_2) oxygen saturations.

The Svo_2 is the hemoglobin saturation obtained through a blood sample from the pulmonary artery; the normal value is >65%. It requires placement of a pulmonary artery catheter. Hankins and colleagues demonstrated that Svo_2 did not vary significantly during pregnancy when compared with non-pregnant subjects [24].

The $Scvo_2$ is the hemoglobin saturation of a blood sample obtained from the junction of the superior vena cava and the right atrium. To obtain it, the clinician only needs a central venous catheter. The normal value is >70%. To our knowledge, normal values during pregnancy have not been described.

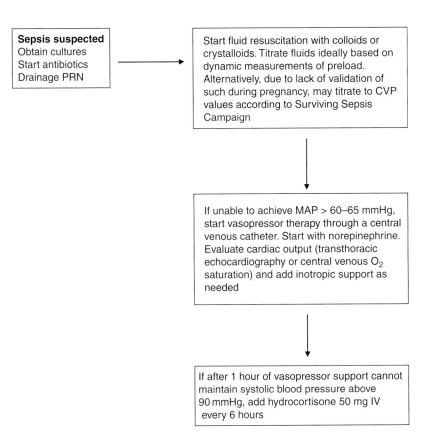

Figure 31.1. Simplified algorithm for the resuscitation of the pregnant septic patient. CVP, central venous pressure; MAP, mean arterial blood pressure; PRN, as needed.

Patients with tissue hypoperfusion will extract more oxygen in an attempt to increase aerobic metabolism. Such increased extraction will lead to a decrease in the saturation of hemoglobin returning to the central circulation. Low values of either Svo_2 or $Scvo_2$ may warrant an attempt to increase oxygen delivery by volume expansion, blood transfusions, or the use of inotropes. Figure 31.1 summarizes the main components of resuscitation in the pregnant septic patient.

Glucose control

A decade ago, studies from Europe showed that strict glucose control (maintaining blood glucose 80–100 mg/dL) in ICU patients was associated with a significant decrease in mortality. Subsequent investigators were unable to replicate the findings. The largest trial available so far actually documented that strict glucose control was associated with increased mortality. Current recommendations are to maintain glucose control in ICU patients (including patients with severe sepsis) between 140 and 180 mg/dL [25]. We recommend maintaining these same values in the pregnant septic patient.

Septic coagulopathy and transfusion requirements

As discussed above, sepsis is characterized by inflammation-mediated activation of the clotting cascade. This hypercoagulable state leads to consumption of both clotting factors and platelets. The manifestations of such coagulopathy range from silent biochemical changes to frank DIC with multiple organ failure.

Activation and consumption of clotting factors is paralleled by consumption of natural anticoagulants such as protein C, protein S, and antithrombin III. Protein C acts not only as an anticoagulant but also promotes fibrinolysis and has anti-inflammatory properties. Although an initial study showed a 6.1% decrease in mortality in patients with severe sepsis after early administration of drotrecogin-alfa (recombinant activated protein C), more recent studies could not confirm this and the drug was recently withdrawn because of severe adverse bleeding events [26].

In the absence of bleeding, platelet transfusions in the septic patient should be withheld until a count <10 × 10^9/L is reached [7]. Similarly, in non-bleeding stable patients in the ICU (including patients with sepsis), red blood cell transfusions should be avoided unless the hemoglobin concentration falls below 7 g/dL. The latter recommendation applies to septic patients after the first 6 hours of evolution (once early goal-directed therapy has been completed).

We discourage the transfusion of blood products such as fresh frozen plasma or cryoprecipitates for the sole purpose of correcting laboratory values unless an invasive procedure is planned or active bleeding is present.

When termination of pregnancy is anticipated, higher thresholds should be aimed for because of the risk of excessive bleeding during spontaneous or operative delivery or evacuation.

Mechanical ventilation

A detailed discussion about mechanical ventilation during pregnancy can be found in Chapter 18.

Conclusions

Sepsis is the leading cause of mortality in the critically ill patient in general, and one of the leading causes of maternal mortality worldwide. The pregnant septic patient should be managed in a multidisciplinary fashion with active participation of the maternal–fetal medicine specialist and the intensivist. Most of the key interventions used to treat sepsis should also be applied during pregnancy taking into consideration pregnancy-induced physiology. The cornerstone of fetal survival is optimizing maternal condition.

References

1. Nduka OO, Parrillo JE. The pathophysiology of septic shock. *Crit Care Clin* 2009;**25**:677–702.

2. Cantwell R, Clutton-Brock T, Cooper G, *et al.* Saving Mothers' Lives: Reviewing Maternal Deaths to make Motherhood Safer 2006–2008. The Eighth Report of the Confidential Enquiries into Maternal Deaths in the United Kingdom. *BJOG* 2011;**118**(Suppl 1):1–203.

3. Naccasha N, Gervasi M, Chaiworapongsa T, *et al.* Phenotypic and metabolic characteristics of monocytes and granulocytes in normal pregnancy and maternal infection. *Am J Obstet Gynecol* 2001;**185**:111–118.

4. American College of Chest Physicians and Society of Critical Care Medicine. Consensus conference: definitions of sepsis and multiple organ failure and guidelines for the use of innovative therapies in sepsis. *Crit Care Med* 1992;**20**:864–874.

5. Angus DC, Linde-Zwirble WT, Lidicker J, *et al.* Epidemiology of severe sepsis in the United States: analysis of incidence, outcome, and associated costs of care. *Crit Care Med* 2001;**29**:1303–1310.

6. Levy MM, Fink MP, Marshall JC, *et al.* 2001 SCCM/ ESICM/ACCP/ATS/SIS International Sepsis Definitions Conference. *Crit Care Med* 2003;**31**:1250–1256.

7. Dellinger RP, Levy MM, Rhodes A, *et al.* Surviving Sepsis Campaign: international guidelines for management of severe sepsis and septic shock:2012. *Crit Care Med* 2013;**41**:580–637.

8. Khan KS, Wojdyla D, Say L, *et al.* WHO analysis of causes of maternal death: a systematic review. *Lancet* 2006;**367**:1066–1074.

9. Kramer HMC, Schutte JM, Zwart JJ, *et al.* Maternal mortality and severe morbidity from sepsis in the Netherlands. *Acta Obstet Gynecol* 2009;**88**:647–653.

10. Smaill FM, Gyte GML. Antibiotic prophylaxis versus no prophylaxis for preventing infection after cesarean section. *Cochrane Database Syst Rev* 2010: CD007482.

11. van Dillen J, Zwart JJ, Schutte JM, van Roosmalen J. Maternal sepsis: epidemiology, etiology and outcome. *Curr Opin Infect Dis* 2010;**23**:249–254.

12. Marshall JC, Naqbi A. Principles of source control in the management of sepsis. *Crit Care Clin* 2009: 753–768.

13. Varghese JM, Roberts JA, Lipman J. Antimicrobial pharmacokinetic and pharmacodynamic issues in the critically ill with severe sepsis and septic shock. *Crit Care Clin* 2011: 19–34.

14. American College of Obstetricians and Gynecologists. Practice Bulletin 120: use of prophylactic antibiotics in labor and delivery. *Obstet Gynecol* 2011;**117**:1472–1479.

15. Tamma PD, Putcha N, Suh YD, Van Arendonk KJ, Rinke ML. Does prolonged beta-lactamic infusions improve clinical outcomes compared to intermittent infusions? A meta-analysis and systematic review of randomized, controlled trials. *BMC Infect Dis* 2011;**11**:181.

16. The Saline Versus Albumin Fluid Evaluation (SAFE) Study Investigators. A comparison of albumin and saline for fluid resuscitation in the intensive care unit. *N Engl J Med* 2004;**350**:2247–2256.

17. Delaney AP, Dan A, McCaffrey J, *et al.* The role of albumin as a resuscitation fluid for patients with sepsis: a systematic review and meta-analysis. *Crit Care Med* 2011;**39**:386–391.

18. Rivers E, Nguyen B, Havstad S, *et al.* Early goal directed therapy in the treatment of severe sepsis and septic shock. *N Engl J Med* 2001;**345**:1368–1377.

19. National Heart, Lung, and Blood Institute Acute Respiratory Distress Syndrome (ARDS) Clinical Trials Network. Comparison of two fluid management strategies in acute lung injury. *N Engl J Med* 2006;**354**:2564–2575.

20. Preau S, Saulnier F, Dewavrin F, Durocher A, Chagnon JL. Passive leg raising is predictive of fluid responsiveness in spontaneously breathing patients with severe sepsis or acute pancreatitis. *Crit Care Med* 2010;**38**:819–825.

21. De Backer D, Aldecoa C, Njimi H, Vincent JL. Dopamine versus norepinephrine in the treatment of septic shock: a meta-analysis. *Crit Care Med* **40**:725–730.

22. Russell JA, Walley KR, Singer J, *et al.* Vasopressin versus norepinephrine infusion in patients with septic shock. *N Engl J Med* 2008;**358**:877–887.

23. Annane D, Bellissant E, Bollaert PE, *et al.* Corticosteroids in the treatment of severe sepsis and septic shock in adults: a systematic review. *JAMA* 2009;**301**:2362–2375.

24. Hankins GD, Clark SL, Uckan E, *et al.* Maternal oxygen transport variables during the third trimester of normal pregnancy. *Am J Obstet Gynecol* 1999;**180**:406–409.

25. Kavanagh BP, McCowen KC. Glycemic control in the ICU. *N Engl J Med* 2010;**363**:2540–2546.

26. Martí-Carvajal AJ, Solà I, Lathyris D, Cardona AF. Human recombinant activated protein C for severe sepsis. *Cochrane Database Syst Rev* 2011:CD004388.

Chapter 32

Trauma

Andrew Tang, Bellal Joseph, Charles Cox, and Peter Rhee

Introduction

Trauma is a leading cause of maternal mortality and morbidity worldwide, with the majority resulting from motor vehicle or road traffic accidents. Effective care for pregnant trauma patients requires not only a thorough understanding of general trauma principles but also knowledge of alterations of maternal physiology during pregnancy and the interplay between maternal and fetal interests. The basic principle in caring for the pregnant trauma patient is "what is good for the mother is good for the baby." Fetal status can reflect the cardiovascular state of the mother, as fetal distress may be a sign of maternal hypovolemia. The best results for resuscitation will be achieved by the Advanced Trauma Life Support (ATLS) approach of airway, breathing, and circulation, plus disability and exposure (ABC-DE), with the early involvement of other specialties (e.g. anesthesia, acute care surgery, and, where needed, other surgical subspecialists such as orthopedists or neurosurgeons) in addition to emergency medicine physicians and obstetricians. The optimal outcome is most likely to be achieved through an algorithm-based care plan that is well coordinated between multiple disciplines.

The first part of this chapter deals with trauma while the second part discusses the specific issue of burns.

Epidemiology

Worldwide, trauma is the leading cause of death for those under the age of 45 years [1]. In the USA, it is estimated that 148 000 deaths are attributable to trauma on an annual basis, among which 42 000 are the result of traffic accidents. According to data by the US National Highway Traffic Safety Administration, there are approximately 115 traffic deaths per day [2].

Trauma is also a leading cause of non-obstetric maternal morbidity and mortality, complicating approximately 6% of all pregnancies: 4 out of every 1000 pregnancies will require hospitalization following trauma for further monitoring and treatment. The incidence of fetal death exceeds maternal death by more than 3 to 1. It is estimated that there are 3.7 trauma-precipitated fetal deaths per 100 000 live births.

In the UK, trauma is the leading cause of hospitalization among women. Trauma is one of the top three causes of death amongst people of reproductive age throughout the Western world, pregnant women being included in these statistics. Major categories of trauma are road traffic accidents (55%), domestic abuse (20%), and falls (20%).

In the UK, of 261 women who died in the triennium 2006–2008 (for a maternal mortality rate of 11.39 per 100 000), 17 died as a result of road traffic accidents. Of the four women who underwent perimortem cesarean between 24 and 41 weeks, no baby survived.

Ikossi *et al.* [3] analyzed 1195 pregnant patients with trauma in the American College of Surgeons National Trauma Database and found that motor vehicle accidents accounted for 70% of all trauma, followed by interpersonal violence (11.6%), and falls (9.3%). It is important to be aware that assault-related injuries during pregnancy are grossly under-reported. Available data suggest that such injuries are twice as prevalent among US racial/ethnic minorities than in white Americans. Multiple US studies have found that pregnant trauma victims tend to be younger, of lower socioeconomic status, more likely to belong to a minority group, and more likely to be uninsured or underinsured. Disturbingly, reports indicate that approximately 20% of pregnant trauma victims test positive for alcohol and drugs.

Maternal Critical Care: A Multidisciplinary Approach, ed. Marc Van de Velde, Helen Scholefield, and Lauren A. Plante.
Published by Cambridge University Press. © Cambridge University Press 2013.

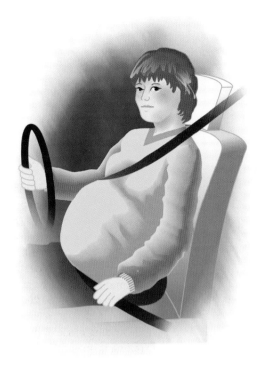

Figure 32.1. Correct use of a seatbelt in pregnancy.

The proper seatbelt application in pregnancy is shown in Figure 32.1. The shoulder belt is placed across the shoulder and between the breasts. The lap belt is positioned as low as possible below the gravid abdomen and across the hips. The lap belt should never be placed directly across the gravid abdomen as this predisposes the uterus, placenta, and fetus to compressive and shear injury during collision.

Considering that motor vehicle crashes account for over 55% of trauma in pregnancy in the UK and 70% of trauma in pregnancy in the USA, the proper use of seatbelts can be life saving. It is estimated that the correct use of seat belts reduces the risk of injury to the unborn child by 70%. While it is true that pregnant women are more likely to wear seatbelts than their age-matched non-pregnant counterparts, US studies have shown that only 73% demonstrate the correct seatbelt application. Discomfort and forgetfulness (53% and 37%, respectively) are the two most common reasons for the lack of seatbelt use, and 10% of pregnant females surveyed in a prenatal clinic believed that seatbelts are actually harmful to the pregnancy [4].

Diagnosis

The care of pregnant patients after trauma revolves around the concept of "what is good for the mother is good for the fetus." The diagnostic workup and treatment approach to the injured pregnant patient follows the ATLS algorithm of the American College of Surgeons Committee on Trauma [5]. Although multiple facets of trauma care occur concurrently in an organized resuscitation bay, the sequence of prioritization begins with ABC-DE (Table 32.1), followed by the secondary survey, comprising detailed physical examination and diagnostic adjuncts such as radiography, ultrasound (specifically focused assessment with sonography for trauma (FAST)), and CT.

It is not uncommon that a patient first learns she is pregnant during her evaluation for trauma. The evaluation of every female within the potential age range for pregnancy should include a urinary or serum human beta-chorionic gonadotropin. The knowledge of a patient's pregnancy and gestational age will guide subsequent workup, particularly in regards to radiographic studies and fetal–maternal monitoring.

As with all trauma patients, care of the injured pregnant patient takes a multidisciplinary approach. This often involves coordinated input from the trauma, anesthesia, obstetrics, and surgical subspecialty services in order to deliver the most efficient and comprehensive care. In addition to providing standard monitoring for the mother, fetal (cardiotocographic) monitoring should be performed for those who are at or beyond the gestational age at which extrauterine survival is possible: this may reflect local guidelines but in the USA is commonly considered to be 24 weeks of gestation. While there is no high level of evidence guiding the duration of maternal–fetal monitoring before safe discharge, common American practice is for maternal and fetal monitoring for at least 4 hours after minor trauma and 24 hours after major trauma. During this time, the clinician should be vigilant in monitoring for vaginal bleeding, preterm labor, premature rupture of the membranes, or any manifestation of maternal hemodynamic instability or suspicion of fetal compromise that mandates further monitoring or intervention.

Clinical features of pregnancy affecting trauma assessment

Pregnancy is associated with physiological changes in every body organ system, all of which impact the

Table 32.1. The airway, breathing, circulation, disability, and exposure sequence in resuscitation

Primary survey	Signs/symptoms	Management options
Airway maintenance and c-spine protection	Direct injury to the airway Edema or foreign body Depressed level of consciousness	Chin lift/jaw thrust Suctioning Establish patent airway (endotracheal intubation) Surgical airway (cricothyroidotomy, tracheostomy)
Breathing	Depressed respiratory function/absence of spontaneous breathing Asymmetrical breath sounds (pneumothorax) Altered respiratory mechanics (flail chest)	Supplemental oxygen Tube thoracostomy Mechanical ventilation
Circulation	Active hemorrhage Hypotension/shock Depressed level of consciousness	Control active hemorrhage Rapid intravenous infusion via large-bore lines Reassess patient
Disability	Glasgow Coma Scale Pupillary response Hemiplegia (impending herniation) Spinal cord injury	Early and emergency treatment of intracranial hypertension Avoid hypoxia/hypotension Urgent neurosurgical consult
Exposure/environment	Completely undress patient to faciliate examination Avoid hypothermia	Warm intravenous fluids Blankets Evaluate for missed injuries

maternal–fetal response to injury. We review them briefly here and refer to Chapter 10 for more detailed information.

Cardiovascular changes

Plasma volume is expanded by an additional 45% above pre-pregnancy levels, and peripheral vascular resistance declines by 30%; resting heart rate gradually rises by 10–15 beats/min, contributing to an overall cardiac output increase by 1.5 L/min, a 25% increase above the normal pre-pregnancy state. The increased plasma volume also results in "physiological anemia of pregnancy," and a hematocrit of 31–35% is within normal limits.

The cardiovascular physiological changes confound the interpretation of vital signs of the pregnant trauma patient. The clinician must be astute in understanding that hemorrhagic shock may have a delayed presentation because of the expanded maternal physiological reserve. Baseline relative tachycardia can be dismissed only after excluding sources of shock. Likewise, a "stable" blood pressure must be interpreted with caution as the expanded plasma volume creates a deceptive scenario that manifests hypotension only after significant blood loss has occurred. The first sign of shock may be fetal heart rate changes as the placental circulation is hypoperfused.

During the second half of the pregnancy, the enlarging uterus may compress the inferior vena cava, causing decreased vascular return to the right heart and, therefore, decreased cardiac output. The resultant "supine hypotension" can be alleviated by elevating the right hip by at least 15°. If there is concern about a possible spinal injury, the patient should be kept on a spine board to be tilted. If this is not possible, the uterus should be manually displaced to alleviate compression on the inferior vena cava.

Respiratory changes

Noticeable respiratory changes during pregnancy include an increase in minute ventilation and a compensated respiratory alkalosis with a decrease in serum bicarbonate. This ultimately leads to a reduction in the patient's total buffering capacity against systemic acidosis.

Gastrointestinal changes

Gastrointestinal secretion and motility are inhibited; competence of the lower esophageal sphincter declines because of hormonal and mechanical effects.

Every trauma patient is suspected of having a full stomach and should be approached with every attempt to minimize the risk of aspiration: this is a particularly important assumption to maintain while caring for the pregnant patient as they are at an even higher aspiration risk. Liberal use of antiemetics, nasogastric tubes, and expedient spinal clearance so patients can be positioned semirecumbent rather than flat are important maneuvers to minimize aspiration. If the need for intubation arises, rapid sequence intubation should be employed. This technique preoxygenates the patient without bag-valve mask ventilation; weight-based induction agent and paralytics are used instead of titrating for effect, and cricoid pressure is applied.

Renal changes

Renal blood flow increases by 30% over pre-pregnant levels, which results in increased glomerular filtration. Clearance of creatinine, urea, and uric acid is increased, leading to decreased serum creatinine and blood urea nitrogen.

A mild degree of hydronephrosis and hydroureter is normal during the late stages of pregnancy because of the gravid uterus compressing the urinary tract.

Hematologic changes

Trauma is generally associated with hypercoagulability unless in the end stages of shock, when massive blood loss and coagulation factor consumption result in profound coagulopathy. Pregnancy is also associated with hypercoagulability through increased production of fibrinogen and coagulation factors plus a decrease in fibrinolytic activity. The interplay between pregnancy, trauma, and coagulopathy has not been specifically studied. While it is plausible that pregnancy-associated hypercoagulability may be protective in early stages of hemorrhage, it may also predispose the patient to increased risk of venous thromboembolism.

Investigations

Primary survey

The primary survey in pregnant patients is done in the same manner as in non-pregnant patients. Primary survey includes assessment and maintenance of the ABCs.

If intubation is required, the initial, weight-based dose of a paralytic agent (neuromuscular-blocking agent or muscle relaxant) is the same for pregnant as non-pregnant patients. Pregnant women are, however, more susceptible to these agents, so the block may last longer. A limited amount may cross the placenta, so if

delivery occurs shortly after the mother has been administered one of these drugs, the pediatrician must be prepared to manage flaccidity or apnea in the newborn.

Because airway edema is more common in pregnant women, a smaller endotracheal tube should generally be selected.

In pregnancy, the risk for aspiration and hypoxia increases because the diaphragm is displaced cranially by the gravid uterus and because of the combined maternal–fetal oxygen demand. Therefore, supplemental oxygen is essential in these patients. The supine position should be avoided after mid-pregnancy in order to avoid inferior vena cava compression; if the spine has not been cleared, the lateral tilt can be supported on a spine board. Because the diaphragm is elevated by up to 4 cm by the late-term gravid uterus, entry into the thoracic cavity during thoracostomy tube placement should be one or two intercostal spaces higher than the usual recommended fifth intercostal location.

A pregnant patient may lose a large volume of blood (30–35%) before there is a change to the vital signs. Early replacement of blood and blood products should be implemented, as lessons learned from recent military campaigns have emphasized the survival advantage of early replacement of blood lost by the previously fit young person. While hypotensive or targeted resuscitation is commonly employed in trauma situations, the optimal hypotensive resuscitation goal in pregnancy has not been defined, particularly given concerns of fetoplacental hypoperfusion under these circumstances. Limited late gestational rabbit models in hemorrhagic shock do show a maternal survival benefit with hypotensive resuscitation [6].

Secondary survey

The uterus is out of the pelvis at 12 weeks and palpable at the umbilicus at 20 weeks; thereafter fundal height increases by 1 cm per week and roughly matches the gestational age. Fetal crown–rump length is used to provide a more objective measure of gestational age during the first trimester. Fetal biparietal diameter, head circumference, and femur length more accurately reflect gestational age after the first trimester. Accurate fetal gestational age critically impacts the management of the mother and the fetus.

The secondary survey comprises a complete history and physical examination along with diagnostic adjuncts such as ultrasound and CT. Gestational age can be estimated from the last menstrual period or, if known, the estimated date of delivery, by abdominal examination, or by ultrasonography. Pelvic examination is an important part of the secondary survey. If there is suspicion of vaginal injury (accidental or deliberate) or pelvic fracture, the examination may be better carried out under an anesthesia.

Pelvic examination

Pelvic and rectal examinations should be routinely performed as a part of the secondary survey in pregnant trauma patients. Perineal trauma, a bulging perineum, vaginal bleeding, or ruptured membranes should be noted and an urgent specialist obstetric opinion sought. A tender or hard uterus and vaginal bleeding suggest placental abruption, but in most cases of vaginal bleeding ultrasound will be indicated prior to pelvic examination.

Focused assessment with sonography for trauma

The FAST approach is a standard diagnostic adjunct employed in the trauma resuscitation bay for the detection of intra-abdominal blood and pericardial tamponade. Goodwin et al. [7] studied the clinical usefulness of FAST in 177 pregnant women with blunt trauma, 85% of whom were in the second and third trimester. The sensitivity and specificity was 83% and 98%, respectively, which are similar to values in the non-pregnant counterparts. The standardization of FAST has decreased CT utilization and has also largely replaced diagnostic peritoneal lavage apart from rare cases (such as the hemodynamically unstable patient with a negative FAST). If diagnostic peritoneal lavage is carried out in the pregnant patient, the catheter insertion site should be supraumbilical to avoid injury to the uterus.

Fetal ultrasound

Ultrasound is the most common imaging modality in evaluating the fetus. It confirms gestational age, fetal well-being, and position of the placenta. The advantages of ultrasound include portability, repeatability, and minimal radiation exposure. Ultrasound does have some limitations and these are important to keep in mind; in trauma when placental abruption is a concern, sensitivity of ultrasound in detecting placental abruption in the acute phase is poor.

Cardiotocography

Cardiotocography is a technical means of recording fetal heart rate and uterine contractions. Because extrauterine survival is feasible at about 24 weeks, it is common practice in the USA to employ cardiotocography after trauma for women who have reached this stage. More than 90% of women with major trauma after 20 weeks of gestation will demonstrate uterine activity within the first hour, decreasing with time; by 4 hours fewer than 30% are still contracting. The persistence of contractions at 24 hours is associated with worse perinatal outcomes. Late decelerations or loss of fetal heart tone variability may signal fetal compromise.

Kleihauer–Betke test for rhesus immunoglobulin

A Kleihauer–Betke test allows identification of the number of fetal cells present in a given volume of maternal blood. It identifies the amount of fetomaternal blood exchange and guides the appropriate dose of rhesus immunoglobulin needed to immunize rhesus-negative mothers. The test is indicated in all rhesus-negative pregnant patients after trauma. Some have advocated using the Kleihauer–Betke test in all pregnant patients after trauma because there is an association between a positive result and a higher risk of preterm labor or placental abruption, but specificity is poor [8].

Diagnostic imaging

The pregnant uterus should be shielded for X-rays whenever possible. Concerns about radiation exposure should not preclude the necessary imaging for the timely identification of injuries. Irradiation of the fetus carries little risk compared with the dangers of undiagnosed maternal trauma. The American College of Obstetricians and Gynecologists recommends keeping total fetal radiation dose to <50 mGy (<5 rads). However, when possible, alternative imaging modalities such as ultrasound and MRI may be used (see Chapter 22).

Types of trauma

Blunt trauma

Blunt trauma accounts for the majority of trauma sustained during pregnancy. Motor vehicle accidents are the most common cause of blunt trauma in pregnant women (55–70%) followed by assault (11–21%) and falls (9%) [1–3]. Traumatic brain injury and uncontrolled maternal hemorrhage account for the majority of maternal deaths. The gravid uterus alters the pattern of injury in the pregnant female compared with non-pregnant counterparts. Direct blunt abdominal trauma is associated with uterine rupture, and 75% of cases involve the fundus. Fetal mortality from uterine rupture associated with blunt trauma approaches 100%. Although uterine rupture is not the direct contributing factor to maternal demise in the majority of cases, it is associated with a 10% maternal mortality through associated abdominal and orthopedic injuries. Severe pelvic fractures are associated with a 30% incidence of intra-abdominal injuries, most commonly to the bladder and small bowel [9–11]. In the pregnant woman, the added risk of uterine and fetal trauma must be considered, including the risk of fetal head trauma when the fetal head is fixed in the maternal pelvis. It is important to note that a pelvic fracture is not a definitive contra-indication to vaginal delivery. However, if the fracture is significantly displaced, unstable, or narrows the pelvic passages, cesarean delivery will likely be required.

The incidence of falls in pregnant women approaches that of women over 70 years of age (27% and 28%, respectively) [12]. Falls increase with progression of pregnancy as a result of the altered center of gravity and biomechanics. The degree of injury is proportional to the force and body part impacted, and can range from simple sprains to fetal loss.

Penetrating trauma

Penetrating trauma accounts for a minority of trauma sustained during pregnancy. The prognosis for the fetus compared with the mother is much worse when penetrating trauma has occurred. Fetal demise can occur through direct injury to fetus, placenta, or the umbilical cord. In mothers, however, since the gravid uterus displaces the abdominal organs superiorly, visceral injury is less likely after penetrating injury to the lower abdomen.

The management of penetrating trauma is essentially the same as in non-pregnant patients. Most stab wounds that enter the thorax or abdomen should be evaluated for the extent of the wound. Exploration may be done in deep penetration, hemodynamic instability, excessive bleeding, or suspicion of injury to an underlying organ. A chest radiograph can be performed if needed to evaluate for traumatic pneumothorax, hemo-thorax, or free air under the diaphragm.

Gunshot wounds require more aggressive management. Upright chest radiographs with radiopaque markers at the site of injury are obtained to identify the bullet trajectory and look for free air under the diaphragm. An amniocentesis under ultrasound guidance may be considered for gunshot wounds to the abdomen: frankly bloody amniotic fluid would indicate fetal injury. Where indicated (e.g. late preterm or near term), amniotic fluid may be sent for indices of fetal lung maturity if it would be helpful in a decision about delivery. An exploratory laparotomy is performed for gunshot wounds to the abdomen with suspicion of hollow viscus or hemodynamically compromising solid organ injuries. The uterus should be examined for a penetrating injury. If the fetus is older than 24–25 weeks of gestation (or the local and customary gestational age at which the perinate has a reasonable chance at extrauterine survival) and fetal injury or distress is evident, an immediate cesarean should be performed. Where there is no suspicion of fetal injury or compromise and the fetal lungs are immature, the uterus may be repaired and the fetus left alone. Labor may take place subsequently after recovery from surgery and anesthesia. In the absence of vaginal bleeding or fetal distress, preterm labor may be suppressed with a tocolytic agent at the discretion of the obstetrician. Penetrating uterine injury at less than 24–25 weeks of gestation should be treated conservatively. Cesarean is indicated in severe maternal hemorrhage or fetal death in association with a uterine rupture or injury that would preclude labor. However, fetal death alone is not an indication for cesarean delivery [13–15]. In some cases it may be necessary to empty the uterus to gain access and complete a trauma laparotomy. There is a place for peri-mortem cesarean in some cases (see Chapter 13).

Domestic and sexual abuse

The incidence of domestic violence complicating pregnancies ranges from 5 to 20% in various series; 20% is the estimate quoted in the most recent UK triennial report 2006–2008 [16]. However, these figures may underestimate the problem. Sexual abuse against pregnant women has been reported to be as high as 17%. Unfortunately, signs and symptoms of both domestic and sexual violence often go unrecognized by the unsuspecting medical professional. Frequent visits to antenatal clinic, emergency department, or primary care physician offices, or discrepancy between injuries and history given, are important clues. When suspected, social and law enforcement agencies should be involved to protect the mother and the unborn fetus from further harm. In many institutions, contact numbers for relevant agencies are put in the ladies' lavatory, usually the one place a controlling partner may not have access to. It may be difficult for the woman to leave the relationship. Treatment ideally would involve the removal of the pregnant mother and any other children from the abusive situation.

Pregnancy-related effects of trauma

Preterm labor

Preterm labor may be precipitated by trauma and is associated with waxing and waning abdominal pain, back pain, pelvic pain, or pressure, and it is associated with vaginal discharge, uterine tenderness, and/or vaginal spotting. Vaginal examination reveals effacement and dilatation of the cervix.

Abruption

Placental abruption refers to the premature separation of the placenta from the uterus after 20 weeks of gestation. Maternal and fetal impact depends on the severity of the abruption and the fetal gestational age. Abruption involving more than 50% of the placenta is frequently associated with fetal demise. Maternal sequelae may include coagulopathy and shock. Placental abruption is suspected when a pregnant woman complains of abdominal pain with or without vaginal bleeding. The uterus may be tender, hard, or contracting without enough relaxation time. Ultrasound should be performed before a vaginal examination to exclude placenta previa. Mild degrees of placental abruption, with a stable mother and a fetus remote from term, may be managed expectantly. Assuming both mother and fetus are stable, or in the setting in which fetal demise has already occurred, vaginal delivery is often recommended over cesarean section because of increased incidence of disseminated intravascular coagulopathy in such patients.

Fetomaternal hemorrhage

It is estimated that <1 mL of fetal blood is lost into maternal circulation during normal pregnancy. Increased transmission of fetal blood into the maternal circulation may be precipitated by trauma to the uterus itself, abruption of the placenta, or labor. Rhesus-negative mothers may develop antibody against rhesus-positive fetal blood and this isoimmunization may complicate the current pregnancy or any future rhesus-positive pregnancies.

Uterine rupture

Uterine rupture is reported to occur in up to 0.6% of blunt abdominal trauma in pregnancy [17]. The risk for uterine rupture increases with increasing gestational age and the force of the trauma. Patients may complain of severe abdominal pain and chest pain (because of the escaped blood irritating the diaphragm), along with loss of uterine contours. During abdominal examination, fetal parts may also be easily palpable, indicating uterine rupture. Uterine rupture is associated with a very high risk of fetal mortality.

Emergency cesarean

The indication for an emergency cesarean in trauma is not well defined; the decision is dependent on both maternal and fetal conditions. It may be considered in pregnant trauma patients with gestational age >24 weeks (assuming appropriate neonatal care resources are available) who are hemodynamically unstable, or with suspicion of significant fetal distress even in a stable mother. It is usually not performed before 24 weeks of gestation as the fetus is not capable of independent survival; the gestational age at which delivery may be considered, of course, will depend heavily on the neonatal resources available. In a multi-institutional retrospective cohort study, 32 emergency cesareans were performed over a period of 8 years, with a mean estimated gestational age of 33 weeks (22–40 weeks); for those over 26 weeks of gestation with fetal heart tones present at the time of emergency cesarean, 75% fetal survival was achieved [18].

Resuscitative thoracotomy

The indications for resuscitative thoracotomy in pregnant patients are the same as in the general population. It is generally accepted that patients arresting within 10 minutes from penetrating trauma and 5 minutes from blunt trauma may be candidates for this last resort in salvage. The objectives of resuscitative thoracotomy include relief of cardiac tamponade, control of cardiac or intrathoracic hemorrhage, performance of open cardiac massage, and the ability to temporarily cross-clamp the thoracic aorta to preserve blood flow to the heart and brain. Resuscitative thoracotomy should be considered in a pulseless pregnant trauma patient when the proper indications are met. If the gestational age is over 24 weeks, then a concomitant perimortem cesarean section should be performed. Case reports exist documenting successful deliveries of neurologically intact fetuses from perimortem cesarean sections. However, infant survival and neurological outcome is directly related to the time lapsed between maternal distress and delivery. Case reports also exist documenting preserved pregnancies with term deliveries after successful resuscitative thoracotomies without crash cesarean sections. There may be a place for delivery at an even earlier gestational age as an adjunct to maternal resuscitation, although perinatal survival is unlikely (see Chapter 12.)

Burns

The skin is the largest organ of the human body and serves to protect against fluid and electrolyte loss, external pathogens, and mechanical trauma. The patient's systemic response to thermal injuries is directly proportional to the size and depth of the burn. It can range from first-degree burns resulting in only temporary discomfort to extensive full-thickness burns resulting in multisystem organ failure and death. The care of the burned patient is a multi-disciplinary endeavor critically anchored on the principles of rapid fluid resuscitation, early nutrition replacement, early excision and skin grafting, and intense physical rehabilitation.

Epidemiology

The World Health Organization estimates there are 195 000 deaths resulting from fires annually [19]. Over 95% of fatal fire-related burns occur in low- and middle-income countries [20]. Southeast Asia alone accounts for over half of all burn-related fatalities. In the USA, 450 000 burn patients received medical treatment in 2011, 10% warranting hospital admission [21].

Diagnosis and treatment

Burn management and outcome is dependent on the size and depth of thermal injury. Even in experienced hands, accurate differentiation between burn depths can be challenging. In addition, burns can also convert to deeper injuries as a consequence of both the initial degree of thermal insult and the appropriateness of resuscitation.

First degree burns

Sunburns are the characteristic first-degree burns. The depth of thermal injury is limited to the epidermis, while all elements of dermal appendages remain intact. The skin is painful, erythematous, blanches, and does not blister. Care is largely aimed at providing a moist and comfortable environment with moisturizing cream and non-steroidal anti-inflammatory medications (not in pregnancy). Healing takes place within a few days as the sloughing damaged skin is replaced by new skin.

Second-degree burns

Second-degree burns are further classified as superficial or deep, for both treatment and prognostic purposes. The cutaneous nerve endings and dermal appendages where the skin's regenerative capacity reside remain intact in superficial second-degree burns. Therefore, these burns are erythematous, blanch, blister, and painful. Spontaneous re-epithelialization takes place from the rete ridges, hair follicles, and sweat glands and is typically completed by 14 days. Tissue response to thermal injury is a dynamic process and superficial second-degree burns can convert to deep second-degree burns. Deep second-degree burns extend to the deep dermal layers with destruction of the dermal appendages. These wounds are typically less sensate, and the quality of healing is poor, with a high propensity of conversion to full-thickness burns. Depending on the size of the wound, small deep second-degree burns can be left for spontaneous healing, but large areas are best treated with tangential excision and split-thickness skin grafting.

Third-degree burns

Third-degree burns extend into the subcutaneous fat with destruction of overlying dermal elements. These wounds are dry, leathery, and insensate. Third-degree burns uniformly have poor spontaneous healing, as healing only takes place from the viable wound edges by the process of contracture after the central wound eschar has separated from the underlying subcutaneous tissue. Poor cosmetic and functional outcome and a high infectious risk result from spontaneous healing. The standard of care is to perform early tangential excision and split-thickness skin grafting.

Fourth-degree burns

Fourth-degree burns involve extensive destruction beyond the skin to the underlying fat, muscle, and bone. Care involves complex reconstruction and, in certain cases, amputation.

General burn care

Approximately 90% of burns can be treated as outpatient. It is important to recognize that burns may result from flame, scalds, chemicals, or electricity. The incidence of severe burns in pregnancy is low, with much of the data coming from third-world countries where heavier reliance on kerosene, lack of housing fire code, and lack of reliable prehospital fire response are contributing factors. Because of its low incidence, standardized management guidelines for pregnancy-related burns have not been established. The care algorithm is extrapolated from knowledge in the general burn and trauma populations.

The seriousness of the burn depends on the surface area involved, the depth of the burn and the presence or absence of inhalation injury. The immediate first aid involves extinguishing the flames by fire retardant or water. Small burns can be treated with cold water immersion of the affected extremity.

The priorities in the pregnant burn patient are the same as that established for all trauma patients based on ATLS. Airway patency and the patient's ability to spontaneously breathe and oxygenate is the first priority. Inhalation injury, such as those suffered in close-quarter household fires, can cause rapid airway edema, leading to hoarseness, stridor, and airway obstruction. A high index of suspicion should be raised when the above signs are present in addition to evidence of facial burns, singed facial hair, and coughing of carbonaceous sputum. In addition to the thermal injury, the toxic byproducts of combustion such as hydrogen cyanide, ammonia, and aldehydes, are inhaled into the alveoli and cause chemical injuries that can progress to acute lung injury and acute respiratory distress syndrome. When such injuries are suspected, early intubation is recommended for both airway protection and supplemental oxygen administration, which shortens the half-life of carboxyhemoglobin from 4.5 hours to 50 minutes.

Burn patients are predictably hypovolemic because of the large losses of interstitial and intracellular fluid. The assessment of burn areas can be estimated using the "Rule of Nines": 9% for head and neck, 9% for each arm, 18% front of trunk, 18% back of trunk, 18% for each lower limb, and 1% perineum. The gravid abdomen would make up more than 18%. The area of the patient's palm represents 1%. Patients suffering from over 20% total body surface area partial-thickness burn should be aggressively resuscitated using the Parkland formula as a guide, and the hourly fluid infusion titrated based on urine output. This resuscitation strategy uses Ringer's lactate infused at 4 mL/%e total body surface area affected per kg body weight. Half of this volume is given in the first 8 hours and the rest given over the next 16 hours.

Burns should be kept moist with silver sulfadiazine as the main stay for wound coverage. Mafenide acetate has superior cartilage penetration and is used for burns over cartilaginous areas such as the nose and ear. Operative management of burns is largely based on early tangential excision and split-thickness skin grafting.

Survival after burns has improved over the past several decades through advancements in critical care management, artificial wound coverage, nutrition support, and early surgical intervention. Data for maternal burn survival are lacking because of its low incidence. Certain authorities advocate for delivery if the maternal total body surface area affected is >50% and the fetus is viable. It is believed that maternal and perinatal mortality is increased if >50% of the body surface is burned. If <30% of the body surface area is burned, maternal and fetal survival is comparable to the general population.

Key learning points

1. Pregnant trauma patients are more likely to be of younger age and lower socioeconomic status.
2. The incidence of fetal loss exceeds maternal loss by a ratio of 3:1.
3. The knowledge of a patient's pregnancy status and fetal gestational age guides workup, management, fetal monitoring, and choice of imaging.
4. Fetal cardiotocography should be considered in all pregnancies admitted after maternal trauma at or past the gestational age of viability.
5. Pregnant patients suffering minor trauma should be monitored for at least 4 hours and up to 24 hours for major trauma.
6. Baseline relative tachycardia can be dismissed only after excluding a source of shock.

7. Every pregnant trauma patient is suspected to have a full stomach; every attempt to minimize the risk of aspiration must be employed.

8. Both pregnancy and trauma are associated with hypercoagulability, predisposing pregnant trauma patients to higher risks of thromboembolic events.

9. Ultrasound effectively confirms gestational age, fetal cardiac activity, and placental location.

10. The Kleihauer–Betke test identifies the amount of fetal blood that has entered the maternal circulation and guides the appropriate dose of rhesus immunoglobulin needed for rhesus-negative mothers.

11. Road traffic accidents are the most common cause of blunt trauma in pregnant women, followed by assault and falls.

12. Placental abruptions are associated with maternal coagulopathy and shock; placental abruption has been reported even after less than major maternal trauma.

13. All pregnant patients with a gestational age >24 weeks, hemodynamically unstable, and exhibiting fetal distress should undergo an emergency cesarean section.

14. Resuscitative thoracotomy should be considered in all pulseless pregnant trauma patients.

15. Patients with partial thickness burns of >20% total body surface area should be resuscitated with the Parkland formula, and the hourly fluid administration titrated based on urine output.

16. Patients with inhalation injuries should be expediently intubated because of the potential for worsening airway edema.

References

1. World Health Organization. *Injury: A Leading Cause of the Global Burden of Disease*. Geneva: World Health Organization, 1999.

2. National Highway Traffic Safety Administration. Fatality Analysis Reporting System. Washington, DC: National Highway Traffic Safety Administration, 2009 (http://www.nhtsa.gov/FARS, accessed 29 January 2013).

3. Ikossi DG, Lazar AA, Morabito D, Fildes J, Knudson MM. Profile of mothers at risk: an analysis of injury and pregnancy loss in 1,195 trauma patients. *J Am Coll Surg* 2005;**200**:49–56.

4. McGwin G, Russell SR, Rux RL, *et al.* Knowledge, beliefs, and practices concerning seat belt use during pregnancy. *J Trauma* 2004;**56**:512–517.

5. American College of Surgeons. *Advanced Trauma Life Support for Doctors Student Manual*, 8th edn. Chicago, IL: American College of Surgeons, 2008.

6. Yu Y, Gong SP, Sheng C, *et al.* Increased survival with hypotensive resuscitation in a rabbit model of uncontrolled hemorrhagic shock in pregnancy. *Resuscitation* 2009;**80**:1424–1430.

7. Goodwin H, Holmes JF, Wisner DH. Abdominal ultrasound examination in pregnant blunt trauma patients. *J Trauma* 2001;**50**:689–693.

8. Muench MV, Baschat AA, Reddy UM, *et al.* Kleihauer–Betke testing is important in all cases of maternal trauma. *J Trauma Inj Infect Crit Care* 2003;**57**:1094–1098.

9. Ali J, Yeo A, Gana TJ, McLellan BA. Predictors of fetal mortality in pregnant trauma patients. *J Trauma* 1997;**42**:782–785.

10. Kissinger DP, Rozycki GS, Morris JA, *et al.* Trauma in pregnancy: predicting pregnancy outcome. *Arch Surg* 1991;**126**:1079–1086.

11. Schiff MA, Holt VL. The injury severity score in pregnant trauma patients: predicting placental abruption and fetal death. *J Trauma* 2002;**53**:946–949.

12. Dunning K, LeMasters G, Levin L, *et al.* Falls in workers during pregnancy: risk factors, job hazards, and high risk occupations. *Am J Ind Med* 2003;**44**:664–672.

13. Chames MC, Pearlman MD. Trauma during pregnancy: outcomes and clinical management. *Clin Obstet Gynecol* 2008;**51**:398–408.

14. Muench MV, Canterino JC. Trauma in pregnancy. *Obstet Gynecol Clin North Am* 2007;**34** 555–583.

15. Kuhlmann RS, Cruikshank DP. Maternal trauma during pregnancy. *Clin Obstet Gynecol* 1994;**37**:274–293.

16. Cantwell R, Clutton-Brock T, Cooper G, *et al.* Saving Mothers' Lives: Reviewing Maternal Deaths to make Motherhood Safer 2006–2008. The Eighth Report of the Confidential Enquiries into Maternal Deaths in the United Kingdom. *BJOG* 2011;**118**(Suppl 1):1–203.

17. Weintraub AY, Leron E, Mazor M. The pathophysiology of trauma in pregnancy: a review. *J Matern Fetal Neonatal Med* 2006;**19**:601–605.

18. Morris JA Jr., Rosenbower TJ, Jurkovich GJ, *et al.* Infant survival after cesarean section for

trauma. *Ann Surg* 1996;**223**:481–488; discussion 488–491.

19. World Health Organization. *Violence and Injury Prevention: Burns*. Geneva: World Health Organization, 2012 (http://www.who.int/violence_injury_prevention/other_injury/burns/en/index.html, accessed 29 January 2013).

20. Maghsoudi H, Samnia R, Garadaghi A, Kianvar H. Burns in pregnancy. *Burns* 2006; **32**:246–250.

21. American Burn Association. *Burn Incidence Fact Sheet*. 2011. Washington, DC: American Burn Association, 2012 (http://www.ameriburn.org/resources_factsheet.php, accessed 29 January 2013).

Chapter 33

Malaria, bites, and stings during pregnancy

Carlo Missant

Introduction

The topic of bites and stings during pregnancy is a very diverse and sometimes exotic one. There are large regional differences, depending on the species living in a particular area. Symptoms can range from mild and almost unnoticed to extremely serious, and the effects on the fetus are not always clear. A review of all possible insects is beyond the scope of this chapter and the interested reader is referred to specific literature focusing on infectiology and tropical diseases. This chapter will focus on mosquitoes (including malaria), ticks and Lyme disease, Hymenoptera (bees and wasps), snakebites, and scorpion and jellyfish stings.

Mosquitoes and malaria

Mosquitoes are a member of the Culicidae insect family. Blood-sucking mosquitoes inject saliva into the bodies of their blood source. This saliva serves as an anticoagulant and is also the main route by which mosquitoes offer passenger pathogens access to the hosts' interior. Visible and irritating mosquito bites are caused by an immune response resulting from the binding of IgG and IgE antibodies to antigens present in the mosquito's saliva. Both immediate and delayed hypersensitivity reactions to mosquito bites may occur, resulting in itching, redness, and swelling. Immediate anaphylactic reactions to mosquito bites are extremely rare.

Effective prevention measures against mosquito bites include the use of mosquito nets and insect repellants. A whole variety of products are commercially available but the most effective repellants contain DEET (*N,N*-diethyl-*m*-toluamide). In the Guidelines for Malaria Prevention in Travellers from the UK, the UK Health Protection Agency states that products containing up to 50% DEET are safe to use

during pregnancy [1]. Other useful repellents are picaridin, oil of eucalyptus, and IR3535 (3-(*N*-butyl-*N*-acetyl)-aminopropionic acid) [2]. Although they can be quite annoying, mosquito bites do not require any medical treatment. In severe cases, several medications are commercially available to decrease symptoms, including oral or topically applied antihistamines. Modern H_1 receptor antihistamines have not shown any teratogenic effects so far, but the general rule applies that oral antihistamines should be avoided in the first trimester of pregnancy. If an antihistamine must be used, chlorpheniramine is generally considered to be safe during pregnancy [3].

Mosquitoes can act as a vector for many disease-causing viruses and parasites as they carry these organisms from person to person without exhibiting symptoms themselves. One specific genus of mosquitoes, *Anopheles*, can cause malaria when they carry the parasitic genus of *Plasmodium*. Currently, over 200 species of *Plasmodium* are recognized and new species continue to be described. At least 11 species infect humans, with the most serious ones being *P. falciparum* and *P. vivax*.

Malaria during pregnancy

It is estimated that 10 000 women and 200 000 infants die as a result of malaria infection during pregnancy each year. Severe maternal anemia, prematurity, and low birth weight contribute to more than half of these deaths [4,5].

Human malaria is caused by five species of *Plasmodium*: *P. falciparum*, *P. vivax*, *P. ovale*, *P. malariae*, and *P. knowlesi*. Most infections are with *P. falciparum* or *P. vivax*, but infections with more than one malarial species also occur. Both *P. falciparum* and *P. vivax* malaria can pose problems for the fetus, with the latter being more serious. The prenatal and neonatal mortality

Maternal Critical Care: A Multidisciplinary Approach, ed. Marc Van de Velde, Helen Scholefield, and Lauren A. Plante.
Published by Cambridge University Press. © Cambridge University Press 2013.

is reported to vary from 15 to 70%. Spontaneous abortion, premature birth, still birth, placental insufficiency and intrauterine grow restriction, low birth weight, and fetal distress are the different problems observed in the growing fetus [4].

One of the unique features of malaria in pregnancy is the ability of *P. falciparum*-parasitized erythrocytes to sequester within the intervillous space of the placenta. These parasites express a specific class of variant surface antigens that mediate adhesion of parasite-infected erythrocytes to the syncytiotrophoblast lining the intervillous space. Once these parasites adhere to the surface of the trophoblastic villi, they induce accumulation of inflammatory leukocytes, necrotizing the adjacent placental tissue. Histopathology of placentae with active malaria infection shows adhesion of infected erythrocytes to syncytiotrophoblast, syncytial degradation, increased syncytial knotting, and, in rare cases, localized destruction of the villi [6].

Clinical manifestations

The clinical presentation of malaria varies according to the underlying endemicity of the region (Figure 33.1) [7].

In holoendemic regions (regions where nearly every individual of a population is infected), most malarial infections in pregnant women are asymptomatic, but the risk for maternal anemia and low birth weight remains. However, for women residing in meso-endemic areas (area with regular seasonal transmission), malaria is more likely to result in febrile illness, severe symptomatic disease, preterm birth, and the death of mother or fetus. In areas of low or unstable malaria transmission, where pregnant women have acquired little immunity, symptomatic malarial disease is the rule and serious complications may occur. Observational studies have shown that parasitemia is highest in the second trimester in both primigravidas and multigravidae and the risk for pregnancy-associated malaria persists for 60 days postpartum [5,8]. Puerperal infection is mostly caused by a new infection, rather than by the release of placental parasites into the maternal blood at delivery. The reason for the high susceptibility to infection postpartum may be related to postpartum changes in the maternal immune system or maternal behavioral changes [9,10].

The clinical manifestations of malaria are non-specific and variable. Virtually all non-immune individuals will experience fever, chills, sweats, headache, myalgias, fatigue, nausea, abdominal pain, vomiting, diarrhea, jaundice, and cough. Pregnant women are

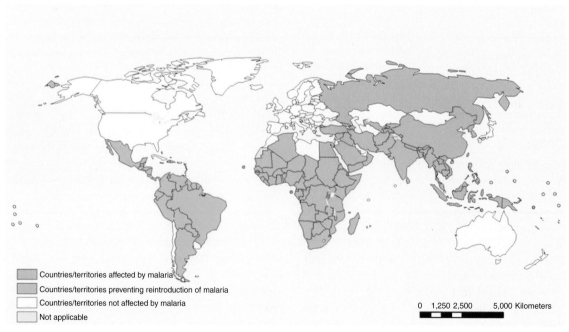

Countries/territories affected by malaria
Countries/territories preventing reintroduction of malaria
Countries/territories not affected by malaria
Not applicable

0   1,250 2,500   5,000 Kilometers

Figure 33.1. Malaria endemicity map. Note that this map is not a definitive source of information about malaria endemnicity. (© World Health Organization, 2011 [7].)

particularly vulnerable to malaria; compared with non-pregnant women, pregnant women experience more severe disease, more fever, more hypoglycemia, and more respiratory complications (pulmonary edema and acute respiratory distress syndrome). In addition to anemia linked to the physiological changes of pregnancy, approximately 60% of pregnant women presenting with malarial infection are anemic, and anemia may be one of the few signs of the disease [11].

Erythrocytes infected with *P. falciparum* are able to sequester within the intervillous space of the placenta. This is known as placental malaria and the median prevalence in holoendemic areas has been reported to be 26%. Erythrocytes infected with *P. vivax* do not sequester in the placenta [12]. Note that placental infection may be detected in absence of peripheral parasitemia. Parasites adhered to the trophoblastic villi will attack leukocytes, causing an inflammatory reaction, leading to necrosis of adjacent placental tissue, placental thickening, and fibrin deposition.

Severe malaria is defined as acute malaria with high levels of parasitemia (>5% red blood cells infected) and/or major signs of organ dysfunction: altered consciousness with or without convulsions, respiratory distress, metabolic acidosis, circulatory collapse, pulmonary edema or acute respiratory distress syndrome, renal failure, hemoglobinuria, disseminated intravascular coagulation, and severe anemia [13,14].

The clinical manifestations of severe malaria vary with age and region. Seizures and severe anemia are relatively more common in children, whereas acute renal failure and jaundice are more common in adults. Cerebral malaria (with coma), shock, acidosis, and respiratory arrest may occur at any age [13,14].

Diagnosis

The diagnosis of malaria should be considered in any febrile woman who has resided in or has traveled to a region with endemic malaria. Standard methods that detect peripheral parasitemia can be used in pregnant women (thick and/or thin peripheral blood smears or rapid diagnostics; Figure 33.2).

It is important to point out that women may have placental parasites without having any circulating in the peripheral blood, making the blood film negative. No reliable peripheral biomarker for the presence of placental malaria has been identified so far; the diagnosis is made by histological examination after delivery.

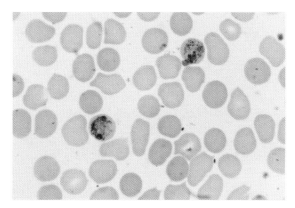

Figure 33.2. Two *Plasmodium malariae* schizonts in a thin blood smear. (Copyright Public Health Library, US Center for Disease Control.)

Treatment

Safety and efficacy data to guide treatment during pregnancy are unfortunately limited. Death can occur within hours after infection so prompt clinical assessment and initiation of therapy are essential.

General clinical management

Supportive therapy (antipyretics, oxygen, ventilatory support, hemodynamic support) must be initiated when needed. Clinical assessments of the patient should be repeated every 2 hours for fast detection and management of complications. In addition, laboratory test for parasitemia, hemoglobin, glucose, and lactate should be repeated with 6 hour intervals. Daily fluid intake and output must be closely monitored [15].

Hypoxemia

Hypoxemia is not a common finding in the setting of severe malaria. In addition to a lower respiratory tract infection, pulmonary edema (resulting from renal impairment) or acute respiratory distress syndrome can be the cause of hypoxia and should be treated accordingly. Management requirements depend on the specific situation and vary from supplemental oxygen delivery to full mechanical ventilation.

Hematological complications

Hematological complications include severe anemia and coagulopathy. Whether the patient requires transfusion must be individualized, but transfusions are mostly reserved for patients with altered consciousness, heart failure, respiratory distress, lactate acidosis, high-density parasitemia, or very low hemoglobin levels (4–5 g/dL). Clinically evident disseminated intravascular coagulation in the setting of severe malaria is rare (< 5%), but profound thrombocytopenia is common and the microcirculation in many organs is occluded by fibrin thrombi [16,17]. Until now, there is no evidence to support platelet transfusion in patients without any sign of bleeding or who are not at high risk for bleeding. Patients with a thrombocytopenia (< 50 × 10^9/L) and serious bleeding should receive platelet transfusion.

Hypoglycemia

Traditionally hypoglycemia is defined as blood glucose < 40 mg/dL. Hypoglycemia is a common complication of malaria and a marker of severe disease. It should be suspected in any comatose patient or in patients who deteriorate suddenly. Hypoglycemia is thought to result from parasite glucose consumption and/or impaired host gluconeogenesis. In addition to primary hypoglycemia, administration of quinine or quinidine can cause iatrogenic hypoglycemia. Hypoglycemia following artesunate therapy (part of the artemisinin group of antimalarial drugs) is less common. Clinical manifestations of hypoglycemia include seizure and altered consciousness, although these are not reliable clinical indicators and blood glucose concentration should be assessed and repeated as part of routine evaluation. Hypoglycemic patients should have intravenous access established promptly, followed by administration of a bolus of dextrose (0.25 g/kg body weight). This is usually achieved with 2.5 mL/kg 10% dextrose solution, since extravasation of higher concentrations of glucose can cause severe tissue damage. Blood glucose measurement should be repeated after 15 minutes, with administration of repeat boluses until the patient is normoglycemic. Maintenance intravenous fluids should contain at least 5% dextrose. Normoglycemic patients can develop hypoglycemia during the course of treatment. In addition, those managed promptly for hypoglycemia at presentation can have subsequent recurrent hypoglycemia [18,19].

Seizures

Seizures can be generalized or focal and may differ from nystagmus to coma. Other causes of neurological symptoms or coma should be excluded (e.g. hypoglycemia, meningitis) and treatment should be started promptly. Benzodiazepines are the first-line agents for seizure treatment. Diazepam 0.4 mg/kg can be administered intravenously or per rectum.

Lorazepam 0.1 mg/kg is an alternative. These doses can be repeated once in seizures that do not cease. If benzodiazepines are not successful, phenobarbital or phenytoin are alternatives. Patients with severe malaria should not receive routine seizure prophylaxis in the absence of clinical seizure activity [20].

High fever

High fever is common in pregnant patients with malaria infection and reflects the host response to endogenous pyrogens released at the time of schizont rupture. The use of antipyretics in patients with high fever is appropriate as high fever can cause convulsions. Acetaminophen is a reasonable antipyretic agent and can be administered orally, rectally, or intravenously. Fetal temperature is 1°C higher than the maternal temperature.

Fluid management

The management of intravascular volume in patients with severe malaria remains difficult, especially in pregnancy where intravascular volume normally is increased. There is only little margin between hypovolemia (and associated renal impairment) and hypervolemia with the risk for pulmonary or cerebral edema. Markers of intravascular volume depletion in patients with severe malaria include cool peripheries, delayed capillary refill, and low urine output. Lactate acidosis may also be a sign of intravascular hypovolemia. Aggressive fluid resuscitation and treatment of acidosis are beneficial in these settings. However, hypervolemia is associated with poor outcome and should be avoided by all means [21,22].

Treatment in pregnancy

In general, the newer the drug, the more likely it is to be effective, but fewer data will be available on safety during pregnancy. In addition, the choice of drug depends on the clinical severity and epidemiological resistance patterns [23].

Chloroquine is the product of choice for first-line therapy for uncomplicated *P. falciparum* infections during pregnancy in chloroquine-sensitive regions. In chloroquine-resistant areas, the combination of quinine and clindamycin is recommended with adequate safety data and low cost. However, quinine is associated with hypoglycemia even in uncomplicated infections, which may increase risks for both mother and fetus [24].

For severe *P. falciparum* malaria in chloroquine-sensitive areas, intravenous quinine is recommended in the first trimester of pregnancy and intravenous artesunate in the second and third trimesters. Artesunate should be used for severe chloroquine-resistant *P. falciparum* malaria at all stages.

For uncomplicated non-falciparum malaria, pregnant women can be treated with chloroquine. Chloroquine-resistant *P. vivax* infections during pregnancy can also be treated with mefloquine. Following treatment of infection with *P. vivax* or *P. ovale*, non-pregnant patients are treated with primaquine to prevent relapse by eradicating the hypnozoite forms that may remain in the liver. Primaquine is contraindicated in pregnancy and, therefore, pregnant women should receive chloroquine once weekly until after delivery, when primaquine can be administered.

A comprehensive overview of treatments is given in Boxes 33.1 and 33.2.

There is growing concern about the emergence and spread of *P. falciparum* resistance to artemisinins, as defined by delayed parasite clearance times. In April 2012, the World Health Organization (WHO) published an update on artemisinin resistance, particularly in the Greater Mekong region (Cambodia, Vietnam, Myanmar, and Thailand) [25]. It is not known whether these foci represent spread or de novo emergence of artemisinin resistance. In response, containment projects were started in the affected regions and cross-border coordination between national programs and projects are urgently needed. Routine monitoring in these affected regions must be continued to be sure that artemisinins are effective and to be able to make changes in treatment policies.

Prophylactic use of antimalarial drugs during pregnancy

Pregnant women should avoid travel to malaria-endemic areas if possible. However, if necessary, measures to prevent mosquito bites along with an effective chemoprophylaxis regimen should be used. Chloroquine or hydroxychloroquine are considered safe to use in all trimesters of pregnancy. Mefloquine is the agent of choice for chloroquine-resistant areas and evidence suggests it is not associated with an increased risk to the fetus. Although the atovaquone–proguanil drug combination is not currently recommended for use during pregnancy, limited data suggest that it is not harmful to the fetus. Doxycycline and primaquine are not recommended during pregnancy.

Box 33.1. Treatment of *Plasmodium falciparum* malaria in pregnancy

Uncomplicated chloroquine-sensitive infections
Chloroquine is the product of choice for first-line therapy: chloroquine 600 mg orally immediately, followed by chloroquine 300 mg orally at 6, 24, and 48 hours

Uncomplicated chloroquine-resistant malaria
First trimester of pregnancy: quinine sulfate 650 mg orally three times per day for 3 to 7 days plus clindamycin 20 mg/kg per day orally divided in three doses for 7 days

Second trimester of pregnancy: artemisinin derivative (artesunate, artemether, artelinic acid) or the quinine plus clindamycin combination can be used

Severe chloroquine-sensitive malaria
First trimester: quinine dihydrochloride 20 mg/kg (in 5% dextrose) intravenous loading dose over 4 hours, 10 mg/kg (over 2 hours) intravenous at intervals of 8 or 12 hours (maximum daily dose 1800 mg)

Second and third trimesters: 2.4 mg/kg loading dose intravenous plus 2.4 mg/kg intravenous at 12 and 24 hours, followed by 2.4 mg/kg once daily

Severe chloroquine-resistant malaria
Artesunate 2.4 mg/kg loading dose intravenous plus 2.4 mg/kg intravenous at 12 and 24 hours, followed by 2.4 mg/kg once daily

Follow-up treatment
After severe acute illness has been treated with intravenous drugs, complete therapy with oral antimalarial drugs selected on the known parasite drug susceptibility and national treatment guidelines should be initiated

---

Box 33.2. Treatment of non-falciparum malaria in pregnancy

Uncomplicated chloroquine-sensitive infection
Chloroquine 1000 mg salt orally immediately, followed by 500 mg salt orally at 6, 24, and 48 hours

Chloroquine-resistant *P. vivax* infections
Mefloquine 750 mg salt orally as initial dose, followed by 500 mg salt orally given 6–12 hours after initial dose

Continuous prophylaxis for pregnant women living in endemic areas is not practical worldwide. An alternative to reduce the risk for malaria infection during pregnancy in women with prior immunity is the program "intermittent preventive treatment during pregnancy" (IPTp). The optimal agent, dose, and frequency depend on the regional differences in transmission intensity and drug resistance, but for areas with medium and high malaria transmission, the WHO recommends IPTp with two doses of sulfadoxine–pyrimethamine at least 1 month apart during the second and third trimesters [26].

Management of labor

Anemia, hypoglycemia, pulmonary edema, and secondary infections in malaria in pregnancy lead to problems for both mother and fetus. Severe *P. falciparum* malaria in pregnancy carries a very high mortality as maternal and fetal distress might be difficult to recognize in these patients.

Falciparum malaria induces uterine contractions, which can result in preterm labor. The frequency and intensity of contractions appear to be related to the height of fever. Fetal distress is common but often unrecognized. Therefore, monitoring of uterine contractions and fetal heart rate is required. All efforts should be made to rapidly bring the temperature under control by direct application of cold or the use of antipyretic drugs.

Careful fluid management is also very important. Dehydration as well as fluid overload should be avoided, because both could be detrimental to the mother and/or the fetus. If there is very high parasitemia, exchange transfusion may have to be carried out.

If necessary, induction of labor may have to be considered. Once the patient is in labor, fetal or maternal distress may indicate the need to shorten the second stage by forceps or vacuum extraction. Cesarean section must sometimes be considered.

Outcome

Adverse perinatal outcomes associated with malaria include miscarriage, fetal growth restriction, preterm birth, low birth weight, perinatal death, and congenital malaria. Factors related to increased severity of malarial infection during gestation include low parity, young maternal age, non-immune immunological status, *P. falciparum* or *P. vivax* species, a high degree of parasitemia, and placental infection. In addition, the

patient's socioeconomic background, place of residency (rural or urban), and season of acquisition has also been shown to have an effect [27]. The increased incidence of preterm deliveries in women infected with *P. falciparum* may be mediated by alterations in cytokine production. Increased levels of tumor necrosis factor-alpha are reported in the intervillous circulation and its concentration correlates with the density of *P. falciparum*-infected erythrocytes [28].

Impaired fetal growth is correlated with the evidence of parasites in the placenta and the corresponding inflammatory infiltrate. Placental malarial infection leads to placental thickening and fibrin deposition, decreasing placental oxygen and nutrient transport [5].

Perinatal and fetal mortality are higher in malaria endemic regions than in non-endemic countries (maternal mortality 61.1/1000 and 25.8/1000, respectively, and fetal mortality 40.1/1000 and 20/1000, respectively). The WHO estimates that 10 000 maternal deaths each year are associated with malaria infection during pregnancy. During the malaria season, maternal mortality rates have been reported to increase by 168%. Younger maternal age has been associated with higher rates of anemia and poorer maternal and fetal outcomes [29].

Congenital malaria from transplacental or peripartum infection of the fetus is being increasingly reported. Numbers vary between 1 and 10% of pregnancies from both malaria-endemic and non-endemic areas following maternal infections with all four species of *Plasmodium* known to infect humans, but most cases are reported following *P. falciparum* or *P. vivax* infection. Placental infection is a prerequisite for but does not predict congenital disease. Congenital malaria usually manifests between the second and eighth week of life. Symptoms include fever, anorexia, lethargy, anemia, and hepatosplenomegaly. In addition, irritability, poor feeding, regurgitation, loose stools, and jaundice may also be seen. The diagnosis of congenital malaria can be confirmed by a smear for malarial parasite from cord blood or blood collected during the heel prick within a week after birth. Differential diagnoses include rhesus incompatibility, cytomegalovirus infection, herpesvirus infection, rubella, toxoplasmosis, and syphilis [30].

There are very few documented studies on *P. vivax* malaria infections in pregnancy. It appears to be more common in primigravidae than multigravidae. Parasite densities are similar in pregnant and non-pregnant states. It may be associated with mild anemia and increased risk of low birth weight and not associated with abortion, stillbirth, or a reduction of the duration of pregnancy [31].

Ticks

Ticks are small arachnids in the order Ixodida. They are vectors of a number of diseases, including Lyme disease, Colorado tick fever, Rocky Mountain spotted fever, African tick bite fever, tularemia, tick-borne relapsing fever, babesiosis, ehrlichiosis, tick paralysis, and tick-borne meningoencephalitis. Of all these diseases, Lyme disease is the most common tick-borne disease above the equator, followed by Rocky Mountain spotted fever [32].

Lyme disease is an emerging infectious disease caused by at least three species of bacteria belonging to the genus *Borrelia*. *B. burgdorferi* is the main cause of Lyme disease in the USA, whereas *B. afzelii* and *B. garinii* are increasingly causing most European cases. Responsible ticks carrying the *Borrelia* bacteria are *Ixodes* species and *Amblyomma americanum* [33].

Lyme disease can affect multiple body systems and produce a wide range of symptoms. Typical lesions of the first phase of borreliosis are erythema chronicum migrans, pain in muscles and joints, fatigue, headache, fever, and general malaise. In the second phase of the disease (weeks to months after infection), pericarditis, myocarditis, atrioventricular conduction problems, meningoencephalitis, and other peripheral neuropathies may occur. After several months, untreated or inadequately treated patients may develop severe and chronic symptoms that affect many parts of the body, including the brain, nerves, eyes, joints, and heart. Lyme arthritis usually affects the knees but in a minority of patients, arthritis can occur in other joints, including the ankles, elbows, wrist, hips, and shoulders [34,35].

Besides protective clothing, early detection of attached ticks and their prompt removal (within 36 hours) is the cornerstone in prevention of Lyme disease.

Lyme spirochetes have been found in semen and breast milk [36]. Transmission across the placenta during pregnancy has not been demonstrated, and no consistent pattern of teratogenicity or specific "congenital Lyme borreliosis" has been identified. Once symptoms arise, antibiotics are the primary treatment for Lyme disease. As with a number of other spirochetal diseases, adverse pregnancy outcomes are possible with untreated infection, and prompt treatment with antibiotics reduces or eliminates this risk. Pregnant women with Lyme disease cannot be treated with the first-choice antibiotic, tetracycline, as it is potentially harmful for the fetus (bone growth). Instead, erythromycin for 10 to 28 days is usually given; it is less effective against the disease but harmless for the fetus [37].

Hymenoptera

Hymenoptera is one of the largest orders of insects, comprising the sawflies, wasps, bees, and ants. Hymenoptera stings are the leading cause of venomous animal-related deaths in the USA and a major cause of animal-related deaths worldwide. Allergic reactions are the most common clinical problem, causing approximately 25 deaths a year. In the general population, 0.4% is at risk for a serious allergic reaction such as anaphylaxis or toxic venom effects [38]. Particularly in pregnant women, impaired blood circulation following anaphylaxis may impair the fetus and lead to premature birth or to malformations of the central nervous system [39].

Local reactions after Hymenoptera stings include a sharp burning pain, itching, and edema. Note that rather extensive reactions may involve an entire extremity and that stings to the tongue or throat may cause loss of airway. Besides local reactions, immediate and delayed systemic reactions can also occur. Systemic reactions include diffuse itching, urticaria, swelling at a distant from the sting site, and flushing, but also more severe symptoms such as laryngeal edema, severe bronchospasm, or profound hypotension.

Immediate treatment of severe anaphylactic reactions/shock in pregnant patients is absolutely required and does not differ from action undertaken in non-pregnant patients: removal of the stinger, airway management, oxygen supply, blood pressure support with fluid and/or epinephrine, intravenous antihistamines, and intravenous steroids [40]. Most steroids are classified as category C medication (probably safe during pregnancy but risks cannot be ruled out in humans) by the US Food and Drug Administration. Prednisone does not represent a major teratogenic risk in humans at therapeutic doses, but it does increase the risk of cleft palate and cleft lip 3.4-fold [41]. There is some evidence in case reports on the use of tranexamic acid in the treatment of severe anaphylactic shock as this antifibrinolytic agent is also a potent inhibitor of the complement cascade [42]. The use of tranexamic acid is incorporated in the Dutch guidelines for treatment of severe anaphylaxis. More details on the treatment of anaphylactic shock can be found in other chapters of this book.

Hyposensitization therapy is useful in the treatment of allergic disease and in the prophylaxis of anaphylaxis to Hymenoptera stings. Most allergic disease results from the patient's production of excessive immunoglobulin (Ig) E directed against a specific antigen. The aim of the therapy is to reduce the excessive antigen-specific IgE production. IN addition to the induction of antigen-specific IgG antibodies, hyposensitization increase the production of the deficient antigen-specific suppressor T-cells, which can then exercise their normal function of inhibiting the IgE-producing B-cells [43]. Hyposensitization therapy administered in pregnancy does not adversely affect the expectant mother or the fetus. However, since an anaphylactic reaction to the therapy could initiate uterine contractions, caution is advised and allergists tend to be reluctant to carry out hyposensitization therapy during pregnancy.

Snakebites

Every year, 1.2–5.5 million people are bitten by a snake, with envenomation occurring in 420 000 to 1 841 000, resulting in 20 000 to 94 000 deaths [44]. Although the available literature about snakebites in pregnant females is scarce, Seneviratne *et al.* [45] reported that pregnant women account for 0.4–1.8 % of hospitalized snakebite victims in South Africa, India, and Sri Lanka. Several publications have reported very high overall fetal death rates, ranging from 38 to 43%, while maternal deaths occurred in 10% after a venomous snakebite. Most recent reports indicate the overall fetal loss at around 20% and maternal death at around 4–5% [46].

In a recent literature review, 213 cases of snakebite in pregnant women were identified in the period between 1966 and 2009 [46]. Snake venoms can be broadly classified as having inflammatory, cytotoxic, neurotoxic or hemotoxic actions. Most snakebites will cause some degree of local effect, such as pain, swelling, bleeding, and redness (local envenomation). In addition, systemic effects may also appear, such as nausea, abdominal pain, hypotension and tachycardia, coagulopathy, rhabdomyolyis, and renal failure (systemic envenomation). It has been reported that a few mothers had systemic envenomation without signs of local envenomation.

The composition and effect of venom varies with the species of snake, age of the snake, geographic locality, and time of year. Other factors influencing the effect of venom on humans include the amount of venom injected and the age and health of the victim.

Several mechanisms have been proposed to explain fetal deaths or abortions after snakebite [46]:

- fetal anoxia associated with maternal shock after envenomation
- direct effect of the venom on the fetus after placental transfer
- hemorrhage into the placenta (caused by direct toxic of the venom)
- hemorrhage in the uterine wall causing placental abruption
- premature uterine contractions initiated by the venom (either via a direct action on uterine muscle or indirectly by bradykinin release)
- pyrexia and cytokine release after tissue damage
- maternal hemorrhage, with acute fetal anemia causing fetal death
- supine hypotension syndrome.

Some components of snake venom may cross the placenta and adversely affect the fetus. The venom of *Vipera aspis* has been shown to cause congenital anomalies in the form of cleft palate and facial deformities in pregnant mice. *Naja nigricollis* venom injected into pregnant mice caused hepatic and myocardial damage as well as pulmonary vascular congestion and extravasation of blood in the intestinal lumen of the fetuses. Arvin, the active defibrinating fraction of the Malayan pit viper (*Calloselasma rhodostoma*) caused high rates of fetal death and resorption during early organogenesis in pregnant rabbits [47,48].

Envenomed patients should be admitted to hospital and observed for a period of at least 24 hours, depending on the clinical circumstances. Supportive therapy can vary from local analgesia and supplemental oxygen via face mask to full hemodynamic and respiratory support and mechanical ventilation. Renal failure may be treated with volume replacement and diuretics, but hemodialysis may occasionally be required. Hyperkalemia secondary to rhabdomyolysis may be treated with calcium, insulin, and glucose. All patients should receive appropriate tetanus prophylaxis and consideration should be given to antibiotic prophylaxis if the bite wound is contaminated. The administration of antivenom is the only required treatment for severe systemic snakebite envenomation. When no antivenom is immediately available, all measures must be taken to delay systemic absorption of the venom and expediting the transport to a hospital with experience in treatment of snakebite victims. The pressure immobilization technique (application of a pressure of 55 mmHg on the immobilized affected limb) has been used to delay systemic absorption after envenomation by snakes with a neurotoxic venom. It cannot be used for bites of snakes with locally necrotic venom, such as the cobra or the viper. The effect of antivenom on the fetus remains unclear. Antivenoms may be used in pregnant patients, but anaphylactic reactions can cause harm to mother and fetus and are not rare. Fetal death rates up to 58% have been reported in mothers given antivenom. However, while the safety of antivenom in pregnancy is unclear, the risks of not administering it outweigh the risks of administering it in correct clinical scenarios.

Scorpion stings

Although all scorpion species possess venom and use it primarily to kill and paralyze their pray so it can be eaten, only 25 have a venom that is dangerous to humans. The venom is a variable mixture of compounds such as neurotoxins and enzyme inhibitors. Symptoms and maternal or fetal effects depend on the specific species and venom.

A sting may immediately result in sweating, pallor, severe local skin reaction, pain, breathing difficulty and respiratory collapse, tachycardia and hypertension, blurred vision, slurred speech, drowsiness, and neurological collapse. Advanced symptoms may include motor hyperactivity, chest pain, vomiting, diarrhea, and abdominal cramps. Certain scorpion species have venom that result in seizure; respiratory, cardiac and nervous failure; paralysis; coma; and death [49].

In contrast to snake and mosquito bites, reports of scorpion stings and evenomation during pregnancy are scarce in medical literature. No obvious similarities are found between various species. For example, no adverse fetal or maternal outcome has been reported after a sting from the North American scorpion, while Kankonkar et al. [50] reported that a number of pregnant women died after a red scorpion sting in the Konkan region in India. In addition, stings from Leiurus quinquestriatus have resulted in abortion

in pregnant women during the first trimester. In general, while the pathophysiology of snake venom on the uterus, placenta, and fetus is well described, the effects of scorpion venom remain unclear [50].

First aid for scorpion stings is generally symptomatic, including analgesia, either systemic (opiates or acetaminophen) or locally applied (such as a cold compress). Hypertensive crises are treated with anxiolytics, antihypertensive drugs, and vasodilators.

Administration of species-specific antivenom is sometimes required if there are near-fatal symptoms. To date, no adverse fetal or maternal effects of scorpion antivenom have been reported.

Jelly fish

Most jellyfish stings are not deadly, but stings of some species of the class Cubozoa (box jellyfish), such as the toxic Irukandji jellyfish, can be deadly. In addition, stings may cause anaphylaxis, which also can be fatal. Medical care may include administration of an antivenom. In a literature review, only one case report of a serious envenomation by the Northern Australian box jellyfish was found. A pregnant women at 34 weeks of gestation was stung by Chironex fleckeri while sitting in water about 50 cm deep. After a few moments, she became unconscious and stopped breathing. Cardiorespiratory resuscitation was immediately started and approximately 30 minutes after envenomation, specific therapy including antivenom was administered. After 4 days of hospitalization, the victim was discharged and 9 weeks later, she delivered a healthy baby by cesarean delivery [49].

Clinical presentation of a patient after a jellyfish sting varies according to the type of jellyfish and the individual patient. Patients usually experience immediate pain at the time of the sting, followed by liner red urticarial lesions. These typical skin lesions burn and itch intensely [49].

Some jellyfish found in Northern Australian waters, such as Caruka barnesi, can cause the so-called Irukandji syndrome [51]. This typically involves a mild to moderate painful sting followed by severe back–chest and abdominal pain, gastrointestinal symptoms, agitation, hypertension, and tachycardia. At a later stage, myocardial injury and pulmonary edema might develop [52,53]. Major box jellyfish (Chironex fleckeri) stings have caused several deaths in Australia, with the venom having cardiotoxic, neurotoxic, and dermonecrotic effects in vivo and hemolytic effects in vitro [54,55]. Patients with a large

375

tenticular contact can experience rapid onset of cardiac arrest. Rare adverse events have been reported with the Atlantic Portuguese man-of war, a jellyfish causing numerous stings around the world. However, cardiovascular or respiratory arrest have been reported in rare cases in addition to drowning because of limb paralysis [56].

Jellyfish tentacles must be removed promptly, as nematocysts continue to administer toxins to the skin. Tentacles can be brushed off using a plastic object and seawater. Fresh water should be avoided as the osmotic pressure can cause the nematocysts to fire. Also vigorous rubbing can stimulate the nematocysts [57].

Acetic acid has been found to inhibit the discharge of nematocysts from Australian box jellyfish and is commonly used for Hawaian box jellyfish stings (but not for the Portuguese man-of-war). In general, local application of acetic acid is best used where there is a risk of life-threatening effects [58]. Local application of heat (hot water, 40–45°C) appears to be an effective treatment for some jellyfish stings as it alters the protein structure of jellyfish toxins. However, it is not appropriate to extrapolate these results in one jellyfish species to another. At least for stings from Hawaiian box jellyfish and Portuguese man-of war, hot water application after removal of all tentacles is recommended. Ice or fresh water should not be applied to the sting as this may help the nematocysts to continue to release toxin [57].

Antivenom is available for severe Australian box jellyfish stings. It is indicated for cardiopulmonary instability and cardiac arrest. It should be given intravenously soon after the sting, since most deaths occur within 5–20 minutes. Pretreatment with magnesium sulfate improves the efficacy of antivenom [59].

Conclusions

Venomous animal bites and stings during pregnancy are rarely reported. However, they can cause serious problems to both mother and fetus. Unfortunately, from cases described in the literature, the occurrence of fetal death is frequent (30–40%) in malaria and snakebite victims. The frequency of fetal deaths after other venomous bites or stings is not known.

Malaria continues to be a worldwide problem affecting millions of pregnant women each year. Prompt diagnosis and adequate treatment is essential to obtain a good outcome for mother and fetus. Regional differences in occurrence and resistance must be taken into account to establish adequate treatment.

Envenomations during pregnancy should continually be reported in medical literature (case reports, case series, etc.) so that information on medical management and fetal outcomes can be evaluated. No formal epidemiological studies of the effects of antivenom on fetal development have been performed. Whereas a large percentage of fetal deaths occurred in mothers who received snake antivenom, it is likely that these deaths were related to the severity of the venom poisoning as opposed to the antiserum. It is generally felt that the risks of significant venom poisoning to the mother and fetus outweigh any concerns about the safety of antivenom to the unborn child. More studies and human investigations are required to evaluate the risk–benefit profiles of snake and scorpion antivenoms on pregnant mothers, embryos, and fetuses.

References

1. Chiodini P, Hill D, Lalloo D, *et al. Guidelines for Malaria Prevention in Travellers from the United Kingdom.* London: Health Protection Agency, 2010.

2. Gamble C, Ekwaru JP, ter Kuile FO. Insecticide-treated nets for preventing malaria in pregnancy. *Cochrane Database Syst Rev* 2006:CD003755.

3. Fradin MS. Mosquitoes and mosquito repellents: a clinician's guide. *Ann Intern Med* 1998;**128**:931–940.

4. Cox-Singh J, Davis TM, Lee KS, *et al.* Plasmodium knowlesi malaria in humans is widely distributed and potentially life threatening. *Clin Infect Dis* 2008;**46**:165–171.

5. McGregor IA. Epidemiology, malaria and pregnancy. *Am J Trop Med Hyg* 1984;**33**:517–525.

6. Ismail MR, Ordi J, Menendez C, *et al.* Placental pathology in malaria: a histological, immunohistochemical, and quantitative study. *Hum Pathol* 2000;**31**:85–93.

7. World Health Organization. *Malaria Endemicity Map.* Geneva: World Health Organization (http://gamapserver.who.int/mapLibrary/Files/Maps/malaria_003.jpg, accessed 7 January 2013).

8. Brabin BJ. An analysis of malaria in pregnancy in Africa. *Bull World Health Org* 1983;**61**:1005–1016.

9. Diagne N, Rogier C, Sokhna CS, *et al.* Increased susceptibility to malaria during the early postpartum period. *N Engl J Med* 2000;**343**:598–603.

10. Ramharter M, Grobusch MP, Kiessling G, *et al.* Clinical and parasitological characteristics of puerperal malaria. *J Infect Dis* 2005;**191**:1005–1009.

11. Whitty CJ, Edmonds S, Mutabingwa TK. Malaria in pregnancy. *BJOG* 2005;**112**:1189–1195.

12. McGready R, Davison BB, Stepniewska K, *et al.* The effects of *Plasmodium falciparum* and *P. vivax* infections on placental histopathology in an area of low malaria transmission. *Am J Trop Med Hyg* 2004;**70**:398–407.

13. White NJ. The treatment of malaria. *N Engl J Med* 1996;**335**:800–806.

14. Crawley J, Chu C, Mtove G, Nosten F. Malaria in children. *Lancet* 2010;**375**:1468–1481.

15. Orton LC, Omari AA. Drugs for treating uncomplicated malaria in pregnant women. *Cochrane Database Syst Rev* 2008:CD004912.

16. Bojang KA, Palmer A, van Boele HM, Banya WA, Greenwood BM. Management of severe malarial anaemia in Gambian children. *Trans R Soc Trop Med Hyg* 1997;**91**:557–561.

17. Taylor TE, Fu WJ, Carr RA, *et al.* Differentiating the pathologies of cerebral malaria by postmortem parasite counts. *Nat Med* 2004;**10**:143–145.

18. White NJ, Miller KD, Marsh K, *et al.* Hypoglycaemia in African children with severe malaria. *Lancet* 1987; **i**:708–711.

19. Taylor TE, Molyneux ME, Wirima JJ, Fletcher KA, Morris K. Blood glucose levels in Malawian children before and during the administration of intravenous quinine for severe falciparum malaria. *N Engl J Med* 1988;**319**:1040–1047.

20. Crawley J, Waruiru C, Mithwani S, *et al.* Effect of phenobarbital on seizure frequency and mortality in childhood cerebral malaria: a randomised, controlled intervention study. *Lancet* 2000;**355**:701–706.

21. Maitland K, Levin M, English M, *et al.* Severe *P. falciparum* malaria in Kenyan children: evidence for hypovolaemia. *Q J Med* 2003;**96**:427–434.

22. Planche T, Onanga M, Schwenk A, *et al.* Assessment of volume depletion in children with malaria. *PLoS Med* 2004;**1**:e18.

23. World Health Organization. *Malaria Country Profiles.* Geneva: World Health Organization (http://www.who.int/malaria/publications/country-profiles/en/index.html, , accessed 7 January 2013).

24. Taylor WR, White NJ. Antimalarial drug toxicity: a review. *Drug Saf* 2004;**27**:25–61.

25. Phyo AP, Nkhoma S, Stepniewska K, *et al.* Emergence of artemisinin-resistant malaria on the western border of Thailand: a longitudinal study. *Lancet* 2012;**379**:1960–1966.

26. Menendez C, Bardaji A, Sigauque B, *et al.* Malaria prevention with IPTp during pregnancy reduces neonatal mortality. *PLoS One* 2010;**5**:e9438.

27. Espinoza E, Hidalgo L, Chedraui P. The effect of malarial infection on maternal–fetal outcome in Ecuador. *J Matern Fetal Neonatal Med* 2005;**18**:101–105.

28. Suguitan AL Jr., Cadigan TJ, Nguyen TA, *et al.* Malaria-associated cytokine changes in the placenta of women with pre-term deliveries in Yaounde, Cameroon. *Am J Trop Med Hyg* 2003;**69**:574–581.

29. Van Geertruyden JP, Thomas F, Erhart A, D'Alessandro U. The contribution of malaria in pregnancy to perinatal mortality. *Am J Trop Med Hyg* 2004;**71**(Suppl):35–40.

30. Lee WW, Singh M, Tan CL. A recent case of congenital malaria in Singapore. *Singapore Med J* 1996;**37**:541–543.

31. Nosten F, ter Kuile FF, Maelankirri L, Decludt B, White NJ. Malaria during pregnancy in an area of unstable endemicity. *Trans R Soc Trop Med Hyg* 1991;**85**:424–429.

32. Grubhoffer L, Golovchenko M, Vancova M, *et al.* Lyme borreliosis: insights into tick–host–borrelia relations. *Folia Parasitol* 2005;**52**:279–294.

33. Cairns V, Godwin J. Post-Lyme borreliosis syndrome: a meta-analysis of reported symptoms. *Int J Epidemiol* 2005;**34**:1340–1345.

34. Cairns V. Post-Lyme disease symptoms. *Am J Med* 2010;**123**:e21.

35. Puius YA, Kalish RA. Lyme arthritis: pathogenesis, clinical presentation, and management. *Infect Dis Clin North Am* 2008;**22**:289.

36. Schmidt BL, Aberer E, Stockenhuber C, *et al.* Detection of *Borrelia burgdorferi* DNA by polymerase chain reaction in the urine and breast milk of patients with Lyme borreliosis. *Diagn Microbiol Infect Dis* 1995;**21**:121–128.

37. Walsh CA, Mayer EW, Baxi LV. Lyme disease in pregnancy: case report and review of the literature. *Obstet Gynecol Surv* 2007;**62**:41–50.

38. Langley RL, Morrow WE. Deaths resulting from animal attacks in the United States. *Wilderness Environ Med* 1997;**8**:8–16.

39. Habek D, Cerkez-Habek J, Jalsovec D. Anaphylactic shock in response to wasp sting in pregnancy. *Zentralbl Gynakol* 2000;**122**:393–394.

40. Krishna MT, Ewan PW, Diwakar L, *et al.* Diagnosis and management of hymenoptera venom allergy: British Society for Allergy and Clinical Immunology (BSACI) guidelines. *Clin Exp Allergy* 2011;**41**:1201–1220.

41. Park-Wyllie L, Mazzotta P, Pastuszak A, *et al.* Birth defects after maternal exposure to corticosteroids:

prospective cohort study and meta-analysis of epidemiological studies. *Teratology* 2000;**62**:385–392.

42. Hoste S, Van AH, Stevens E. Tranexamic acid in the treatment of anaphylactic shock. *Acta Anaesthesiol Belg* 1991;**42**:113–116.

43. Krishna MT, Huissoon AP. Clinical immunology review series: an approach to desensitization. *Clin Exp Immunol* 2011;**163**:131–46.

44. White J. Bites and stings from venomous animals: a global overview. *Ther Drug Monit* 2000;**22**:65–8.

45. Seneviratne SL, de Silva CE, Fonseka MM, *et al.* Envenoming due to snake bite during pregnancy. *Trans R Soc Trop Med Hyg* 2002;**96**:272–274.

46. Langley RL. Snakebite during pregnancy: a literature review. *Wilderness Environ Med* 2010;**21**:54–60.

47. Dao B, Da E, Koalaga AP, Bambara M, Bazie AJ. Snake bite during pregnancy. *Med Trop* 1997;**57**:100–101.

48. James RF. Snake bite in pregnancy. *Lancet* 1985;**ii**:731.

49. Langley RL. A review of venomous animal bites and stings in pregnant patients. *Wilderness Environ Med* 2004;**15**:207–215.

50. Kankonkar RC, Kulkurni DG, Hulikavi CB. Preparation of a potent anti-scorpion-venom-serum against the venom of red scorpion (*Buthus tamalus*). *J Postgrad Med* 1998;**44**:85–92.

51. Burnett JW, Calton GJ, Burnett HW, Mandojana RM. Local and systemic reactions from jellyfish stings. *Clin Dermatol* 1987;**5**:14–28.

52. Macrokanis CJ, Hall NL, Mein JK. Irukandji syndrome in northern Western Australia: an emerging health problem. *Med J Aust* 2004;**181**:699–702.

53. Little M, Pereira P, Mulcahy R, *et al.* Severe cardiac failure associated with presumed jellyfish sting. Irukandji syndrome? *Anaesth Intensive Care* 2003;**31**:642–647.

54. Ramasamy S, Isbister GK, Seymour JE, Hodgson WC. The in vitro effects of two chirodropid (*Chironex fleckeri* and *Chiropsalmus* sp.) venoms: efficacy of box jellyfish antivenom. *Toxicon* 2003;**41**:703–711.

55. Ramasamy S, Isbister GK, Seymour JE, Hodgson WC. The in vivo cardiovascular effects of box jellyfish *Chironex fleckeri* venom in rats: efficacy of pre-treatment with antivenom, verapamil and magnesium sulphate. *Toxicon* 2004;**43**: 685–690.

56. Kaufman MB. Portuguese man-of-war envenomation. *Pediatr Emerg Care* 1992;**8**:27–8.

57. Fenner PJ, Williamson JA, Burnett JW, Rifkin J. First aid treatment of jellyfish stings in Australia. Response to a newly differentiated species. *Med J Aust* 1993;**158**:498–501.

58. Thomas CS, Scott SA, Galanis DJ, Goto RS. Box jellyfish (*Carybdea alata*) in Waikiki. The analgesic effect of sting-aid, Adolph's meat tenderizer and fresh water on their stings: a double-blinded, randomized, placebo-controlled clinical trial. *Hawaii Med J* 2001;**60**:205–7, 210.

59. Currie BJ. Marine antivenoms. *J Toxicol Clin Toxicol* 2003;**41**:301–308.

Chapter 34

Pregnancy and liver disease

Chris Verslype and Michael P. Plevyak

Introduction

Up to 5% of all pregnancies are complicated by liver pathology [1,2]. The challenge for the clinician is to diagnose and treat liver disorders before conception in order to minimize fetal and maternal morbidity and mortality.

This chapter proposes a general approach to the pregnant woman with suspected liver disease before reviewing liver diseases that are related and unrelated to pregnancy. The management of clinically significant portal hypertension during pregnancy will be discussed, as well as guidelines regarding pregnancy in patients who have undergone liver transplantation or who have liver cell adenomas.

General approach to the pregnant woman with suspected liver disease

Clinical assessment

The clinical assessment of patients with liver disease during pregnancy is challenging because of the physiological changes during pregnancy that can be mistaken for liver dysfunction. The hyperdynamic cardiovascular state (rise in cardiac output, fall in blood pressure and systemic vascular resistance) seen in normal pregnancy may resemble the situation in a patient with advanced liver disease. Moreover, increased splanchnic blood flow and compression of the inferior vena cava in the supine position by the gravid uterus may induce transient portal hypertension [3,4]. Increased blood volume, particularly in the azygous system, can lead to the development of esophageal varices in healthy pregnant women.

The hyperestrogenic state of pregnancy induces palmar erythema and spider nevi, which are typical clinical signs of patients with alcoholic hepatitis and cirrhosis. During pregnancy, blood flow to the liver remains constant and microscopic liver architecture appears normal [5].

Cholestasis, portal hypertension, and liver failure are major clinical entities that should be recognized in any patient as soon as possible and particularly in the pregnant woman because of the prognostic implications for mother and child. Cholestatic liver disease should be suspected in a patient with pruritus without rash and/or jaundice. The presence of ascites or varices in the upper (esophagus, stomach) or lower gastrointestinal tract or a history of gastrointestinal bleeding may point to clinically significant portal hypertension. Hepatic encephalopathy, which may range from mild confusion to deep coma, is often preceded or accompanied by jaundice and is indicative of liver failure. In some patients, a combination of these clinical entities may exist.

Biochemical tests

A number of blood tests are commonly used to screen for liver disease, confirm its presence, estimate severity, assess prognosis, and evaluate therapy. In most centers, liver function tests include aminotransferases (aspartate transaminase (AST), alanine transaminase (ALT)), alkaline phosphatase, gamma-glutamyltransferase (GGT), and serum bilirubin. Strictly speaking, these tests do not assess liver function but indicate the presence of hepatocellular necrosis, cholestasis, and hyperbilirubinemia. The prothrombin time (after vitamin K) and, to a lesser extent, serum albumin are more indicative of hepatic synthetic capacity.

The serum levels of the aminotransferases reflect the amount of hepatocellular injury and death on a day-by-day basis. Serum aminotransferase levels can rise to over 10 times the upper limit of normal (ULN)

Maternal Critical Care: A Multidisciplinary Approach, ed. Marc Van de Velde, Helen Scholefield, and Lauren A. Plante.
Published by Cambridge University Press. © Cambridge University Press 2013.

in hepatic hypoxia, acute viral hepatitis, toxin-induced necrosis, and acute bile duct obstruction. In chronic hepatitis, the levels are generally <5× ULN [6,7]. Serial assessment of transaminases can be used to monitor progress in an individual patient but correlation is poor between absolute values and the extent of necrosis. Serum ALT activity, but not AST, is slightly higher in the second trimester of pregnancy compared with non-pregnant women, but remains below the ULN [8]. Increased serum AST and ALT noted during labor may be secondary to contractions of uterine muscle [9]. In conclusion, serum AST and ALT levels remain normal during pregnancy prior to labor, and increased values should lead to further investigation.

Serum alkaline phosphatase rises in cholestasis and to a lesser extent with hepatocyte injury. Serum alkaline phosphatase increases significantly in late pregnancy as a result of placental and bone production. This limits the utility of alkaline phosphatase as a test to diagnose cholestasis of pregnancy. Hepatic and non-hepatic causes of alkaline phosphatase elevation can be differentiated by determination of its isoenzymes, or more easily by testing for GGT, which rises in liver disease but not in bone disease. Known inducers of GGT are bile acids (cholestasis), prolonged regular abuse of alcohol, and, particularly, antiepileptic drugs (phenytoin, carbamazepine). A decline in GGT can be observed during estrogen administration or during the second and third trimester of pregnancy [8]. Fasting total bile acid concentrations are unaltered in normal pregnancy and are, therefore, a specific test for the diagnosis of cholestasis.

Conjugated bilirubin can be elevated in cholestatic and hepatocellular disease and is associated with a rise in the serum enzymes discussed above. An isolated rise in serum bilirubin (without enzyme elevation) may be familial (Gilbert phenomenon) or result from hemolysis. Conjugated bilirubin concentrations are significantly lower during the second and third trimesters compared with non-pregnant women. This can be partially explained by hemodilution because albumin is the bilirubin-transporting protein [8].

The hepatocyte is the principal site of synthesis of the majority of coagulation proteins. The prothrombin time (after vitamin K administration) represents a good indicator of liver synthetic function because of the short half-life of factor VII (100–300 minutes). Estimation of individual clotting factors is rarely necessary, although the level of factor V (not vitamin K dependent) is related to outcome in acute liver failure. Serum albumin [10] provides some indication of hepatic synthetic capacity. However, serum albumin levels may be normal with acute liver failure because the half-life of albumin is approximately 22 days. Because of hemodilution, serum albumin levels are significantly lower during all trimesters of pregnancy compared with non-pregnant women [8].

Several scoring systems have been developed to asses liver function (Table 34.1). The Child–Pugh score reflects the severity of chronic liver disease according to the degree of ascites, the prothrombin time, the plasma concentrations of bilirubin and albumin, and the degree of encephalopathy. A total score of 5–6 is considered grade A (well-compensated disease), 7–9 is grade B, and 10–15 is grade C (decompensated disease). These grades correlate with 1- and 2-year patient survival. More recently, the MELD (Model of End Stage Liver Disease) has been introduced in clinical practice to predict prognosis in patients with cirrhosis and to guide listing for liver transplantation

Table 34.1. Assessment of liver function with the Child–Pugh classification

Factor	Units	1 point	2 points	3 points
Serum bilirubin	μmol/L	<34	34–51	>51
	mg/dL	<2.0	2.0–3.0	>3.0
Serum albumin	g/L	>35	30–35	<30
	g/dL	>3.5	3.0–3.5	<3.0
Prothrombin time or	Seconds prolonged	0–4	4–6	>6
international normalized ratio		<1.7	1.7–2.3	>2.3
Ascites		None	Moderate	Severe
Hepatic encephalopathy		None	Mild	Severe

The score is calculated by adding the scores of the 5 factors to give a grade: A, 5–6; B, 7–9; C, >9.

(Box 34.1). This score uses the prothrombin time, serum bilirubin, and creatinine as input values.

Imaging of the liver

Real-time ultrasonography represents the most widely used imaging method in clinical hepatology, to evaluate biliary tract obstruction, to identify collateral vessels and splenomegaly in portal hypertension, and to examine tumor vascularity. It is also valuable in diagnostic assessment of portal vein or hepatic vein thrombosis. More recently, liver elastography is used by many hepatologists to evaluate liver stiffness. This non-invasive technique uses both ultrasound (5 MHz) and low-frequency (50 Hz) elastic waves, whose propagation velocity is directly related to elasticity [11]. Unfortunately, there is no published experience yet in pregnancy.

If ultrasound is inconclusive, MRI is a safe imaging modality during pregnancy. No contrast injection is needed for blood vessel or bile duct visualization. Image quality has improved to such a degree that MR cholangiography has replaced diagnostic endoscopic retrograde cholangiopancreatography [12]. Contrast agents (e.g gadolinium) should be avoided during pregnancy because of transplacental transfer and unknown fetal effects [13]. More recently, diffusion-weighted imaging has been introduced allowing characterization of liver lesions, without contrast administration [14].

Liver disorders during pregnancy

Liver disease in pregnancy is generally separated into disorders that develop only in pregnancy and those that present coincidentally with pregnancy. We recommend a systematic approach that focuses on the major differential diagnostic characteristics of the pregnancy-related liver diseases (Table 34.2) [2,15]

Box 34.1. Model of end-stage Liver disease (MELD)

Survival probability of a patient with end-stage liver disease is estimated from

$[(0.957 \times \log_e$ Creatinine (mg/dL)) $+ 0.378 \times (\log_e$ Bilirubin (mg/dL)) $+ (1.120 \times \log_e$ INR) $+ 0.643] \times 10$

where INR is the international normalized ratio

An online calculator for MELD is available at http://www.mayoclinic.org/meld/mayomodel6.html

---

Table 34.2. Major differential diagnostic characteristics of pregnancy-related liver diseases in the second half of pregnancy

	Intrahepatic cholestasis of pregnancy	Acute fatty liver of pregnancy	HELLP-syndrome
Trimester	(2)–3	3	(2)–3
Symptoms	Pruritus	Tiredness, vomiting	Abdominal pain
Jaundice (bilirubin)	<5 mg/dL	Variable, >5 mg/dL if severe	Rare, and if present 5 mg/dL
Liver failure	No	Yes	No
Hypoglycemia	No	Yes	No
Mental status	Normal	Hepatic encephalopathy (ammonia ↑)	Headache, seizures, signs of disseminated intravascular coagulation
Cause of increased prothrombin time	Low vitamin K	Liver dysfunction	
Thrombocytopenia	No	No	Per definition
Transaminases	Variable, 2–20× ULN	Variable, up to10×ULN	Per definition, up to 10× ULN
Hemolysis	No	No	Per definition
Arterial hypertension	No	25–50%	85%
Imaging	Normal	Fatty changes	Hepatic infarction, hematoma
Liver histology	Cholestasis, limited inflammation	Microvesicular steatosis (zone 3)	Patchy necrosis, sinusoidal thrombi, and hemorrhage

ULN, upper limit of normal; HELLP, hemolysis, elevated liver enzymes, low platelets.

Table 34.3. Non-invasive evaluation of patients with clinical or biochemical suspicion of liver disease

	Evaluation
1. Clinical history and physical examination	Include medications
2. Liver disease	
Hepatobiliary imaging	Liver ultrasound (or if in doubt MRI)
Liver synthetic and excretory function	Prothrombin time, albumin, bilirubin
3. Specific tests	
Viral infection (hepatitis viruses A–E, cytomegalovirus, herpes simplex virus, Epstein–Barr virus)	Test for hepatitis B, C, D; for others only relevant to test if there is markedly elevated serum aminotransferases (>10× ULN)
Autoimmune disease	Anti-nuclear antibody, anti-mitochondrial antibody, smooth muscle cell antibody, liver–kidney microsomal antibodies, immunoglobulins
Alpha-1-antitrypsin deficiency	Protein electrophoresis (genetic testing)
Wilson disease	Serum ceruloplasmin, urinary copper excretion
4. Exclude non-hepatic causes of elevated aminotransferases	
Thyroid disorders	Thyroid-stimulating hormone
Coeliac disease	Tissue transglutaminase antibodies
Muscle pathology	Creatine kinase

ULN, upper limit of normal.

and a limited battery of additional tests for pregnancy-unrelated liver diseases (Table 34.3). The most frequent liver diseases that can be encountered during pregnancy are reviewed below.

Pregnancy-related liver diseases

Hyperemesis gravidarum

Hyperemesis gravidarum occurs in 0.3–2% of pregnancies and is characterized by intractable vomiting in the first half of pregnancy resulting in dehydration, electrolyte imbalance, weight loss, and ketosis [2,15,16]. Thiamine deficiency may lead to Wernicke's encephalopathy. The etiology is poorly understood and likely involves a combination of hormonal, genetic, immunological, and psychological factors. Serum ALT and AST are usually mildly elevated, although levels up to 20× ULN have been reported. Jaundice is uncommon and there is no risk of liver failure. Liver biopsy is not indicated and when done shows steatosis, focal necrosis, or bile plugs. Therapy involves frequent small low-fat meals, intravenous fluids, thiamine and folate supplementation, and antiemetic medication. Liver test abnormalities usually return to normal levels within a few days

of volume expansion and the cessation of vomiting. Persistently elevated transaminases are indicative of an alternative diagnosis such as acute viral hepatitis. Other pregnancy-related conditions such as acute fatty liver of pregnancy and the HELLP syndrome (hemolysis, elevated liver enzymes, and low platelets) typically present in the third trimester of pregnancy and are as such easily distinguished from hyperemesis gravidarum.

Intrahepatic cholestasis of pregnancy

Intrahepatic cholestasis of pregnancy is characterized by generalized pruritus (particularly affecting the soles and palms and is worse at night) and high fasting serum bile acid levels (>10 mmol/L) in the late second or third trimester [15,16]. Mild jaundice (serum bilirubin <5 mg/dL) is present in 10–25% of women and appears 1–4 weeks after the start of pruritus [15, 16]. Aminotranferase levels may be normal to mildly elevated with levels 10–20× ULN in rare cases. There is no evolution to liver failure. Diagnosis is made based on these clinical and biochemical findings. Liver imaging is rarely necessary. A liver biopsy may show signs of cholestasis and inflammatory changes but is not required for the diagnosis. The incidence of intrahepatic cholestasis of pregnancy varies among different geographic areas and populations: 0.1–0.5% in the USA and Australia to 10–16% in Scandinavia and Chile. The condition is associated with a relatively high rate of fetal morbidity, from premature birth and meconium-stained amniotic fluid, and intrauterine fetal death (0.4–1.6%) from fetal anoxia [2]. The risk of adverse fetal outcome appears to increase with increasing bile acid levels, particularly once a level of >40 μmol/L is achieved [17].

Prognosis for the mother is excellent, despite the pruritus and an increased risk for postpartum hemorrhage (because of cholestasis-induced vitamin K malabsorption). The rapid and complete recovery following delivery (within 2 weeks) is a typical feature. Risk factors include multiparity; advancing maternal age and multiple gestation and recurrence rates are high. Women with a history of intrahepatic cholestasis of pregnancy have more gallstone-related disease (pancreatitis, cholecystitis) and cholestasis from oral contraceptive use.

The pathogenesis of the disease is only partially understood. Hormonal changes in estrogen and progesterone metabolites, together with genetically determined mutations in bile transporter proteins, such as multidrug resistance glycoprotein-3 and bile salt export pump, play a role [18]. The link between high bile salt concentrations and fetal morbidity is possibly related to induction of myometrial contractions and placental vasoconstriction [16].

Intrahepatic cholestasis of pregnancy is associated with an approximately 1% risk of fetal death, which occurs at a median gestational age of 38 weeks [2]. Delivery at 37–38 weeks is commonly performed to minimize perinatal morbidity and mortality. Fetal monitoring is recommended despite the inability to prevent cases of sudden fetal death. Ursodeoxycholic acid is considered the drug of choice for the treatment of intrahepatic cholestasis of pregnancy. In a double-blind placebo-controlled study, 130 Swedish women were randomized to ursodeoxycholic acid (1 g/day, 3 weeks) or dexamethasone (12 mg/day, 1 week). The patients that were treated with ursodeoxycholic acid had significant improvement of pruritus and biochemical parameters of cholestasis [19]. There was no difference in fetal complications, but this may be because of the small group of patients (34) with bile salt levels >40 mmol/L.

Acute fatty liver of pregnancy

Acute fatty liver of pregnancy (also discussed in Chapter 37) affects approximately 5 in 100 000 pregnancies and is associated with a 1–2% maternal mortality rate and 10% perinatal mortality rate [20]. In rare cases, it can be associated with beta-oxidation defects in the fetus. The characteristic microscopic alteration is microvesicular steatosis [21]. Patients usually present in the third trimester and may exhibit acute liver failure with hepatic encephalopathy, jaundice, marked elevation of transaminases, prolonged prothrombin time, and hypoglycemia. The differential diagnosis includes acute viral hepatitis and the HELLP syndrome (Table 34.2). Management of acute fatty liver of pregnancy involves intensive supportive care and prompt delivery. The clinical condition may deteriorate further within the first 48 hours following delivery and liver transplant may be indicated in the absence of liver regeneration [2]. According to a retrospective evaluation of 54 admissions with pregnancy-related liver disease, the classical King's College criteria were not effective in predicting outcome. Instead, a serum lactate of 2.8 mg/dL and the presence of encephalopathy had sensitivity of 90% and a specificity of 86% to predict liver transplant or death [22].

Liver diseases unrelated to pregnancy

Several viruses may induce hepatitis. The natural history of the disease is dependent upon the host's immune response to the virus. Most cases of acute hepatitis are characterized by malaise, nausea, anorexia, and vomiting. Jaundice may develop and biochemically there may be a marked elevation of transaminases. The occurrence of hepatic encephalopathy and prolongation of prothrombin time is indicative of acute liver failure. Several viruses (e.g. hepatitis A (HAV) and E (HEV), herpes simplex virus (HSV), cytomegalovirus, Epstein–Barr viruses) that usually cause an acute self-limited hepatitis may occasionally result in acute liver failure.

Infections with hepatitis B virus (HBV), C virus (HCV), or delta virus may run a chronic course and the viral genome can be detected in the serum more than 6 months after infection. Most of these patients are asymptomatic and are only diagnosed after detection of liver tests abnormalities. A long-standing infection can induce cirrhosis, which may lead to fibrosis, nodular regeneration, vascular shunt formation, and clinically significant portal hypertension. In addition to viruses, the pregnant woman may develop autoimmune, drug-induced (including toxins), or metabolic liver disease.

Hepatitis A

Hepatitis A virus is transmitted via the fecal–oral route and the incidence of acute HAV during pregnancy is less than 1 in 1000. Diagnosis is made by detection of antibodies to HAV of the IgM type. The clinical presentation and disease course is similar to nonpregnant patients. Acute HAV infection in the third trimester of pregnancy is associated with preterm labor in approximately 60% of patients [15,23]. In acute liver failure, liver transplantation may be indicated. Perinatal HAV transmission is uncommon and most remain subclinical. A safe and effective vaccine against HAV is available. After birth, children of mothers with HAV infection in the last trimester should receive the vaccine, and some experts also recommend administration of immunoglobulin.

Hepatitis B and delta

Hepatitis B virus is highly infectious and transmitted parenterally by percutaneous or mucosal exposure, sexually, and from mother to infant. The clinical presentation and course of the disease is similar to nonpregnant infected individuals. Diagnosis of HBV infection is made by detection of hepatitis B surface antigen (HBsAg) in the serum. It is difficult to determine, in the absence of previous serology, if a patient acquired a new infection or has a flare of a chronic hepatitis B. Although intrauterine infection has been reported, the intrapartum period is the time of greatest risk. The risk of vertical transmission is 10–20% in women positive for HBsAg but negative for hepatitis e antigen (HBeAg; found in the blood only when there are viruses also present). Women with a high HBV viral load or those positive for HBeAg have an 80–90% chance of transmitting the virus to their infant [15,24]. Perinatal infection commonly progresses to chronic infection, which is associated with an increased risk of developing cirrhosis and liver cancer. Because of the risk of vertical transmission, HBsAg status should be assessed early in pregnancy and unimmunized high-risk patients should be vaccinated, even during pregnancy. Administration of HBV human immunoglobulin and the HBV vaccine within 12 hours of birth to all neonates born to HBsAg-positive women reduces the vertical transmission rate by 85–95% [16]. The use of antiviral drugs such as lamivudine or tenofovir during the third trimester in women with a high viral load appears to be safe during pregnancy and may further reduce the risk of vertical transmission [25]. However, there is no consistency about

definition of high viral load among different studies. The vertical transmission rate does not appear to be affected by mode of delivery or breastfeeding.

Hepatitis delta virus is a subviral satellite dependent upon the presence of HBV for replication. Its diagnosis is established by serological testing. Vertical transmission is possible but preventable by using the measures to prevent HBV infection.

Hepatitis C

Hepatitis C virus is transmitted through the parenteral route and is mainly a disease of intravenous drug users. Following a mostly asymptomatic acute infection, more than 80% of patients will develop chronic hepatitis and are at risk for developing cirrhosis or primary liver cancer over the following two to three decades. The incidence of chronic HCV infection in pregnant women is similar to that of the general population and ranges from <1% up to 2.4% [2,26]. Diagnosis of HCV infection is confirmed by the detection of HCV RNA in serum. The antibodies that are detectable are not protective and an effective vaccine is not available. Transaminase activity levels may fall in the second half of pregnancy with a concurrent rise in serum HCV RNA levels, but this is not clinically significant. Women with chronic HCV infection usually experience an uneventful pregnancy except when advanced fibrosis and portal hypertension is present.

Unlike HBV infection, vertical transmission of HCV is generally below 10%. Factors that increase this risk include HIV coinfection, high viral load ($>10^6$ copies/mL), and membrane rupture >6 hours [2]. Risk of transmission is unaffected by mode of delivery or breastfeeding. The presence of serum HCV RNA at 6 months of age is indicative of congenital HCV infection. Vertically acquired neonatal HCV infection usually manifests as mild liver disease, although spontaneous clearance later on is possible. Antiviral therapy is generally postponed until young adulthood. Current antiviral therapy for HCV includes interferon and ribavirin, which are contraindicated during pregnancy.

Hepatitis E

Hepatitis E virus is endemic to large areas of Africa, Asia, and Central America and shares the same fecal–oral transmission route as HAV. Sporadic cases are increasingly diagnosed in developed countries. Pregnant women are particularly susceptible to this viral infection and HEV infection during the last two trimesters of pregnancy is associated with up to 60% risk of fulminant hepatic failure, resulting in high maternal (41–54%) and fetal (69%) mortality rates [15,27]. Delivery does not affect maternal outcome and there is no therapy to prevent transmission.

Herpes simplex virus hepatitis

Pregnancy increases susceptibility to HSV hepatitis, which is otherwise rarely seen in adults. Maternal and neonatal mortality rates may be as high as 40%. Mucocutaneous lesions are not always present. The high level of transaminases and coagulopathy in the absence of jaundice ("anicteric" hepatitis) should raise suspicion of HSV hepatitis, for which intravenous therapy with acyclovir is effective [28].

Autoimmune hepatitis

Autoimmune hepatitis has a prevalence of 0.1–1.2 per 100 000 in the Caucasian population. The clinical manifestations of this condition vary widely and include asymptomatic patients, those with acute fulminant hepatitis, and those with chronic hepatitis and cirrhosis. Although autoimmune hepatitis is typically associated with infertility, a patient with well-controlled disease can become pregnant. Autoimmune hepatitis is classically treated with corticosteroids as induction therapy and azathioprine in maintenance. More recently, budenoside was shown to control the disease with fewer systemic side effects than dexamethasone. Autoimmune hepatitis tends to run a highly variable course in pregnancy. Postpartum flares are common, which is similar to other autoimmune conditions. The risk of fetal loss, preterm birth, and fetal growth restriction appears to be increased in women with autoimmune hepatitis. However, successful pregnancy outcome is anticipated in women with well-controlled disease [29–31]. Treatment commonly consists of corticosteroids and/or azathioprine. Corticosteroids are considered safe during pregnancy, although there is some debate concerning azathioprine (US Food and Drug Administration pregnancy category D), but data suggest low risk.

In patients with cholestatic autoimmune liver diseases, such as primary sclerosing cholangitis or primary biliary cirrhosis, limited data are available concerning pregnancy outcome [32]. In patients with primary sclerosing cholangitis, concomitant inflammatory bowel disease may pose specific problems that are beyond the scope of this chapter. For both diseases, ursodeoxycholic acid is a standard treatment and is considered safe during pregnancy (US Food and Drug Administration pregnancy category B).

Non-alcoholic fatty liver disease

Non-alcoholic fatty liver disease (NAFLD) is becoming the most frequent liver disease in the Western world, with at least 20% prevalence in unselected populations [33,34]. It is a spectrum of liver disease, ranging from steatosis to steatohepatitis, with advanced fibrosis and eventually cirrhosis. Non-alcoholic fatty liver disease is the hepatic manifestation of the metabolic syndrome, which includes obesity, arterial hypertension, hyperlipidemia, and type 2 diabetes mellitus. The influx of free fatty acids together with insulin resistance on a susceptible genetic background is a driving mechanism, but the pathogenesis remains poorly understood [35]. Patients may remain asymptomatic for decades. The diagnosis is made by the combination of abnormal liver tests (typically with the ALT:AST ratio >2:1), the suggestion of liver steatosis on imaging, and (rarely) a liver biopsy. The histological findings are similar to alcoholic liver disease; therefore, the differential diagnosis can only be made in patients who abstain from alcohol. Therapy includes control of the components of the metabolic syndrome and lifestyle changes. Despite the supposed high prevalence of NAFLD in the general population, there are virtually no data in the literature concerning NAFLD and pregnancy [36]. Despite the lack of data, an increased risk of pre-eclampsia is expected in women with NAFLD because of its associated comorbidities, such as obesity and hypertension.

Hepatic vein thrombosis (Budd–Chiari syndrome)

Pregnancy, along with other hypercoagulable states (i.e. myeloproliferative disorders and inherited thrombophilia), are risk factors for the rare condition of hepatic vein thrombosis [37]. The clinical picture is dependent upon the number of veins involved. Prognosis is poor in patients with painful hepatomegaly and marked ascites. Therapy consists of low-molecular-weight heparin and the timely placement of a transjugular portosystemic shunt to decompress the liver. Liver transplant may be indicated in case of overt liver failure.

Treatment in pregnancy involves anticoagulation, although thrombosis may occur despite therapy. Maternal outcome is generally favorable but an increased rate of miscarriage and preterm delivery have been reported [37].

Wilson disease

Wilson disease is a rare autosomal recessive disorder of copper metabolism characterized by deposition of excess copper in the liver, brain, and kidney. Patients may present with jaundice, elevated transaminases, and hemolytic anemia, which may be mistaken for the HELLP syndrome.

Pregnant patients should continue anticopper therapy throughout pregnancy to prevent disease flare and acute liver failure. The dose of D-penicillamine (US Food and Drug Administration category D drug) should be decreased by 25–50% in pregnancy [38]. An excellent outcome for 12 pregnancies in patients with Wilson disease was demonstrated using D-penicillamine [39]. Zinc may potentially represent an alternative treatment [40].

Drug-induced liver disease, including alcohol

The liver is susceptible to damage by drugs and toxins as it has an important role in metabolizing xenobiotics. The degree of drug-induced liver injury can vary from mild transient elevation of liver tests to severe injury and acute failure. Hepatotoxicity is a result of multiple factors and is difficult to predict. A few drugs that cause liver injury have a predictable, dose-dependent toxic mechanism of action, the most widely recognized being acetaminophen. When acetaminophen overdose is excluded, most cases of drug-induced liver injury result from rare, unpredictable reactions to commonly used drugs [41]. The drug itself or its metabolite may be inherently hepatotoxic. The level of exposure, environmental factors, and genetic factors could play a role in hepatotoxicity. During pregnancy, the liver remains vulnerable to these toxic drug reactions. Catastrophic cases of drug-induced liver injury have been reported in pregnancy, even with drugs that were presumed "safe" in pregnancy [42].

Ethanol ingestion in pregnancy may be associated with dangerous consequences for mother and child. In non-pregnant women, the intake of more than two units a day and particularly binge drinking, is associated with many health risks, including but not limited to liver disease. The liver disease caused by alcohol represents the same histological spectrum as discussed for NAFLD. The histological liver changes caused by alcohol are similar to those seen with NAFLD. In contrast with NAFLD, patients with alcoholic hepatitis (without cirrhosis) may present with the clinical picture of acute liver failure (marked jaundice, prolonged prothrombin time, encephalopathy, portal hypertension, and moderately

elevated serum transaminases), with a high risk of death (up to 50%). The pathogenesis of liver disease relates to ethanol metabolism with generation of acetaldehyde, which is highly toxic because of the formation of protein and DNA adducts that promote glutathione depletion, lipid peroxidation, and mitochondrial damage [43].

Alcohol ingestion may have several negative effects on pregnancy. The age-adjusted relative risk of second trimester spontaneous abortions (15–27 weeks) was 1.03 (non-significant), 1.98 ($p < 0.01$), and 3.53 ($p < 0.01$) for women taking fewer than 1, one to two, and more than three units daily, compared with non-drinkers [44]. Alcohol exposure in pregnancy may lead to fetal alcohol spectrum disorder, which includes craniofacial, cardiac, growth, and behavioral abnormalities. Fetal injury may occur with alcohol exposure at any time in pregnancy, although the risk of birth defects is highest with first trimester consumption. Abstinence from alcohol is recommended during pregnancy because a safe level of consumption has not been determined [45].

Management of clinically significant portal hypertension

Portal hypertension may arise in the context of liver disease (most often cirrhosis from the various causes discussed above) or in non-cirrhotic disorder (most often portal vein thrombosis). Fertility is unaffected in women with non-cirrhotic portal hypertension. Cirrhosis is associated with a high incidence of amenorrhea, making pregnancy less likely to occur [46]. The spontaneous abortion rate can be as high as 40% of pregnancies in women with cirrhosis.

Clinically significant portal hypertension is defined by the presence of esophagogastric varices and/or ascites that correlate with an invasively measured hepatic venous pressure gradient of >10 mmHg. The increased blood volume that occurs during pregnancy may worsen portal hypertension and increase the risk of variceal bleeding, which develops in 20–25% of patients [2]. Pregnancy outcome in women with cirrhosis and portal hypertension is variable. Fetal and maternal mortality rates up to 50% were reported in older studies. In a recent retrospective series of 62 pregnancies in 29 women with cirrhosis, maternal complications (ascites, encephalopathy, or variceal hemorrhage) occurred in 10% of patients and one mother died [47]. The reduction in complications in recent studies likely reflects the implementation of evidence-based treatments for portal hypertension, such as the use of non-selective beta-blockers and/or endoscopic band ligation of the varices. Mortality rates are higher in cirrhotic (<10–50%) than in non-cirrhotic (10%) patients [48].

The existing prognostic models of cirrhosis severity are useful in determining outcomes in pregnant women with cirrhosis. Higher MELD and Child–Pugh scores (discussed above) are associated with poorer outcomes for mother and newborn. In the study of Westbrook et al. [47], a MELD score at the time of conception ≥10 predicted, with 83% sensitivity and 83% specificity, which patients were likely to have significant, liver-related complications. No patient who had a MELD score ≤6 at the time of conception developed significant hepatological complications.

Women with a MELD score of ≥10 should be advised against pregnancy.

Every patient with suspicion of cirrhotic or non-cirrhotic portal hypertension (history of liver disease and upper gastrointestinal bleeding, imaging suggestive of cirrhosis, low platelets) who is pregnant or considering pregnancy should undergo upper endoscopy to evaluate for varices. The best timing would be the second trimester. Primary prophylaxis with a non-selective beta-blocker may be indicated. If there is intolerance to beta-blockers or if gastrointestinal bleeding does occur during pregnancy, urgent endoscopic ligation of the varices is indicated [49]. The administration of vasoactive drugs such as terlipressin is contraindicated because of uterine ischemia and ischemia of fetal digits (Table 34.4) [2].

Table 34.4. Indication and safety of drugs for liver disease during pregnancy

	Medication	FDA category	Remarks	Breastfeeding
Autoimmune hepatitis, post–liver transplant	Prednisone	C	Safe	No, except low dose
	Azathioprine	D	Safe	No
	Cyclosporine	C	Safe	No
	Tacrolimus	C	Safe	No
	Mycophenolate mofetil	Undetermined	Not recommended, limited data	Not recommended, limited data
	Everolimus	Undetermined	Not recommended, limited data	Not recommended, limited data
Intrahepatic cholestasis of pregnancy	Ursodeoxycholic acid	B	Indicated for, and safe	Yes
Hepatitis B virus	Lamivudine	C	Safe	No
	Entecavir	C	Not recommended	No
	Tenofovir	C	Safe	No
Hepatitis B and C virus	Interferon	C	Not recommended, high dose may induce abortion	No
Hepatitis C virus	Ribavirin	X	Contraindicated, fetal toxicity	Unknown
Wilson disease	Pencillamine	D	Embryopathy, but need to continue therapy	No
	Zinc	C	Safe	Yes
Esophageal varices	Beta-blockade	C (first trimester)/D (second/third trimester)	Risk of fetal bradycardia and intrauterine growth retardation, but necessary to prevent variceal bleeding	Yes
Variceal bleeding	Terlipressin	X	Contraindicated, uterine ischemia	No data

FDA, US Food and Drug Administration.

In patients with known varices on a stable and well-tolerated regimen of beta-blockers before pregnancy, it is not known whether endoscopy should be repeated during pregnancy.

Patients with portal hypertension may have significant varicose veins on the abdominal wall and in the epidural space. Visualization of these collaterals by MRI may minimize risks in regional anesthesia or cesarean delivery [50]. An additional reason to perform an MRI in pregnant patients with portal hypertension is to look for splenic artery aneurysms. These vascular abnormalities are prone to rupture during the third trimester, with high fetal and maternal mortality rates [51]. Preconceptional screening and treatment (coiling) of splenic aneurysms in patients with known portal hypertension is recommended [52]. Operative vaginal delivery following passive fetal descent is suggested to avoid the valsalva maneuver and minimize the risk of variceal bleeding.

Special situations

Pregnancy in women after liver transplant

Nearly 90% of women of childbearing age return to a fertile state by 7 months after liver transplant. Women are generally advised to delay conception for at least 1 year to stabilize graft function and immunosuppressant dose and optimize control of comorbid conditions [15]. A 2012 meta-analysis that included 450 pregnancies in 306 liver transplant recipients revealed a live birth rate of nearly 77% and a miscarriage rate of 15.6%. The risk of pre-eclampsia (21.9%), preterm delivery (39.4%), and cesarean delivery (44.6%) were increased compared with the general US population [53]. The risk of gestational diabetes and low birth weight is also increased in the liver transplant recipient [15]. Variable rates of rejection during pregnancy (2–10%) and graft loss directly attributable to pregnancy (0–10%) have been reported [53].

The safety of the immunosuppressive drugs is given in Table 34.4. Most data are available for corticosteroids, azathioprine, cyclosporine, and tacrolimus-based regimens. Mycophenolate mofetil and everolimus should be avoided in pregnancy. Breastfeeding is contraindicated in women taking immunosuppressive drugs.

Hepatocellular adenomas and bleeding risk

Hepatocellular adenomas are a rare but important problem with some having a tendency for malignant transformation. However, during pregnancy they may cause life-threatening bleeding. The lesion typically develops in women and most often in long-term users of oral contraceptives. The annual incidence has been estimated in (older) case–control studies to be <5 per 100 000 long-term (>5 years) oral contraceptive users.

Hepatocellular adenomas arise in a normal liver, while a similar lesion in a cirrhotic liver is called a regenerative or dysplastic nodule. The composing cells closely resemble normal hepatocytes, often contain fat or glycogen, and are arranged in regular plates up to three cells thick, without acinar architecture. Portal tracts containing bile ducts are absent [54].

Studies that correlate lesional genotype with phenotype form the basis of a new histological/molecular classification of hepatocellular adenomas. Based on molecular criteria (mutations in genes encoding hepatocyte nuclear factor-1α and β-catenin) and histological criteria (the presence/absence of inflammation, cytological and architectural atypia, steatosis, sinusoidal congestion, and mild ductular reaction), subgroups of hepatocellular adenoma can be defined with variable risks of bleeding and malignant transformation. The occurrence of hemorrhage seems to cluster with the inflammatory hepatocellular adenoma [55]. There are two types of hemorrhage: internal bleeding, usually admixed with necrotic changes (this type is mostly observed in adenomas >4 cm); and spontaneous rupture, which causes subcapsular hematoma and possible hemoperitoneum. Mortality rates of 44% and 38%, respectively, for mother and fetus have been described when rupture occurred during pregnancy [56].

The diameter of bleeding adenomas in the literature varies between 6.5 and 19 cm. These tumors are prone to bleed in the third trimester, but one third rupture in the postpartum period. Other benign lesions, such as focal nodular hyperplasia or hemangiomas, have no bleeding risk [56].

Preconceptional detection of hepatocellular adenoma by ultrasound, contrast-enhanced CT, and, particularly, MRI allow for a specific diagnosis. Resection of a hepatocellular adenoma before pregnancy is necessary with large tumors (≥4–5 cm) or when there are factors that suggest malignant transformation, such as rapid growth, change in radiological characteristics, or elevated serum alpha-fetoprotein. Hepatocellular adenomas that are discovered during pregnancy should be followed by ultrasound at monthly intervals and should be treated according to the criteria above.

Conclusions

The management of liver disease during pregnancy requires a multidisciplinary collaboration between obstetrician, hepatologist, anesthesiologist, and pediatrician in order to optimize outcome for mother and child.

It is challenging for the clinician to interpret abnormal liver tests in the context of the normal physiological changes during pregnancy. The timely recognition of cholestasis, clinically significant portal hypertension, and liver failure is essential to minimize fetal and maternal morbidity and mortality. The differentiation of diseases related or unrelated to pregnancy is important and determines the management.

References

1. Ch'ng CL, Morgan M, Hainsworth I, Kingham JG. Prospective study of liver dysfunction in pregnancy in Southwest Wales. *Gut* 2002;**51**:876–880.

2. Hay JE. Liver disease in pregnancy. *Hepatology* 2008;**47**:1067–1076.

3. Scott DB, Kerr MG. Inferior vena caval pressure in late pregnancy. *J Obstet Gynaecol Br Commonw* 1963;**70**:1044–1049.

4. Britton RC. Pregnancy and esophageal varices. *Am J Surg* 1982;**143**:421–425.

5. Perez V, Gorodisch S, Casavilla F., *et al.* Ultrastructure of human liver at the end of normal pregnancy. *Am J Obstet Gynecol* 1971;**110**:428–431.

6. Kuntz E. Laboratory diagnostics. In Kuntz E, Kuntz HD (eds.) *Hepatology, Principles and Practice.* Heidelberg: Springer-Verlag, 2001, pp. 78–112.

7. Pratt DS, Kaplan MM. Evaluation of abnormal liver-enzyme results in asymptomatic patients. *N Engl J Med* 2000;**342**:1266–1271.

8. Bacq Y, Zarka O, Bréchot JF, *et al.* Liver function tests in normal pregnancy: a prospective study of 103 pregnant women and 103 matched controls. *Hepatology* 1996;**23**:1030–1034.

9. David AL, Kotecha M, Girling JC. Factors influencing postnatal liver function tests. *BJOG* 2000;**107**:1421–1426.

10. Rothschild MA, Oratz M, Schreiber SS. Serum albumin. *Hepatology* 1988;**8**:385–401.

11. Sandrin L, Fourquet B, Hasquenoph JM, *et al.* Transient elastography: a new noninvasive method for assessment of hepatic fibrosis. *Ultrasound Med Biol* 2003;**29**:1705–1713.

12. Van Hoe L, Vanbeckevoort D, Van Steenbergen W. *Atlas of Cross-sectional and Projective MR Cholangio-pancreatography.* Berlin: Springer-Verlag, 1999.

13. Shellock FG, Kanal E. Safety of magnetic resonance imaging contrast agents. *J Magn Reson Imaging* 1999;**10**:477–484.

14. Vandecaveye V, De Keyzer F, Verslype C, *et al.* Diffusion-weighted MRI provides additional value to conventional dynamic contrast-enhanced MRI for detection of hepatocellular carcinoma. *Eur Radiol* 2009;**19**:2456–2466.

15. Joshi D, James A, Quaglia A, Westbrook RH, Heneghan MA. Liver disease in pregnancy. *Lancet* 2010;**375**:594–605.

16. Lee N, Brady C. Liver disease in pregnancy. *World J Gastroenterol* 2009;**15**:897–906.

17. Glantz A, Marschall HU, Mattsson LA. Intrahepatic cholestasis of pregnancy: relationships between bile acid levels and fetal complication rates. *Hepatology* 2004;**40**:467–474.

18. Wasmuth HE, Glantz A, Keppeler H, *et al.* Intrahepatic cholestasis of pregnancy: the severe form is associated with common variants of the hepatobiliary phospholipid transporter ABCB4 gene. *Gut* 2007;**56**:265–270.

19. Glantz A, Marschall HU, Lammert F, Mattsson LA. Intrahepatic cholestasis of pregnancy: a randomized controlled trial comparing dexamethasone and ursodeoxycholic acid. *Hepatology* 2005;**42**:1399–1405.

20. Knight M, Nelson-Piercy C, Kurinczuk JJ, Spark P, Brocklehurst P; UK Obstetric Surveillance System. A prospective national study of acute fatty liver of pregnancy in the UK. *Gut* 2008;**57**:951–956.

21. Rolfes DB, Ishaj KG. Liver disease in pregnancy. *Histopathology* 1986;**10**:555–570.

22. Westbrook RH, Yeoman AD, Joshi D, *et al.* Outcomes of severe pregnancy-related liver disease: refining the role of transplantation. *Am J Transplant* 2010;**10**:2520–2526.

23. Elinav E, Ben-Dov IZ, Shapira Y, *et al.* Acute hepatitis A infection in pregnancy is associated with high rates of gestational complications and preterm labor. *Gastroenterology* 2006;**130**:1129–1134.

24. Lee C, Gong Y, Brok J, Boxall EH, Gluud C. Effect of hepatitis B immunisation in newborn infants of mothers positive for hepatitis B surface antigen: systematic review and meta-analysis. *BMJ* 2006;**332**:328–336.

25. Sookoian S. Liver disease during pregnancy: acute viral hepatitis. *Ann Hepatol* 2006;**5**:231–236.

26. Sookoian S. Effect of pregnancy on pre-existing liver disease: chronic viral hepatitis. *Ann Hepatol* 2006;**5**:190–197.

27. Banait VS, Sandur V, Parikh F, *et al.* Outcome of acute liver failure due to acute hepatitis E in pregnant women. *Ind J Gastroenterol* 2007;**26**:6–10.

389

28. Kang AH, Graves CR. Herpes simplex hepatitis in pregnancy: a case report and review of the literature. *Obstet Gynecol Surv* 1999;**54**:463–468.

29. Heneghan MA, Norris SM, O'Grady JG., *et al.* Management and outcome of pregnancy in autoimmune hepatitis. *Gut* 2001;**48**:97–102.

30. Candia L, Marquez J, Espinoza LR. Autoimmune hepatitis and pregnancy: a rheumatologist's dilemma. *Semin Arthritis Rheum* 2005;**35**:49–56.

31. Buchel E, Van Steenbergen W, Nevens F., *et al.* Improvement of autoimmune hepatitis during pregnancy followed by flareup after delivery. *Am J Gastroenterol* 2002;**97**:3160–3165.

32. Heathcote E. Management of primary biliary cirrhosis. *Hepatology* 2000;**31**:105–113.

33. Browning JD, Szczepaniak LS, Dobbins R, *et al.* Prevalence of hepatic steatosis in an urban population in the United States: impact of ethnicity. *Hepatology* 2004;**40**:1387–1395.

34. Bedogni G, Miglioli L, Masutti F, *et al.* Prevalence of and risk factors for nonalcoholic fatty liver disease: the Dionysos Nutrition and Liver Study. *Hepatology* 2005;**42**:44–52.

35. Cohen JC, Horton JD, Hobbs HH. Human fatty liver disease: old questions and new insights. *Science* 2011;**24**; 332: 1519–1523.

36. Page L, Girling J. A novel cause for abnormal liver function tests in pregnancy and the puerperium: non-alcoholic fatty liver disease. *BJOG* 2011;**118**:1532–1535.

37. Rautou PE, Angermayr B, Garcia-Pagan JC, *et al.* Pregnancy in women with known and treated Budd–Chiari syndrome: maternal and fetal outcomes. *J Hepatol* 2009;**51**:47–54.

38. Roberts EA, Schilsky ML. A practice guideline on Wilson disease. *Hepatology* 2003;**37**:1475–1492.

39. Lowette KF, Desmet K, Witters P, *et al.* Wilson's disease: long-term follow-up of a cohort of 24 patients treated with D-penicillamine. *Eur J Gastroenterol Hepatol.* 2010;**22**:564–571.

40. Brewer GJ, Johnson VD, Dick RD, *et al.* Treatment of Wilson's disease with zinc. XVII: treatment during pregnancy. *Hepatology* 2000;**31**:364–370.

41. Björnsson E. Drug-induced liver injury: Hy's rule revisited. *Clin Pharmacol Ther* 2006;**79**:521–528.

42. Sequeira E, Wanyonyi S, Dodia R. Severe propylthiouracil-induced hepatotoxicity in pregnancy managed successfully by liver transplantation: A case report. *J Med Case Rep* 2011;**5**:461.

43. Joenje H. Metabolism: alcohol, DNA and disease. *Nature* 2011;**475**:45–46.

44. Anokute CC. Epidemiology of spontaneous abortions: the effect of alcohol consumption and cigarette smoking. *Natl Med Assoc* 1996;**78**: 771–775.

45. de Sanctis L, Memo L, Pichini S, Tarani L, Vagnarelli F. Fetal alcohol syndrome: new perspectives for an ancient and underestimated problem. *J Matern Fetal Neonatal Med* 2011;**24**(Suppl 1):34–37.

46. Cundy TF, O'Grady JG, Williams R. Recovery of menstruation and pregnancy after liver transplantation. *Gut* 1990;**31**:337–338.

47. Westbrook RH, Yeoman AD, O'Grady JG, *et al.* Model for end-stage liver disease score predicts outcome in cirrhotic patients during pregnancy. *Clin Gastroenterol Hepatol* 2011;**9**:694–699.

48. Kochhar R, Kumar S, Goel RC, *et al.* Pregnancy and its outcome in patients with noncirrhotic portal hypertension. *Dig Dis Sci* 1999;**44**:1356–1361.

49. Starkel P, Horsmans Y, Geubel A. Endoscopic band ligation: A safe technique to control bleeding esophageal varices in pregnancy. *Gastrointest Endosc* 1998;**48**:212–214.

50. Hirabayashi Y, Shimizu R, Fukuda H, Saitoh K, Igarashi T. Effects of the pregnant uterus on the extradural venous plexus in the supine and lateral positions, as determined by magnetic resonance imaging. *Br J Anaesth* 1997;**78**:317–319.

51. Barrett JM, Caldwell BH. Association of portal hypertension and ruptured splenic artery aneurysm in pregnancy. *Obstet Gynecol* 1981;**57**:255–257.

52. Sunagozaka H, Tsuji H, Mizukoshi E, *et al.* The development and clinical features of splenic aneurysm associated with liver cirrhosis. *Liver Int* 2006;**26**:291–297.

53. Deshpande NA, James NT, Kucirka LM, *et al.* Pregnancy outcomes in liver transplant recipients: a systematic review and meta-analysis. *Liver Transpl* 2012;**18**:621–629.

54. Verslype C, Libbrecht L. The multidisciplinary management of gastrointestinal cancer. The diagnostic and therapeutic approach for primary solid liver tumours in adults. *Best Pract Res Clin Gastroenterol* 2007;**21**:983–996.

55. Zucman-Rossi J, Jeannot E, Nhieu JT, *et al.* Genotype-phenotype correlation in hepatocellular adenoma: new classification and relationship with HCC. *Hepatology* 2006;**43**:515–524.

56. Cobey FC, Salem RR. A review of liver masses in pregnancy and a proposed algorithm for their diagnosis and management. *Am J Surgery* 2004;**187**:181–191.

Chapter 35

Autoimmune disease in pregnancy

Karim Djekidel and Bob Silver

Introduction

It is unclear why many autoimmune conditions have a predilection for women. However, there is considerable evidence that estrogen increases the risk and androgens may decrease the risk of autoimmune disease. Pregnancy is associated with a dramatic increase in estrogen and other hormones; consequently, there is the potential for autoimmune disease to worsen during pregnancy (see Clinical case 35.1). The actual story is more complicated. Some conditions typically improve during pregnancy while others remain stable or worsen. In some cases, maternal disease becomes so severe that critical care and admission to an intensive care unit (ICU) is required. This is particularly so for lupus nephritis or a flare with neurological complications, scleroderma renal crisis, myasthenia, and adrenal crises. Other autoimmune disorders such as rheumatoid arthritis may be the source of technical or diagnostic challenges in ICU.

> **Clinical case 35.1.** Critical care presentation of autoimmune disease in pregnancy
>
> A 26-year-old nulliparous woman at 26 weeks of gestation is admitted to the ICU with acute renal failure, hypertension, and pulmonary edema. She also has thrombocytopenia. During checkups in her first trimester her blood pressure was been normal and she had no proteinuria on urinalysis. She has known systemic lupus erythematosus and this seems likely to be a lupus flare with nephritis. However, these features also are characteristic of severe pre-eclampsia. Distinguishing between lupus nephritis and pre-eclampsia is critical because pre-eclampsia requires delivery whereas lupus flare does not. This has dramatic consequences for the fetus given the very early gestational age.

Systemic lupus erythematosus

Systemic lupus erythematosus (SLE) is considered to be the "prototypical" autoimmune disease. It is a chronic, multisystem disorder that primarily affects women of childbearing age. The condition affects about 1 in 200 individuals and is about three times more common in African-Americans than Caucasians.

The condition is a syndrome and patients must have both clinical criteria and confirmatory laboratory studies to be considered to have SLE. Common symptoms include fatigue, arthralgias, fever, and rash (Table 35.1). The disease may affect numerous organ systems such as joints, skin, kidneys, lungs, nerves, and other organs. In order to be considered to have SLE, patients must meet at least 4 of the 11 criteria established by the American College of Rheumatology (Box 35.1) [1].

The laboratory features of SLE can be confusing. Antibodies to double-stranded DNA (anti-dsDNA) fluctuate with disease activity and can be used to assess lupus flares. They are particularly associated with nephritis. In contrast anti-nuclear antibodies (ANA) are not very specific and do not correlate with disease activity (despite fluctuations over time). Accordingly, there is little benefit to serial assessment of ANA levels. Other antibodies such as anti-Ro (SSA), anti-La (SSB), anti-ribonucleoprotein, and anit-smooth muscle do not fluctuate much and are not useful for monitoring disease status.

The effect of pregnancy on systemic lupus erythematosus

Flares are estimated to occur during pregnancy in over half of pregnant women. Factors that increase the risk for flare include active disease at the time of conception, lupus nephritis, an SLE Active Disease Activity Index score of ≥ 5, or acute cessation of hydroxychloroquine.

Maternal Critical Care: A Multidisciplinary Approach, ed. Marc Van de Velde, Helen Scholefield, and Lauren A. Plante.
Published by Cambridge University Press. © Cambridge University Press 2013.

Table 35.1. Frequency of clinical symptoms in patients with systemic lupus erythematosus

Symptom	Frequency (%)
Fatigue	80–100
Fever	80–100
Arthritis	80–95
Myalgias	70
Weight loss	60
Photosensitivity	60
Raynaud phenomenon	60
Malar rash	50
Nephritis	50
Mouth ulcers	50
Pleurisy	50
Lymphadenopathy	50
Pericarditis	30
Neuropsychiatric	20–30

Box 35.1. American College of Rheumatology revised criteria for the diagnosis and classification of systemic lupus erythematosus

Must meet at least four of the following for diagnosis:

- malar rash
- discoid rash
- photosensitivity
- oral ulcers
- arthritis
- serositis (pleuritis or pericarditis)
- nephritis (proteinuria ≥3+ (500 mg/24 hours), or cellular casts in urine
- neurological disorder (seizures, psychosis, or stroke)
- hematological disorder (hemolytic anemia, thrombocytopenia, leukopenia, or lymphopenia)
- immunological disorders (anti-double-stranded DNA, anti-smooth muscle, anti-cardiolipin antibodies, or lupus anticoagulant)
- antinuclear antibodies

Source: Tan et al., 1982 [1].

Ideally, patients should be in remission for 6–12 months prior to becoming pregnant.

Other maternal risks include thrombocytopenia, which occurs in one quarter of women with SLE. Risk factors for thrombocytopenia include anti-phospholipid antibodies, active disease, and pre-eclampsia. Chronic pain from joints damaged by lupus arthritis may worsen during pregnancy because of the increased weight bearing and relaxation of ligaments. Rashes may appear to worsen because of the increased blood volume associated with normal pregnancy.

Flares during pregnancy can be treated with hydroxychloroquine and corticosteroids. Intravenous immunoglobulin (IVIG) may be beneficial in the treatment of lupus nephritis. Patients with acute lupus nephritis who do not respond to the above options may require cyclophosphamide. If there is no response to medical therapy and the serum creatinine levels are >3.5 mg/dL, patients should be started on dialysis (sooner if indicated) to avoid potential adverse fetal effects.

Lupus nephritis

Renal disease is a major concern during pregnancy. There is increased risk of accelerating a decrease in renal function if the pre-pregnancy serum creatinine is ≥1.5 mg/dL. The decline is thought to be caused by the development of pre-eclampsia with acute tubular necrosis. Conversely, women with serum creatinine levels <1.5 mg/dL are not at increased risk for permanent decrease in renal function caused by pregnancy [2,3].

Nephritis is characterized by increased levels of anti-dsDNA, decreased complement, and erythrocyte casts in the urine. In contrast, pre-eclampsia may be associated with elevated liver function tests. Features that may be useful in distinguishing between lupus flare (particularly nephritis) and pre-eclampsia are shown in Table 35.2. Pre-eclampsia rarely occurs before 20 weeks of gestation whereas lupus nephritis can present at any time. Renal biopsy may be useful but is rarely performed during pregnancy because of the theoretical increased risk of bleeding with the increased blood volume.

Overall, the rate of pre-eclampsia is 30% in patients with SLE. However, the rate is much higher (over 60%) in women with underlying renal disease [4]. Other conditions that increase the risk for developing pre-eclampsia include hypertension and antiphospholipid syndrome (APS; see below).

Severe lupus flare with central nervous system involvement

Rarely, patients may have central nervous system complications of SLE. These include headaches, seizures, stroke, chorea, peripheral neuropathy, psychosis, and mood disorders. It is crucial to exclude other potential causes (other than SLE flare) with assessment of

Table 35.2. Laboratory tests that may be used to distinguish pre-eclampsia from a lupus flare

Test	Pre-eclampsia	Lupus flare
Decreased complement levels	+	+++
Increased anti-double-stranded DNA	–	+++
Antithrombin III deficiency	++	+/–
Microangiopathic hemolytic anemia	++	–
Coombs-positive hemolytic anemia	–	++
Thrombocytopenia	++	++
Leukopenia	–	++
Urinary cellular casts/ hematuria	–	+++
Increased serum creatinine	+/–	++
Hypocalcuria	++	+/–
Increased liver transaminases	++	+/–
Elevated uric acid levels	++	–

infection, intracranial lesions such as tumor or bleeding, and metabolic abnormalities. In fact, it is typically a diagnosis of exclusion. The most common cause seems to be diffuse cerebritis caused by autoantibodies. Symptoms and signs are either diffuse or, if focal, shifting in location and not explained by other organic causes. Central nervous system SLE most commonly occurs during the first 2 years after the onset of SLE. Helpful studies may include spinal tap, brain imaging, and electroencephalography. Treatment is similar to other types of lupus flare. It is important to be cognizant of the risk for thrombotic stroke in women with anti-phospholipid antibodies.

Medical therapy during pregnancy

Fortunately, many medical therapies for SLE are safe to use during pregnancy. Ideally, women should appropriately modify their medical regimens prior to conception. Issues regarding these drugs are summarized in Table 35.3.

Obstetric management

Although of unproven efficacy, intensive fetal surveillance may reduce the risk of adverse fetal outcomes in pregnancies complicated by SLE (see Chapter 13 for details regarding fetal surveillance). Ideally, patients

Table 35.3. Medications used for the treatment of systemic lupus erythematosus in pregnancy

Drug/class of drug	FDA pregnancy class	Safety in pregnancy
NSAIDs	B (D in third trimester)	Avoid for periods longer than 48 hours for tocolysis; may cause fetal renal damage, closure of the ductus arteriosus, pulmonary hypertension, necotizing enterocolitis
Aspirin	D (high dose)	Avoid high-dose aspirin (>100 mg/day); higher risk in the third trimester; similar risks as NSAIDs, bleeding
Corticosteroids	B	Non-fluorinated corticosteroids are safe (e.g. prednisone, prednisilone, hydrocortisone); avoid fluorinated steroids such as dexamethasone and betamethasone unless the intent is to treat the fetus; dosing should be minimized because of maternal and obstetric effects
Hydroxychloroquine	C	Increasing experience in pregnancy with no adverse fetal effects reported; abrupt cessation in pregnancy is associated with flares
Cyclosporine	C	Increasing experience in pregnancy with no adverse fetal effects reported; long-term follow-up is limited
Azathioprine	D	Increasing experience in pregnancy with no adverse fetal effects reported with daily doses 2 mg/kg
Cyclophosphamide	D	Avoid if possible, teratogenic
Mycophenolate mofetil	D	Avoid if possible, tertatogenic; associated with facial cleft and face and ear abnormalities
Methotrexate	X	Contraindicated

NSAIDs, non-steroidal anti-inflammatory drugs.

Box 35.2. Management protocol for patients with systemic lupus erythematosus

Priorities
- Avoid medications that are harmful to the fetus
- Prompt detection of pre-eclampsia and uteroplacental insufficiency
- Discern between lupus exacerbations and pre-eclampsia
- Appropriate detection and treatment of lupus flares

Preconception counseling
- Discuss potential pregnancy complications including pre-eclampsia, preterm labor, miscarriage, fetal death, fetal growth restriction, and neonatal lupus
- Clinically evaluate lupus *activity*; delay pregnancy until remission of 6–12 months
- Evaluate patient for nephritis, hematological abnormalities, and anti phospholipid antibodies
- Discontinue non-steroidal anti-inflammatory drugs and cytotoxic agents

Antenatal care
- Frequent *visits* to assess systemic lupus erythematosus status and to screen for hypertension
- Serial ultrasounds to *evaluate* interval fetal growth
- Antenatal surveillance at 32 weeks or earlier if indicated

Treatment of mild to moderate exacerbations
- If the patient is taking glucocorticoids, increase the dose to at least 20–30 mg/day
- If the patient is not taking glucocorticoids, start 15–20 mg prednisone daily; alternatively, intravenous methylprednisolone (1000 mg daily) for 3 days may *avoid* the need for daily maintenance doses of steroids
- If the patient is not taking hydroxychloroquine, initiate 200 mg twice daily

Treatment of *severe* exacerbations without renal or CNS manifestations
- Rheumatology consultation and consider hospitalization
- Glucocorticoid treatment 1.0–1.5 mg/kg; expect clinical improvement in 5–10 days
- Taper the glucocorticoids once the patient demonstrates clinical improvement
- If the patient cannot be tapered off high doses of glucocorticoids, consider starting cyclosporine or azathioprine

Treatment of *severe* exacerbations with renal or CNS involvement
- Hospitalization and rheumatology consultation
- Initiate intravenous glucocorticoid treatment, 10–30 mg/kg methylprednisolone daily for 3–6 days
- Maintain patient on 1.0–1.5 mg/kg oral prednisone
- When the patient responds, taper the glucocorticoid
- For unresponsive patients, consider plasmapheresis

---

with SLE should be managed during pregnancy by both an obstetrician and a rheumatologist. Management of SLE pregnancies is summarized in Box 35.2.

Antiphospholipid syndrome

Antiphospholipid syndrome is characterized by thrombosis and pregnancy complications [5]. It is a syndrome and, like SLE, requires both clinical features and confirmatory laboratory studies for a diagnosis (Table 35.4). There is considerable overlap with SLE. It is estimated that 15–20% of women with SLE

have APS. Individuals with APS but no other autoimmune condition are considered to have primary APS. This includes more than half of the individuals with APS. Those with APS and SLE or another autoimmune or "rheumatic condition" are termed as having secondary APS.

Clinical features

Between 30 and 55% of patients with APS will have at least one thrombosis. The most common are venous thromboses, accounting for 70% of cases. Up to 50%

Table 35.4. Criteria for the classification of the antiphospholipid syndrome[a]

Criteria	Features
Clinical criteria	
Vascular thrombosis	One or more episodes of arterial, venous, or small vessel thrombosis in any tissue or organ confirmed by imaging, Doppler studies, or histopathology; superficial venous thromboses are excluded
Pregnancy morbidity	One or more unexplained deaths of a morphological normal fetus at or beyond the 10th week of gestation, with normal morphology documented by ultrasound or direct examination of the fetus *or* One or more premature births of a morphologically normal neonate prior to 34 weeks of gestation because of severe pre-eclampsia, eclampsia, or severe placental insufficiency *or* Three or more unexplained consecutive spontaneous miscarriages prior to the 10th week of gestation, with maternal anatomical or hormonal abnormalities, and paternal and maternal chromosome causes excluded
Laboratory criteria	
Lupus anticoagulant	Present in plasma on two or more occasions at least 12 weeks apart, detected according to the guidelines of the International Society on Thrombosis and Hemostasis
Anti-cardiolipin of IgG and/or IgM isotype	Present in blood in medium or high titer (>40 GPL, >40 MPL, or >99th percentile) on two or more occasions at least 12 weeks apart, measured by standardized ELISA
Anti-β2-glycoprotein-1 antibody of IgG and/or IgM isotype	Present in blood (titer >99th percentile) on two or more occasions at least 12 weeks apart, measured by standardized ELISA

ELISA, enzyme-linked immunosorbent assay; MPL and GPL, arbitrary units of IgM and IgG isotypes, respectively.
[a] Definite antiphospholipid syndrome is present if a patient meets at least one of the clinical criteria and one of the laboratory criteria.

of these are pulmonary embolisms. Patients with APS are more likely to have venous thromboses in unusual locations, such as the hepatic vein or mesentery. It is estimated that 2% of individuals with unexplained thrombosis will have APS. There is also an increased risk for arterial thrombosis. The most common are cerebrovascular accidents, but arterial thromboses may occur in coronary arteries or other uncommon locations. Approximately 4–5% of patients with unexplained arterial thrombosis will have anti-phospholipid antibodies.

Autoimmune thrombocytopenia also is common in women with APS. It is impossible to distinguish it from the thrombocytopenia associated with SLE alone or idiopathic thrombocytopenic purpura (ITP). Other medical disorders associated with anti-phospholipid antibodies include hemolytic anemia, livedo reticularis, chorea gravidarum, transverse myelitis, pyoderma-like leg ulcers, and aseptic heart valve vegetations.

The most frequent obstetric complication of APS is pregnancy loss. In patients with lupus anticoagulant (see below), the rate of pregnancy loss in untreated women is 90%. Up to half of all losses in women with APS occur in the second or third trimesters. Either fetal death occurring after 10 weeks of gestation

or recurrent early pregnancy loss (defined as three or more losses at before 10 weeks of gestation) are criteria for APS. It is critical that the losses be unexplained.

Pregnancies resulting in live births are often complicated by pre-eclampsia, small for gestational age fetus, abnormal fetal heart rate tracings, and preterm birth [6,7]. Pre-eclampsia affects 25–50% of APS pregnancies. It often is severe and occurs relatively early in gestation. These complications result in "medically indicated" preterm birth in one third of women with APS [6,7].

Laboratory features

Anti-phospholipid antibodies are a heterogeneous group of antibodies that bind to some combination of proteins and phospholipids. Although many anti-phospholipid antibodies have been described, there are three that are recommended for clinical use [8]. These include lupus anticoagulant, anti-cardiolipin antibodies, and anti-β2-glycoprotein antibodies. Each of these antibodies may be transiently elevated, particularly in the setting of infection. Therefore, positive results should be confirmed on two occasions at least 12 weeks apart.

Lupus anticoagulant is detected in plasma using phospholipid-dependent clotting assays. Lupus anticoagulant interferes with the assay, causing a prolonged clotting time. Since there are other causes of prolonged clotting assays, such as clotting factor deficiencies and specific inhibitors, the presence of lupus anticoagulant must be confirmed with additional testing.

Anti-cardiolipin and anti-β_2-glycoprotein-1 antibodies assays are standardized using standard sera and the results are reported in a semiquantitative fashion (low, medium, or high titers). Low-positive results are common in normal individuals and are not criteria for APS. Higher titers are uncommon in healthy people and are more strongly associated with the clinical features of the disease.

Catastrophic antiphospholipid syndrome

Rarely, unfortunate patients with APS will suffer microvascular thromboses (arterial and venous) in multiple organs, leading to severe illness and sometimes death [9]. This is in contrast to the usual large vessel thrombosis seen with typical APS, and the condition has been termed "catastrophic" APS. Organs typically affected include the lungs, kidneys, and gastrointestinal tract. Less commonly, adrenal glands, liver, brain, and heart also may be involved. The condition often occurs postpartum. A typical presentation is a patient presenting with severe dyspnea 1 or 2 days after delivery. They may have acute respiratory distress syndrome and pulmonary embolus and their kidneys are affected by microangiopathy and, sometimes, renal infarctions. Central nervous system involvement may include confusion, stupor, drowsiness, seizures, and infarctions. Abdominal pain may occur from thrombosis in mesenteric vessels. Common triggers include infection, trauma, surgery, and discontinuation of anticoagulation therapy. It also may present in patients without a history of prior thrombosis.

The differential diagnosis includes lupus nephritis, disseminated intravascular coagulation, and thrombocytopenic thrombotic purpura. Making a diagnosis can be tricky because titers of anti-cardiolipin antibodies may actually decrease at the time of thrombosis [10]. Nonetheless, over 95% of patients with catastrophic APS will have lupus anticoagulant, high titers of anti-cardiolipin antibodies, or both. They may have anti-dsDNA if they have SLE.

No treatment has been proven to be efficacious for catastrophic APS. Typical treatment includes full-dose anticoagulation and high-dose steroids, often in association with plasmapheresis and/or IVIG. Thrombolytics also may be considered in life-threatening situations. The patient should receive aggressive supportive care. It is important to appropriately utilize ventilatory support, dialysis, vasopressors, and antihypertensive therapy as appropriate.

Obstetric management

Obstetric complications of APS are, in part, thought to be caused by thrombosis and infarction in the uteroplacental circulation. In addition, there is increasing evidence that inflammation is important to the pathophysiology. The mainstay of medical treatment during pregnancy is unfractionated heparin or low-molecular-weight heparin and low-dose aspirin (75–100 mg/day). These drugs may improve uteroplacental blood flow, decrease inflammation and improve placental growth. The optimal dose of unfractionated heparin or low-molecular-weight heparin is uncertain and controversial. Women with prior thromboembolism should receive full anticoagulant dosing throughout pregnancy. Those without prior thrombosis may receive thromboprophylactic dosing during pregnancy and through 6 weeks postpartum (Box 35.3). Since pregnancy alters the pharmacokinetics of heparin metabolism, dosing is slightly increased compared with non-pregnant individuals. See Chapter 25 for details.

Other treatments remain experimental. Intravenous immunoglobulin reduces the severity of the autoimmune disease or inflammatory state, and successful pregnancies have been reported in women with APS refractory to heparins. However, IVIG is expensive and a small, randomized trial showed no benefit compared with heparin and aspirin alone [11]. Accordingly, it is not advised for first-line therapy. Hydroxychloroquine, specific complement inhibitors, and tumor necrosis-alpha inhibitors are being evaluated as potential therapies for APS but are of unproven efficacy. If possible, prednisone should be avoided in women taking heparins. Both prednisone and heparins cause osteopenia and the risk is compounded in patients taking both drugs.

Systemic sclerosis

Systemic sclerosis is a rare chronic multiorgan autoimmune disease characterized by widespread fibrosis

---

Box 35.3. Management protocol for patients with antiphospholipid syndrome

Goals of therapy
- Embryonic and fetal survival
- Prompt detection of uteroplacental insufficiency and pre-eclampsia
- Prevention of thrombosis

Preconception counseling
- Review pregnancy risks such as miscarriage, fetal death, pre-eclampsia, fetal growth restriction, uteroplacental insufficiency, and preterm birth
- Evaluate the accuracy of the diagnosis; confirm the presence of anti-phospholipid antibodies if necessary

Antenatal care
- When a live embryo is detected, start subcutaneous unfractionated heparin 10 000–20 000 U/day in divided doses or the equivalent dose of LMWH (prophylactic); higher doses (therapeutic) should be used in patients with prior thrombosis
- Calcium supplementation and weight-bearing exercise
- Frequent assessment for the development of pre-eclampsia
- Serial ultrasounds to evaluate interval fetal growth
- Fetal surveillance starting at 32 weeks, or earlier if complications arise
- If a patient has a history of a thromboembolic event or suffers an acute episode during pregnancy, start therapeutic doses of heparin to maintain the partial thromboplastin time at 1.5–2.5 times normal, or use LMWH (enoxaparin) 1 mg/kg twice a day
- If using LMWH, anti-factor Xa levels should be checked every trimester in order to maintain levels of 0.5–1.1 U/mL

LMWH, low-molecular-weight heparin.

---

and vasculopathy. It has the highest case-specific mortality of any of the autoimmune rheumatic diseases [12]. The major determinant of poor outcomes is the extent of the underlying visceral vasculopathy. Pregnancy should only be considered in patients with stable disease (3–5 years) and minimal vasculopathy. While pregnancy in and of itself does not appear to significantly affect disease activity, expectant mothers and their fetuses remain at risk for life-threatening complications, which frequently require intensive care.

Scleroderma renal crisis

Scleroderma renal crisis is responsible for most maternal deaths in pregnancies with systemic sclerosis [13]. Malignant hypertension, proteinuria, acute kidney injury, microangiopathic changes, and the pathognomonic "onion skin" appearance of the renal arteries on pathology are its typical features [14]. Early (within 5 years of disease) onset and diffuse disease are major risk factors for the development of this complication; as a consequence, women with these characteristics should be advised against pregnancy. High-dose corticosteroid therapy has also been associated with scleroderma renal crisis in a large, retrospective case–control study [15].

As scleroderma renal crisis shares many traits with pre-eclampsia – which has a higher incidence in patients with scleroderma – these two disorders may be difficult to differentiate. Worsening of renal function and the absence of proteinuria in the early stages support a diagnosis of renal crisis [16]. In addition, characteristic fibrosis on skin biopsy; pulmonary fibrosis; and elevated ANA, anti-centromere and anti-topoisomerase I (anti-SCL-70) suggest scleroderma. Whereas delivery of the fetus is therapeutic in pre-eclampsia, it has no effect on renal crisis of scleroderma. In difficult cases, renal biopsy may facilitate a clear diagnosis [17].

The mainstay of treatment is angiotensin-converting enzyme (ACE) inhibitors. These should be instituted without delay at the first suspicion of renal crisis as they are potentially life saving and organ preserving [18]. Use of ACE inhibitors is relatively contraindicated during pregnancy. However, in this circumstance, the benefits likely outweigh the risks and ACE inhibitors should not be withheld as successful pregnancies can occur in women taking ACE inhibitors and treatment may save the life of the mother [3].

Additional antihypertensive agents may be needed for optimal blood pressure control. Renal replacement therapy may be required, but ACE inhibitors must be continued as renal recovery and liberation from hemodialysis may occur up to 18 months following the episode [19]. Life-long ACE inhibitor use is usually required following an episode of renal crisis, and future pregnancies need to be judiciously planned. One study of long-term outcomes in a cohort of 145 patients with scleroderma renal crisis noted either death or the need for permanent dialysis in 39% [20]. Normotensive renal crisis can be encountered and should strongly be suspected in early diffuse scleroderma with unexplained rapidly deteriorating renal function and microangiopathic hemolytic anemia with thrombocytopenia. Although technically "normal," blood pressure may actually be higher than ideal for these select patients. Accordingly, they may also benefit from low-dose ACE inhibitors [19].

Pulmonary arterial hypertension

Pulmonary arterial hypertension is a common complication in women with systemic sclerosis. Morbidity and mortality in pregnant women remains excessively high, with reported death rates between 25 and 50%. Pregnancy should, therefore, be strongly discouraged or terminated if already present. Chapter 23 has details on the diagnosis and management of pulmonary hypertension in pregnancy.

Aspiration

Gastroesophageal reflux is an inherent part of systemic sclerosis and frequently worsens during pregnancy, thus increasing the risk of acute large volume aspiration. This can result in aspiration pneumonitis or pneumonia as well as the devastating acute respiratory distress syndrome [21]. Aggressive antacid treatment, avoiding meals at bedtime, wearing loose clothing, and elevating the head of the bed (not sitting up or propped up as this may increase the intra-abdominal pressure and aggravate the reflux) might minimize the danger.

Primary immune thrombocytopenia

Idiopathic thrombocytopenic purpura is an autoimmune disease characterized by immune-mediated destruction of platelets. It leads to thrombocytopenia and mucocutaneous bleeding. It affects about 1 per 1000 pregnancies and accounts for about 5% of cases of thrombocytopenia in pregnancy. Most cases are easily managed but sometimes serious maternal hemorrhage may occur.

The diagnosis of ITP is one of exclusion (see Clinical case 35.2). The complete blood count is typically normal other than thrombocytopenia (platelet count $<100 \times 10^9$/L) [22]. Peripheral smear may show an increased percentage of enlarged platelets and bone marrow biopsy (gold standard but not required for a diagnosis) may show increased immature megakaryocytes. Tests for anti-platelet antibodies are not diagnostic for, or useful, in most cases of ITP. It is very difficult to distinguish ITP from gestational thrombocytopenia. This is a common, mild thrombocytopenia (platelet count $>70 \times 10^9$/L) that is of no clinical consequence [23] and which accounts for over 70% of thrombocytopenia during pregnancy. If thrombocytopenia occurs outside of pregnancy, is severe ($<50 \times 10^9$/L), or is associated with bleeding it is likely ITP. Other causes of thrombocytopenia are HELLP syndrome (hemolysis, elevated liver enzymes, and low platelets), pre-eclampsia, drug-induced thrombocytopenia, or pseudo-thrombocytopenia; in addition, SLE; APS; infections with HIV, hepatitis C or hepatitis B virus; thrombotic thrombocytopenic purpura; hereditary thrombocytopenias; and disseminated intravascular coagulation also should be excluded.

> **Case 35.2. A woman in the third trimester with severe headache**
>
> A 22-year-old nulliparous woman presents at 32 weeks of gestation with a severe headache. She is noted to have an intracranial hemorrhage on CT scan. Her only other abnormalities are numerous petechiae and echymosis. She is noted to have a platelet count of 4×10^9/L and there is suspicion for pre-eclampsia. However, she has normal blood pressure, no proteinuria, and normal liver function tests. She has never had thrombocytopenia before. There is no evidence of infection, HIV serology is negative, and she has not received any medications. She has primary immune thrombocytopenia and should be treated with steroids and intravenous immunoglobulin.

Maternal treatment

The primary goal is the avoidance of serious bleeding. Treatment is recommended when (1) there is mucocutaneous bleeding, (2) the platelet count is $<10 \times 10^9$/L at any time during pregnancy, or (3) platelet count is $<30 \times 10^9$/L in the late second or third trimesters [24].

The first-line therapy for ITP during pregnancy is corticosteroids, typically prednisone. It is important to use a non-fluorinated corticosteroid (prednisone, prednisolone, methylprednisolone, or hydrocortisone) that has little activity after crossing the placenta. A typical daily dose is 1–1.5 mg/kg based on pre-pregnancy body weight. Another option is to use a "pulse dose" of 15.0 mg/kg daily (up to 1 g/day) for 3 days followed by a rapid taper. Improvement in the platelet count occurs in about 50–70% of women and should be apparent within 2–3 weeks. If the platelet count is acceptable, the dose can be slowly tapered by 10–20% per week until the lowest dose required to maintain an acceptable platelet count is reached. Using the minimal effective dose helps to minimize untoward side effects of high-dose steroids.

It is also common to use IVIG to treat pregnant women with ITP. It is quite safe but is inconvenient and expensive. Consequently, it is usually reserved for ITP that is refractory to steroids or in urgent circumstances (e.g. platelet count $<10 \times 10^9$/L during the third trimester). The optimal dose is uncertain but is usually 0.5–2.0 mg/kg per day for 2–5 days. Khellaf and colleagues [25] have developed a scoring system utilizing age and cutaneous, mucosal, gastrointestinal, urinary, gynecological, and central nervous system bleeding. A score ≥8 is predictive of a high risk of bleeding and considered an indication for the use of IVIG.

Intravenous rhesus-D immunoglobulin also has been successful in treating ITP, at a dose of 75 mg/kg [24]. Although there are theoretical concerns about causing fetal hemolysis, this has not occurred, perhaps because the antibody binds to maternal blood cells prior to reaching the fetal circulation. Use is restricted to RhD-positive women. Other cytotoxic agents such as cyclophosphamide, danazol, alkaloids, and cochicine should be avoided because of adverse fetal effects. There are increasing data regarding the safety of azathioprine during pregnancy and this drug may be considered for refractory cases.

Platelet transfusions are not very effective because of their rapid destruction. However, it is an excellent temporizing measure in someone who is bleeding or requires surgery. A transfusion of one unit of apheresed platelets is usually adequate, although the rise in platelet count is usually less than the 40 000 cells/unit noted in patients without ITP. Splenectomy can be safely accomplished during pregnancy, particularly in the second trimester. Nonetheless, it is usually avoided because of an increased risk for bleeding and other complications during pregnancy.

Myasthenia gravis

Characterized by fluctuating muscular weakness and fatigue, myasthenia gravis is a consequence of autoantibodies directed at the acetylcholine receptor. This leads to impaired neuromuscular transmission. Reflex, sensory, and coordination abilities are spared. The weakness improves with rest or injection of the short-acting acetylcholinesterase inhibitor edrophonium (tensilon confirmatory test). The presence of autoantibodies against the acetylcholine receptor in up to 85% of patients (seropositive) confirms clinical suspicion. In seronegative patients, electrophysiological testing may show progressive decreases in the muscle action potential following repetitive nerve stimulation [26]. Other less common antibodies such as the anti-muscle-specific tyrosine kinase may aid in the diagnosis of patients without acetylcholine receptor antibodies [27]. Thymomas can be found in 10% of patients and other autoimmune diseases often coexist. The course of the disease during pregnancy is variable and unaffected by the pregestational clinical state. Remission, exacerbation, disease stability, or life-threatening myasthenic crisis are all possibilities. As in systemic sclerosis, the risk of a complication is highest the first few years following disease onset and lowest 7 years or more after diagnosis [28]. Pregnancy should, therefore, be postponed following the diagnosis and as with other autoimmune diseases, women with myasthenia gravis desiring children should ideally be counseled prior to planning a pregnancy.

Treatment rests on either increasing the availability of acetylcholine at the neuromuscular junction via long-acting acetylcholinesterase inhibitors such as pyridostigmine for mild to moderate disease or immunosuppression with corticosteroids, azathioprine, and cyclosporine for more advanced disease. Pyridostigmine at the approved dose of less than 600 mg/day is considered safe during pregnancy. Thymectomy if indicated should be performed prior to or after pregnancy because of the surgical risk and its delayed results [26].

Myasthenic crisis

A potentially deadly complication of myasthenic crisis is acute respiratory failure requiring mechanical support, and this may occur in almost one quarter of patients with myasthenia gravis [29]. It can be a consequence of diaphragmatic, accessory respiratory muscle, oropharyngeal, or vocal cord weakness, but it can also arise from an inability to clear secretions [30].

Recognition of impending respiratory failure is critical in order to initiate ventilator assistance electively rather than as an emergency. Although effort dependent, indicators of respiratory muscle insufficiency include a vital capacity 20 mL/kg, a maximal inspiratory pressure 30 cmH$_2$O, and a maximal expiratory pressure 40 cmH$_2$O – the so-called 20/30/40 rule (typically performed in the pulmonary function laboratory). A reduction by 30% of these measurements from their baseline is also worrisome. Hypoxia, hypercarbia, and paradoxical breathing are ominous signs. Intubation by an experienced provider is preferred as non-invasive positive pressure ventilation with bilevel positive airway pressure carries an increased risk of aspiration in the pregnant patient owing to impaired gastric emptying. Once stabilized, infection, which is a common trigger, should be aggressively sought and treated. Other potential triggers include surgery, emotional stress, general anesthesia, certain medications, and pregnancy itself.

The cornerstone of treatment of myasthenic crisis is to remove circulating antibodies via plasma exchange or to inactivate these antibodies with IVIG, which are both considered to be safe in pregnancy. While there is a lack of clear evidence of superiority, plasmapheresis is favored over IVIG because of a faster response. It is not readily available at all centers and is more expensive than IVIG. Other potential complications of plasmapheresis include hypotension, infection, thrombosis (catheter related), and coagulopathy. Use of IVIG is contraindicated in IgA deficiency and it has been associated with renal failure, anaphylactic reactions, and aseptic meningitis. Hyperviscosity and volume overload should be taken into consideration when contemplating use of IVIG.

Cesarean delivery should be reserved for the usual obstetric indications, and epidural, spinal, or combined spinal–epidural anesthesia is recommended in order to minimize the administration of systemic analgesics. These have the potential of depressing respiration in a patient already susceptible to hypoventilation. Epidural anesthesia is also helpful in reducing fatigability and normalizing breathing. Given its reliance on striated muscle, the second stage of labor may be affected and obstetricians should be prepared for forceps or vacuum extraction. The pushing phase may be supported with intravenous or intramuscular neostigmine, the anticholinesterase inhibitor of choice during labor and delivery [31]. Women with myasthenia gravis are not at increased risk of developing pre-eclampsia. However,

should it occur, magnesium sulfate is relatively contraindicated in myasthenia gravis. Phenytoin has been used for eclampsia prophylaxis in such cases, although efficacy is unproven and phenytoin also may exacerbate myasthenia gravis. Numerous other drugs may worsen myasthenia gravis and should be avoided when possible.

Rheumatoid arthritis

Rheumatoid arthritis is a systemic autoimmune disease marked by chronic joint inflammation. It can be difficult to diagnose; a symmetrical pattern of articular involvement and a positive rheumatoid factor suggest the disorder. Approximately 75% of women will experience a meaningful remission during pregnancy. Conversely, a disease flare within 9 months of delivery is extremely common [32]. Rarely, maternal disability from the disease may inhibit vaginal delivery and/or make caring for the infant difficult. However, fetal outcomes in pregnancies to women with rheumatoid arthritis are excellent and similar to the general population. The primary management is medical therapy. The reader is referred to a recent review for details [33].

Failed intubation in rheumatoid arthritis

Endotracheal intubation can be difficult in women with rheumatoid arthritis. It is already difficult in pregnancy. Indeed, pregnant women are 10-fold more likely to have a failed intubation than non-pregnant individuals [34]. Patients with rheumatoid arthritis often have cervical spine instability, particularly in the atlantoaxial area. This makes intubation even harder, striking fear into the informed intensivist or anesthesiologist. The traditional "sniffing position" during intubation can have disastrous consequences. A careful and thorough assessment of the airway as well as guidance with fiberoptic devices or videolaryngoscopes in the hands of the most qualified person may optimize the chances of a successful intubation.

Adrenal crisis

Adrenal crisis (acute adrenocortical insufficiency or Addisonian crisis) may occur during pregnancy. Typically, this results from physiological stress (e.g. urinary tract infection or labor) in someone with chronic adrenal insufficiency from chronic glucocorticoid use (as is often the case with autoimmune diseases) or pituitary neoplasm. However, primary adrenal insufficiency also may occur. This can be precipitated by acute adrenal hemorrhage from obstetric bleeding in association with postpartum hemorrhage, disseminated intravascular coagulation, placental abruption, and so on. Symptoms often include nausea, vomiting, weakness, lightheadedness, and abdominal pain. The patient is usually in shock and may have hyponatremia, hyperkalemia, hypoglycemia, seizures, and increased pigmentation.

Diagnosis can be difficult in pregnancy because cortisol and adrenocorticotropic hormone responses to corticotropin-releasing hormone are blunted in pregnancy. Also, cortisol levels are lower in normal pregnancy than in non-pregnant women and the placenta produces adrenocorticotropic hormone. Therefore, the corticotropin-releasing hormone stimulation test is unreliable in pregnancy. Early morning cortisol levels of ≤3.0 mg/dL confirm the diagnosis, while levels >19 mg/dL exclude the diagnosis in the first half of pregnancy. Assessment for anti-adrenal antibodies may facilitate the diagnosis.

It is appropriate to treat critically ill patients empirically with steroids and supportive care. Treatment is initiated with 75–100 mg intravenous hydrocortisone, followed by the same dose every 6–8 hours [35]. Aggressive hydration and glucose replacement with a 50 g glucose infusion also is advised. In patients with long-standing Addison disease, mineralocorticosteroid requirements are usually stable in pregnancy.

References

1. Tan EM, Cohen AS, Fries JF, et al. The 1982 revised criteria for the classification of systemic lupus erythematosus. *Arthritis Rheum* 1982;**25**:1271–1277.

2. Burkett G. Lupus nephropathy and pregnancy. *Clin Obstet Gynecol* 1985;**28**:310–323.

3. Imbasciati E, Tincani A, Gregorini G, et al. Pregnancy in women with pre-existing lupus nephritis: predictors of fetal and maternal outcome. *Nephrol Dial Transplant* 2009;**24**:519–525.

4. Lockshin MD, Reinitz E, Druzin ML, et al. Lupus pregnancy. Case–control prospective study demonstrating absence of lupus exacerbation during or after pregnancy. *Am J Med* 1984;**77**:893–898.

5. Miyakis S, Lockshin M D, Atsumi D, et al. International consensus statement on an update of the classification criteria for definite antiphospholipid syndrome (APS). *Thromb Haemost* 2006;**4**:295–306.

6. Branch DW, Silver RM, Blackwell JL, et al. Outcome of treated pregnancies in women with antiphospholipid syndrome: an update of the Utah experience. *Obstet Gynecol* 1992;**80**:614–620.

7. Lima F, Khamashta MA, Buchanan NM, et al. A study of sixty pregnancies in patients with the antiphospholipid syndrome. *Clin Exp Rheumatol.* 1996;**14**:131–136.

8. Branch DW, Khamashta MA. Antiphospholipid syndrome: obstetric diagnosis, management, and controversies. *Obstet Gynecol* 2003;**101**:1333–1344.

9. Asherson RA, Cervera R, Piette JC, et al. Catastrophic antiphospholipid syndrome. Clinical and laboratory features of 50 patients. *Medicine* 1998;**77**:195–207.

10. Drenkard C, Sanchez-Guerrero J, Alarcon-Segovia D. Fall in antiphospholipid antibody at time of thromboocclusive episodes in systemic lupus erythematosus. *Rheumatology* 1989;**16**:614–617.

11. Branch DW, Peaceman AM, Druzin M, et al. A multicenter, placebo-controlled pilot study of intravenous immune globulin treatment of antiphospholipid syndrome during pregnancy. The Pregnancy Loss Study Group. *Am J Obstet Gynecol* 2000;**182**:122–127.

12. Khanna D, Denton CP. Evidence-based management of rapidly progressing systemic sclerosis. *Best Pract Res Clin Rheumatol.* 2010;**24**:387–400.

13. Steen VD. Pregnancy in scleroderma. *Rheum Dis Clin North Am* 2007;**33**:345–358, vii.

14. Chakravarty EF. Vascular complications of systemic sclerosis during pregnancy. *Int J Rheumatol.* 2010;**201**: doi:10.1155/2010/287248.

15. Steen VD, Medsger TA Jr. Case–control study of corticosteroids and other drugs that either precipitate or protect from the development of scleroderma renal crisis. *Arthritis Rheum* 1998;**41**:1613–1619.

16. Gayed M, Gordon C. Pregnancy and rheumatic diseases. *Rheumatology* 2007;**46**:1634–1640.

17. Mok CC, Kwan TH, Chow L. Scleroderma renal crisis during pregnancy. *Scand J Rheumatol* 2003;**32**:55–57.

18. Steen VD, Costantino JP, Shapiro AP, et al. Outcome of renal crisis in systemic sclerosis: relation to availability of angiotensin converting enzyme (ACE) inhibitors. *Ann Int Med* 1990;**113**:352–357.

19. Steen VD. Scleroderma renal crisis. *Rheum Dis Clin N Am* 2003;**29**:315–333.

20. Steen VD, Medsger TA. Long-term outcomes of scleroderma renal crisis. *Ann Int Med* 2000;**133**:600–603.

21. Cossio M, Menon Y, Wilson W, et al. Life threatening complications of systemic sclerosis. *Crit Care Clin* 2002;**18**:819–839.

22. George JN, Woolf SH, Raskob GE, et al. Idiopathic thrombocytopenic purpura: a practice guideline

developed by explicit methods for the American Society of Hematology. *Blood* 1996;**88**:3–40.

23. Burrows RF, Kelton JG. Thrombocytopenia at delivery: a prospective survey of 6715 deliveries. *Am J Obstet Gynecol* 1990;**162**:731–734.

24. Provan D, Stasi R, Newland AC, *et al.* International consensus report on the investigation and management of primary immune thrombocytopenia. *Blood.* 2010;**115**:168–186.

25. Khellaf M, Michel M, Schaeffer A, *et al.* Assessment of a therapeutic strategy for adults with severe autoimmune thrombocytopenic purpura based on a bleeding score rather than a platelet count. *Haematologica* 2005;**90**:829–832.

26. Ciafaloni E, Massey JM. Myasthenia gravis and pregnancy. *Neurol Clin* 2004;**22**:771–782.

27. Meriggioli MN, Sanders DB. Autoimmune myasthenia gravis: emerging clinical and biological heterogeneity. *Lancet Neurol* 2009;**8**:475–490.

28. Kalidindi M, Ganpot S, Tahmesebi F, *et al.* Myasthenia gravis and pregnancy. *J Obstet Gynaecol* 2007;**27**:30–32.

29. Murthy JM, Meena AK, Chowdary GV, *et al.* Myasthenic crisis: clinical features, complications and mortality. *Neurol India* 2005;**53**:37–40.

30. Lacomis D. Myasthenic crisis. *Neurocritical Care* 2005;**03**:189–194.

31. Stafford I, Dildy G. Myasthenia gravis and pregnancy. *Clin Obstet Gynecol* 2005;**48**:48–56.

32. Keeling S, Oswald A. Pregnancy and rheumatic disease: "by the book" or "by the doc." *Clin Rheumatol.* 2009;**28**:1–9.

33. Partlett R, Roussou E. The treatment of rheumatoid arthritis during pregnancy. *Rheumatol Int* 2011;**31**:445–449.

34. Hawthorne L, Wilson R, Lyons G, *et al.* Failed intubation revisited:17-yr experience in a teaching maternity unit. *Br J Anaesth* 1996;**76**:680–684.

35. Ambrosi B, Barbetta L, Morricone L. Diagnosis and management of Addison's disease during pregnancy. *J Endocrinol Invest* 2003;**26**:698–702.

Chapter

36

Pre-eclampsia

Leiv Arne Rosseland, Helen Ryan,
Laura A. Magee, and Peter von Dadelszen

Introduction

Pre-eclampsia (proteinuric gestational hypertension) accounts for approximately half of admissions for critical care on the basis of a direct obstetric cause [1,2]. The number of delivery hospitalizations resulting from pregnancy hypertension is increasing in the USA [3], and morbidity, complications, and death attributed to substandard care are documented [4]. The optimal treatment of patients with pre-eclampsia and with which level of care these patients are best helped is under debate [5].

Epidemiology

Pre-eclampsia complicates 2–8% of pregnancies [6], and the reported incidence of eclampsia varies between 2.7 to 8.2 per 10 000 births [6]. The incidence of the pre-eclampsia related syndrome of hemolysis, elevated liver enzymes, and low platelets (HELLP) is difficult to estimate because of the lack of internationally accepted diagnostic criteria.

Pathogenesis and consequences of pre-eclampsia

Figure 36.1 shows the pathogenesis of pre-eclampsia.

Risk factors

Risk factors for pre-eclampsia represent a bewildering array of causative antecedents that reflect the complexity of the maternal syndrome. They can be loosely categorized into broad groups: familial/genetic factors, primipaternity and sperm exposure, pre-existing medical conditions, smoking, and miscellaneous factors [6].

Etiology

Pre-eclampsia is a multifactorial disorder that begins with inadequate placental function and, consequently, a mismatch of fetal demands compared with placental blood supply [7]. Why it occurs early in the minority of pregnancies affected by mismatch, and close to term in most affected pregnancies, remains uncertain. Maternal factors predisposing to a pro-inflammatory state, such as obesity, chronic infection, and autoimmune disease, probably contribute to early-onset or severe pre-eclampsia [8]. Whether the shedding of placental proteins and vasoactive and inflammatory mediators is the consequence of chronic placental ischemia, ischemia–reperfusion injury, oxidative stress, or a combination of all of these factors is not clear; however, the ultimate result is diffuse endothelial dysfunction with consequent maternal end-organ damage similar to that in the systemic inflammatory response syndrome [7]. The endothelial dysfunction and associated increased vascular reactivity precede the onset of symptomatic clinical disease and the loss of endothelial integrity that contributes to derangements of sodium–volume homoeostasis and reversal of many of the cardiovascular changes (e.g. increased cardiac output and intravascular volume) that accompany normal pregnancy. As a result, pre-eclampsia is a low-output, high-resistance state [7]. Eclampsia, convulsions during pregnancy or after delivery, is a common cause of maternal death and severe morbidity [9].

The HELLP syndrome is most commonly regarded as related to severe pre-eclampsia. As the etiology remains unknown, there is still a debate as to whether or not HELLP syndrome represents a separate disease entity. It is described as a placenta-induced disease but with a more acute and predominant inflammatory process targeting the liver and with a major activation of the coagulation system.

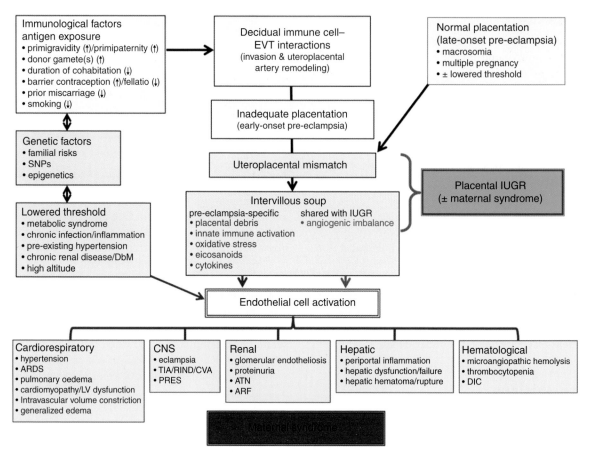

Figure 36.1. The origins and consequences of pre-eclampsia. In this model of pre-eclampsia, the maternal syndrome develops from a number of pathways, leading to uteroplacental mismatch, in which the fetoplacental demands outstrip the maternal circulatory supply. In response to the mismatch, and probably caused, in part, by recurrent ischemia–reperfusion injury within the intervillous (maternal blood) space of the placenta and accelerated placental apoptosis and aponecrosis, a soup of endothelium-damaging substrates is released, with resulting endothelial cell activation and consequent development of the maternal syndrome of pre-eclampsia. Some elements of the soup – activated peripheral blood leukocytes – can cause direct end-organ damage. ARDS, acute respiratory distress syndrome; ARF, acute renal failure; ATN, acute tubular necrosis; CVA, cerebrovascular accident; DbM, diabetes mellitus; DIC, disseminated intravascular coagulation; EVT, extravillous cytotrophoblast; IUGR, intrauterine growth restriction; LV, left ventricle; PRES, posterior reversible encephalopathy syndrome; RIND, reversible ischemic neurological deficit; SNP, single nucleotide polymorphism; TIA, transient ischemic attack.

Normal pregnancy leads to a reduction in vascular systemic resistance and a mid-trimester fall in blood pressure [10]. Physiologically reduced angiotensin II responsiveness in parallel with increased production of vasodilatory prostaglandins and nitrous oxide are probably central mechanisms. Consequently, the autonomic nervous system is of increased importance in pregnancy for the homeostatic regulation of blood pressure. The situation is quite different in pre-eclampsia, and the reduced importance of sympathetic basal activity is clearly demonstrated by the increased tolerance of neuraxial sympathetic blockade [11,12]. A lack of the mid-trimester fall in blood pressure has been observed in patient populations developing pre-eclampsia [13]. Observational studies of women with pre-eclampsia have shown that variance in hemodynamic measures is large, and this may complicate scientific analyses of antihypertensive drugs and intravenous volume therapy. A better understanding of the enhanced vascular reactivity [14] combined with clinical studies [12,15,16] have changed the management before and after delivery in women with pre-eclampsia. Implementation of less invasive hemodynamic monitoring devices has increased the possibility of individualized treatment guided by more precise estimates of preload, afterload, cardiac output, and invasively measured arterial pressures. The level of evidence for this physiological approach in order to prevent organ failure is low and more clinical research data are required.

Diagnosis

Pre-eclampsia is generally defined as new hypertension (diastolic blood pressure ≥90 mmHg) and substantial proteinuria (≥300 mg in 24 hours) at or after 20 weeks of gestation [7]. However, how best to define the maternal syndrome of pre-eclampsia, and how to differentiate mild from severe disease, is an area of active research [17].

A comparison of current international classification systems for the hypertensive disorders of pregnancy is presented in Table 36.1 [18].

Although perinatal risks in pre-eclampsia have long been recognized to be highest remote from term, the 20-fold increase in maternal mortality that is associated with pre-eclampsia arising earlier than 32 weeks of gestation (compared with that at 37 weeks or later) [19] seems not to have been as noted, emphasizing the importance of early-onset pre-eclampsia as a severity criterion.

The debate between setting the systolic blood pressure definition of severe hypertension at either 160 mmHg or 170 mmHg needs to be resolved

Table 36.1. Classification of hypertensive disorders of pregnancy

	NICE (2010)	SOMANZ (2008)	SOGC (2008)	ASH (2008)
Pre-existing or chronic hypertension (BP ≥140/90 mmHg before 20⁺⁰ weeks of gestation)	Chronic hypertension: before 20 weeks of gestation or being treated at time of referral for primary or secondary etiology	Chronic hypertension: essential secondary white coat ± superimposed pre-eclampsia	Pre-existing hypertension: ± comorbid conditions ± superimposed pre-eclampsia	Chronic hypertension: ± superimposed pre-eclampsia
Gestational hypertension (BP ≥ 140/90 mmHg after 19⁺⁶ weeks of gestation)	Gestational hypertension: without significant proteinuria	Gestational hypertension: without significant proteinuria returning to normal within 12 weeks postpartum	Gestational hypertension: ± comorbid conditions ± superimposed pre-eclampsia	Gestational hypertension or transient hypertension: BP returning to normal within 6 weeks of birth Late postpartum hypertension: BP rise developing up to 6 months postpartum and normalized by 1 year postpartum
Pre-eclampsia (clinical definition)	New hypertension (BP ≥140/90 mmHg) presenting after 20 weeks of gestation with clinically relevant proteinuria (see significant proteinuria, below)	Gestational hypertension + one or more of the following: proteinuria (dipstick then confirmed by either random spot protein–creatinine ratio >30 mg/mmol or 0.3 g/24 h); serum/plasma creatinine >90 μmol/L); oliguria; hematological involvement (thrombocytopenia, hemolysis, disseminated intravascular coagulation); liver involvement (raised serum transaminases, severe epigastric or right upper quadrant pain); neurological involvement (convulsions, hyper-reflexia with sustained clonus, severe headache, persistent visual disiurbances, stroke); pulmonary edema; fetal growth restriction; placental abruption	Pre-existing hypertension and resistant hypertension, new proteinuria, or adverse condition (see severity criteria, below) Gestational hypertension plus proteinuria (spot protein–creatinine ratio >30 mg/mmol l or 0.3 g/24 h) or adverse condition	Gestational hypertension or Chronic hypertension with proteinuria (dipstick ≥ +1, spot protein–creatinine ratio ≥30 mg/mmol, or ≥0.3 g/24 h)

Table 36.1. (*cont.*)

	NICE (2010)	SOMANZ (2008)	SOGC (2008)	ASH (2008)
Pre-eclampsia (research definition)	Not defined	De novo hypertension ≥2 weeks, returning to normal postpartum, with properly documented proteinuria	Not defined	Not defined
Severe hypertension (mmHg)	160/110	170/110	160/110	160/110
Significant proteinuria	>300 mg/day or spot protein–creatinine ratio >30 mg/mmol	Not defined	> 300 mg/day or spot protein–creatinine ratio >30 mg/mmol	>300 mg/day or spot protein–creatinine ratio >30 mg/mmol
Severity criteria	Severe hypertension: maternal symptoms (vision problems, severe headache, epigastric pain, vomiting, papiledema); biochemical abnormalities or hematological impairment (platelet count 100×10^9/L or AST/ALT >70 U/L, elevated serum creatinine)	Not defined	Gestational age at onset 34^{+0} weeks, heavy proteinuria Maternal symptoms: persistent, new or unusual headache; visual disturbances; persistent abdominal or right upper quadrant pain; severe nausea or vomiting; chest pain or dyspnea Maternal signs of end-organ dysfunction: eclampsia, severe hypertension, pulmonary edema, or suspected placental abruption Abnormal maternal laboratory tests: elevated serum creatinine, elevated AST, ALT or LDH with symptoms, platelet count 100×10^9/L or serum albumin 20 g/L Fetal morbidity: oligohydramnios, intrauterine growth restriction, absent or reversed end-diastolic flow in the umbilical artery by Doppler velocimetry, intrauterine fetal death	Gestational age 35 weeks Maternal symptoms: headache, visual disturbances, abdominal pain, severe diastolic hypertension (>110 mmHg) Abnormal maternal laboratory tests: significant proteinuria or oliguria, increased serum creatinine, decreased glomerular filtration rate, increased AST or LDH Fetal morbidity: non-reassuring cardiotogography

ALT, alanine transaminase; ASH, American Society of Hypertension; AST, aspartate transaminase; BP, blood pressure; LDH, lactate dehydrogenase; NICE, UK National Institute for Health and Clinical Excellence; SOMANZ, Society of Obstetric Medicine of Australia and New Zealand; SOGC, Society of Obstetricians and Gynecologists of Canada.
Source: adapted from Payne *et al.*, 2011 [18].

because of rising concerns about lethal maternal stroke risks at the lower threshold for blood pressure [4,7]. None of the classification systems seems to have been independently assessed for the ability to identify women and fetuses at heightened risk of the adverse events that make pre-eclampsia so important.

Differential diagnosis of severe pre-eclampsia

Table 36.2 [7] summarizes the differential diagnosis for women presenting with severe pre-eclampsia.

The HELLP syndrome is defined in varying ways in the literature, and each clinician should refer to local

Table 36.2. Differential diagnosis of severe pre-eclampsia

Organ system	Diagnoses
Vasculature	Pheochromocytoma Hyperaldosteronism Cushing disease Thyrotoxicosis Coarctation of the aorta
Renal system	Lupus nephritis Acute and chronic glomerulonephritis Interstitial nephritis Pyelonephritis
Liver and pancreas	Acute fatty liver of pregnancy Pregnancy cholestasis Hyperemesis gravidarum Cholecystitis, cholangitis Viral hepatitis Acute pancreatitis Gastritis, gastric ulcer

Hemostasis	Benign thrombocytopenia of
	    pregnancy
	Thrombotic thrombocytopenic
	    purpura
	Hemolytic–uremic syndrome
	Idiopathic thrombocytopenic
	    purpura
	Antiphospholipid syndrome
	Folate deficiency
	Systemic lupus erythematosus
	Septic or hemorrhagic shock

Respiratory system	Pneumonia Pulmonary embolus (Catastrophic) antiphospholipid syndrome
Cardiovascular system	Peripartum cardiomyopathy Myocardial ischemia or infarction
Brain	Cerebral systemic lupus erythematosus Epilepsy Brain tumor Cerebrovascular accident Hypertensive encephalopathy Metabolic disease
Eyes	Retinal arterial or venous thrombosis Retinal ischemia Retinal detachment Persistent spasm of retinal vessels Central serous retinopathy Uveal melanoma Choroidal osteoma

Source: Steegers *et al.,* 2010 [7].

definitions. Hemolysis can be documented in peripheral blood smear, which typically shows schiztocytes, or by elevated plasma lactate dehydrogenase, low haptoglobin, and increased bilirubin concentration. Elevated liver enzymes (aspartate or alanine aminotransferase) and low platelets ($<100 \times 10^9$/L) should be present; if not

all these laboratory values are abnormal, it will often be described as a partial HELLP syndrome.

Differential diagnoses of HELLP syndrome are listed in Table 36.3 [20].

Clinical features

Pre-eclampsia may be asymptomatic and apart from being diagnosed as having hypertension and proteinuria patients may have few complaints. Symptoms such as headache, nausea, epigastric pain, visual disturbance, restlessness, and irritability indicate increased severity, HELLP syndrome, or imminent eclampsia. In a Scandinavian cohort, 89% had at least one physical complaint before the first eclamptic seizure, severe headache being the most common [9].

Severity assessment and prognostics

Maternal mortality rates in critically ill obstetric patients is reported to be <5%, but the variance is great [21]. Scoring systems routinely used in intensive care units (ICUs) have documented positive predictive value in mortality risk assessment in the general ICU population. The Acute Physiological and Chronic Health Evaluation (APACHE) scoring system, the Simplified Acute Physiological Score (SAPS), and the Mortality Prediction Model all performed well in the prediction of obstetric patients' ICU outcome compared with non-obstetric female age-matched ICU patients [22]. None of the existing models to predict critical care outcomes appears to have utility in predicting ICU-related maternal mortality. For example, the APACHE score can overestimate maternal mortality by up to 12-fold [23–28]. For APACHE-II, the observed/estimated mortality rate of obstetric ICU patients ranges from 0.08 to 0.93; for APACHE-III, mortality rate is 0.43. In studies of the Simplified Acute Physiological Score version II, the rate varies from 0.43 to 1.40 [22,29]. Therefore, novel critical care clinical prediction tools to ascribe maternal risks are required because of the unique physiology of the pregnant/postpartum state. For example, maternal cardiac output increases by 30–50% in pregnancy, with further increases up to 50% during labor and 80% in the immediate postpartum period.

In response to the understanding of the origins and end-organ consequences of pre-eclampsia (Figure 36.1), von Dadelszen *et al.* [17] undertook the Pre-eclampsia Integrated Estimate of RiSk (PIERS) study. They developed and internally validated the

Table 36.3. Differential diagnoses of HELLP syndrome: frequency of signs, symptoms, and laboratory findings

	Thrombotic thrombocytopenic purpura	Hhemolytic–uremic syndrome	HELLP syndrome
Abdominal pain	++	++	++
ADAMST13 activity	+/++	–	–
Anemia	++	++	+
Elevated lactic dehydrogenase	++ very high values	++ very high values	++
Elevated transaminases	–/+	–/+	++
Fever	+	–	–
Headache or visual disturbance	++	-	++
Hypertension	+/++	++	++
Jaundice	–	–	+
Nausea and vomiting	++	++	++
Proteinuria	+ and hematuria	++	++
Thrombocytopenia	++	++	++
von Willebrand factor	++	++	–

HELLP, hemolysis, elevated liver function tests, low platelets; + indicates prevalence of finding in affected patients.
Source: adapted from Stella *et al.*, 2009 [20].

fullPIERS model in a prospective, multicenter study in women who were admitted to tertiary obstetric centers with pre-eclampsia or who developed pre-eclampsia after admission. The outcome of interest was maternal mortality or other serious complications of pre-eclampsia. Routinely reported and informative variables were included in a stepwise backward elimination regression model to predict the adverse maternal outcome. The model performance was assessed using the area under the curve (AUC) of the receiver operating characteristic and stratification capacity. They observed that 261 of 2023 women with pre-eclampsia had adverse outcomes at any time after hospital admission (106 (5%) within 48 hours of admission). Predictors of adverse maternal outcome included gestational age, chest pain or dyspnea, oxygen saturation, platelet count, and serum creatinine and aspartate aminotransferase concentrations. The fullPIERS model predicted adverse maternal outcomes within 48 hours of study eligibility (AUC, 0.88; 95% confidence interval (CI), 0.84–0.92). Moreover, the fullPIERS model performed well (AUC, >0.7) up to 7 days after eligibility, and accurate risk stratification was achieved. However, external validation of the model has not been performed. Once externally validated, the fullPIERS model should identify women at increased risk of adverse outcomes up to 7 days before complications arise and thereby modify direct patient care (e.g. timing of delivery, place of care), improve the design of clinical trials, and inform biomedical investigations related to pre-eclampsia.

The modified early obstetric warning system has been validated in an obstetric population, including patients with pre-eclampsia [30]. The aim of this system is early recognition and treatment of acute morbidity based on systematic observations of maternal physiological variables. Singh *et al.* reported a sensitivity of 89%, specificity of 79%, but a positive predictive value of only 39%, and concluded that the trigger parameters have to be adjusted [30].

Management

Monitoring

Assessment of cerebral function via continuous communication with the awake patient is essential and provides important hemodynamic information. Novel methods based on analyses of the arterial pulse wave have proven accurate in cardiac output trending compared with pulmonary artery catheter data [31]. These minimally invasive and non-invasive monitoring systems have become available since the late 1990s.

Measuring flow, and not only blood pressure and heart rate as surrogates for cardiac output, is now implemented in clinical practice [32]. There is lack of agreement between values obtained from central venous pressure and pulmonary capillary wedge pressure in pre-eclampsia [33], and the use of pulmonary artery catheter in maternal critical care should be limited to pulmonary hypertension in patients for whom ongoing treatment aiming at a reduction of pulmonary arterial pressure within a few days necessitates continuous monitoring. The need for measurements of cardiac output, volume status, systemic vascular resistance, or arterial blood pressure are better solved by transthoracic echocardiography or minimally invasive monitoring systems, alone or in combination [16]. Invasive arterial catheters are often utilized in the ICU, both for continuous monitoring and for frequent blood sampling. Frequent arterial blood gas analyses give information about trends in oxygenation, circulation, and hemolysis. Measurements of platelet counts, liver enzymes, and hemolysis variables should be repeated daily, or even more frequently if HELLP syndrome or disseminated intravascular coagulation is diagnosed (up to every 4 hours, depending on acuity).

Transcranial Doppler measurements have given interesting insight in cerebral hemodynamics in pre-eclampsia [34]. To date, it is unclear how this knowledge can be put into clinical practice, and transcranial Doppler is not a part of routine monitoring.

Blood pressure control

There is consensus that sustained severe hypertension in pregnancy should be treated as it is considered to be a risk factor for maternal end-organ complications (such as stroke), independent of pre-eclampsia [7,35]. In fact, many of the serious maternal (e.g. pulmonary edema, placental abruption) and perinatal (e.g. preterm delivery and perinatal death) complications are more common among women with severe gestational hypertension without proteinuria than in those women with non-severe gestational hypertension with proteinuria [35].

A systolic blood pressure threshold of 160 mmHg has been suggested as more appropriate for defining severe maternal hypertension, based on a case series of 28 women with pre-eclampsia and stroke [35]. In this series, 96% of women had a systolic blood pressure ≥160 mmHg immediately prior to their stroke, but only 13% had a diastolic blood pressure ≥110 mmHg. This series has been criticized for its potentially biased ascertainment of cases and its small sample size, which precludes use of a statistical model that could confirm the independent importance of systolic blood pressure by adjusting for diastolic blood pressure and other important covariates.

The three most recent UK Confidential Enquiries into Maternal Deaths have found that the second most common cause of maternal death was pre-eclampsia/eclampsia, of which the majority related to stroke and failure of effective antihypertensive therapy. Therefore, the reports have concluded that systolic blood pressures ≥160 mmHg must be treated and this recommendation has been reflected in recently published Canadian and UK guidelines (Table 36.1)[18]. In addition, a diastolic blood pressure of ≥110 mmHg must be treated even when systolic blood pressure is <160–170 mmHg [35].

Almost all severe hypertension in pregnancy is without clear hypertension-related end-organ dysfunction and, as such, most episodes are classified as hypertensive "urgencies." It is unclear how to classify the seriousness of headache and visual symptoms. Both are very common among women admitted to hospital with pre-eclampsia (i.e. 30% and 19%, respectively), yet, the incidence of adverse central nervous system outcomes in this group is rare (0.3%) [17]. Also, headache is a well-recognized side effect of medications used in pre-eclampsia, such as nifedipine.

Most episodes of severe hypertension in pregnancy can be managed without an arterial line. Based on extrapolation of the approach outside pregnancy, mean arterial blood pressure should be lowered by no more than 25% over minutes to hours, and then further lowered if necessary to 160/100 mmHg over hours. In selected cases, hypertensive urgencies may be treated with oral agents, which have peak drug effects in 1–2 hours (e.g. oral labetalol or intermediate-acting nifedipine). However, recognizing that gastric emptying may be delayed or unreliable among women in active labor [28], intravenous antihypertensives may be required. Magnesium sulfate infusion will often be indicated for seizure prophylaxis or control when a patient is admitted to a high dependency unit or ICU. Invasive hemodynamic monitoring should be considered. The risk and discomfort of a peripheral arterial line is minor, but the information gained may help the critical care physician in optimizing treatment [25]. Pain during insertion of an arterial line can be minimized by local infiltration of lidocaine 1% or, if time allows it, topical anesthesia with lidocaine/prilocaine cream. Ultrasound-guided technique may reduce patient stress during insertion of the cannula.

Additional associated factors that may be contributing to severe hypertension should be addressed. These include pain, upset, and inadequate levels of antihypertensive therapy related to delayed gastric emptying in labor. In addition, epidural analgesia may be beneficial by producing peripheral vasodilatation [35]. The efficacy of sympathetic block is limited in pre-eclamptic patients [15], and most clinicians perform neuraxial techniques only for labor analgesia or anesthesia during cesarean section.

As the uteroplacental circulation may not autoregulate blood flow in term pre-eclampsia, precipitous falls in maternal blood pressure may be associated with fetal heart rate abnormalities, and monitoring is prudent [35]. This may be even more important in early-onset disease where uteroplacental modification is usually incomplete (Figure 36.1), leaving uterine precapillary arterioles able to constrict as part of a generalized splanchnic response to hypotension. There are limited data on the pharmacological effects of antihypertensives on fetal heart rate or pattern in human pregnancy [36].

In a manner similar to the uteroplacental circulation, the maternal cerebral vasculature may not autoregulate blood flow in the setting of severe hypertension, particularly when mean arterial pressure exceeds 140 mmHg (e.g. blood pressure of 180/120 mmHg) in the previously normotensive patient [35]. The effects of each antihypertensive agent on myocardial performance, cerebral blood flow, and the fetus are not very well established in the pre-eclamptic population. The choice of antihypertensive agent should be guided by local experience and continuous monitoring of blood pressure and flow, both for the mother and the baby. The basic principle to apply in clinical practice is "start low" (with regards to dose) and "go slow" (in terms of repeating doses) [35].

Agents for treatment of severe hypertension

Thirty trials (3446 women) have compared one antihypertensive drug with another. These trials have been systematically reviewed in two high-quality publications [37,38], and there have been three recently published trials [39].

Most trials have compared parenteral hydralazine with either labetalol (six trials) or oral calcium channel blockers (nine trials). Another trial has compared intravenous labetalol with oral nicardipine. These are the medications used most commonly to treat severe hypertension in pregnancy and, as such, these data are most informative for clinical practice (Table 36.4).

When hydralazine was compared with other antihypertensives together, parenteral hydralazine was associated with more adverse effects, including maternal hypotension, cesarean section, and fetal

Table 36.4. Antihypertensive drugs for severe pregnancy hypertension

Agent	Dosage	Comments
Labetalol	Start with 20 mg i.v.; repeat 20–80 mg i.v. every 30 min Alternative: i.v. infusion of 1–2 mg/min to a maximum of 300 mg (then switch to oral)	Best avoided in women with asthma; parenteral labetalol may cause neonatal bradycardia but this is not a major problem in clinical practice
Nifedipine	5–10 mg capsule to be bitten and swallowed, or just swallowed, every 30 min; 10 mg intermediate-release tablets every 45 min to a maximum of 80 mg/day	There are three types of nifedipine preparations (capsules, intermediate-release tablets, and slow-release tablets) with which all staff must be familiar; nifedipine capsules cause a reflex increase in sympathetic tone, which is best avoided in women for whom increased myocardial oxygen demands could be dangerous (e.g. coronary artery disease) or in the setting of fixed valvular obstruction
Hydralazine	Start with 2–5 mg i.v., repeat every 30 min in doses up to 10 mg, or 0.5–10 mg/h i.v., to a maximum of 20 mg i.v. (or 30 mg i.m.)	May increase the risk of maternal hypotension; hydralazine causes a reflex increase in sympathetic tone, which is best avoided in women for whom increased myocardial oxygen demands could be dangerous (e.g. coronary artery disease) or in the setting of fixed valvular obstruction

i.v., intravenous; i.m., intramuscular.
Source: adapted from Payne *et al.*, 2011 [18].

heart rate abnormalities (21 trials, 1085 women) [37]. When compared with parenteral labetalol specifically in a subgroup analysis, hydralazine was a more effective antihypertensive [37]. A subsequently published trial found no between-group difference in persistent severe hypertension (5% in each group) but maternal hypotension occurred in 2/100 women treated with hydralazine compared with 0/100 treated with labetalol [39]. It should be noted that labetalol was associated with more neonatal bradycardia, which required intervention in one of six affected babies in the relevant trial [37], and a similar result was seen in a subsequently published trial of labetalol versus hydralazine [39]. When hydralazine has been compared with calcium channel blockers (nine trials), hydralazine was a less effective antihypertensive [37,38]. Hydralazine was also associated with more fetal heart rate abnormalities [37]. There have been no new relevant trials. When labetalol has been compared with calcium channel blockers (one trial, 60 women), no between-group differences in outcomes have been seen. There have also been case reports of neuromuscular blockade with contemporaneous use of nifedipine and magnesium sulfate, but the risk was estimated to be <1% in a single center, controlled study and complete data synthesis [40]; blockade is reversed with 10 g intravenous calcium gluconate, which is immediately available in all delivery suites and ICUs.

Low dose diazoxide (15 mg intravenous), an arterial vasodilator, compared favorably with hydralazine 5 mg intravenous in a randomized controlled trial of 124 women [28].

Intravenous nicardipine may be an alternative. Sixty consecutive pregnant women with severe hypertension (systolic blood pressure ≥170 mmHg and/or diastolic blood pressure ≥110 mmHg) were randomized to either intravenous nicardipine (10 mg/5 min) or intravenous labetalol (1 mg/min per kg body weight bolus) [41]. Labetalol and nicardipine equally achieved a 20% lowering in blood pressure, with nicardipine causing a significantly greater decrease in systolic and diastolic blood pressure. No women had hypotensive episodes. The length of time to achieve the blood pressure goal was also similar (12 and 11 minutes, respectively). Both drugs were well tolerated (more tachycardia with nicardipine). Other non-randomized data have supported intravenous nicardipine with varying regimens [42–44]. In addition, in a randomized controlled trial of 100 women with non-severe hypertension of pre-eclampsia, oral nicardipine (20 mg three times

daily) was more effective than oral metoprolol in reducing both systolic and diastolic blood pressure [45].

Nitroglycerin (glyceryl trinitrate) is primarily venodilatory. Since women with pre-eclampsia are usually intravascularly volume depleted, and increased systemic vascular resistance is the major pathophysiological finding [15], nitroglycerin would not be a logical choice of antihypertensive agent in women with severe hypertension and pre-eclampsia [28].

In the context of ICU, sodium nitroprusside can be used [28]. The theoretical concerns are well known: light sensitive, requires careful monitoring, and has the potential to cause fetal cyanide toxicity. A published review of case reports (22 women, 24 fetuses) documented stillbirths among 5 of 18 women treated antenatally (27.8%) with nitroprusside, although the authors could not attribute these deaths to fetal cyanide toxicity [37]. After delivery of the baby, sodium nitroprusside has the advantage of being efficacious, the critical care staff are familiar with the titration of doses, and the half-life is short. A continuous invasive measurement of arterial blood pressure is recommended.

A comment should be made regarding the choice of antihypertensive agent and its potential to cause cerebral vasodilatation. In posterior reversible encephalopathy syndrome, of which eclampsia (and possibly pre-eclampsia with neurological symptoms) is thought to be a form, acute elevations in blood pressure result in forced dilatation of vascular smooth muscle (of cerebral arteries and arterioles) and increased blood–brain barrier permeability, promoting edema [35,46]. Theoretically, it may be prudent to choose an antihypertensive agent that does not cause cerebral vasodilatation outside pregnancy, such as labetalol and nicardipine, rather than hydralazine or nifedipine [35]. However, basing antihypertensive choice on such considerations is not recommended. First, there are no data from pregnancy; second, as mentioned above, magnesium sulfate may actually dilate the cerebral vasculature although magnesium prevents and treats eclampsia in human pregnancy [35].

Table 36.4 lists the doses of the most commonly used antihypertensive drugs for severe hypertension in pregnancy. Following treatment of severe hypertension, oral antihypertensive therapy should usually be started to maintain blood pressure unless there was a clear, modifiable precipitant (such as the pain of labor). During labor, gastric emptying may be unreliable.

Postpartum, blood pressure peaks on days 3–6 in previously normotensive women [47]; normalization of elevated blood pressure occur later in pre-eclampsia (mean 16 days; SD, 9.5) compared with gestational hypertension (mean 6 days; SD, 5.5) [48]. Consideration should be given to restarting antihypertensive therapy after delivery, particularly in women with pre-eclampsia, in whom postpartum hypertension and pulmonary edema are more common, which is possibly related to mobilization of extravascular fluid into the intravascular space. Captopril, enalapril, and other angiotensin-converting enzyme inhibitors may be used for severe postpartum hypertension without precluding breastfeeding. Breastfeeding information is available free of charge in the Lactmed database [49]. Management issues around postpartum hypertension and breastfeeding are discussed in detail in the UK NICE guidelines [39]. In the critical care setting it is important to have in mind before delivery that antihypertensive treatment may affect the uteroplacental flow rate and may affect the fetus negatively.

In summary, there is consensus that severe hypertension in pregnancy should be treated to decrease maternal risk. Parenteral hydralazine and labetalol and oral nifedipine have been best studied in randomized trials for this indication. No agent is clearly superior to others, although parenteral hydralazine may be associated with more maternal hypotension and adverse fetal heart rate effects.

Fluid management

Intravascular volume depletion has been considered the norm in women with pre-eclampsia [7,50]. In response to this, there was a period of enthusiasm for plasma volume expansion [51–53], but the clinical effectiveness of this strategy is not supported by the results [54]. Studies have not been able to establish a goal-directed volume therapy, and current practice is to administer intravenous fluids carefully because of the risk of pulmonary edema. Thornton et al. [55] devised a set of clinical indicators to benchmark outcomes for women suffering from the hypertensive disorders of pregnancy. Seven clinical indicators were designed and applied retrospectively to data collected from two tertiary referral centers, Royal Prince Alfred Hospital (RPA), Sydney, Australia and British Columbia Women's Hospital and Health Centre (BCW), Vancouver Canada. Comparisons were made using the established clinical indicators. There were significantly more episodes of maternal pulmonary edema at BCW than at RPA (1.2% and 0.1%, respectively; $p < 0.001$).

Therefore, in follow-up, the investigators sought to determine rates of and potential causative factors for acute pulmonary edema in hypertensive pregnant women [56]. A retrospective individual-patient data review was conducted for a calendar year (2005) at RPA and BCW. There were 472 women at RPA and 408 women at BCW diagnosed with one of the four presentations of hypertension in pregnancy. During this period, there were no cases of acute pulmonary edema at RPA and 19 cases at BCW. None of the women had any known pre-existing cardiac abnormality. Antenatal pharmacological management of hypertension and steroid treatment for fetal lung maturity was significantly more frequent at the center reporting no cases of pulmonary edema. Further, smoking was less frequent in the population at this center. The 19 women with acute pulmonary edema at BCW received larger quantities of intravenous fluids. Therefore, the development of acute pulmonary edema in women with hypertension during pregnancy was associated with high levels of intravenous fluid administration.

The Pre-Eclampsia Trial Amsterdam (PETRA), a two-center Dutch randomized controlled trial, tested whether or not plasma volume expansion combined with a more advanced antihypertensive treatment protocol would benefit both mother and child as temporizing management of severe and early-onset pre-eclampsia [52]. Of 216 women with a gestational age of 24^{+0}–33^{+6} weeks with severe pre-eclampsia and HELLP syndrome or severe intrauterine growth retardation with gestational hypertension, and/or pre-eclampsia, 111 women were randomly allocated to the treatment group (plasma volume expansion and a diastolic blood pressure target of 85–95 mmHg) and 105 to the control group (intravenous fluid restriction and diastolic blood pressure target of 95–105 mmHg). There was no statistically difference in major maternal morbidity (total 11%). There were more cesarean sections in the treatment group than in the control group (98% and 90%, respectively; $p < 0.05$). The authors concluded that addition of plasma volume expansion in temporizing treatment does not improve maternal or fetal outcome in women with early preterm hypertensive complications of pregnancy. Based on a retrospective review of 62 917 pregnancies among which 51 women were diagnosed with acute pulmonary edema, Sciscione *et al.* [57] found that the most common causes were the use of tocolytic agents, underlying cardiac disease, fluid overload, and pre-eclampsia. The pre-eclamptic population was not uniform within or between the analyzed samples. None of the studies took into consideration the great variance in hemodynamic status in the pre-eclamptic population [12]. There is a growing interest in hemodynamic pathophysiology in pre-eclamptic patients and increasing scientific data to support cardiac output monitoring rather than blood pressure monitoring [58]. The development of minimal-invasive hemodynamic monitoring devices providing continuous patient data has opened a new research era and changed anesthetic practice [16]. Whether new therapy protocols directed by defined goals in physiological variables actually can improve maternal and fetal outcome has to be tested in controlled clinical trials.

Normally, pregnancy leads to an approximately 40% increase in plasma volume. In an observational trial of 29 patients with eclampsia, Zeeman *et al.* [59] documented a significant hemoconcentration compared with subsequent normal pregnancies in the same subjects. Increased hemoglobin concentration is an independent risk factor for stillbirth [60]. Women with pre-eclampsia have decreased blood volume and significantly increased hemoglobin concentration prior to delivery [61], and elevated hemoglobin concentration is inversely correlated with fetal growth. In general, high hemoglobin concentration is associated with stillbirth, preterm birth, and growth retardation [62].

In the absence of pre-existing renal disease that mandates an urine output of 30 mL/h, urine output ≥15 mL/h should be accepted as normal in pregnancy [39,63]. Acute renal failure is very uncommon in this population and diuretic therapy is not documented to reduce the risk. There have been no renal failure-related maternal deaths in the UK since the late 1980s, and, since a policy of "running women with pre-eclampsia dry" (80 mL/h total input in women with severe pre-eclampsia) has become widespread, there has not been a pre-eclampsia maternal death related to pulmonary edema in the UK since the late 1990s.

Even if the typical woman with pre-eclampsia has a reduced circulating blood volume, it is also common to develop generalized edema. When this body water goes into circulation during the first few days after delivery, diuretics may be given to speed the elimination of excess water and thereby minimize the risk of severe pulmonary edema. Therapy can be guided by echocardiography and hemodynamic monitoring of intrathoracic blood volume or the amount of extravascular lung water. Low urine output is quite common in the first days after delivery and should be interpreted neither as an indication for diuretics nor one for intravenous volume expansion.

If a woman with pre-eclampsia requires supplemental oxygen therapy, has an increasing respiratory rate, or suffers from shortness of breath, echocardiography should be performed to diagnose coexistence of cardiac diseases or pre-eclampsia-related cardiac dysfunction and to evaluate preload and cardiac output. Continuous minimally invasive monitoring of hemodynamic variables may be useful.

Neuroprotection

Prevention of pre-eclampsia-related cerebral complications is one of the major indications for observation and treatment in ICU. Stroke may be ischemic or hemorrhagic, and ischemic infarction may turn into hemorrhagic stroke. In patients with chronic hypertension, hemorrhage in the striatocapsular area is more common. Aneurysmal bleeding must also be considered, although it is rare in this population [46,64]. Minor infarction and bleeding may not be fatal, but morbidity may be substantial. Treatment should follow guidelines for neurointensive care medicine (Table 36.5) [65] and strict control of the systolic blood pressure is necessary to prevent sudden hemorrhage in a brain region with ischemic infarction. The latest UK Confidential Enquiries into Maternal Deaths and Child Health has suggested that systolic blood pressure should be kept 150 mmHg to avoid unobserved and sustained spikes in systolic blood pressure to >160 mmHg [4], which is stricter than in the current guidelines and not pertinent to women receiving critical care (Table 36.1) [18].

Magnesium sulfate

Prevention and management of eclamptic seizures is based upon giving magnesium sulfate [7,39,63]. The exact mechanism is still not established. Women with severe pre-eclampsia should be considered for magnesium sulfate prophylaxis. Findings from randomized controlled trials support a regimen of magnesium sulfate given as a 4 g intravenous loading dose during a 15–20 minutes period, followed by an infusion of 1 g/h, with a first or recurrent seizure

Table 36.5. American Heart Association/American Stroke Association class I recommendations for treatment of intracerebral hemorrhage

	Recommendations	Class/level of evidence[a]
Emergency diagnosis and assessment of ICH and its causes	Rapid neuroimaging with CT or MRI is recommended to distinguish ischemic stroke from ICH (unchanged from the previous guideline)	Class 1, level A
Medical treatment for ICH	Patients with a severe coagulation factor deficiency or severe thrombocytopenia should receive appropriate factor replacement therapy or platelets, respectively (new recommendation)	Class I, level B
Hemostasis/antiplatelets/deep vein thrombosis prophylaxis	Patients with ICH whose INR is elevated because of oral anticoagulant use should have their warfarin withheld, receive therapy to replace vitamin K-dependent factors and correct the INR, receive intravenous vitamin K (revised from the previous guideline)	Class I, level C
	Patients with ICH should have intermittent pneumatic compression for prevention of venous thromboembolism in addition to elastic stockings (unchanged from the previous guideline)	Class I, level B
Inpatient management and prevention of secondary brain injury		
General monitoring	Initial monitoring and management of ICH patients should take place in ICU, preferably with physician and nursing neuroscience intensive care expertise (unchanged from the previous guideline)	Class I, level B
Management of glucose	Glucose should be monitored and normoglycemia is recommended	Class I, level C
Seizures and antiepileptic drugs	Patients with clinical seizures should be treated with antiepileptic drugs (revised from previous guideline)	Class I, level A
	Patients with a change in mental status who are found to have eletrographic seizures on electroencephalography should be treated with antiepileptic drugs	Class I, level C
Procedures/surgery, clot removal	Patients with cerebellar hemorrhage who are deteriorating neurologically or who have brainstem compression and/or hydrocephalus from ventricular obstruction should undergo surgical removal of the hemorrhage as soon as possible (revised from the previous guideline)	Class I, level B
Prevention of recurrent ICH	After the acute ICH and with no medical contraindications, blood pressure should be well controlled, particularly for patients with ICH location typical of hypertensive vasculopathy (new recommendation)	Class I, level A

ICH, intracerebral hemorrhage; INR, international normalized ratio.
[a] Based on the American Heart Association's Stroke Council's levels of evidence grading algorithm.
Source: from Morgenstern *et al.*, 2010 [65].

treated with another 2–4 g intravenous loading dose. This regimen does not need testing of blood concentrations of magnesium sulfate because clinical effect can be monitored with deep tendon reflexes. Additionally, this regimen provides a wider therapeutic index between effect and toxicity risk than does the historical 2 g/h regimen.

In a Scandinavian cohort, 89% had at least one physical complaint before the first seizure, severe headache being the most common [9], and nearly half of patients received substandard care. Imminent eclampsia (headache, hyper-reflexia, blurred vision, and epigastric pain) necessitates continuous monitoring, magnesium sulfate prophylaxis, and a high level of care. The risk of seizure decreases 12 hours after birth [53]. Not all seizures or altered mental state is eclampsia, and since subarachnoidal hemorrhage is more frequent in women with pre-eclampsia, emergency cerebral CT or MRI will often be indicated.

Hematological changes/HELLP syndrome

Patients with HELLP syndrome have an increased risk of venous thromboembolism and bleeding. Normal pregnancy is physiologically hypercoagulable and this is pathologically enhanced in pre-eclampsia. The inter-related risk of pre-eclampsia and thrombophilia is not well characterized. Probably, coagulation and microembolization in the liver is important in the pathophysiology of HELLP [66]. Point of care monitors of coagulation have been implemented in clinical practice. Thromboelastography has been validated in the pregnant population and relevant reference values described [67]. Patients with severe pre-eclampsia with platelet count <100 × 10⁹/L may even be hypocoagulable [68]. The clinical impact of coagulation monitors remains to be documented. The use of corticosteroids (dexamethasone) may be justified in clinical situations in which an increased rate of recovery in platelet count is considered clinically worthwhile prior to delivery, surgery, or anesthetic procedures because of the considerable bleeding risk [69].

Pain relief and stress reduction

Women with pre-eclampsia who are managed in a high dependency unit or ICU may have fear, anxiety, and concerns about the possibility of death or harm to the baby. Abdominal pain may indicate liver pathology (HELLP syndrome) and headache may represent imminent eclampsia. Labor pain and pain after cesarean delivery should be treated with neuraxial techniques if not contraindicated by low platelet counts [57]. Analgesic choice may be complicated because acetaminophen (paracetamol) is contraindicated in the setting of liver disease, non-steroidal anti-inflammatory drugs may worsen hypertension or affect bleeding risk (particularly when platelet counts are low or falling), and opioids may potentiate magnesium-induced respiratory depression. Incremental dosing of intravenous opioids is usually safe, both for the mother and breastfed baby. If opioid analgesics are given for longer than 2–3 days, the breastfed baby should be monitored for opioid-related effects. Breastfeeding and early skin-to-skin contact between mother and baby is important for the baby [70], and probably also for the mother's well-being; it should be given high priority, even in a high dependency unit. Corticosteroid treatment (often administered prior to a preterm delivery) can relieve pain and nausea.

Acknowledgements

Beth Payne and Paul Yong, Vancouver, contributed to the data review upon which much of this chapter is based.

References

1. Lapinsky S, Kruczynski K, Seaward G, Farine D, Grossman R. Critical care management of the obstetric patient. *Can J Anesth* 1997 Mar 1;**44**:325–329.

2. Keizer JL, Zwart JJ, Meerman RH, *et al.* Obstetric intensive care admissions: A 12-year review in a tertiary care centre. *Eur J Obstet Gynecol Reprod Biol* 2009;**128**:152–156.

3. Kuklina EV, Ayala C, Callaghan WM. Hypertensive disorders and severe obstetric morbidity in the United States. *Obstet Gynecol* 2009;**113**:1299.

4. Cantwell R, Clutton-Brock T, Cooper G, *et al.* Saving Mothers' Lives: Reviewing Maternal Deaths to make Motherhood Safer 2006–2008. The Eighth Report of the Confidential Enquiries into Maternal Deaths in the United Kingdom. *BJOG* 2011;**118**(Suppl 1):1–203.

5. Wheatly S. Maternal critical care: what' in a name? *Int J Obstet Anesth* 2010;**19**:353–355.

6. Hutcheon JA, Lisonkova S, Joseph KS. Epidemiology of pre-eclampsia and the other hypertensive disorders of pregnancy. *Best Pract Res Clin Obstet Gynaecol* 2011;**25**:391–403.

7. Steegers EA, von Dadelszen P, Duvekot JJ, Pijnenborg R. Pre-eclampsia. *Lancet* 2010;**376**:631–644.

8. Eastabrook G, Brown M, Sargent I. The origins and end-organ consequence of pre-eclampsia. *Best Pract Res Clin Obstet Gynaecol* 2011;**25**:435–447.

9. Andersgaard AB, Herbst A, Johansen M, *et al.* Eclampsia in Scandinavia: incidence, substandard care, and potentially preventable cases. *Acta Obstet Gynecol Scand* 2006;**85**:929–936.

10. Grindheim G, Estensen ME, Langesaeter E, Rosseland LA, Toska K. Changes in blood pressure during healthy pregnancy: a longitudinal cohort study. *J Hypertens* 2012;**30**:342–350.

11. Assali NS, Prystowsky H. Studies on autonomic blockade. I. Comparison between the effects of tetraethylammonium chloride (TEAC) and high selective spinal anesthesia on blood pressure of normal and toxemic pregnancy. *J Clin Invest* 1950;**29**:1354–1366.

12. Dyer RA, Piercy JL, Reed AR, *et al.* Hemodynamic changes associated with spinal anesthesia for cesarean delivery in severe preeclampsia. *Anesthesiology* 2008;**108**:802–811.

13. Hermida RC, Ayala DE, Iglesias M. Predictable blood pressure variability in healthy and complicated pregnancies. *Hypertension* 2001;**38**:736–741.

14. Mishra N, Nugent WH, Mahavadi S, Walsh SW. Mechanisms of enhanced vascular reactivity in preeclampsia. *Hypertension* 2011;**58**:867–873.

15. Sharwood-Smith G, Drummond GB. Hypotension in obstetric spinal anaesthesia: a lesson from pre-eclampsia. *Br J Anaesth* 2009;**102**:291–294.

16. Langesaeter E. Is it more informative to focus on cardiac output than blood pressure during spinal anesthesia for cesarean delivery in women with severe preeclampsia? *Anesthesiology* 2008;**108**:771.

17. von Dadelszen P, Payne B, Li J, *et al*. Prediction of adverse maternal outcomes in pre-eclampsia: development and validation of the fullPIERS model. *Lancet* 2011;**377**:219–227.

18. Payne B, Magee LA, von Dadelszen P. Assessment, surveillance and prognosis in pre-eclampsia. *Best Pract Res Clin Obstet Gynaecol* 2011;**25**:449–462.

19. Mackay AP, Berg CJ, Atrash HK. Pregnancy-related mortality from preeclampsia and eclampsia. *Obstet Gynecol* 2001;**97**:533–538.

20. Stella CL, Dacus J, Guzman E, *et al*. The diagnostic dilemma of thrombotic thrombocytopenic purpura/hemolytic uremic syndrome in the obstetric triage and emergency department: lessons from 4 tertiary hospitals. *Am J Obstet Gynecol* 2009;**200**:381.

21. Martin SR, Foley MR. Intensive care in obstetrics: an evidence-based review. *Am J Obstet Gynecol* 2006;**195**:673–689.

22. El-Solh AA, Grant BJ. A comparison of severity of illness scoring systems for critically ill obstetric patients. *Chest* 1996;**110**:1299–1304.

23. Muench MV, Baschat AA, Malinow AM, Mighty HE. Analysis of disease in the obstetric intensive care unit at a university referral center: a 24-month review of prospective data. *J Reprod Med* 2008;**53**:914.

24. Afessa B, Morales IJ, Scanlon PD, Peters SG. Prognostic factors, clinical course, and hospital outcome of patients with chronic obstructive pulmonary disease admitted to an intensive care unit for acute respiratory failure. *Crit Care Med* 2002;**30**:1610.

25. Hazelgrove JF, Price C, Pappachan VJ, Smith GB. Multicenter study of obstetric admissions to 14 intensive care units in southern England. *Crit Care Med* 2001;**29**:770.

26. Karnad DR, Lapsia V, Krishnan A, Salvi VS. Prognostic factors in obstetric patients admitted to an Indian intensive care unit. *Crit Care Med* 2004;**32**:1294.

27. Mahutte NG, Murphy-Kaulbeck L, Le Q, *et al*. Obstetric admissions to the intensive care unit. *Obstet Gynecol* 1999;**94**:263.

28. Tang LC, Kwok AC, Wong AY, *et al*. Critical care in obstetrical patients: an eight-year review. *Chinese Med J* 1997;**110**:936.

29. Tempe A, Wadhwa L, Gupta S, Bansal S, Satyanarayana L. Prediction of mortality and morbidity by simplified acute physiology score II in obstetric intensive care unit admissions. *Indian J Med Sci* 2007;**61**:179.

30. Singh S, McGlennan A, England A, Simons R. A validation study of the CEMACH recommended modified early obstetric warning system (MEOWS). *Anaesthesia* 2012;**671**:12–18.

31. Hadian M, Kim HK, Severyn DA, Pinsky MR. Cross-comparison of cardiac output trending accuracy of LiDCO, PiCCO, FloTrac and pulmonary artery catheters. *Crit Care* 2010;**14**:R212.

32. Armstrong S, Fernando R, Columb M. Minimally-and non-invasive assessment of maternal cardiac output: go with the flow! *Int J Obstet Anesth* 2011;**20**:330–340.

33. Bolte AC, Dekker GA, van Eyck J, van Schijndel RS, van Geijn HP. Lack of agreement between central venous pressure and pulmonary capillary wedge pressure in preeclampsia. *Hypertens Pregnancy* 2000;**19**:261–271.

34. Belfort MA, Clark SL, Sibai B. Cerebral hemodynamics in preeclampsia: cerebral perfusion and the rationale for an alternative to magnesium sulfate. *Obstet Gynecol Surv* 2006;**61**:655.

35. Magee LA, Abalos E, von Dadelszen P, *et al*. How to manage hypertension in pregnancy effectively. *Br J Clin Pharmacol* 2011;**72**:394–401.

36. Waterman EJ, Magee LA, Lim KI, *et al*. Do commonly used oral antihypertensives alter fetal or neonatal heart rate characteristics? A systematic review. *Hypertens Pregnancy* 2004;**23**:155–169.

37. Magee LA, Cham C, Waterman EJ, Ohlsson A, von Dadelszen P. Hydralazine for treatment of severe hypertension in pregnancy: meta-analysis. *BMJ* 2003;**327**:955.

38. Duley L, Henderson-Smart DJ, Meher S. Drugs for treatment of very high blood pressure during pregnancy. *Cochrane Database Syst Rev* 2006;(**3**): CD001449.

39. National Institute for Health and Clinical Excellence. *Hypertension in Pregnancy (CG107)*. London: NICE, 2010 (http://guidance nice.org.uk/CG107, accessed 29 January 2013).

40. Magee LA, Miremadi S, Li J, *et al*. Therapy with both magnesium sulfate and nifedipine does not increase the risk of serious magnesium-related maternal side effects in women with preeclampsia. *Am J Obstet Gynecol* 2005;**193**:153–163.

41. Elatrous S, Nouira S, Ouanes Besbes L, *et al*. Short-term treatment of severe hypertension of pregnancy: prospective comparison of nicardipine and labetalol. *Intensive Care Med* 2002;**28**:1281–1286.

42. Carbonne B, Jannet D, Touboul C, Khelifati Y, Milliez J. Nicardipine treatment of hypertension during pregnancy. *Obstet Gynecol* 1993;**81**:908.

43. Aya AGM, Mangin R, Hoffet M, Eledjam JJ. Intravenous nicardipine for severe hypertension in pre-eclampsia: effects of an acute treatment on mother and foetus. *Intensive Care Med* 1999;**25**:1277–1281.

44. Hanff LM, Vulto AG, Bartels PA, *et al.* Intravenous use of the calcium-channel blocker nicardipine as second-line treatment in severe, early-onset pre-eclamptic patients. *J Hypertens* 2005;**23**:2319.

45. Jannet D, Carbonne B, Sebban E, Milliez J. Nicardipine versus metoprolol in the treatment of hypertension during pregnancy: a randomized comparative trial. *Obstet Gynecol* 1994;**84**:354.

46. Zeeman GG, Cipolla MJ, Cunningham FG. Cerebrovascular (patho)physiology in preeclampsia/eclampsia. In Marshal D, Lindheimer JM, Roberts FG, Cunningham LC, Chesley LC (eds.) *Chesley' Hypertensive Disorders in Pregnancy*. San Diego, CA: Academic Press-Elsevier, 2009, pp. 227–246.

47. Walters BN, Thompson ME, Lee A, De Swiet M. Blood pressure in the puerperium. *Clin Sci* 1986;**71**:589.

48. Ferrazzani S, De Carolis S, Pomini F, *et al.* The duration of hypertension in the puerperium of preeclamptic women: relationship with renal impairment and week of delivery. *Am J Obstet Gynecol* 1994;**171**:506–512.

49. US National Library of Medicine. *Drugs and Lactation Database (LactMed)*. Bethesda, MD: Specialized Information Services (http://toxnet.nlm.nih.gov/cgi-bin/sis/htmlgen?LACT, accessed 5 December 2012).

50. Visser W, Wallenburg HC. Central hemodynamic observations in untreated preeclamptic patients. *Hypertension* 1991;**17**:1072–1077.

51. Cloeren SE, Lippert TH. Effect of plasma expanders in toxemia of pregnancy. *N Engl J Med* 1972;**287**:1356–1357.

52. Ganzevoort W, Rep A, Bonsel GJ, *et al.* A randomised controlled trial comparing two temporising management strategies, one with and one without plasma volume expansion, for severe and early onset pre-eclampsia. *Br J Obstet Gynaecol* 2005;**112**:1358–1368.

53. Cloeren SE, Lippert TH, Hinselmann M. Hypovolemia in toxemia of pregnancy: Plasma expander therapy with surveillance of central venous pressure. *Arch Gynecol Obstet* 1973;**215**:123–132.

54. Ganzevoort W, Sibai BM. Temporising versus interventionist management (preterm and at term). *Best Pract Res Clin Obstet Gynaecol* 2011;**25**:463–476.

55. Thornton C, Hennessy A, von Dadelszen P, Nishi C, Makris A, Ogle R. An international benchmarking collaboration: measuring outcomes for the hypertensive disorders of pregnancy. *J Obstet Gynaecol Can* 2007;**29**:794–800.

56. Thornton CE, von Dadelszen P, Makris A, *et al.* Acute pulmonary oedema as a complication of hypertension during pregnancy. *Hypertens Pregnancy* 2011;**30**:169–179.

57. Sciscione AC, Ivester T, Largoza M, *et al.* Acute pulmonary edema in pregnancy. *Obstet Gynecol* 2003;**101**:511.

58. Valensise H, Vasapollo B, Novelli GP, *et al.* Maternal and fetal hemodynamic effects induced by nitric oxide donors and plasma volume expansion in pregnancies with gestational hypertension complicated by intrauterine growth restriction with absent end-diastolic flow in the umbilical artery. *Ultrasound Obstet Gynecol* 2008;**31**:55–64.

59. Zeeman GG, Cunningham FG, Pritchard JA. The magnitude of hemoconcentration with eclampsia. *Hypertens Pregnancy* 2009;**28**:127–137.

60. Stephansson O, Dickman PW, Johansson A, Cnattingius S. Maternal hemoglobin concentration during pregnancy and risk of stillbirth. *JAMA* 2000;**284**:2611–2617.

61. Amburgey OA, Ing E, Badger GJ, Bernstein IM. Maternal hemoglobin concentration and its association with birth weight in newborns of mothers with preeclampsia. *J Matern Fetal Neonatal Med* 2009;**22**:740–744.

62. Steer PJ. Maternal hemoglobin concentration and birth weight. *Am J Clin Nutr* 2000;**71**:1285S–7S.

63. Magee LA, Helewa M, Moutquin JM, von Dadelszen P. Diagnosis, evaluation, and management of the hypertensive disorders of pregnancy. *J Obstet Gynaecol Can* 2008;**30**(Suppl):S1–48.

64. Bateman BT, Olbrecht VA, Berman MF, *et al.* Peripartum subarachnoid hemorrhage: nationwide data and institutional experience. *Anesthesiology* 2012;**116**:324–333.

65. Morgenstern LB, Hemphill JC, Anderson C, *et al.* Guidelines for the management of spontaneous intracerebral hemorrhage. *Stroke* 2010;**41**:2108–2129.

66. Barton JR, Sibai BM. *Gastrointestinal Complications of Pre-eclampsia*. Philadelphia, PA: Elsevier, 2009, pp. 179–188.

67. Polak F, Kolnikova I, Lips M, *et al.* New recommendations for thromboelastography reference ranges for pregnant women. *Thromb Res* 2011;**128**: e14–e17.

68. Sharma SK, Philip J, Whitten CW, Padakandla UB, Landers DF. Assessment of changes in coagulation in parturients with preeclampsia using thromboelastography. *Anesthesiology* 1999;**90**:385.

69. Woudstra DM, Chandra S, Hofmeyr GJ, Dowswell T. Corticosteroids for HELLP (hemolysis, elevated liver enzymes, low platelets) syndrome in pregnancy. *Cochrane Database Syst Rev* 2010(9):CD008148.

70. Moore E, Anderson G, Bergman N. Early skin-to-skin contact for mothers and their healthy newborn infants. *Cochrane Database Syst Rev* 2007(2):CD003519.

Chapter 37

Acute fatty liver of pregnancy

Linda Watkins and Mieke Soens

Introduction

Acute fatty liver of pregnancy (AFLP) is a very rare disease characterized first in 1940 by Sheehan in a series of six case reports describing clinical features and postmortem findings [1]. It is characterized histologically by fatty infiltration of liver cells and commonly presents with symptoms of acute liver failure. It classically presents in the third trimester, with vomiting, epigastric pain, and general malaise.

Acute fatty liver of pregnancy clinically has a similar presentation to other causes of liver dysfunction in particular the HELLP syndrome (hemolysis, elevated liver enzymes, and low platelets). There is some debate as to whether AFLP is part of a spectrum of pre-eclampsia-related diseases. Other possible differential diagnoses are hemolytic–uremic syndrome, viral hepatitis, and choleostasis. One of the difficulties is that diseases characterized by liver dysfunction in pregnancy often share clinical characteristics, and women often have features of more than one possible cause. It is often a diagnosis of exclusion and may only be confirmed on liver biopsy, although several attempts have been made to try to characterize the disease clinically and biochemically.

In general, AFLP is reversed by delivery and generally expert opinion agrees that expediting delivery improves the prognosis for mother and baby. Management will usually involve a multidisciplinary team to plan delivery and postnatal care, which may include the obstetrician, maternal medicine specialist, anesthesiologist, hematologist, and hepatologist.

Morbidity and outcomes

In the past there was a high mortality and morbidity for mother and baby. Recent case series and population reviews have shown this to be significantly reduced; however, cases of maternal and fetal death are still reported [2,3]. The UK Obstetric Surveillance System (UKOSS) reported their prospective study into AFLP in the UK showing the maternal mortality to be 1.8% in 57 cases [4]. Perinatal mortality rate was 104/1000 births in this cohort. Because of the high rate of intrauterine fetal death, they also report a 60% admission rate to critical care. Cesarean section rates are reported as 60–80% and usually because of fetal distress, which can be very acute in onset.

Epidemiology

Several case series have been reported. To date, the largest two are national population-based studies. The largest retrospective study from the Netherlands over 2 years showed an incidence of severe morbidity caused by AFLP of 3.2 per 100 000 maternities [3]. In the UK, a prospective study carried out over 18 months by the UKOSS group gave an incidence of 5 per 100 000 maternities [4]. There have been several hospital-based case series, usually giving a higher observed incidence, which may be because the patients with severe morbidity are more often referred to as tertiary units. A case series from two large centers in the USA for a Latin-American population estimated an incidence of 15 per 100 000 maternities while a series from Chile estimated a prevalence of 6.3 per 100 000.

Proposed risk factors include primiparity, higher maternal age, and multiple pregnancies. The UKOSS data confirmed an association with twin pregnancies (18% of cases) and found a possible link with low body mass index (<20), which was not statistically significant [4].

Environmental and genetic factors

In the mid 1990s links were made between pregnancy complicated by AFLP and the child subsequently developing a Reye-like syndrome (hypoglycemia and

Maternal Critical Care: A Multidisciplinary Approach, ed. Marc Van de Velde, Helen Scholefield, and Lauren A. Plante. Published by Cambridge University Press. © Cambridge University Press 2013.

abnormal liver enzymes) in a group of families [5,6]. This led to the suggestion of a link with mitochondrial dysfunction caused by defects in oxidation in long-chain fatty acids [7]. There are case series with recurrent AFLP, but numbers are small, partly because of the rarity of the disease; it is also postulated that women may avoid further pregnancy after the first occurrence of AFLP [4,8,]. However there are also reported cases in multiparous women with previously unaffected pregnancies. Possibly because of the rarity of the disease, there is no evidence that it is more common in certain populations.

Etiology

Current theories surround mitochondrial dysfunction and defects in long-chain fatty acid oxidation. Initial suspicion arose in a mother who had recurrent AFLP where both her children died in infancy and were found to have the liver histology changes also found in AFLP. There have since been several reports showing a strong link between fetal long-chain 3-hydroxyacylcoenzyme A dehydrogenase (LCHAD) deficiency and maternal liver disease in pregnancy, particularly AFLP, but also severe pre-eclampsia and HELLP syndrome.

Deficiency of LCHAD is part of a complex group of errors of metabolism called mitochondrial trifunctional protein (MTP) defects. The LCHAD deficiency causes defective mitochondrial fatty acid beta-oxidation. Mitochondrial fatty acid beta-oxidation is particularly important in the creation of energy in skeletal and heart muscle, and it also occurs within the liver at times of fasting or illness. These types of defect have been found to be the cause of sudden infant death syndrome at autopsy in a small proportion of cases. They have also been associated with non-ketotic hypoglycemia and hepatic coma (Reyes-like syndrome).

Children affected by MTP defects can also present with a cardiomyopathy, progressive neuropathy, or skeletal myopathy depending on the mutation. These defects are inherited in an autosomal recessive pattern.

Interestingly, in a follow-up study screening 27 children born following maternal AFLP and 81 after HELLP syndrome, one in five children born to mothers with AFLP were found to be homozygous for a genetic mutation (most commonly G1528C) associated with MTP but none were found in the HELLP group.

In one case series, elevated serum creatine prior to the admission episode was noted and autopsies have shown changes of abnormal fatty acid beta-oxidation in kidneys [8].

The precise mechanism is still unclear even in those found to have a fetus affected by LCHAD deficiency. One postulated mechanism is hepatotoxicity caused by the build up of toxic metabolites created through incomplete breakdown of long-chain fatty acids. Up to now, there are several theories postulated as to how a defect in fatty acid oxidation may be implicated in the pathogenesis of AFLP (Table 37.1).

Table 37.1. Etiological theories for acute fatty liver of pregnancy

Etiology	Evidence	Potential therapy
Genetic susceptibility in fetus: fatty acid oxidation defect in the fetus and placenta leading to increased toxic metabolites in the mother	Link between LCHAD affected fetus and maternal AFLP; evidence of long-chain fatty acid beta-oxidation within the placenta	Screening children of affected mothers to enable treatment of child and guide genetic counseling
Genetic susceptibility in the mother: reduced capacity for fatty acid oxidation	Mothers who are heterozygous for gene defects affecting LCHAD/MTP can be affected by AFLP	
Metabolic changes of pregnancy: increased lipolysis and decreased B oxidation in third trimester	Theory only	
Environmental stress; high-fat diet	Theory only; diet low in long-chain fatty acids useful in treating children affected by LCHAD	Low fat diet
Female sex hormones	Treating female mice liver mitochondria with estrogen and progestogen caused a decrease in oxidation of fatty acids	

AFLP, acute fatty liver of pregnancy; LCHAD, long-chain 3-hydroxyacylcoenzyme A dehydrogenase; MTP, mitochondrial trifunctional protein.

Diagnosis

Acute fatty liver of pregnancy is rare and can present in a similar way to other causes of liver function abnormality both in pregnancy and non-pregnancy related (Table 37.2). It may present in a very non-specific manner and may only be recognized in retrospect. Symptoms often reported include vomiting and nausea, abdominal pain, and general malaise. Classically it presents in the third trimester but cases have been recognized as early as 22 weeks. The prodromal illness may go on for up to 2 weeks before presentation and hence it may be mistaken for a viral illness by both patients and clinicians if further investigations are not done [2,8].

Ch'ng et al. [9] devised diagnostic criteria for AFLP based on previous reports to help them analyse abnormal liver function tests to prospectively in a large patient cohort in South Wales. These have come to be known as the Swansea criteria (Box 37.1) and were used by the UKOSS group to objectively confirm diagnosis of AFLP in conjunction with case note review by experienced clinicians. Another group in India then went on to validate the Swansea criteria with a retrospective cohort of patients who had undergone liver biopsy in pregnancy.

When considering the differential diagnosis, it is worth bearing in mind the wide causes of liver function abnormality both in pregnancy and non-pregnancy related (Table 37.2). Investigations and history may help to form a positive diagnosis of an alternative cause, particularly as AFLP is usually a diagnosis of exclusion.

Clinical features

Typically, AFLP presents in a non-specific way. It may present with signs and symptoms of acute hepatitis, classically nausea, vomiting, and abdominal pain. There may or may not be hypoglycemia.

Most women with AFLP present with symptoms in the third trimester, usually around 36 weeks of gestation in most case series (Table 37.3). It is rarely the diagnosis on admission, but studies suggest it is

---

Box 37.1. Diagnostic criteria for acute fatty liver of pregnancy: the Swansea criteria

Six or more of the following features in the absence of another explanation:

- vomiting
- abdominal pain
- polydipsia/polyuria
- encephalopathy
- elevated bilirubin
- hypoglycemia
- elevated urate
- leukocytosis
- ascites or bright liver on ultrasound
- elevated transaminases
- elevated ammonia
- renal impairment
- coagulopathy
- microvesicular steatosis on liver biopsy

Source: from Ch'ng et al., 2002 [9]

Table 37.2. Differential diagnosis of acute fatty liver of pregnancy

	Disorder
Pregnancy specific	HELLP Severe pre-eclampsia Obstetric choleostasis Hyperemesis gravidarum
Infections	Hepatitis A, B, C, E viruses Malaria Sepsis Other viral (HIV, cytomegalovirus)
Hematological	Hemolytic–uremic syndrome
Autoimmune	Autoimmune hepatitis Primary billary cirrhosis Sclerosis cholangitis
Metabolic	Wilsons disease Hemachromatosis
Toxic	Acetaminophen overdose
Structural	Blocked bile duct (gallstones)

Table 37.3. Signs and symptoms found in acute fatty liver of pregnancy

System	Signs/symptoms
Abdominal	Nausea, vomiting, abdominal pain
Hepatic	Jaundice
Pancreatic	Polydipsia/polyuria
Neurological	Encephalitis
Hematological	Coagulopathy
General	Often a general feeling of non-specific malaise

diagnosed antenatally in 50–75% of cases and before a week postpartum in the remainder.

Investigations

Clinically, AFLP is a disease that presents with symptoms and signs of general liver dysfunction and often required the exclusion of other causes. The Swansea criteria (Box 37.1) have been shown to be useful in making a diagnosis of AFLP without resorting to liver biopsy, which carries risks of morbidity and mortality.

There is often a cross-over with the features of HELLP (Table 37.4). Two of the most distinctive features of AFLP are profound hypoglycemia and hyperuricemia, which is more marked than the presenting pre-eclamptic features. In the 2006–2008 UK Confidential Enquiries into Maternal Deaths and Child Health report, one case had unexpected histological findings of AFLP with clinical features of pre-eclampsia [10]. This was also the finding in one of the patients reviewed by Castro et al.[8], who had a liver biopsy because of uncertain diagnosis.

Table 37.5 give the laboratory tests that will help in diagnosis.

Management

The general principles of management of AFLP include:

- multidisciplinary input (obstetric, anaesthesia, hepatology, haematology, neonatal team, critical care)
- maternal monitoring and one-to-one nursing by a midwife qualified for high dependency care
- monitoring the fetus
- plan for delivery with aggressive treatment of hypoglycemia and coagulopathy prior to delivery
- high dependency care
- admission to ICU in severe AFLP
- transfer to liver unit if there is fulminant liver failure
- postnatal thromboprophylaxis.

Timing and method of delivery

Early delivery is indicated to improve prognosis for mother and baby. Most case series show delivery is usually within 4 days of presentation. In addition,

Table 37.4. Differential diagnosis of HELLP syndrome and acute fatty liver of pregnancy

Symptoms/presentation	HELLP	Acute fatty liver of pregnancy
Epigastric pain	++	+
Vomiting	+/−	++
Hypertension	++	+
Proteinuria	++	+
Elevated liver enzymes	+	++
Hypoglycemia	+/−	++
Hyperuricemia	+	++
Elevated creatinine	+/−	+
Disseminated intravascular coagulation	+	++
Thrombocytopenia (without disseminated intravascular coagulation)	++	+/−
Raised white blood cell count	+	++
Ultrasound/CT	Normal/hepatic hematoma	Normal/echobright liver/ascites
Multiple pregnancy	−	+
Primiparous	++	+
Male fetus	50%	70% (M:F, 3:1)

Source: adapted from Nelson-Piercy, 2006 [11].

Table 37.5. Laboratory tests

	Test	Possibly identified
Essential investigations		
Tests of diagnostic value	Full blood count, urea and electrolytes, ammonia, clotting studies, blood glucose, liver transaminases, bilirubin	Leukocytosis, renal impairment, coagulopathy (often in presence of platelet count >100 × 10^9/L), hypoglycemia
Tests required to exclude other pathology	C-reactive protein, septic screen and viral serology, urinalysis	Hepatitis B,C E viruses, cytomegalovirus, proteinuria
Abdominal ultrasound	May show echobright liver and/or ascites	Only seen in about one third of patients with AFLP; useful for excluding obstructive causes of jaundice (e.g. gallstones)
Possible further investigations		
CT	Limited role antenatally	May pick up fatty infiltration not seen on ultrasound
MRI	No evidence of diagnostic benefit	
Liver biopsy	AFLP is characterized by microvesicular fatty infiltration (steatosis)	Considered in the past as gold standard for diagnosis but not without risks; often not done because of associated coagulopathy and should only be considered if there is diagnostic uncertainty

- coagulopathy may influence urgency and mode of delivery
- delivery should ideally be planned in advance with appropriate monitoring *in situ* and senior staff available
- the least traumatic mode of delivery should be aimed for to reduce the risk of tissue trauma and subsequent bleeding
- the need for clotting factor replacement should be anticipated and pre-empted if surgery is anticipated in patients with coagulopathy
- induction of labor may be considered.
- cesarean section is often performed for fetal distress, which may be acute.

Anesthesia

Anesthesia requirements for labor or cesarean section include:

- regional anesthesia
- general anesthesia
- uterotonics
- non-steroidal anti-inflammatory drugs (NSAIDs).

Box 37.2 provides the key points for anesthesia in AFLP.

Anesthesia for labor

When considering labor analgesia for patients with AFLP, the anesthesiologist should be aware that the patient may have impaired metabolic activity, which

> **Box 37.2. Key points for anesthesia in acute fatty liver of pregnancy**
>
> - AFLP is often associated with metabolic impairment and severe coagulopathy and the condition is unpredictable
> - Large-bore intravenous access should be obtained
> - Cross-matched blood should be immediately available
> - Neuraxial anesthesia should only be performed if hemostasis is unimpaired or carefully corrected; however, coagulation may deteriorate rapidly
> - Remifentanil patient-controlled analgesia is the preferred alternative for labor analgesia
> - The half-life of amide type local anesthetics may be significantly prolonged
> - General anesthesia may contribute to neurological deterioration in the postoperative period; documentation of mental status before and after general anesthesia is crucial
> - Postoperative analgesia may be complicated by impaired renal and hepatic function

may quickly progress to liver failure. Special attention should be paid to the often severe coagulopathic state. A prolonged prothrombin time is an early feature of AFLP, often followed by thrombocytopenia. Furthermore, AFLP is often complicated by disseminated intravascular coagulation (DIC) and significant antithrombin III deficiency [12]. Epidural or combined spinal–epidural analgesia may be safe if hemostasis is unimpaired or has been carefully corrected; however, it is important to keep in mind that coagulation may deteriorate rapidly. In addition, patients with severe hepatic failure may have increased intracranial pressure secondary to cerebral edema. The incidence of this life-threatening complication in patients with AFLP of pregnancy is unknown, and careful neurological monitoring is essential. Alternatives for neuraxial analgesia include patient-controlled analgesia with parenteral opioids. However, clearance of most opioids, apart from remifentanil, may be significantly delayed in patients with AFLP. Remifentanil is rapidly metabolized by non-specific plasma esterases and is, therefore, the preferred choice for patients with severe liver disease. The anesthesiologist should anticipate postpartum hemorrhage for any parturient with AFLP. Adequate intravenous access should be secured and cross-matched blood should be immediately available. Profound hypoglycemia, resulting from impaired gluconeogenesis and glycogenolysis, is a very common feature of AFLP. Glucose levels should be checked frequently.

Anesthesia for cesarean delivery

Although cesarean delivery offers no clear advantage over expeditious vaginal delivery, many patients with AFLP will undergo cesarean delivery, most often dictated by rapid maternal deterioration and/or fetal distress. When considering anesthetic options for cesarean delivery in patients with AFLP, it is important to balance the potential negative effect of general anesthesia on hepatic encephalopathy against the risks associated with regional anesthesia in the setting of coagulopathy.

Regional anesthesia

Cesarean delivery may be complicated by hemorrhage secondary to coagulopathy and large-bore intravenous access should be obtained.

Because AFLP is an unpredictable condition and hepatic function may deteriorate quickly with development of severe coagulopathy, many anesthesiologists avoid regional anesthesia in all but the mildest cases.

Neuraxial anesthesia may reduce hepatic blood flow, but the impact of this on the course of AFLP is unknown [13].

Amide type local anesthetics undergo hepatic biotransformation and their half-life may be significantly prolonged [14].

Patients may require transfusions and administration of fresh frozen plasma or cryoprecipitate.

General anesthesia

General anesthesia is frequently preferred for patients with AFLP, given the often severe coagulopathy. If general anesthesia is employed, neurological deterioration in the postoperative period may be caused by the residual effects of anesthetic agents, progressive encephalopathy, or raised intracranial pressure. Documentation of the mental status before and after a general anesthetic is crucial.

Volatile anesthetic agents with faster washout times, such as sevoflurane or desflurane, may be preferable. Volatile anesthetics decrease hepatic oxygen delivery, but the relevance of this to AFLP is not known. Frink et al. [15] found that hepatic oxygen delivery was reduced to the following levels of control at 1.0 minimum alveolar concentration: 86% by sevoflurane, 81% by isoflurane, 57% by enflurane, and 57% by halothane. Kanaya et al. [16] confirmed that isoflurane has a more favorable effect than halothane on liver perfusion.

Gentle laryngoscopy with direct visualization of the airway during profound neuromuscular blockade is key in minimizing airway trauma and bleeding. Succinylcholine is still recommended as the muscle relaxant for rapid sequence induction, despite the reduced levels of plasma cholinesterase in pregnancy and hepatic disease. Remifentanil, as discussed above, is eliminated independently of hepatic function. It can be used as an initial dose to prevent hemodynamic responses to intubation.

Postoperative analgesia may also be complicated by impaired renal and hepatic function.

Use of uterotonics

Occurrence of AFLP is not a contraindication to uterotonic drugs, and it is important to treat uterine atony promptly. However ergometrine should be used with caution particularly if the patient has associated hypertension.

Non steroidal anti-inflammatory drugs

Because of the link between AFLP and Reyes syndrome in children and the epidemiological evidence linking aspirin taken during viral illness in children as a precipitating cause of Reyes syndrome, it has been suggested that NSAIDs should be avoided in pregnancy. The theory is that aspirin-like medications inhibit residual long-chain fatty acid oxidation and so could trigger AFLP in a susceptible woman. Because of the risk to the fetus of reduced renal function and premature closure of the ductus arteriosus in the third trimester, NSAIDs are now rarely used during pregnancy. Although NSAIDs are only used in exceptional circumstances during pregnancy, they are commonly used postnatally. It would seem prudent to avoid their use in any women with suspected AFLP even if there is no evidence of coagulopathy or renal impairment.

Management of coagulopathy

Disseminated intravascular coagulation may develop antenatally and may only be recognized on laboratory tests [2,8]. Morbidity from AFLP is often related to severe coagulopathy and the need for repeated surgery to control postpartum bleeding [11]. It is, therefore, important to recognize and treat coagulopathy prior to any planned surgery and anticipate that clotting factors may be needed when vaginal delivery is planned. Clinical bleeding in AFLP is usually associated with cesarean delivery, uterine atony, and genital tract trauma [8]. Castro and colleagues [8] advised aiming for the least traumatic mode of delivery by avoiding episiotomy if possible and using less sharp dissection at cesarean section, essentially advocating a Cohen type entry technique. In their case series of 28 patients, they concluded that if delivery is atraumatic then coagulopathy may not need to be treated.

During labor and in the immediate postnatal period, it is advisable to assess prothrombin times every 6 hours [17].

In AFLP, DIC is associated with anti thrombin III deficiency, and so anti thrombin III infusions have been tried to reverse DIC in patients with AFLP, but no clinical benefit was found in a small case series [18].

It is important to treat DIC in the presence of clinical bleeding aggressively under the guidance of the hematologist. Close liaison with the hematology laboratory is required as multiple blood products providing clotting factors may be needed. Fresh frozen plasma contains all clotting factors required to replace consumed clotting factors and, in particular, contains antithrombin III; however, cryoprecipitate may also be required if a consumptive coagulopathy develops as this will provide more fibrinogen [19]. Ward-based devices that test and measure clot strength and function may be useful to provide timely information to guide clotting factor replacement.

Management of hypoglycemia

Hypoglycemia results from reduced vasopressinase degradation in the dysfunctional liver; this significantly increases circulating concentrations of vasopressinase and consequently increases clearance of antidiruetic hormone, leading to a diabetic insipidus effect. In suspected AFLP, it is imported to check for and aggressively treat hypoglycemia. Two hourly glucose assessments should be made. Infusions of 10% dextrose may not be adequate, and hypoglycemia often requires infusions of large volumes of high concentration (50%) glucose via a long line [17].

Management of multiorgan dysfunction syndrome

Patients who develop severe AFLP are at risk of developing dysfunction in multiple organs: liver, kidneys, pancreas.

The multiple organ dysfunction syndrome can be defined as the development of potentially reversible physiological derangement involving two or more organ systems not involved in the disorder that resulted in ICU admission, and arising in the wake of a potentially life-threatening physiological insult [20].

Renal and respiratory failure as well as liver failure, encephalopathy and coagulopathies are seen in AFLP. There are also several case reports of associated pancreatitis. Patients who develop multiorgan dysfunction should be managed in an advanced critical care setting with multidisciplinary input [17] to facilitate appropriate supportive measures.

Management of severe liver dysfunction

Early liaison with hepatologists is advised. Early communication with the nearest liver transplant unit may be advisable, particularly if no hepatologist available locally. This is to provide expert advice on investigations and management and to facilitate transfer and notification of the transplant team if required after delivery [17].

The majority of women will recover very quickly following delivery. Women who develop fulminant hepatic failure and encephalopathy require transfer to a specialist liver unit.

Management of renal failure

Acute renal necrosis has been associated with women who have sustained major hemorrhage [8]. It is likely that hypotension associated with hemorrhage aggravates existing renal impairment. Women who develop renal failure will require optimal fluid resuscitation guided by invasive monitoring in conjunction with treatment for associated morbidity [21]. Nephrology input may be needed. Generally, renal function recovers with supportive measures but temporary dialysis is sometimes needed [4,8,21].

Plasmaphoresis or plasma exchange has been used in specialist centers to allow time for cellular regeneration in women who were developing renal failure as a result of severe AFLP [22]. One case report describes using a molecular absorbent recirculatory system to reduce the amount of albumin-bound toxins in a patient affected by AFLP [23].

Management of pancreatitis

Several patients with severe AFLP have developed pancreatitis. This is thought to be inflammatory in nature and is reversible [8]. Resulting hyperglycemia can require treatment with insulin infusions.

Liver transplantation

The majority of patients will recover completely with supportive measures following delivery. There has been recent success with the use of plasma exchange. Liver transplant may be required in women with severe liver failure and for those who show signs of irreversible liver failure despite delivery and intensive supportive care. There are no reliable data for survival in transplanted patients. In the UKOSS AFLP data, only one patient who received a transplant subsequently died [4].

Thromboprophylaxis

The risk of bleeding and of venous thromboembolism needs to be balanced. Once coagulopathy has corrected, then prophylactic anticoagulation with low-molecular-weight heparin needs to be considered on a case-by-case basis.

Neonatal follow-up

The risk of the fetus carrying an *MTP* mutation and leading to LCHAD deficiency in one study of 27 women affected by AFLP was 1 in 5 [24]. It would seem reasonable to screen all babies born to mothers with AFLP for MTP mutations. This would allow affected babies to have the correct dietary restrictions to minimize the risk of metabolic dysfunction. It also allows mothers to seek genetic counseling and prenatal diagnosis [7].

Prognosis

Over the last 50 years, case fatality rates have fallen drastically: from 70% in the 1960s down to 1.8% in the UKOSS study [4]. Following recovery from AFLP, maternal prognosis is excellent. Perinatal mortality rates have also fallen (104 per 1000 still births and live births) but still remain more than 10 times higher than the back ground population (8 per 1000 in 2006) [4].

Subsequent pregnancies

It is difficult to give a precise figure regarding incidence of AFLP in a future pregnancy. In early studies, there was a high rate of maternal mortality and of those who did survive few went on to have further babies. There have been case reports of recurrent AFLP but also of women who have gone on to have a subsequent normal pregnancy. However, if the baby is found to have LCHAD deficiency the rate of developing AFLP in a subsequent pregnancy with the same partner could be as high as 25% [7]. If the baby does not have AFLP then recurrence is hard to predict.

Key learning points

1. AFLP is a very rare cause of liver dysfunction presenting in the third trimester.
2. Patients commonly present with nausea, vomiting, abdominal pain, and prodromal illness.
3. AFLP may be related to the spectrum of pre-eclamptic diseases.
4. Diagnostic features include hypoglycemia and hyperuricemia out of proportion to pre-eclamptic features.
5. Early delivery improves maternal and neonatal outcome.
6. Management requires multidisciplinary input and clear plans should be developed for delivery as fetal distress is the commonest reason for cesarean delivery.

7. Coagulopathy is common; clinical bleeding is related to tissue trauma and uterine atony.
8. Mode of delivery should be the least traumatic to the mother, induction of labor may be considered.
9. Large-bore intravenous access should be obtained in all patients and cross-matched blood should be immediately available.
10. Neuraxial anesthesia should only be performed if hemostasis is unimpaired or carefully corrected; coagulation may deteriorate rapidly.
11. AFLP is often associated with encephalopathy and careful neurological monitoring is essential.
12. General anesthesia is frequently preferred for cesarean delivery but documenting mental status before and after a general anesthetic is crucial.
13. Profound hypoglycemia is a very common feature of AFLP and glucose levels should be checked frequently.
14. Care should be one to one in an obstetric high dependency unit HDU; transfer to ICU is needed in 60% after delivery.
15. Multidisciplinary supportive care is needed until recovery of organ function.
16. Prompt transfer to specialist liver units is required if there is fulminant hepatic failure and hepatic encephalopathy.
17. Hepatic function will normally recover fully after delivery.

References

1. Sheehan HL. The pathology of acute yellow atrophy and delayed chloroform poisoning. *J Obstet Gynecol* 1940;**47**:49–62.

2. Castro MA, Goodwin TM, Shaw KJ, Ouzounian JG, McGehee WG. Disseminated intravascular coagulation and antithrombin III depression in acute fatty liver of pregnancy. *Am J Obstet Gynecol* 1996;**174**:211–216.

3. Dekker RR, Schutte JM, Stekelenburg J, Zwart JJ, van Roosmalen J. Maternal mortality and severe maternal morbidity from acute fatty liver of pregnancy in the Netherlands. *Eur J Obstet Gynecol Reprod Biol* 2011;**157**:27–31.

4. Knight M, Nelson-Piercy C, Kurinczuk JJ, Spark P, Brocklehurst P. UK Obstetric Surveillance System. A prospective national study of acute fatty liver of pregnancy in the UK. *Gut* 2008;**57**:951–956.

5. Sims HF, Brackett JC, Powell CK, *et al.* The molecular basis of pediatric long chain 3-hydroxyacyl-CoA dehydrogenase deficiency associated with maternal acute fatty liver of pregnancy. *Proc Natl Acad Sci USA* 1995;**92**:841–845.

6. Treem WR, Shoup ME, Hale DE, *et al.* Acute fatty liver of pregnancy, hemolysis, elevated liver enzymes, and low platelets syndrome, and long chain 3-hydroxyacyl-coenzyme A dehydrogenase deficiency. *Am J Gastroenterol* 1996;**91**:2293–2300.

7. Ibdah JA. Acute fatty liver of pregnancy: an update on pathogenesis and clinical implications. *World J Gastroenterol* 2006;**12**:7397–7404.

8. Castro MA, Fassett MJ, Reynolds TB, Shaw KJ, Goodwin TM. Reversible peripartum liver failure: a new perspective on the diagnosis, treatment, and cause of acute fatty liver of pregnancy, based on 28 consecutive cases. *Am J Obstet Gynecol* 1999;**181**:389–395.

9. Ch'ng CL, Morgan M, Hainsworth I, *et al.* Prospective study of liver dysfunction in pregnancy in Southwest Wales. *Gut* 2002;**51**:876–880.

10. Cantwell R, Clutton-Brock T, Cooper G, *et al.* Saving Mothers' Lives: Reviewing Maternal Deaths to make Motherhood Safer 2006–2008. The Eighth Report of the Confidential Enquiries into Maternal Deaths in the United Kingdom. *BJOG* 2011;**118**(Suppl 1):1–203.

11. Nelson-Piercy C. *Handbook of Obstetric Medicine*, 3rd edn, Ch. 11: Liver disease. London: Informa Healthcare, 2006.

12. Knox TA, Olans LB. Liver disease in pregnancy. *N Engl J Med* 1996;**335**:569–576.

13. Kenedy WF Jr. Effects of spinal and peridural blocks on renal and hepatic functions. *Clin Anesth* 1969;**2**:109–121.

14. Thomson PD, Melmon KL, Richardson JA, *et al.* Lidocaine pharmacokinetics in advanced heart failure, liver disease and renal failure in humans. *Ann Intern Med* 1973;**78**:499–508.

15. Frink EJ Jr., Morgan SE, Coetzee A, Conzen PF, Brown PR Jr. The effects of sevoflurane, halothane, enflurane and isoflurane on hepatic blood flow and oxygenation in chronically instrumented greyhound dogs. *Anesthesiology* 1992;**76**:85–90.

16. Kanaya N, Iwasaki H, Namiki A. Noninvasive ICG clearance test for estimating hepatic blood flow during halothane and isoflurane anaesthesia. *Can J Anaesth* 1995;**42**:209–212.

17. Williamson C, Girling J. Hepatic and gastrointestinal disease. In James DK, Steer PJ, Weiner CP, Gonk B (eds.) *High Risk Pregnancy, Management Options*, 3rd edn. Philadelphia, PA: Elsevier-Saunders, 2006, pp. 1511–1550.

18. Castro MA, Ouzounian JG, Colletti PM, *et al.* Radiologic studies in acute fatty liver of pregnancy. A review of the literature and 19 new cases. *J Reprod Med* 1996;**41**:839–843.

19. Johansen R, Cox C, Grady K, Howell C. *Managing Obstetric Emergencies and Trauma, The MOET Course Manual*, Ch. 16: Massive obstetric haemorrhage. London: RCOG Press, 2003.

20. Marshall JC. The multiple organ dysfunction syndrome. In Holzheimer RG, Mannick JA (eds.) *Surgical Treatment: Evidence Based and Problem-Oriented*. Munich: Zuckschwerdt, 2001.

21. Williams D. Renal disease. In James DK, Steer PJ, Weiner CP, Gonk B (eds.) *High Risk Pregnancy, Management Options*, 3rd edn. Philadelphia, PA: Elsevier-Saunders, 2006, pp. 1098–1124.

22. Martin JN Jr., Briery CM, Rose CH, *et al.* Postpartum plasma exchange as adjunctive therapy for severe acute fatty liver of pregnancy. *J Clin Apher* 2008;**234**:138–143.

23. de Naeyer S, Ysebaert D, van Utterbeeck M, *et al.* Acute fatty liver of pregnancy and molecular absorbent recirculating system (MARS)-therapy: a case report. *J Matern Fetal Neonatal Med* 2008;**21**:587–589.

24. Yang Z, Yamada J, Zhao Y, Strauss AW, Ibdah JA. Prospective screening for pediatric mitochondrial trifunctional protein defects in pregnancies complicated by liver disease. *JAMA* 2002;**288**:2163–2166.

Chapter 38

Peripartum cardiomyopathy

Michelle Walters, Marc Van de Velde, Steven Dymarkowski, and Helen Scholefield

Introduction

Peripartum cardiomyopathy (PPCM) is a rare and potentially fatal cause of left ventricular heart failure that occurs during pregnancy or postpartum. Patients have no pre-existing cardiac pathology and no other causes of heart failure are identified. It is a diagnosis of exclusion. Peripartum cardiomyopathy differs from other dilated cardiomyopathies and should not be confused with idiopathic dilated cardiomyopathy caused by relative volume overload and presenting in pregnancy.

Diagnosis of PPCM is often delayed as the clinical features of the disease can overlap with normal physiological signs of pregnancy or with other complications of pregnancy, for example pre-eclampsia. Management of PPCM requires prompt multidisciplinary care in order to minimize morbidity and mortality associated with the disease. Outcome varies from complete recovery of left ventricular function to persistent ventricular dysfunction requiring heart transplantation or leading to death.

Epidemiology

The true incidence of PPCM is not known. Reported incidences vary geographically. The USA estimates PPCM to occur in 1 in 3000–4000 live births; however, smaller case series suggest higher incidences in South Africa (1 in 1000) and Haiti (1 in 300) [1–3]. Differences in study design, the use of different diagnostic criteria, and difficulties excluding other causes of heart failure may explain some of the geographical variation seen.

Patient risk factors may be advanced maternal age, multiparity, multiple pregnancy, and African or African-American race. Pre-eclampsia and gestational hypertension are also associated with PPCM. High incidences of PPCM in specific communities and familial clustering suggest a genetic or environmental predisposition [1,4,5].

Etiology

Many mechanisms for the development of PPCM have been proposed (Table 38.1) [6–10]. Multifactorial causes and a genetic susceptibility are likely. Recent research suggests apoptotic or defective antioxidative defence mechanisms may be responsible for the development of PPCM [6].

Diagnosis and definitions

Peripartum cardiomyopathy is a form of cardiac failure secondary to left ventricular systolic dysfunction. It is clinically difficult to distinguish from other types of cardiac failure and consequently remains a diagnosis of exclusion (see Table 38.2 for differential diagnosis). Patients with pre-existing cardiac pathology tend to decompensate during the second trimester when the hemodynamic changes of pregnancy are at a maximum. In patients with PPCM this is not the case; they most often (but not exclusively) present in the third trimester or postpartum.

The initial diagnosis can be delayed as the signs and symptoms of cardiac failure can be confused with normal physiological changes occurring in pregnancy. Delay in diagnosis may lead to a poor outcome. The Confidential Enquiries into Maternal and Child Health in the UK from for the period 2003–2005 reported 12 late deaths from PPCM [11]. In many, the diagnosis had not been made early enough and appropriate treatment was delayed. The following triennium 2006–2008 reported 15 probable deaths from PPCM, six of these women dying several weeks after delivery [12]. Commonly the signs and symptoms of pulmonary edema were wrongly attributed to other causes of breathlessness and inadequately investigated.

Diagnostic criteria for PPCM were first established by Demakis and Rahimtoola in 1971 [13] and have since

Maternal Critical Care: A Multidisciplinary Approach, ed. Marc Van de Velde, Helen Scholefield, and Lauren A. Plante. Published by Cambridge University Press. © Cambridge University Press 2013.

Table 38.1. Pathophysiological theories for peripartum cardiomyopathy

Etiology	Evidence	Potential therapy
Abnormal maternal autoimmune response	High circulating titers of autoantibodies against selective cardiac tissue proteins [7]	Immunosuppression
Inflammatory or viral myocarditis	Lymphocytic infiltrate on endomyocardial biopsy [8]	Anti-inflammatory agents; immunoglobulin therapy
	Elevated serum C-reactive protein, interleukins, and tumor necrosis factor-alpha [9]	
Oxidative stress.	Pregnancy-induced oxidative stress triggering prolactin cleavage; the resulting derivative exhibits cardiotoxicity and apoptotic actions [6]	Prolactin suppression with dopamine D_2-receptor antagonist bromocriptine [10]

Table 38.2. Differential diagnosis of peripartum cardiomyopathy

	Disorders
Complications of pregnancy	Massive pulmonary embolism Amniotic fluid embolism Severe pre-eclampsia or HELLP syndrome
Cardiac disorder	Hypertensive heart disease Myocardial ischemia Congenital heart disease Valvular disease Pre-existing idiopathic or familial dilated cardiomyopathy Restrictive or hypertrophic cardiomyopathy Volume overload Diastolic dysfunction
Respiratory	Pulmonary embolism Lower respiratory tract infection
Infection	Sepsis Acquired immunodeficiency syndrome cardiomyopathy Viral, bacterial, or fungal cardiomyopathy
Metabolic/toxic	Thyroid disease Selenium, thiamine, or phosphate disturbance Alcoholic cardiomyopathy Cocaine abuse
Systemic disease	Sarcoidosis Systemic lupus erythematosus

HELLP, hemolysis, elevated liver enzymes, and low platelets.

been adapted to include echocardiographic evidence of new left ventricular systolic dysfunction (Box 38.1) [1,13].

More recently, an alternative classification has been proposed in order to reduce underdiagnosis. This includes women with PPCM who present outside of the time period set by the original classification (Box 38.1) [14].

Clinical features

Presentation of PPCM is typically with signs and symptoms of acute cardiac failure towards the end of pregnancy or postpartum (Table 38.3).

Investigations

Investigations are required to exclude alternative causes of heart failure and assess disease severity (Table 38.4) [14,15]. No investigation has successfully been used as a prognostic tool or as a predictor of outcome. Following discharge, investigations should be repeated regularly to assess recovery of left ventricular function. Cardiovascular MRI can demonstrate PPCM (Figure 38.1).

Management

General management principles are:

- multidisciplinary care (obstetrics, cardiology, anesthesia, neonatology, critical care)
- early diagnosis and treatment
- a clear plan for delivery, potential obstetric emergencies, and acute clinical decompensation
- medication decisions, which may be influenced by pregnancy or breastfeeding; however, in critically ill women, maternal well-being over-rides that of the fetus and the most optimal therapy is used
- medical management principles similar to those of other causes of heart failure
- reduce preload to reduce circulatory overload and pulmonary congestion
- reduce afterload to reduce myocardial work and improve cardiac output
- improve contractility as required
- invasive monitoring may be necessary to assess hemodynamic status and guide management
- intensive care admission in severe cases
- thromboprophylaxis.

429

> **Box 38.1.** Diagnostic criteria for peripartum cardiomyopathy
>
> **US National Institutes of Health**
> - New-onset cardiac failure in last months of pregnancy or in the 5 months following delivery
> - Absence of another determinable cause for the cardiac failure
> - Absence of pre-existing heart disease prior to the last months of pregnancy
> - Left ventricular systolic dysfunction demonstrated on echocardiography, such as depressed ejection fraction and/or M-mode fractional shortening
>
> *Source*: US National Institutes of Health, 2000 [1]
>
> **European Society of Cardiology**
> - Idiopathic cardiomyopathy, diagnosis of exclusion
> - Heart failure secondary to left ventricular systolic dysfunction
> - Presents towards end of pregnancy or in the months following delivery
> - Left ventricle may not be dilated, but ejection fraction nearly always reduced to 45%
>
> *Source*: European Society of Cardiology Working Group on PPCM, 2010 [14]

Table 38.3. Signs and symptoms of peripartum cardiomyopathy

	Signs and symptoms
Cardiac	Tachycardia, arrhythmias, palpitations, normal or raised blood pressure, low blood pressure in late disease with low cardiac output state, displaced apex beat, gallop rhythm, third heart sound, edema, elevated jugular venous pressure, precordial discomfort, hemoptysis, increased pulmonary capillary wedge pressure, new murmurs consistent with atrioventricular regurgitation, sudden cardiac arrest
Vaculature: peripheral emboli	Acute limb or bowel ischemia, cerebral vascular accident.
Respiratory	Exertional dyspnea, orthopnea, paroxysmal nocturnal dyspnea, cough, tachypnea, oxygen desaturation, crepitations and crackles on lung auscultation
Abdominal	Hepatosplenomegaly, abdominal discomfort secondary to organ congestion
Neurological	Dizziness, fatigue

Obstetric management

Only a small proportion of women with PPCM will be diagnosed antenatally. Uteroplacental perfusion may be compromised either by the cardiomyopathy or by drug therapy, and ongoing fetal surveillance is indicated in the form of fetal growth assessment and cardiotocography.

Elective preterm or early delivery is not associated with improvement in maternal clinical status or ventricular function. However, in cases of decompensated heart failure or to allow advanced or novel therapies, delivery may simplify maternal management.

With either induced or spontaneous labor, early analgesia is desirable and a prolonged second stage should be avoided. The preferred delivery method is vaginal unless other factors preclude. Labor and delivery should be conducted in a setting in which appropriate staffing and resources are available, both personnel and technological. Attempts should be made to minimize hemodynamic derangements in the process.

After delivery of the neonate and placenta, preload increases (autotransfusion once the placental circulation is abolished) and the risk of pulmonary edema is particularly high. Judicious diuretics may be administered at this time.

Uterotonic drugs are administered after delivery of the placenta in order to decrease the potential for hemorrhage, or treat hemorrhage once it occurs. These drugs, however, must be used with caution in PPCM. High or bolus doses of oxytocin given intravenously can precipitate hypotension or arrhythmias and should, therefore, be avoided. The drug should be given instead as a slow intravenous infusion or as an intramuscular injection. Ergot drugs (methylergonovine, ergometrine) should be avoided in all patients with cardiac dysfunction because they provoke vasoconstriction and can produce hypertension, myocardial ischemia, and pulmonary edema. The F-series prostaglandins (e.g. carboprost, tromethamine) are best avoided because of the potential for vasoconstriction. The E-series prostaglandins, however (e.g. misoprostol), may be used with awareness of their tendency to cause vasodilation.

When treating hemorrhage caused by atony in a patient with PPCM, the obstetrician may proceed sooner to mechanical methods such as uterine balloon or hemostatic suturing, simply because the options for medical therapy are limited. Box 38.2 gives the key points of obstetric management.

Table 38.4. Investigations in peripartum cardiomyopathy

	Tests	Possible significance
Essential tests		
Exclusion of other pathology	Full blood count, urea and electrolytes, clotting studies, C-reactive protein, blood glucose, cardiac enzymes, lactate, liver transaminases, D-dimers	
	Septic screen and viral serology	Infectious etiology
	Urinalysis	Pre-eclampsia may occur in conjunction with PPCM)
	Arterial blood gas sample	Evaluation oxygenation
	Plasma B-type natriuretic peptide or *N*-terminal pro-B-type natriuretic peptide	Released from the myocardium in response to raised left ventricular end-diastolic pressures; found to be elevated in patients with PPCM [14]
Evaluation of pulmonary congestion	Chest radiograph	Cardiomegaly, pulmonary edema, pleural effusions, increased pulmonary vascularity, basal infiltrates
Evaluation of heart function	Electrocardiography; changes are common but mostly non-specific for PPCM	Sinus tachycardia, arrhythmias, atrial fibrillation, ST or T wave abnormalities, axis deviation, intraventricular block patterns, left ventricular hypertrophy Changes may remain after treatment [14,15]
Diagnosis and monitoring	Echocardiography is essential for diagnosis, assessing disease severity, response to treatment, monitoring recovery	Excludes thrombus in either ventricles or atria particularly left ventricular thrombus, assesses systolic ventricular function, ejection fraction, fractional shortening, ventricular dilatation, valvular dysfunction, left ventricular hypertrophy Estimate pulmonary artery pressures to aid excluding pulmonary embolus
Further investigations to consider		
Differential diagnosis and monitoring recovery	Cardiovascular MRI (Figure 38.1)	Non-invasive reference technique that accurately measures left ventricular function and dimensions Higher specificity for detecting left ventricular thrombus than with echocardiography [16] No pattern exclusive to PPCM. Specific MRI enhancement techniques can be used to differentiate pathologies, e.g. myocardial fibrosis, myocarditis, myocardial infarction
Identification of cellular changes, lymphocytic myocarditis	Endomyocardial biopsy	Controversial invasive procedure with relatively high complication rate; rationale is in order to commence immunosuppressive therapy, although sensitivity of biopsies for myocarditis is at best 50% [17] Usually reserved for patients awaiting cardiac transplantation or those failing to improve despite maximum medical therapy

PPCM, peripartum cardiomyopathy.

Anaesthetic management

Regional anesthesia

Regional anesthesia may be performed for labor analgesia or cesarean delivery. In labor, early analgesia is recommended to minimize the hemodynamic stress associated with labor pain and to reduce the risk of acute maternal decompensation. The sympathectomy induced by regional anesthesia causes a fall in systemic vascular resistance, which in moderation can improve ventricular function. Both epidural and combined spinal–epidural techniques are safe when used

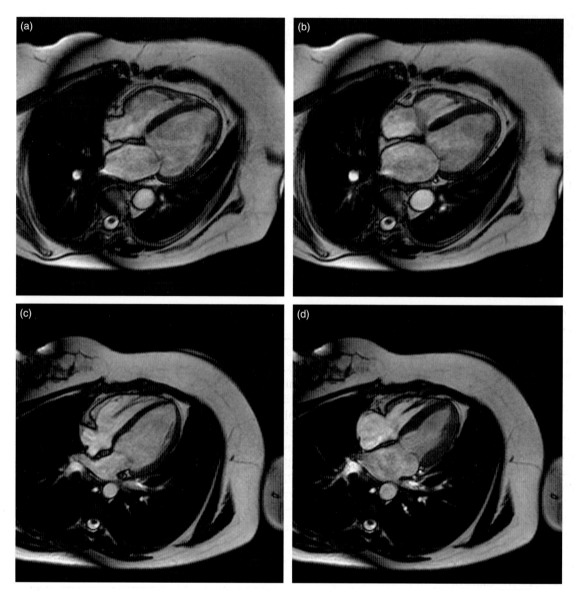

Figure 38.1. Peripartum cardiomyopathy. Computed tomography in a 32-year-old woman 4 weeks after delivery who presented with protracted disproportionate fatigue and dyspnea. Horizontal long axis images at end-diastole (a) and at end-systole (b) show ventricular dilatation and strong decrease in contractile function. There was no specific enhancement pattern on the postcontrast images (not shown). Similar images in age-matched volunteer (c,d) for comparison.

cautiously. The anesthetic block should be titrated incrementally in order to maintain hemodynamic stability and prevent rapid reductions in systemic vascular resistance and preload. Single-shot spinal techniques are avoided because they potentially can cause dramatic falls in systemic vascular resistance. Even small doses of intrathecal local anesthetic have been associated with severe hypotension in patients with PPCM.

Large-bore intravenous access is essential and invasive arterial blood pressure monitoring may be needed,

depending on severity. Fluid preload or concurrent load should be avoided if congestive cardiac failure is present. Vasopressors may be necessary and pure alpha-agonists (e.g. phenylephrine) should be used in preference to mixed alpha- and beta-adrenergic agonists in order to avoid tachycardia.

General anesthesia

Traditionally, general anesthesia was considered the technique of choice for cesarean delivery in high-risk

> **Box 38.2.** Key points in obstetric management of peripartum cardiomyopathy
>
> - Develop a plan for the delivery
> - Regional pathways for multidisciplinary management are useful with clear lines of communication and escalation to specialist centers at the appropriate time
> - Early delivery does not improve outcome but may be necessary for appropriate management
> - Vaginal delivery is preferred, consider instrumental
> - Early labor analgesia
> - Minimize hemodynamic derangements
> - Beware of increase in preload after autotransfusion
> - Caution with the hemodynamic effects uterotonic drugs

> **Box 38.3.** Key points in anesthetic management of peripartum cardiomyopathy
>
> - Avoid rapid changes in hemodynamic status
> - Early labor analgesia is recommended to reduce cardiovascular stress
> - Regional anesthesia may be an appropriate alternative to general anesthesia for cesarean section
> - Use gradual incremental techniques, e.g. epidural or combined spinal–epidural
> - Avoid single-shot spinal agent
> - Invasive monitoring can guide fluid and vasopressor management
> - Consult a cardiac anesthesiologist
> - Beware of the cardiac depressant effect of general anesthetic agents and use a modified rapid sequence and cardiac anesthetic techniques

parturients with cardiac dysfunction. The risk of hemodynamic instability at induction has led increasingly to regional anesthesia becoming an appropriate alternative, assuming that cardiovascular stability can be preserved. General anesthesia may still be required because of acute maternal cardiorespiratory decompensation or fetal emergencies. Cardiovascular collapse at induction of general anesthesia has been reported in women with undiagnosed PPCM and suggests a need for modification to standard anesthetic techniques. A modified rapid sequence induction is recommended, using a "cardiac anesthetic" technique, with high doses of opioids to avoid precipitant drops in systemic vascular resistance. Anesthetic agents with myocardial depressant effects are best avoided. Cardiac anesthesiologists should be consulted and pediatricians made aware of opioid administration. Invasive pressure monitoring and transesophageal echocardiography can be used perioperatively to optimize the cardiovascular status. Box 38.3 gives the key points in anesthetic management.

Management of secondary heart failure

Managing heart failure in PPCM follows the same principles as treating heart failure from other causes, and the reader should be guided by available guidelines [18]. Treatment goals are to relieve pulmonary congestion, reduce preload and afterload, increase contractility, and improve outcome by encouraging left ventricular remodeling and recovery.

During pregnancy, it is necessary to consider the effects of hemodynamic therapy on uterine blood flow;

cardiotocography may be useful to ascertain these effects. Some medications for heart failure may be contraindicated in pregnancy or breastfeeding. An alternative is usually available, such as angiotensin-converting enzyme inhibitors, or angiotensin receptor blockers can be substituted with nitrates or hydralazine. In all cases, the most optimal therapy should be used regardless of the pregnancy, and fortunately dilemmas are infrequent as critically ill patients with PPCM are more likely to have an expedited delivery or be already postpartum. Boxes 38.4 and 38.5 give the management of acute decompensated heart failure and chronic stable heart failure, respectively.

Thromboprophylaxis

Occurrence of PPCM increases the risk of cardiac thrombosis and systemic thromboembolism [17]. At increased risk are women with cardiac arrhythmias, a previous history of thromboembolism, mural thrombus on echocardiography, a reduced ejection fraction, or a severely dilated left ventricle. Prophylactic anticoagulation should be considered in all women with PPCM, and those with additional risk factors require anticoagulation at therapeutic levels. The implications of antenatal anticoagulation and the possible use of regional anesthesia need to be considered and timing and mode of delivery planned accordingly. After delivery, it is imperative to continue anticoagulation as soon as safely possible. It is not clear how long this should be continued in the postnatal period; it

> **Box 38.4.** Management of acute decompensated heart failure in peripartum cardiomyopathy
>
> - Supplemental oxygen
> - Fluid restriction and loop diuretics to relieve pulmonary congestion
> - Non-invasive ventilation, positive-end expiratory pressure or endotracheal intubation and positive pressure ventilation as required
> - Vasodilators to reduce preload and afterload; use cautiously in patients with low systolic blood pressure
> - Inotropes in low cardiac output states, guided by invasive hemodynamic monitoring
> - Monitor uteroplacental perfusion indirectly with electronic fetal monitoring
> - Extracorporeal membrane oxygenation and mechanical cardiovascular support with ventricular assist devices or intra-aortic balloon pumps may be necessary if refractory to medical therapy or as a therapeutic bridge while awaiting cardiac transplantation [19]
> - Venovenous hemofiltration may assist volume offloading in patients unable to produce a diuresis
> - Thromboprophylaxis (see text)

> **Box 38.5.** Managing chronic stable heart failure in peripartum cardiomyopathy
>
> - Angiotensin-converting-enzyme inhibitors improve outcome; start these once the patient is stabilized but before hospital discharge and continue until left ventricular function has normalized
> - Initiate beta-blockade early, preferably at diagnosis unless in acute decompensation; continue until left ventricular function has recovered
> - Consider temporary or permanent insertion of an implantable cardiodefibrillator in patients with persistent left ventricular dysfunction at risk of arrhythmias or sudden death [20]
> - Thromboprophylaxis (see text)

might be necessary until left ventricular function has normalized.

New or experimental therapeutic developments

Levosimendan

The inotrope levosimendan sensitizes cardiac myofilaments to intracellular calcium and additionally mediates vascular smooth muscle dilatation through opening of ATP-sensitive potassium channels. The subsequent increase in cardiac output and reduction in pulmonary and systemic vascular resistance are favorable in acute heart failure, and levosimendan has successfully been used in PPCM [21,22]. Although trials have shown benefits in outcomes with the use of levosimendan in acute heart failure from other causes, this has not yet been specifically demonstrated in PPCM.

Bromocriptine

Unbalanced oxidative stress in pregnancy is thought to trigger cleavage of prolactin into a pro-apoptotic antiangiogenic derivative, resulting in cell death.

Bromocriptine, a dopamine D_2-receptor antagonist, blocks the production of prolactin and hence the cytotoxic derivative. In pilot studies, the addition of bromocriptine to standard heart failure treatment has demonstrated significant improvement in recovery of left ventricular ejection fraction [10]. Patients taking bromocriptine are unable to breastfeed and are at increased risk of thromboembolic events. Further evaluation of bromocriptine is needed before it can be recommended [20].

Intravenous immunoglobulin therapy

Intravenous immunoglobulin has been administered to patients with PPCM based on the theory that PPCM develops after an autoimmune response to a recent viral infection. One retrospective study found improvement in ejection fraction at follow-up compared with patients treated with conventional heart failure therapy [23]. This has not yet been demonstrated prospectively in PPCM.

Immunosuppressive therapy

Immunosuppressive therapy (prednisolone, cyclosporine, azathioprine) may be advocated if no improvement occurs in symptoms after 2 weeks of standard medical therapy [1].

Pentoxifylline

Pentoxifylline is a xanthine anti-inflammatory agent that inhibits the production of tumor necrosis factor-alpha, levels of which have been shown to be elevated in PPCM. A single study has found improved outcome in patients given pentoxyfylline in addition to conventional heart failure therapy [24].

Cardiac transplantation

Cardiac transplantation is an important therapy for a small number of patients for whom maximal medical management has failed and who remain in refractory symptomatic heart failure with poor systolic ventricular function. Because the rate of recovery of PPCM is higher than with other dilated cardiomyopathies, mechanical bridge therapy to recovery should be attempted before referral for cardiac transplantation [20]. Long-term survival after cardiac transplant for PPCM is similar to that of males requiring transplantation for idiopathic dilated cardiomyopathy and may be improved compared with women with idiopathic dilated cardiomyopathy [25]. It is not clear if there is any difference in rejection and infection rates [25–27]. Successful pregnancy is possible after cardiac transplantation.

Prognosis

Although the incidence of chronic morbidity and mortality is high when compared with progressive heart failure, there is a higher likelihood of left ventricular recovery compared with other forms of non-ischemic dilated cardiomyopathy. Over 50% of patients with PPCM are likely to regain normal ventricular function, although this may take up to 2 years from diagnosis. Most accurate predictors of prognosis are left ventricular size and function at diagnosis and 6 months after delivery. Fractional shortening <20%, left ventricle end-diastolic diameter >5.5–6 cm, and/or an ejection fraction <27% at diagnosis are associated with persistent left ventricular dysfunction [20]. The incidence of complications is higher in non-Caucasian women [28].

The risk of death within 4 years of diagnosis ranges from 9 to 30% in various studies [2,14]. In patients with persistent left ventricular dysfunction, mortality may be as high as 85% at 5 years [29]. Many of the mortality data are derived from the era before the angiotensin-converting enzyme inhibitors and beta-blockers became available, and with contemporary medical management the prognosis is improved [30]. The main causes of death are progressive left ventricular failure, thromboembolism, arrhythmias, and sudden death.

It is important to recognize that even in recovered patients with normal left ventricular function on echocardiography, there may be a persistent decreased contractile reserve that can be unmasked on dobutamine stress testing, suggesting a potential suboptimal response to future hemodynamic stress [31].

Subsequent pregnancies

The likelihood of developing PPCM in a subsequent pregnancy depends on whether left ventricular function has normalized before the beginning of the second pregnancy. On a background of persistent left ventricular dysfunction, a recurrence of PPCM in a subsequent pregnancy may occur in approximately 45%, compared with only 17% of women with normalized left ventricular function [32].

In addition to the increased risk of recurrence, mothers with persistent left ventricular dysfunction who become pregnant again have an increased risk of premature delivery, fetal loss, and maternal mortality [33]. Consequently, patients with persistent left ventricular dysfunction are usually advised against subsequent pregnancies.

Women with normalized left ventricular function are less likely to redevelop PPCM if their ejection fraction remains >55% following discontinuation of heart failure medication and if adequate contractile reserve is demonstrated on stress echocardiography [32]. Women with a history of PPCM are best assessed and counseled individually by obstetricians and cardiologists as to their level of risk.

Because of the increased risk of thromboembolism, combined oestrogen–progesterone contraceptive preparations are contraindicated. Progesterone-only preparations or intrauterine devices are considered safe [14].

Key learning points

1. PPCM is a rare cause of left ventricular systolic failure presenting in late pregnancy or in the postpartum period.
2. PPCM is a diagnosis of exclusion. Initial presentation may be confusing because of overlap with normal physiological signs and symptoms of late pregnancy.
3. Ejection fraction is 45% and associated with dilated left ventricular end-diastolic dimensions.
4. Management requires multidisciplinary input and clear plans should be developed for the delivery and possible obstetric emergencies.

5. Timing of delivery depends on maternal and fetal well-being. Early delivery does not improve maternal condition but may be necessary to appropriately manage the mother and prevent fetal compromise.

6. Vaginal delivery is recommended, with epidural or combined spinal–epidural analgesia and avoiding a prolonged second stage.

7. A rapid decline in blood pressure should be avoided. Gradual incremental regional anesthesia is advised, for labor analgesia or cesarean section.

8. If cesarean section is performed under general anesthesia, a modified rapid sequence and cardiac anesthesia technique is necessary.

9. Pharmacological management of heart failure is similar to managing heart failure from other causes.

10. In severe heart failure, invasive monitoring is advised to guide fluid and drug management. Fetal well-being should be closely monitored because of the potential changes in uterine blood flow following maternal hemodynamic therapy.

11. Thromboprophylaxis is required until normalization of left ventricular function.

12. Approximately 50% of women fully recover left ventricular function. Women who have not regained normal ventricular function suffer increased morbidity and mortality and are advised against a subsequent pregnancy.

References

1. Pearson GD, Veille J-C, Rahimtoola S, *et al.* Peripartum Cardiomyopathy. National Heart, Lung and Blood Institute and Office of Rare Diseases (National Institutes of Health) Workshop Recommendations and Review. *JAMA* 2000;**283**:1183–1188.

2. Desai D, Moodley J, Naidoo D. Peripartum cardiomyopathy: experiences at King Edward VIII Hospital, Durban, South Africa and a review of the literature. *Trop Doct* 1995;**25**:118–123.

3. Fett JD, Christie LG, Carraway RD, Murphy JG. Five-year prospective study of the incidence and prognosis of peripartum cardiomyopathy at a single instition. *Mayo Proc* 2005;**80**:1602–1606.

4. Sliwa K, Fett J, Elkayam U. Peripartum cardiomyopathy. *Lancet* 2006;**368**:687–693.

5. van Spaendonck-Zwarts K, van Tintelen J, van Veldhuisen DJ, *et al.* Peripartum cardiomyopathy as a part of familial dilated cardiomyopathy. *Circulation* 2010;**121**:2169–2175.

6. Hilfiker-Kleiner D, Kaminski K, Podewski E, *et al.* A cathepsin D-cleaved 16 kDa form of prolactin mediates peripartum cardiomyopathy. *Cell* 2007;**128**:589–600.

7. Lamparter S, Pankuweit S, Maisch B. Clinical and immunological characteristics in peripartum cardiomyopathy. *Int J Cardiol* 2007;**118**:14–20.

8. Rizeq MN, Rickenbacher PR, Fowler MB, Billingham ME. Incidence of myocarditis in peripartum cardiomyopathy. *Am J Cardiol* 1994;**74**:474–444.

9. Sliwa K, Skudicky D, Bergemann A, *et al.* Peripartum cardiomyopathy: analysis of clinical outcome, left ventricular function, plasma levels of cytokines and Fas/Apo-1. *J Am Coll Cardiol* 2000;**35**:701–705.

10. Sliwa K, Blauwet L, Tibazarwa K, *et al.* Evaluation of bromocriptine in the treatment of acute severe peripartum cardiomyopathy: a proof of concept pilot study. *Circulation* 2010;**121**:1465–1473.

11. Lewis G (ed.) *Saving Mothers' Lives: Reviewing Maternal Deaths to Make Motherhood Safer, 2003–2005. The Seventh Report on Confidential Enquiries into Maternal Deaths in the United Kingdom.* London: CEMACH, 2007.

12. Cantwell R, Clutton-Brock T, Cooper G, *et al.* Saving Mothers' Lives: Reviewing Maternal Deaths to make Motherhood Safer 2006–2008. The Eighth Report of the Confidential Enquiries into Maternal Deaths in the United Kingdom. *BJOG* 2011;**118**(Suppl 1):1–203.

13. Demakis JG, Rahimtoola SH. Peripartum cardiomyopathy. *Circulation* 1971;**44**:964–968.

14. Sliwa K, Hilfiker-Kleiner D, Petrie MC, *et al.* Current state of knowledge on aetiology, diagnosis, management and therapy of peripartum cardiomyopathy: a position statement from the Heart Failure Association of the European Society of Cardiology Working Group on peripartum cardiomyopathy. *Eur J Heart Fail* 2010;**12**:767–778.

15. Tibazarwa K, Lee G, Carrinton M, Stewart S, Sliwa K. The 12-lead ECG in peripartum cardiomyopathy. *Cardiovasc J Afr* 2012;**23**:1–8.

16. Srichai MB, Junor C, Rodriguez LL. Clinical, imaging and pathological characteristics of left ventricular thrombus: a comparison of contrast-enhanced MRI, transthoracic and transoesophageal echocardiogram. *Am Heart J* 2006;**152**:75–84.

17. Tidswell M. Peripartum cardiomyopathy. *Crit Care Clin* 2004;**20**:777–788.

18. Dickstein K, Cohen-Solal A, Gerasimos F, *et al.* ESC guidelines for the diagnosis and treatment of acute and chronic heart failure 2008. *Eur Heart J* 2008;**29**:2388–2442.

19. Gevaert S, Van Bellghem Y, Bouchez S, *et al.* Acute and criticaly ill peripartum cardiomyopathy and 'bridge to' therapeutic options: a single center experience with

intra-aortic balloon pump, extra corporeal membrane oxygenation and continuous-flow left ventricular assist devices. *Crit Care* 2011;**15**:R93.

20. Elkayam U. Clinical characteristics of peripartum cardiomyopathy in the United States. *J Am Coll Cardiol* 2011;**58**:659–670.

21. Nguyen HD, McKeown B. Levosimendan for post-partum cardiomyopathy. *Crit Care Resus* 2005;**7**:107–110.

22. Benolo S, Lefoll C, Katchatouryan V, Payen D, Mebazaa A. Successful use of levosimendan in a patient with peripartum cardiomyopathy. *Anesth Analg* 2004;**98**:822–824.

23. Bozkurt B, Villnueva FS, Holubkov R, *et al.* Intravenous immune globulin in the therapy of peripartum cardiomyopathy. *J Am Coll Cardiol* 1999;**34**:177–180.

24. Sliwa K, Skudidky D, Candy G, *et al.* The addition of pentoxifylline to conventional therapy improves outcome in patients with peripartum cardiomyopathy. *Eur J Heart Fail* 2002;**4**:305–309.

25. Rasmusson KD, Stehlik J, Brown RN, *et al.* Long-term outcomes of cardiac transplantation for peripartum cardiomyopathy: a multiinstitutional analysis. *J Heart Lung Transplant* 2007;**11**:1097–1104.

26. Keogh A, Macdonald P, Spratt P, *et al.* Outcome in peripartum cardiomyopathy after heart transplantation. *J Heart Lung Transpl* 1994;**2**:202–207.

27. Rickenbacher PR, Rizeg MN, Hunt SA, Billingham ME, Fowler MB. Long-term outcome after heart transplantation for peripartum cardiomyopathy. *Am Heart J* 1994;**5**:1318–1323.

28. Goland S, Modi K, Janmohmaed M, *et al.* Clinical profile and predictors of complications in peripartum cardiomyopathy. *J Card Fail* 2009;**8**:645–650.

29. Demakis JG, Rahimtoola SH, Sutton GC, *et al.* Natural course of peripartum cardiomyopathy. *Circulation* 1971;**6**:1053–1061.

30. Amos AM, Wissam AJ, Russell SD. Improved outcomes in peripartum cardiomyopathy with contemporary. *Am Heart J* 2006;**152**:509–513.

31. Lampert MB, Weinert L, Hibbard J, *et al.* Contractile reserve in patients with peripartum cardiomyopathy and recovered left ventricular function. *Am J Obstet Gynecol* 1997;**176**:189–195.

32. Fett JD, Fristoe KL, Welsh SN. Risk of heart failure relapse in subsequent pregnancy among peripartum cardiomyopathy mothers. *Int J Gynaecol Obstet* 2010;**109**:34–36.

33. Elkayam U. Pregnant again after peripartum cardiomyopathy: to be or not to be? *Eur Heart J* 2002;**23**:753–756.

Obstetric hemorrhage

Sina Haeri, Vicki Clark, and Michael A. Belfort

Introduction

Obstetric hemorrhage remains as one of the top three direct obstetric causes of maternal mortality worldwide, with most deaths occurring within 24–48 hours of delivery. Given that the majority of morbidity and mortality related to hemorrhage is avoidable, the cornerstone of effective prevention strategy will involve risk factor identification, rapid diagnosis, and timely management. The aim of this chapter is to review the epidemiology, etiology, and management measures related to obstetric hemorrhage.

Epidemiology

Historically, hemorrhage has been one of the most common and preventable causes of maternal death. Developing countries shoulder a disproportionate share of these deaths with a hemorrhage-related death risk of 1 in 1000 deliveries, which is approximately 100 times higher than the rates seen in resource-rich nations [1,2]. For example, in Africa and Asia, hemorrhage accounts for more than a third of all maternal deaths [1]. As pointed out in a review by El-Refaey and Rodeck, this higher proportion of hemorrhage-related deaths can be attributed to limited access to care, as well as the higher incidence of multiparity, uterine fibroids, and anemia [3]. Even though overall maternal mortality worldwide is decreasing, this trend has yet to be fully realized in hemorrhage-related deaths.

In the USA, the risk of death from obstetric hemorrhage has remained steady (7.7 per 100 000 deliveries), which accounts for 13–30% of all maternal mortality [1]. Indeed, in a population-based study by Chang and colleagues, hemorrhage was noted to be a more common cause of maternal mortality following stillbirths (22%) and abortions (21%) than following live births [4]. Similarly, the impact of hemorrhage may also vary depending on gestational age. Whereas the majority of first and second trimester deaths are from hemorrhage, the more common causes of maternal death later in the pregnancy include pulmonary embolism and hypertensive complications. The incidence of hemorrhage itself has been increasing in the USA, with a recent population-based study indicating a 26% increase in the incidence of postpartum hemorrhage (PPH) between 1994 and 2006 [5]. Interestingly, the authors attributed this rise predominantly to increased rates of uterine atony (from 1.6% to 2.4%) rather than changes in rates of cesarean delivery, vaginal birth after cesarean delivery, maternal age, multiple birth, or chronic medical illness [5].

Definition of obstetric hemorrhage

Unlike many other obstetric diagnoses, there is no uniformly accepted definition for obstetric hemorrhage. Conventionally, an estimated blood loss >500 mL following a vaginal delivery, and >1000 mL following a cesarean delivery has been arbitrarily used to define PPH in the second and third trimesters. More objective definitions such as a 10% decrease in hematocrit or a need for blood transfusion have also been proposed in the past [6]. However, these suggestions have clinical limitations as postdelivery hematocrit determinations may not be correct, laboratory results may be overtaken by medical emergency, and the degree of decrease may be less meaningful in the physiologically altered patient (e.g. hemoconcentration in pre-eclampsia). Physical examination findings indicative of excessive blood loss are particularly useful in first and early second trimester pregnancies. These include tachycardia hypotension, dizziness, pallor, or oliguria. Overall, and more subjectively, hemorrhage can be defined as blood loss that, if left untreated, may lead to shock and/or death of a mother.

Table 39.1. Classification of hemorrhage based on blood loss volume and maternal physiological response

Class	Blood loss volume (mL)	Blood loss (%)	Maternal response
1	900	15	Asymptomatic
2	1200–1500	20–25	Mild tachycardia (<120 beats/min), mild tachypnea (<30 breaths/min), orthostatic hypotension, narrowing of the pulse pressure, decreased capillary refill
3	1800–2100	30–35	Severe tachycardia (>120 beats/min), severe tachypnea (>30 breaths/min), cool extremities, severe hypotension, confusion
4	≥2400	40	Oliguria, decreased conscious level

Classification of hemorrhage

Regardless of timing or cause, hemorrhage in itself may also be classified according to the acute blood loss quantity and the resultant maternal physiological response (Table 39.1).

Hypovolemic (hemorrhagic) shock

Hemorrhagic shock involves a cascade of physiological events as the body combats and attempts to compensate the acute volume loss. The diagnosis is often made by the presence of hypotension, oliguria, acidosis, and ultimately cardiovascular collapse. The state of shock results from decreased preload in the intravascular volume loss. The decreased preload leads to a diminished cardiac output, which in turns leads to a compensatory rise in the systemic vascular resistance.

As with other types of shock, there is a physiological continuum through preshock (resuscitated or compensated shock), shock (multiorgan dysfunction), and end-organ dysfunction (or death). Volume replacement, restoration of the oxygen-carrying capacity, and definitive treatment of the underlying cause are crucial steps in the management of obstetric-related hemorrhagic shock. Vasopressors generally do not play a primary role in the obstetric setting as they do not correct the primary problem and may, in fact, lead to further decrease in tissue perfusion.

Hemorrhage in early pregnancy

Hemorrhage in the first and early second trimester is often caused by a ruptured extrauterine pregnancy or as a complication of an abortion (spontaneous or induced). For the purpose of this chapter, we will focus on hemorrhage occurring later in the pregnancy.

Hemorrhage in later pregnancy

Placental abruption

Placental abruption is the premature separation of the placenta from the uterus and is implicated in one third of all antepartum hemorrhages. This condition is generally attributed to the rupture of abnormal maternal vasculature within the decidua basalis or interruption of the fetoplacental vessels. The resultant bleeding leads to the formation of a hematoma, which ultimately causes placental separation and diminished maternal–fetal gas and nutrient exchange.

Classically, placental abruption has been described as third trimester vaginal bleeding accompanied by abdominal tenderness. Concurrently, the clinical picture may also include uterine bleeding, contractions, tenderness, non-reassuring fetal heart rate patterns, fetal demise, or because of the formation of the retroplacental clot which consumes coagulation factors, disseminated intravascular coagulation in more severe cases. Abruption can also present in a concealed fashion without overt vaginal bleeding.

Placenta previa

Placenta previa refers to the presence of placental tissue overlying or in proximity to the internal cervical os. Bleeding, which ranges from spotting to hemorrhage, is the main complication. Placenta previa complicates approximately 4 in 1000 pregnancies that are over 20 weeks of gestation. Common risk factors include increased number of prior cesarean deliveries, multiparity, prior uterine instrumentation, and increased maternal age. Previa may be associated with placenta accreta, malpresentation, preterm premature rupture of the membranes, vasa previa, or velamentous insertion of the umbilical cord. Therefore, antepartum search for these coexisting morbidities is advised.

The characteristic clinical presentation of placenta previa is painless vaginal bleeding after 20 weeks of gestation. Bleeding is likely to occur during the third trimester because of development of the lower uterine segment and contraction-associated shearing forces at the inelastic placental attachment site, resulting in placental detachment and bleeding.

If a cesarean delivery is required, three to four units of blood and a hysterectomy tray should be available as placenta previa is often associated with a placenta accreta (10%) and hemorrhage. Caution must be exercised to avoid cutting the placenta during the delivery. An intraoperative ultrasound examination may be helpful in localizing the placental edge and determining the best location for a hysterotomy.

Uterine rupture

The approximate incidence of rupture is 2–8 per 10 000 deliveries [7]. Uterine rupture is rarely encountered in industrialized nations in the absence of previous surgery and, when present, is most often attributed to the use of oxytocics in the setting of a uterine scar [8]. Prolonged obstructed labor, more commonly in the developing world, has also been linked to higher rates of rupture particularly in the setting of grand multiparity, macrosomia, and fetal malpresentation. Most ruptures occur in the lower anterior segment during labor and at the fundus during the period before labor.

Rupture of an unscarred uterus is far less likely and is frequently attributed to obstetric interventions, including the use of uterotonic drugs for induction or augmentation of labor, mid-cavity forceps delivery, or breech extraction with internal podalic version [7].

Fetal bradycardia is the most common clinical signal of a uterine rupture. Consequently, the onset of any fetal heart rate abnormality in a woman undergoing a trial of labor after cesarean should prompt immediate investigation to exclude a rupture. Abdominal pain, abrupt arrest of contractions, and retraction of the fetal presenting part have also been reported but are less commonly seen as the initial sign of a rupture. Intrauterine catheter monitoring has not proven useful for prediction of impending uterine rupture and there is very poor correlation between uterine contractility patterns and rupture [9].

Uterine rupture should be considered in every obstetric patient with hemorrhagic shock in whom the cause is not immediately apparent. Catheterization of the bladder during labor will frequently reveal blood-stained urine, but fresh arterial blood indicates that the rupture actually involves the bladder [10]. Rupture-related bleeding is generally intraperitoneal or retroperitoneal into the broad ligament. Vaginal bleeding may occur; however, it is more commonly seen in woman with obstructed labor but may be hidden above an impacted presenting part. Over 50% of ruptures are first diagnosed after delivery, when intractable hemorrhage follows precipitous, spontaneous, or instrumental vaginal delivery. Alternatively, if bleeding is concealed, profound shock may occur before rupture is suspected.

Treatment options for uterine rupture include surgical repair of the defect or hysterectomy. Most authors consider hysterectomy to be the procedure of choice for uterine rupture. Subtotal hysterectomy may be performed if the rupture is confined to the uterine corpus, as it is associated with decreased operating time, morbidity, mortality, and hospital stay.

Postpartum hemorrhage

The mechanical vasoconstriction caused by contraction of the myometrium is further enhanced by local and systemic hemostatic factors in providing hemostasis [11]. Consequently, hemorrhage can be chiefly attributed to insufficient myometrial contractility, faulty decidualization, or coagulation defect. In the second and third trimesters, hemorrhage following delivery can be classified as primary/early or secondary/late. Primary PPH is more common, occurs within the first 24 hours of delivery, and is predominantly caused by uterine atony [6]. Less common causes of primary PPH include retained placenta (decidualization defect), bleeding diatheses, perineal lacerations, uterine rupture, and uterine inversion. Secondary PPH occurs between 24 hours and 6 weeks after delivery, is generally less severe than primary PPH, and is most commonly secondary to retained placental fragments, subinvolution of the placental site, infection, or coagulation defects.

Primary postpartum hemorrhage

General management strategies

Given the often-preventable nature of significant morbidity from hemorrhage, the foundation of effective morbidity and mortality reduction involves risk factor identification, rapid diagnosis, and timely management. Indeed, two reports examining pregnancy-related deaths in the USA demonstrated that between 73 and 93% of deaths secondary to PPH were preventable [12]. General strategies for the management of obstetric hemorrhage will be described initially and later sections will focus on cause-specific measures.

Although hemorrhage is often idiopathic, identification of risk factors prior to hemorrhage will allow the practitioner adequate preparation, timely diagnosis,

Table 39.2. Risk factors associated with postpartum hemorrhage

Cause	Risk factor(s)
Uterine atony	Polyhydramnios, multifetal gestation, grand multiparity, macrosomia, rapid or prolonged labor, chorioamnionitis, uterine relaxants
Obstetric trauma	Operative delivery, macrosomia, precipitous delivery, episiotomy
Retained placenta	Placenta accreta/increta/percreta, placental succinturiate lobe, prior cesarean delivery, placenta previa
Acquired coagulopathy	Anticoagulant use, placental abruption, amniotic fluid embolism, pre-eclampsia, retained intrauterine fetal demise, gestational thrombocytopenia
Inherited coagulopathy	Von Willebrand disease, hemophilia, idiopathic thrombocytopenia purpura
Uterine rupture	Prior uterine surgery, internal podalic version, prolonged labor, mid-forceps delivery, uterotonic use, high parity
Uterine inversion	Uterine atony, excessive cord traction, macrosomia, fundal placentation, oxytocin use, primaparity, placenta accreta, uterine anomalies
Cesarean delivery	General anesthesia, obesity, pre-eclampsia, chorioamnionitis
General	History of hemorrhage, inadequate prenatal care

and more efficient control of the emergency. Table 39.2 includes risk factors associated with some of the more common causes of PPH. In addition to knowledge of these risks, recognition of factors complicating treatment, such as maternal blood type, antibody status, or specific religious beliefs (Jehovah's Witness) can prove invaluable in planning. Appropriate patient counseling and resource preparation, including such items as medication, equipment, and personnel should follow the risk identification phase.

Early recognition of the signs (e.g. oliguria, hypotension, tachycardia, and tachypnea) and symptoms (e.g. lightheadedness, confusion, pallor, and sweating) of PPH is a provider's best diagnostic ally (e.g. use of a maternal early obstetric warning scoring system).

Assistance from additional staff, including nursing and anesthesiology, ought to be requested expeditiously. Supplemental oxygen should be administered immediately via face mask to enhance oxygen delivery. Adequate intravenous access (two large gauge cannulae) followed by rapid crystalloid administration (3 mL per 1 mL estimated blood loss to compensate for extravascular redistribution) should begin immediately. In extremis, intraosseous administration may be necessary. In severe hemorrhage, the initial resuscitation should begin with rapid infusion of normal saline or colloid followed by blood component therapy. This early volume resuscitation will prevent irreversible tissue damage and the resulting decline in vascular tone, systemic vascular resistance, and response to vasoactive agents. There is mounting evidence in the trauma literature supporting the use of colloid agents as first-line therapy for hemorrhage and hypotension; however, this has yet to be tested in the pregnant population, more specifically involving antepartum hemorrhage or PPH. To that end, in mild to moderate hemorrhage, or where colloid solutions are not readily available, initiation of therapy with crystalloids is recommended. However, as mentioned above, colloid agents should be considered as first line in severe PPH.

Some general strategies are preventative in nature and aimed at those patients deemed as high risk well before the acute event. These include arterial line placement for close monitoring, autologous blood transfusion, and erythropoietin.

The use of an intraoperative autologous transfusion device such as the Cell Saver has been suggested when there is anticipated large blood loss or in patients where religious beliefs preclude the use of blood component therapy. This strategy is discussed in further detail below.

The use of recombinant human erythropoietin has attracted much interest recently, with several trials showing a reduction in allogeneic transfusions following its use in gynecological, orthopedic, and cardiac surgery. Unfortunately, its cost–effectiveness or use in the general population is questioned, and its use is best reserved for patients who would refuse allogeneic transfusion or are too anemic to qualify for autologous transfusions [13]. Much like Cell Saver technology, it has a limited role in the acute setting.

Anti-shock trousers are lower-body counterpressure devices designed to autotransfuse the central circulation. Although some authors have reported success with these trousers in postpartum shock, a randomized trial in the general trauma setting failed to show a survival benefit [14]. Further, as the trousers cover the perineum, this restricts examination of the relevant areas. Anti-shock trousers are hardly used in the USA or Europe and are best reserved for specific scenarios such as patients in remote locations requiring a long transport to a medical facility. The use of non-pneumatic antishock garments in Egypt and Nigeria has had relative success.

Teamwork training

Given the often-identified failures in communication and teamwork during obstetric sentinel events, an area of recent focus has been teamwork training [15]. The evidence supporting the implementation of teamwork training programs, simulation drills, and practice guidelines/protocols is becoming increasingly available. Recently, several training programs have been proposed and implemented including Team STEPPS (Team Strategies and Tools to Enhance Performance and Patient Safety) [15]. PROMPT (PRactical Obstetric Multi-Professional Training) and MOET (Management of Obstetric Emergencies and Trauma) are two similar courses in the UK [16,17]. Despite limited evidence of improved patient safety, maternal or neonatal outcomes simulation drills have demonstrated improvement in knowledge, clinical skills, communication, and team performance in the catastrophic hemorrhage scenario. There is also accumulating evidence supporting the development and implementation of practice guidelines and protocols. Specifically related to hemorrhage, promising results have been reported following the implementation of institution-wide practice guidelines, including decreased incidence of massive hemorrhage, need for transfusions, and intensive care unit admissions [18]. The California Maternal Quality Care Collaborative and the New York State Health Advisory Hemorrhage Guidelines are two examples of widespread protocol dissemination.

Pharmacological management of uterine atony

Oxytocin

Oxytocin binds to specific uterine receptors and intravenous administration (5–10 units) has an almost immediate onset of action. The mean plasma half-life is 3 minutes; therefore, to ensure a sustained contraction a continuous intravenous infusion is necessary. The usual dose is 20–40 U/L crystalloid, with the dose rate adjusted according to response. Plateau concentration is reached after 30 minutes. Intramuscular injection has a time of onset of 3–7 minutes, and the clinical effect is longer lasting, at 30–60 minutes. Most studies find oxytocin alone reduces the need for further medication and is associated with fewer adverse side effects [19]. Compared with other agents,

oxytocin has been found to reduce the need for manual placenta removal in some studies, regardless of route of administration, and is safe [19]. Oxytocin is metabolized by the liver and kidneys. It has approximately 5% of the antidiuretic effect of vasopressin; if given in large volumes of electrolyte-free solution, it can cause water overload (headache, vomiting, drowsiness, and convulsions). These are symptoms that may be mistakenly attributed to other causes. Rapid administration of an intravenous bolus of oxytocin results in relaxation of vascular smooth muscle. Hypotension with a reflex tachycardia may occur. This is important in hemodynamically unstable patients and particularly in patients with cardiac dysfunction where hypotension can be significant. The oxytocin bolus can cause marked increase in cardiac output and decrease in systemic vascular resistance; therefore, caution must be exercised as there are reports of deaths associated with oxytocin bolus administration. Indeed, most experts would agree that the bolus should be ideally delivered over a period of 5–10 minutes. Oxytocin is stable at temperatures up to 25°C, but refrigeration may prolong shelf life. Carbetocin is a newly developed long-acting oxytocin analogue that might be used as an uterotonic agent. It is in use in Canada, but has yet to receive approval for use in the USA or endorsement from the Royal College of Obstetricians in the UK.

Methylergonovine

The ergot alkaloid methylergonovine (methylergometrine) and its parent compound ergometrine result in a sustained tonic contraction of uterine smooth muscle via stimulation of alpha-adrenergic myometrial receptors. The dose is 0.2 mg for methylergonovine and 0.2–0.5 mg for ergometrine and can be repeated after 2–4 hours if necessary. Time of onset of action is 2–5 minutes when given intramuscularly. These agents are extensively metabolized in the liver and the mean plasma half-life is approximately 30 minutes. However, plasma levels do not seem to correlate with uterine effect, since the clinical action of ergometrine is sustained for 3 hours or more. When oxytocin and ergometrine derivatives are used simultaneously, PPH is being controlled by two different mechanisms: oxytocin producing an immediate response and ergometrine a more sustained action. Nausea and vomiting are common side effects. Vasoconstriction of vascular smooth muscle also occurs as a consequence of the alpha-adrenergic action. This can result in elevation of central venous pressure and systemic blood pressure, thus potentially leading to pulmonary edema, stroke, and myocardial infarction. Contraindications include heart disease, autoimmune conditions associated with Raynaud phenomenon, peripheral vascular disease, arteriovenous shunts (even if surgically corrected), and hypertension. Women with pre-eclampsia/eclampsia are particularly at risk of severe and sustained hypertension. With intravenous administration, onset of action with ergot alkaloids is almost immediate but is associated with more severe side effects. This route may be indicated if intramuscular absorption may be delayed (e.g. in shock). The drug should be given over at least 60 seconds with careful monitoring of blood pressure and pulse.

Prostaglandin $F_{2\alpha}$ (carboprost, dinoprost)

Prostaglandin $F_{2\alpha}$ stimulates contraction of smooth muscle cells. Carboprost (15-methylprostaglandin $F_{2\alpha}$) is an established second-line treatment for PPH unresponsive to oxytocic agents. It is available in single-dose vials of 0.25 mg. It may be given by deep intramuscular injection or by direct injection into the myometrium, either under direct sight at cesarean section or transabdominally/transvaginally after vaginal delivery. It is not licenced for the latter route and there is concern about direct injection into a uterine sinus, although it is commonly used in this way (of note, this route is contraindicated in the UK because of reports of inadvertent intravenous injection). Direct injection may be more efficacious in shock, when tissue hypoperfusion may compromise absorption following intramuscular injection. Repeat doses may be given every 15 minutes to a maximum of eight doses (2 mg), with ongoing bimanual compression and fundal massage. The F-class prostaglandins cause bronchoconstriction, venoconstriction, and constriction of gastrointestinal smooth muscle. Associated side effects include nausea, vomiting, diarrhea, pyrexia, and bronchospasm. There are case reports of hypotension and intrapulmonary shunting with arterial oxygen desaturation; therefore, carboprost is contraindicated in patients with cardiac or pulmonary disease. Studies have demonstrated no significant difference between injectable carboprost and ergot compound injections in rates of PPH [19]. Carboprost is expensive and, therefore, unaffordable in many developing countries. Dinoprost (natural prostaglandin $F_{2\alpha}$) is more readily available; intramyometrial injection of 0.5–1.0 mg is effective for uterine atony.

Prostaglandin E_2 (dinoprostone)

Prostaglandin E_2 (dinoprostone) is generally a vasodilatory prostaglandin; however, it causes contraction of smooth muscle in the pregnant uterus. Dinoprostone is widely available on labor wards as an intravaginal pessary for cervical ripening. Rectal administration (2 mg given every 2 hours) has been successful as a treatment for uterine atony, vaginal administration probably being ineffective in the presence of ongoing uterine hemorrhage. Because of its vasodilatory effect, this drug should be avoided in hypotensive and hypovolemic patients. However, it may be useful in women with heart or lung disease in whom carboprost is contraindicated.

Prostaglandin E_1 (misoprostol)

Misoprostol is a synthetic analogue of prostaglandin E_1 and is metabolized in the liver. The tablet(s) can be given orally, vaginally, or rectally. An international multicenter randomized trial reported that oral misoprostol is less successful than parenteral oxytocin as prophylaxis for PPH [20]. Misoprostol may, however, be of benefit in treating PPH. A meta-analysis indicated that oral or sublingual misoprostol at a dose of 600 μg was useful in PPH but did not demonstrate a benefit over other uterotonics [20]. Adverse effects include maternal pyrexia and shivering. Of note, misoprostol is inexpensive, heat and light stable, has a long shelf life, and does not require sterile needles and syringes for administration. It may, therefore, be of particular benefit in developing countries.

Non-pharmacologic management of uterine atony
Uterine tamponade

Historically, uterine tamponade was performed using sterile gauze, with up to 5 m of 5–10 cm gauze introduced into the uterus, either using a specific packing instrument or long forceps. Packs are generally left *in situ* for 24–36 hours, and prophylactic antibiotics given. Uterine packing fell out of use because of concerns about concealed bleeding, infection, trauma, and problems in performing adequate packing. However, there is little documented evidence to support these concerns and it has been suggested that the risks have been overstated. The pelvic pressure pack, also known as the "mushroom" or "umbrella," has been successfully used for control of after hysterectomy hemorrhage in both gynecological and obstetric patients. Pelvic packing may prove useful following a cesarean delivery or hysterectomy in controlling low-pressure bleeding in the pelvis, which is often venous or microvascular in nature. If pelvic packing is successful, after a brief period of observation, no blood will be seen seeping through or around the gauze. There are various techniques for pelvic packing, but regardless, the free end can be brought through the center of a transverse incision or the inferior edge of a vertical scar. The packing should remain in place for 48 hours with the patient on broad-spectrum antibiotics and removed under general anesthesia.

Several inflatable mechanical devices have more recently been employed as alternative means of uterine tamponade. These are rapid and easy procedures to perform and their efficacy can readily be evaluated. Initial experience included tamponade using a Sengstaken–Blakemore tube, gastric balloon, Rusch urological hydrostatic balloon catheter inflated with 400–500 mL saline, and a sterile condom inflated with up to 500 mL of solution tied to a Foley catheter [21]. More recently, the Bakri and Ebb balloons have been employed as tamponade devices. These temporizing agents may allow for correction of coagulopathy in anticipation of surgical intervention. Often they lead to cessation of hemorrhage altogether and should be attempted where future fertility is a consideration or in low-resource areas. A continuous oxytocin infusion and prophylactic antibiotic coverage are advised for these procedures. The Bakri and Ebb balloons have mechanisms in place to monitor for continued bleeding and inadequate tamponade. A vaginal pack is usually required to keep the ballon in place.

Uterine brace suture

The B-Lynch suture (described by B. Lynch in 1997) is a uterine brace suture designed to vertically compress the uterine body when there is diffuse bleeding caused by uterine atony. In order to assess whether the suture will be effective, bimanual compression is applied to the uterus. If bleeding stops, compression with a brace suture should be equally successful. Single or multiple stitches may be inserted at the same time and, according to the shape, they may be called brace suture, simple brace, or square sutures. Normal uterine anatomy and resumption of normal menses has been demonstrated on follow-up [22,23].

Bilateral uterine artery ligation

Bilateral ligation of the ascending branches of the uterine artery is considered a simple, safe, and efficacious alternative to hysterectomy. Published reports indicate a 96% success rate with this procedure, even when the uterus has remained atonic. No long-term effects on menstrual patterns or fertility have been reported [23]. In fact, in those women who have subsequently undergone repeat cesarean section, the uterine vessels appeared to have recanalized. The success rate is substantially decreased when the bleeding is in the lower uterine segment or from a placenta previa. Unilateral or bilateral ligation of the ovarian artery may be performed as an adjunct to ligation of uterine arteries. This is particularly helpful in situations unresponsive to uterine artery ligation. If embolization is to be considered, it must be noted that vascular ligation may make the procedure more difficult.

Bilateral internal iliac artery ligation

Internal iliac artery ligation is a more complex procedure than uterine artery ligation. Incorrect identification of the internal iliac artery may result in accidental ligation of the ureters or of the external or common iliac artery, resulting in lower limb and pelvic ischemia. Femoral or pedal pulses should, therefore, be checked before and after the procedure. Recanalization of ligated vessels may occur, and successful pregnancy has been reported whether or not recanalization has taken place. Success rates are generally reported to be approximately 40%, likely because of the existence of an extensive collateral circulation [24]. Therefore, uterine artery ligation should be considered a more efficacious treatment modality. Given the high complication rate and required expertise for internal iliac artery ligation, there is only a limited role for this procedure in the treatment of PPH, being restricted to hemodynamically stable patients of low parity in whom future fertility is of paramount concern.

Arterial embolization

Uterine devascularization by selective arterial embolization is becoming more popular, particularly in centers with the required radiology resources. Using the femoral artery as an access point, the site of arterial bleeding is located by injection of contrast into the aorta. The bleeding vessel is selectively catheterized, and absorbable gelatin sponge injected thereafter. This procedure affords a temporary blockade, which lasts for approximately 10 days. If the site of bleeding cannot be identified, embolization of the anterior branch of the internal iliac artery or the uterine artery is performed. Uterine atony and pelvic trauma are the major indications for embolization, and overall success rates of 85–100% are reported [25]. Higher failure rates are associated with placenta accreta and procedures performed following failed bilateral internal iliac artery ligation [25]. Subsequent successful pregnancies have been documented.

Compared with surgical devascularization, embolization has several advantages. It is less invasive and generally results in visualization of the bleeding vessel. Occlusion of distal arteries close to the bleeding site is possible, thereby reducing the risk of ongoing bleeding from a collateral circulation. The efficacy of embolization can immediately be assessed, and repeated embolization of the same or different arteries can be performed. Disadvantages are the necessity for rapid availability of specialist equipment and personnel, and the need to transfer a hemorrhaging patient to the radiology suite. Embolization may also be a time-consuming procedure, generally requiring between 1 and 3 hours, but with hemostasis of the major bleeding vessel frequently established in 30–60 minutes.

A similar but alternative approach involves prophylactic placement of inflatable balloon catheters in internal iliac arteries. Generally, in a previously identified high-risk patient such as one with placenta accreta, balloon catheters are placed in the interventional radiology suite prior to surgery but are not inflated. Following delivery of the baby, the catheters can be immediately inflated. Such catheters can be deflated at the completion of surgery and left *in situ* during the next 24–48 hours to be reinflated if required The use of prophylactic occlusion balloons in the internal iliac arteries before selective embolization has shown a greater than 80% success rate for control of PPH [25]. Various reports have confirmed these findings, with normal resumption of menses within 3–6 months and subsequent uncomplicated pregnancies [26].

Hysterectomy

Peripartum hysterectomy is frequently considered the definitive procedure for obstetric hemorrhage, but it is not without complications including postoperative febrile morbidity. In the emergency situation, the major concern is that peripartum hysterectomy can be a complex procedure, because of the ongoing blood loss and the grossly distorted pelvic anatomy from edema, hematoma formation, and trauma. Adequate

hemostasis is not always achieved, and further procedures may be necessary including uterine artery embolization. Experienced operators are required and the attendance of senior colleagues is advised.

Hysterectomy is indicated if conservative procedures such as embolization or uterine devascularization fail to control bleeding. The time lapse between delivery and successful surgery is the most important prognostic factor. If the primary procedure fails, it is recommended that hysterectomy is performed promptly, without attempts at another conservative measure. In severely shocked patients with life-threatening hemorrhage, hysterectomy is in most circumstances the first-line treatment.

A subtotal hysterectomy can generally be performed if bleeding is from the uterine body. It is generally simpler than a total hysterectomy – the cervix and vaginal angles can be difficult to identify in women who have labored to full dilation. There is also less risk of injury to the ureter and bladder. One study reported the incidence of urinary tract injury to be 13% for subtotal hysterectomy compared with 25% for total hysterectomy [27].

Patients with periods of prolonged hypotension during surgery should also be evaluated for Sheehan syndrome in the postoperative period.

Management of uterine inversion

Uterine inversion is the folding of the fundus into the uterine cavity in varying degrees. The main predisposing factors for puerperal inversion are a fundal placenta, flaccid myometrium, and a dilated cervix. It is diagnosed clinically, with early-onset PPH accompanied by the appearance of a vaginal mass followed by various degrees of maternal cardiovascular collapse. In approximately 60–70% of women, the placenta is still attached at the moment of inversion. The extent of the reported bleeding is variable and depends on the degree of prolapse.

Management should be tailored to addressing the main risks of inversion, which are hemorrhage and cardiovascular collapse. Institution of aggressive blood product and fluid replacement, replacement of the uterus, and administration of potent uterotonics to keep the uterus contracted and prevent reinversion are needed. If possible, the placenta should not be removed before uterine replacement since this exacerbates blood loss. Replacement can usually be accomplished manually by placing a hand in the vagina with the fingers placed circumferentially around the prolapsed fundus. The last region of the uterus that inverted should be the first to be replaced. This avoids multiple layers of uterine wall within the cervical ring. Uterine relaxation may be necessary, with beta-sympathomimetic agents, magnesium sulfate, or low-dose nitroglycerin. Caution should be exercised with the use of nitroglycerin, which may exacerbate hypotension and tachycardia, and it may only be useful if the placenta is present. General anesthesia and use of halogenated gases may be needed to provide full uterine relaxation. If there is a tightly contracted cervical ring, which prohibits vaginal replacement of the fundus, surgical options may have to be exercised such as incising the ring via a vaginal approach.

If these measures fail, abdominal procedures have been described using laparotomy.

Once the uterus has been replaced, all uterine relaxant drugs should be stopped and manual removal of the placenta should follow. With early diagnosis and prompt replacement of the fundus, laparotomy and hysterectomy can be avoided. In many cases, delay in definitive management is what leads to increased edema, blood loss, and associated morbidity. Most authorities would recommend antibiotic use after manual replacement although specific evidence of the utility of this is lacking.

Management of retained, trapped, and adherent placenta

Using a diagnostic cut-off of 30 minutes for a prolonged third stage, 42% of retained placentae deliver spontaneously within the next 30 minutes, with very few delivering spontaneously after 60 minutes. Because the incidence of significant PPH rises after 30 minutes in the third stage, manual removal of the placenta when 30–60 minutes into the third stage is advised. Consideration of the potential for placenta accreta or percreta should always precede the attempt, and if there is any real potential appropriate preparations for dealing with this should be put in place

Trapped placenta, which often follows the intravenous administration of ergometrine, results from the closure of the cervix at the same time as placental detachment occurs, thus trapping the placenta. Delivery of a trapped placenta can usually be achieved using controlled cord traction, which encourages cervical dilatation. Intravenous or sublingual nitroglycerin (100–200 µg) is useful as a short-term tocolytic agent, appears efficacious and safe, and may obviate the need for general anesthesia for uterine relaxation.

Releasing the cord clamp to allow blood trapped in the placenta to drain may also help.

With an adherent placenta, the uterine fundus remains broad and high and myometrial contractions may be weak or absent, but there is no bleeding while the placenta remains wholly attached. Adherent placenta is caused by a deficiency in the contractile force exerted by the myometrium underlying the placental site despite normal anatomy (not placenta accreta). When there is active bleeding, immediate active management is necessary.

Management of morbidly adherent placenta (accreta, increta, percreta)

Placenta accreta is a condition in which all or part of the placenta is adherent to the uterine wall because of myometrial invasion by chorionic villi. Three grades are defined according to the depth of myometrial invasion:

- *accreta*: 80% of cases, chorionic villi are in contact with the myometrium, rather than being contained within the decidua
- *increta*: 15% of cases, extensive villous invasion into the myometrium
- *percreta*: 5% of cases, villous invasion extends to (or through) the serosal covering of the uterus.

Multiparity, prior uterine surgery, advanced maternal age, placenta previa, prior uterine curettage and previous cesarean delivery, uterine irradiation for intra-abdominal cancer therapy, and prior endometrial ablation have been identified as risk factors for placenta accreta. The reported incidence of placenta accreta has increased 10-fold since the late 1990s, most likely related to increasing cesarean delivery rates.

All grades of placenta accreta can result in profound PPH; therefore, being alert to this possibility is essential for patients who have a combination of placenta previa and a history of previous uterine surgery. If the diagnosis of placenta accreta can be confirmed, plans for delivery by cesarean section by a surgeon experienced in dealing with such cases, and in a facility where resuscitation and intensive care are available, should be made.

Suspected/known placenta accreta

Known placenta accreta/percreta is best managed by a dedicated team of experienced clinicians including pathology (blood bank), anesthesiology, surgery (gynecological oncology, urology, and vascular), interventional radiology, and neonatology. Preoperative consultation with blood bank personnel is essential because of the very real possibility of massive transfusion. Patients with placenta percreta frequently will require more blood products than the average hospital blood bank has in stock, and when a patient has a rare blood type or antibodies this issue becomes even more important. Elective surgery may require delay until additional units of blood can be located and transported to the blood bank. As mentioned above, availability of options such as Cell Saver technology should be discussed with the patient and the consulting services. Adequate fresh frozen plasma, cryoprecipitate, and platelets are needed with the Cell Saver blood because of the lack of these products in the reconstituted red cells. Although transfusing washed red cells will increase the hematocrit, unless fresh frozen plasma and platelets are transfused simultaneously there will be a risk of dilutional coagulopathy. Preoperative anesthesia consultation is essential to allow appropriate planning and allocation of personnel.

Preoperative pelvic artery occlusion has been proposed as an adjunct to minimize blood loss at the time of hysterectomy. However, there is emerging evidence that preoperative placement of balloon catheters in the internal iliac arteries is not useful and it is no longer recommended [28]. Indeed, inflation of the balloons after delivery may actually complicate the hysterectomy by opening up collateral vessels deeper in the pelvis that are more difficult to control than the immediate branches of the internal iliac artery.

Some authors have reported cases where the placenta is left *in situ* until a later date while administering chemotherapeutic agents to the patient (mono or polyagent therapy); however, this is not routine clinical practice and further discussion is beyond the scope of this chapter.

Unsuspected and/or massively bleeding placenta accreta

Sometimes placenta accreta or percreta is only discovered at the time of delivery. Very occasionally this will be at the time of vaginal delivery (will be heralded by a retained placenta). More usually, the placenta accreta or percreta is discovered at the time of repeat cesarean section. There is often very little time to prepare the patient for controlled surgery, and frequently the massive hemorrhage is already underway at the time of diagnosis. The overarching principle in such cases

should always be to limit the hemorrhage as quickly as possible and to perform definitive surgery before the patient develops coagulopathy, hypothermia, or circulatory instability. A large part of the mortality and morbidity in these situations is related to unnecessary delay compounded by unsuccessful attempts to preserve the uterus. Recognition of the problem and decisive surgical action, combined with aggressive resuscitation and use of blood products, is required to deal with massive hemorrhage from accreta.

After delivery of the fetus, no attempts should be made to remove the placenta if it does not separate with gentle cord traction, as incomplete separation will lead to further bleeding. The umbilical cord should be tied off and replaced within the uterus. The uterus should then be closed in a single layer with a locked suture. It is quite possible to lose a significant amount of blood into the uterine cavity during the surgery without any outward indication and uterine size should be monitored carefully to alert of this occurrence. In some cases, a red rubber catheter can be used as a tourniquet above the level of the placental edge to help to compress the uterus. The hysterectomy should be performed using careful systematic stepwise devascularization. Avoid making any holes in the peritoneal covering of the placenta, which is usually all that covers the highly vascular placental tissue. The most common error in this regard is traction or compression of the lower segment by an assistant, or puncture with a retractor during efforts to expose the lateral pelvic side walls. The inadvertent puncture of the peritoneal covering of the placenta before uterine devascularization can turn a controlled, minimally bloody procedure into a hemorrhagic emergency.

Because of the extreme vascularity (often massively enlarged collateral vessels and neovascularization), the blood supply to the uterus is frequently unrecognizable from that seen in other women. The uterine arteries may not be easily identified, and there may be multiple other arterial feeders to the abnormally implanted placenta via vascular anastomoses originating from the superior and inferior vesical and rectal cascades. This will often require careful dissection of the retroperitoneal space and judicious devascularization well clear of the sides of the uterus to avoid tearing through the friable and highly vascular tissue close to the placenta. The use of supracervical hysterectomy in true placenta previa percreta is to be discouraged because in most such cases the placental tissue invades the cervix, and attempts to remove the corpus of the uterus simply result in the disruption of huge vascular channels supplying the placenta. It is helpful to demarcate the placental edges using ultrasound and, if necessary, utilize a fundal incision to avoid the placenta prior to the delivery of the neonate.

Urogenital tract trauma

Genital tract trauma, often associated with operative vaginal delivery, is also a significant cause of PPH. Trauma may be found anywhere along the urogenital tract, including perineum, vagina, cervix, uterus, and bladder. Hemodynamic instability is often associated with delayed diagnosis and repair. Hematomas may result in postpartum hypotension through concealed blood loss, particularly with those hematomas forming below the level of the levator ani, as they may hold up to 2 L of blood. Unlike infralevator hematomas, which are contained in Colles fascia and fascia lata, supralevator hematomas may extend deep into the retroperitoneal space. The latter are associated with uterine incision dehiscence in the setting of a prior cesarean delivery. Another common cause of hematoma formation is inadequate surgical repair of perineal lacerations. Generally, management is conservative for hematomas <3 cm and evacuation for those that are larger. If the bleeding vessel is seen, then suture ligation is advised. Otherwise, vaginal or tight hematoma cavity packing may be employed. In bleeding unresponsive to these measures, arterial ligation, angiographic embolization, or laparotomy are potential management options.

In retroperitoneal hematomas specifically, the space is large, making the management decision a difficult one. Many patients with a retroperitoneal hematoma require either surgical or angiographic intervention. However, since it is also a confined space, conservative management may suffice as the hematoma in itself may tamponade the slowly bleeding vessels. If surgery is warranted, hemostasis can be achieved after opening the retroperitoneal space by identifying and ligating the lacerated blood vessel. An alternative is hypogastric artery ligation of the ipsilateral vessel, which usually stops the bleeding. As discussed above, pelvic packing is yet another alternative surgical therapy for retroperitoneal bleeding.

Secondary postpartum hemorrhage

Secondary postpartum hemorrhage most commonly occurs 2–3 weeks after delivery and is often attributed to retained placenta, endometritis, genital tract tears,

and, rarely, scar dehiscence or genital tract malignancy. As with PPH, initial approach includes ascertainment of the cause and medical management. If bleeding is not stopped with medical management, surgical intervention, including uterine vascular ligation, hysterectomy, and arterial embolization, may become necessary. Where a specific cause is not found, angiography may prove beneficial in diagnosing vascular causes of the hemorrhage.

Anesthesic considerations

Anesthetic techniques

Because of the well-known risks of failed intubation in the parturient, obstetric anesthesiologists would normally choose a regional technique for operative delivery However, spinal and epidural anesthesia cause sympathetic blockade and the compensatory vasoconstriction normally present to maintain cardiac output is, therefore, lost. Faced then with a bleeding pregnant or postpartum woman for whatever cause, general anesthesia is the technique of choice. Inhalational anesthetic agents used in the past, particularly halothane, could cause uterine relaxation and worsen existing uterine atony, but the newer agents such as sevoflurane [29] are less likely to do so and uterotonics are usually administered concurrently.

There will be instances where a regional technique has been started and unexpected hemorrhage occurs. Conversion to general anesthesia may be required because of the length of the operative procedure, patient discomfort, and also from a practical point of view, because an awake patient and present partner can distract the anesthestist from necessary resuscitative procedures.

There is controversy about anesthesia for patients who may potentially bleed catastrophically, for example with placenta previa or accreta. Many anesthesiologists will induce general anesthesia from the start in anticipation of hemorrhage, but others may perform a combined spinal–epidural technique that can last the course of a hysterectomy if required [30,31]. Personal and patient preference as well as operator experience will undoubtedly influence choice of anesthetic technique.

If the patient has not been seen prior to the hemorrhage, assessment has to be swift. Attention should be paid to airway abnormalities, venous access, and volume status. Tachycardia, cool peripheries, agitation, tachypnea, and oliguria are more accurate reflectors of hypovolemia than hypotension, as the previously healthy woman will vasoconstrict efficiently to maintain her blood pressure. Estimation of blood loss is often a guess but crystalloid should be administered to approximately three times the estimated blood loss or colloid in equal volumes to blood loss [32]. All fluids should be warmed. An arterial line is useful in a bleeding unstable patient as it provides instantaneous blood pressure readings and also can be used for frequent blood sampling. A central venous catheter will provide large-bore access as well as monitoring volume status. A urinary catheter is mandatory. Resuscitation is often "on the hoof" as the definitive treatment is surgery that should not be delayed while fluid/blood is being administered. A rapid infusor device should be available.

Blood component therapy

Blood may be necessary, guided by near patient testing (e.g. the Hemocue), as standard laboratory tests will lag behind the clinical event [33]. Every obstetric unit should have O-negative blood available in the event of catastrophic hemorrhage until matched blood is to hand. Correction of the deficit in blood volume with crystalloid or colloid will generally maintain hemodynamic stability, while transfusion of red cells is used to improve tissue oxygenation. Each unit of packed cells contains approximately 200 mL red cells, and will raise the hematocrit by approximately 3 points unless there is continued bleeding. In a stable obstetric patient, the Royal The UK College of Obstetricians and Gynecologists *Green-top Guideline 47* suggests that transfusion is rarely indicated when the hemoglobin is >10 g/dL and almost always indicated when 6 g/dL [34]. Blood component therapy should also be considered if signs of hemodynamic instability persist (e.g. tachycardia, hypotension).

Massive transfusion is defined as replacement by transfusion of 50% or more of the patient's blood volume in 12–24 hours or transfusion of 8–10 (or more) units of packed red blood cells. With respect to massive transfusions, there are recent data, both from the battlefield and from civilian life, suggesting that early and extensive use of fresh frozen plasma and platelets, in a 1:1:1 ratio with packed red blood cells is of benefit in terms of reducing mortality in patients with massive hemorrhage from trauma. Others have shown that use of a 1:1 ratio of packed red blood cells to fresh frozen plasma before moving the patient to intensive care may result in earlier correction of coagulopathy, decreased

need for packed red blood cells in intensive care, and reduced mortality. It should be emphasized that there are no comparable data for use of this ratio in obstetrics, but the empiric use of such an approach in massive obstetric hemorrhage is potentially a strategy that could be of benefit, and one deserving of investigation. It is highly advised that each institution or healthcare system develop its own specific massive transfusion protocol. There are numerous published protocols that may be used as an example. One resource is the Californian Maternal Quality Care Collaborative's *Obstetric Hemorrhage Toolkit* [35].

The associated potential acute metabolic effects of massive transfusion, including hypothermia, hypocalcemia, and hyperkalemia, should also be kept in mind. Hypocalcemia may be treated with calcium gluconate or calcium chloride. Aside from these acute adverse effects of a massive transfusion, the provider must possess general knowledge of the signs, symptoms, causes, treatment, and prevention of transfusion-related reactions. Table 39.3 outlines several transfusion reactions, associated clinical signs, and treatment recommendations. Table 39.4 includes a summary of blood components and their approximate effects.

Coagulopathy often accompanies major hemorrhage. This can be caused by disseminated intravascular coagulation where the coagulation factors have been consumed pathologically in clot formation, for example in the large retroplacental clot that accompanies an abruption or the microscopic clots that can occur in pre-eclampsia. However, coagulopathy can also be induced iatrogenically by overenthusiastic fluid replacement – the so-called dilutional coagulopathy. Here, the absolute quantity of coagulation factors is normal but the much increased intravascular volume overwhelms the coagulation system and there is a relative paucity of coagulation products.

Coagulopathy

Coagulopathy becomes apparent clinically by lack of clotting in the surgical field but may be lessened by timely administration of coagulation products. Early and rapid detection of impending coagulopathy can be diagnosed with thromboelastometry (TEG calls their technique thromboelastography and ROTEM call their's thromboelastometry), which will also indicate which coagulation products (fresh frozen plasma, cryoprecipitate, or platelets) are required [36]. By comparison, standard laboratory coagulation test results

Table 39.3. Transfusion-related reactions with associated symptoms and treatment

Reaction	Symptoms	Action
Intravascular hemolysis	Fever, shock, acute renal failure, DIC	Stop transfusion, hydrate, support blood pressure and respirations, treat shock and DIC if present
Febrile morbidity	Fever	Stop transfusion, antipyretic, meperidine 25–50 mg i.v. or i.m.
Anaphylaxis	Urticaria, itching, dyspnea, hypotension	Stop transfusion, give antihistamine (oral or i.m.), epinephrine and/or steroids (if severe)
Transfusion-related lung injury	Dyspnea, fever, hypoxia, pulmonary edema, hypotension, normal capillary wedge pressure	Support blood pressure and respirations (may require intubation), transfer to intensive care
Fluid overload	Acute cardiac failure, dyspnea, pulmonary edema	Induce diuresis, support cardiorespiratory systems as needed
Delayed transfusion reactions	Anemia, fever, and jaundice	Identify antiglobulin, observe coagulation tests and urine output
Bacterial contamination	Rigors, fever, chills, shock	Stop transfusion, antibiotics, support blood pressure

DIC, disseminated intravascular coagulation; i.m., intramuscular; i.v., intravenous.

Table 39.4. Blood component therapy summary

Component	Unit volume (mL)	Content	Unit effect
Red blood cells	350	Red cells	Increase hematocrit by 3%
Frozen plasma	200–300	All clotting factors	Increased fibrinogen by 7–10 mg/dL
Cryopercipitate	10–15	Fibrinogen, factors VIII and XIII, von Willebrand factor	Increased fibrinogen by 7–10 mg/dL
Platelets	50	Platelets	Increase platelet count by 30×10^9/L
Whole blood (if available)	500	All components	

can take up to 45 minutes. A low fibrinogen of <2 g/L reflects impending coagulopathy [37]. Calcium should be given in massive transfusion as hypocalcemia will exacerbate coagulopathy.

Recombinant factor VIIa was thought to have a major role in the management of obstetric hemorrhage when coagulopathy was present. However, its use recently has only been advocated in intractable hemorrhage and following hematology advice. It must be emphasized that, prior to the administration of this costly drug, hypothermia, hypocalcemia, and acidosis should be reversed and appropriate coagulation products given. There have been reports of a higher risk of arterial thromboembolism with its use [38]. The dose is 90 µg/kg intravenously over 5 minutes, which can be repeated after 20 minutes [39] if there has been no response.

If there is evidence of fibrinolysis, as diagnosed by the classic tadpole trace in thromboelastometry, there is a role for tranexamic acid, with 1 g given over 1 minute and another 1 g given 30 minutes later if bleeding continues. This is supported by work in trauma patients and following both vaginal delivery and cesarean section [40–42]. An international study, WOrld Maternal ANtifibrinolytic (WOMAN) trial, has been set up to assess the effects of the early administration of tranexamic acid on PPH after vaginal delivery or cesarean delivery. It is due to be completed by 2015. It should be noted that fibrinolysis cannot be diagnosed by standard laboratory tests.

Cell salvage

Cell salvage has been well established in many surgical specialties but the uptake has been slow in obstetrics because of concerns of amniotic fluid embolism and rhesus isoimmunization [43]. There have been no proven cases of amniotic fluid embolism caused by cell salvage, but it is currently recommended that a separate sucker is used for amniotic fluid and another for salvaged blood [44]. When the latter is transfused, this should be done through a leukocyte depletion filter. Recently, there have been reports of hypotension associated with the use of leukocyte depletion filters [45,46]. There is transference of fetal red cells to the mother in salvaged blood as the cell salvage machine cannot differentiate between maternal and fetal red cells, and a Kleihauer–Betke test should be performed in all rhesus-negative mothers and an appropriate dose of anti-D given after birth to reduce the risk of rhesus isoimmunization if the baby is rhesus positive.

Critical care

Facilities to care for a patient following a major hemorrhage vary widely from unit to unit. Some smaller maternity units do not have the resources, beds, staff, or equipment to care for such a patient. Others substitute recovery or labor ward beds and introduce care based on a 1:1 midwife to patient model. The larger units tend to have dedicated high dependency units with appropriate levels of staff and technical resources. Delivery of care remains multidisciplinary, with obstetricians and anesthesiologists working together with midwives. Ward rounds should be done several times a day to ensure care is appropriate in potentially rapidly evolving situations.

Hemorrhage is the commonest cause of admission to intensive care units [47] and becomes necessary either because there are no high dependency unit facilities or the patient requires a higher level of care than can be provided in a particular unit. The latter is usually initiated because of multiorgan dysfunction. Ventilation in intensive care is sometimes necessary after hemorrhage to maximize oxygenation or simply to "rest" the patient if surgery has been prolonged (e.g. following cesarean hysterectomy) or until other pathologies have been resolved (e.g. coagulopathy). If a patient has inherent cardiac disease, then invasive monitoring to detect arrhythmias or cardiac failure is necessary and the intensive care unit is the best place for this. More commonly, cardiac failure can follow overtransfusion, and the ensuing pulmonary edema will result in hypoxia requiring ventilatory support. Definitive treatment is induction of diuresis. Inotropic support may also be required. Renal failure from inadequate resuscitation is now a condition rarely seen in the obstetric patient, but pre-eclamptics and those with chronic renal disease are at risk following hemorrhage. Renal replacement therapy may be required. Hepatic failure is very rare following hemorrhage and again only likely if pre-eclampsia is also present.

Conclusions

Obstetric hemorrhage is a common complication in the peripartum period. It has multiple causes and a successful outcome for both mother and baby is dependent on rapid diagnosis, resuscitation, and definitive treatment, which may involve pharmacological and surgical therapies. Multiple specialties are involved in the care of the hemorrhaging parturient, including obstetricians, anesthesiologists, midwives, hematologists, and occasionally radiologists and intensivists. Good communication is essential and drills improve efficiency of the team. If managed appropriately however, treating a patient with major hemorrhage is one of the most satisfying aspects of obstetrics and anesthetics, as the majority of previously healthy women return from a near-death situation to one of complete resolution from this complication in a relatively short time period.

References

1. Hogan MC, Foreman KJ, Naghavi M, *et al.* Maternal mortality for 181 countries, 1980–2008: a systematic analysis of progress towards Millennium Development Goal 5. *Lancet* 2010;**375**:1609–1623.

2. Abou Zahr C, Royston E. *Global Mortality: Global Factbook.* Geneva: World Health Organization, 1991.

3. El-Refaey H, Rodeck C. Post-partum haemorrhage: definitions, medical and surgical management. A time for change. *Br Med Bull* 2003;**67**:205–217.

4. Chang J, Elam-Evans LD, Berg CJ, *et al.* Pregnancy-related mortality surveillance: United States, 1991–1999. *MMWR Surveill Summ* 2003;**52**:1–8.

5. Callaghan WM, Kuklina EV, Berg CJ. Trends in postpartum hemorrhage: United States, 1994–2006. *Am J Obstet Gynecol* 2010;**202**:353.e1–353e6.

6. Combs CA, Murphy EL, Laros RK Jr. Factors associated with postpartum hemorrhage with vaginal birth. *Obstet Gynecol* 1991;**77**:69–76.

451

7. Eden RD, Parker RT, Gall SA. Rupture of the pregnant uterus. A 53-year review. *Obstet Gynecol* 1986;**68**:671–674.

8. Taylor DR, Doughty AS, Kaufman H, Yang L, Iannucci TA. Uterine rupture with the use of PGE$_2$ vaginal inserts for labor induction in women with previous cesarean sections. *J Reprod Med* 2002;**47**:549–554.

9. Devoe LD, Croom CS, Youssef AA, Murray C. The prediction of 'controlled' uterine rupture by the use of intrauterine pressure catheters, *Obstet Gynecol* 1992;**80**:626–629.

10. Thakur A, Heer MS, Thakur V, *et al.* Subtotal hysterectomy for uterine rupture *Int J Gynecol Obstet* 2001;**74**;29–33.

11. Lockwood CJ, Schatz F. A biological model for the regulation of peri-implantational hemostasis and menstruation. *J Soc Gynecol Invest* 1996;**3**:159–165.

12. Clark SL, Belfort MA, Dildy GA, *et al.* Maternal death in the 21st century: causes, prevention and relationship to cesarean delivery. *Am J Obstet Gynecol* 2008;**199**:36. e1–36e5.

13. Crosby E. Perioperative use of erythropoietin. *Am J Ther* 2002;**9**:371–376.

14. Mattox KL, Bickell W, Pepe PE, Burch J, Feliciano D. Prospective MAST study in 911 patients. *J Trauma* 1989;**29**:1104–1111.

15. PROMPT Maternity Foundation. *UK PROMPT (PRactical Obstetric Multi-Professional Training)*. Bristol: PROMPT Maternity Foundation (http://www. promptmaternity.org/, accessed 29 January 2013).

16. ALSO UK. *Managing Obstetric Emergencies and Trauma Manual and Advanced Life Support in Obstetrics Manual*. Newcastle, UK: ALSO UK (www. also.org.uk, accessed 29 January 2013).

17. Alonso A, Baker DP, Holtzman A. Reducing medical error in the military health system: how can team training help?. *Hum Resource Manag Rev* 2006;**16**:396.

18. Skupski DW, Lowenwirt IP, Weinbaum FI, *et al.* Improving hospital systems for the care of women with major obstetric hemorrhage. *Obstet Gynecol* 2006;**107**:977.

19. McDonald S, Abbott JM, Higgins SP. Prophylactic ergometrine-oxytocin versus oxytocin for the third stage of labour. *Cochrane Database Syst Rev* 2007; (3):CD000201.

20. Gülmezoglu AM, Forna F, Villar J, Hofmeyr GJ. Prostaglandins for preventing postpartum haemorrhage. *Cochrane Database Syst Rev* 2007; CD000494.

21. Katesmark M, Brown R, Raju KS. Successful use of a Sengstaken–Blakemore tube to control massive postpartum haemorrhage. *Br J Obstet Gynaecol* 1994;**101**:259–260.

22. Habek D. Kulas T. Bobi-Vukovi M, *et al.* Successful of the B-Lynch compression suture in the management of massive postpartum hemorrhage: case reports and review *Arch Gynecol Obstet* 2006;**273**:307–309.

23. Hebisch G, Huch A. Vaginal uterine artery ligation avoids high blood loss and puerperal hysterectomy in postpartum hemorrhage. *Obstet Gynecol* 2002;**100**:574–578.

24. Dildy GA III. Postpartum hemorrhage: new management options. *Clin Obstet Gynecol* 2002;**45**:330–344.

25. Pelage JP, Le Dref O, Mateo J, *et al.* Life-threatening primary postpartum hemorrhage: treatment with emergency selective arterial embolization. *Radiology* 1998;**208**:359–362.

26. Clement D, Kayem G, Cabrol D. Conservative treatment of placenta percreta: a safe alternative. *Eur J Obstet Gynecol Reprod Biol* 2004;**114**:108–109.

27. Usta IM, Hobeika EM, Musa AA, Gabriel GE, Nassar AH. Placenta previa-accreta: risk factors and complications. *Am J Obstet Gynecol* 2005;**193**:1045–1049.

28. Bodner LJ, Nosher JL, Gribbin C, *et al.* Balloon-assisted occlusion of the internal iliac arteries in patients with placenta accreta/percreta. *Cardiovasc Intervent Radiol* 2006;**29**:354–361.

29. Yamakagem Mori T, Tsujiguchi N, *et al.* The inhibitory effects of halothane, isoflurane and sevoflurane on contractility and intracellular calcum concentration of pregnant myometrium in rats. *Anesthesiology* 1998;**89**: A1050.

30. Mok M, Heidemann, Dundas K, Gillespie I, Clark V. Interventional radiology in women with suspected placenta accreta undergoing caesarean section. *Int J Obstet Anesth* 2008;**17**:255–261.

31. Lilker SJ, Meyer RA, Downey KN, Macarthur AJ. Anesthetic considerations for placenta accrete. *Int J Obstet Anesth* 2011;**20**:288–292.

32. Bose P, Regan F, Paterson-Brown S. Improving the accuracy of estimated blood loss at obstetric haemorrhage using clinical reconstructions. *Br J Obstet Gynaecol* 2006;**113**:919–924.

33. Richards NA, Boyce H, Yentis SM. Estimation of blood haemoglobin concentration using the Hemocue during caesarean section: the effects of sampling site. *Int J Obstet Anesth* 2010;**19**:67–70.

34. Royal College of Obstetricians and Gynecologists. *Blood Transfusions in Obstetrics (Green-top 47)*. London: Royal College of Obstetricians and Gynecologists, 2008.

35. Shields L, Lee R, Druzin M, for the Californian Maternal Quality Care Collaborative. *Obstetric*

Hemorrhage Toolkit: Obstetric Hemorrhage Care Guidelines and Compendium of Best Practices. Los Angeles, CA: Californian Maternal Quality Care Collaborative, 2009 (www.cmqcc.org/resources/856/download, accessed 7 December 2012).

36. Armstrong S, Fernando R, Ashpole K, Simons R, Columb M. Assessment of coagulation in the obstetric population using ROTEM thromboelastometry. *Int J Obstet Anesth* 2011;**20**:293–298.

37. Charbit B, Mandelbrot L, Samain E, *et al*. The decrease of fibrinogen is an early predictor of the severity of postpartum hemorrhage, *J Thromb Haemost* 2007;**5**:266–273.

38. Levi M, Levy JH, Andersen HF, Truloff D. Safety of recombinant activated factor VII in randomized clinical trials. *N Engl J Med* 2010;**363**:1791–1800.

39. Franchini M, Franchi M, Bergamini V, *et al*. The use of recombinant activated FVII in postpartum haemorrhage. *Clin Obstet Gynecol* 2010;**53**:219–227.

40. Shakur H, Roberts I, Bautista R, *et al*. Effects of tranexamic acid on death, vascular occlusive events, and blood transfusion in trauma patients with significant haemorrhage (CRASH-2): a randomised, placebo-controlled trial. *Lancet* 2010;**376**:23–32.

41. Ducloy-Bouthors A, Broisin F, Keita H, *et al*. Tranexamic acid reduces blood loss in postpartum haemorrhage. *Crit Care* 2010;**14**: P37.

42. Sekhavat L, Tabatabaii A, Dalili M, *et al*. Efficacy of tranexamic acid in reducing blood loss after cesarean section. *J Matern Fetal Neonatal Med* 2009;**22**:72–5.

43. Allam J, Cox M, Yentis SM. Cell salvage in obstetrics. *Int J Obstet Anesth* 2008;**17**:37–45.

44. UK National Institute of Clinical Excellence. *NHS: Intra-operative Blood Cell Salvage in Obstetrics (IPG 144)*. London: National Institute of Clinical Excellence, 2005 (www.nice.org.uk/guidance/IPG144/, accessed 29 January 2013).

45. Kessack LK, Hawkins N. Severe hypotension related to cell salvaged blood transfusion in obstetrics. *Anaesthesia* 2010;**65**:745–748.

46. Sreelakshmi TR, Eldridge J. Acute hypotension associated with leucocyte depletion filters during cell salvaged blood transfusion. *Anaesthesia* 2010;**65**:742–744.

47. Zwart JJ, Dupuis JR, Richers A, Ory F, van Roosmalen J. Obstetric intensive care admission: a 2 year nationwide population-based cohort study. *Intensive Care Med* 2010;**36**:256–263.

Chapter 40

Anaphylactoid syndrome of pregnancy (amniotic fluid embolus)

Derek Tuffnell, Giorgio Capogna, Katy Harrison, and Silvia Stirparo

Introduction

In 1941, Steiner and Luschbaugh described amniotic fluid embolism (AFE) for the first time, after they found fetal debris in the pulmonary circulation of women who had died during labor. Since then, it has commonly been believed that AFE is a rare obstetric emergency in which amniotic fluid, fetal cells, hair, or other debris enter the maternal circulation, causing maternal cardiorespiratory collapse. However, current data suggest that the process is more similar to anaphylaxis than to embolism and, therefore, the term "anaphylactoid syndrome of pregnancy" has been suggested. In fact, in both anaphylaxis and AFE there is entrance into the circulating blood of a foreign substance and the release of mediators, and both have a similar temporal sequence of hemodynamic compensation and recovery.

Although AFE is a rare condition with a poorly understood pathophysiology, it is a condition that causes significant maternal and fetal morbidity and mortality. It presents during labor, delivery, or during the immediate postpartum period with catastrophic maternal collapse or signs of acute fetal compromise such as a bradycardia. Signs and symptoms of AFE are variable and often non-specific, making diagnosis difficult. Confirmation of the diagnosis usually occurs retrospectively or at autopsy, if made at all. Treatment is entirely supportive, and AFE, therefore, presents a truly multidisciplinary challenge.

Outcome is also highly variable. Fetal outcome is excellent if AFE occurs after delivery. Maternal mortality, although improving, is still significant and in those women who do survive neurological morbidity is common.

Epidemiology

The actual incidence of AFE is unknown. This is mainly because of the difficulties in making and confirming the diagnosis. Various studies from across the world have calculated an incidence of 1 in 80 000 pregnancies up to 1 in 8000 pregnancies [1–5], The UK Obstetric Surveillance System and the Confidential Enquiries into Maternal Deaths (CEMACH) attempt to record all UK cases of AFE and maternal deaths as a result. In the 2006–2008 triennium CEMACH report, 13 mothers died from AFE, making it the fourth leading cause of direct maternal deaths [6]. The UK Amniotic Fluid Embolism Register looked at the incidence and outcome of AFE between 1997 and 2004. This suggests that AFE has a mortality of 37% in the UK [7]. However, in the subsequent period (2005–2009) the mortality rate was reduced to 20% [5]. Worldwide, mortality has been found to be as high as 86% but other studies have come up with rates which are similar to those in the UK [2,4,8]. Again, the problems with diagnosis and follow-up make calculation of mortality rates very difficult.

The changing mortality rate is probably the result of two factors: better intensive care and earlier and better recognition of the fact that "milder" cases exist. For example, according to Benson "the mere fact of survival" was generally considered "proof that a given individual did not have an amniotic fluid embolism" [9].

Benson proposed a new clinical definition of AFE that would apply "to patients who survive, as well as to those who die" [9]. Milder AFE tends to present with less dramatic collapse and often only transient hemodynamic change, whereas severe AFE is characterized by collapse with cardiac arrest. In the USA, Clark *et al.* [10] established clinical criteria for AFE for the national registry; these criteria have been followed in the UK since 1997 in an effort to develop a registry of cases [10,11]. These criteria are:

- acute hypotension or cardiac arrest
- acute hypoxia (dyspnea, cyanosis, or respiratory arrest)
- coagulopathy (laboratory evidence of intravascular coagulation or severe hemorrhage)
- onset of all of the above during labor or within 30 minutes of delivery
- no other clinical conditions or potential explanations for the signs and symptoms.

Typically, AFE presents with a cluster of features. This becomes clear when a larger series of cases is considered. In early series reporting a high mortality rate, such as the Morgan series [11], almost all women presented with cardiorespiratory collapse. Other signs and symptoms were breathlessness, hypotension, collapse (e.g. hypovolemic), and seizures. Fetal signs and symptoms did not feature in this series, but in 17% of the US series the abnormal fetal heart rate pattern was bradycardia [10]. Coagulopathy and bleeding were uncommon presenting features [10,11].

Coagulopathy and massive hemorrhage seem to be features that develop later. "Coagulopathy may develop shortly after the event, but becomes clinically apparent only later. However if early coagulation screen is done, it may already be detected early on" [7]. The multiple clinical presentations support the hypothesis that early deaths are caused by direct and "toxic" effects of a bolus of fetal material or amniotic fluid; the women who survive that initial event then become exposed to a cascade of related problems that follow. Most deaths now occur in this acute phase of collapse [12]. It seems likely though that some women are "sensitive" to amniotic fluid whereas other women can have amniotic fluid in the circulation with no ill effect.

Risk factors

Medical inductions of labor, advancing maternal age, particularly in women from ethnic minority groups, cesarean section, and multiple pregnancy have all been demonstrated as risk factors for AFE [4,5,8]. Other proposed risk factors include operative vaginal birth, manual removal of placenta, polyhydramnios, placenta previa and accreta, eclampsia, and cervical laceration and uterine rupture [1–3,5,7,13]. However, at present there is little evidence to either substantiate or refute these suggestions.

Etiology

The two different names for this condition reflect the fact that we do not know the exact pathophysiological mechanism responsible for the syndrome. Autopsy examination of the maternal lungs shows evidence of fetal tissue (e.g. fetal squames or hair) thought to have come from amniotic fluid [1,2,5]. The amniotic fluid is forced into the maternal circulation through vessels in the uterus or cervix when they are damaged or when a pressure gradient is produced. Once the amniotic fluid has entered the maternal circulation, it eventually ends up in the lungs and pulmonary circulation. Here it causes a cascade of events and triggers a two-phase process. In the first phase, pulmonary artery vasospasm with pulmonary hypertension and elevated right ventricular pressure cause hypoxia, which leads to myocardial and pulmonary capillary damage. In the second phase, the left heart fails, and acute respiratory distress syndrome and maternal cardiovascular collapse develop.

There are two proposed mechanisms for these changes. One is that there is a physical blockage of the pulmonary vasculature by the amniotic fluid embolus. The second is that the fetal tissue produces an anaphylactoid reaction within the vessels, releasing immune modulators such as histamine, prostaglandins, and leukotrienes. A combination of both of these is likely to occur [1–3].

If the mother survives the initial collapse, she will then go on to develop left ventricular failure, pulmonary edema, disseminated intravascular coagulation, and neurological impairment (Figure 40.1) [1–3].

The following are factors that are considered to contribute to the pathology:

- pressure gradient favoring the entry of fetal material into maternal circulation
  - small tears in the endocervical and lower uterine vein
  - placental separation site
- pulmonary vascular occlusion: histological evidence of amniotic fluid debris in early reports
- coagulation effects
  - procoagulant substances
  - tissue factors (binding with factor VII and activation of factor X)
  - trophoblastic tissues
  - complement activation

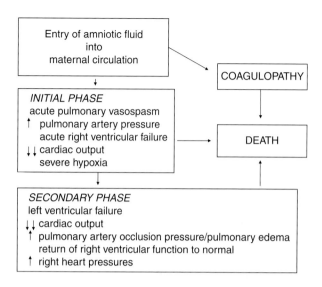

Figure 40.1. Biphasic theory of collapse with amniotic fluid embolus (AFE).

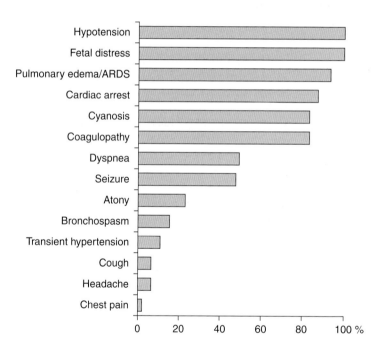

Figure 40.2. Etiology of the effects of amniotic fluid embolus.

- vasoactive effects
  - release of prostaglandins E2 and F2α
  - release of leukotrienes C4 and D4
  - release of endothelin (myocardial depressant, pulmonary artery and coronary constrictor).

Diagnosis

Most women with AFE present with collapse but occasionally, early more subtle signs and symptoms are present, which can rapidly progress to collapse if left untreated. If the woman is still pregnant then fetal distress is usually seen. While Clark *et al.* [10] originally used 30 minutes after birth as a cut-off, there do seem to be cases of AFE that occur up to at least 60 minutes, and later series allow a longer time after birth before the first signs or symptoms as cut-off.

Initial presentation is acute maternal collapse during labor, delivery, or up to 60 minutes after delivery with no other clear cause and with a broad spectrum [10] of initial clinical presentation (Figure 40.2).

Amniotic fluid embolism is a diagnosis of exclusion, or one which is made after the autopsy finding of fetal squames or hair in the maternal lungs, which often require immunochemistry for identification [1,2,5]. However, fetal squamous cells are commonly found in the circulation of laboring patients who do not develop the syndrome. Even in a patient who is critically ill, aspirate of the distal port of a pulmonary artery catheter that contains fetal squamous cells is considered suspicious for but not diagnostic of AFE syndrome.

Most recently, new diagnostic tests have been reported which may help in the diagnosis of AFE, such as immunohistochemical techniques to demonstrate the evidence of amniotic fluid debris [14], monoclonal antibodies to identify amniotic fluid-derived mucin in maternal serum [15], and maternal determination of meconial components (zinc coproporphyrin-1) [16]. However, these new tests appear to be more research tools rather than practical routine diagnostic tests. Tryptase has been reported as elevated or normal so it is not a discriminator in the diagnosis.

Differential diagnosis

Since treatment of AFE is entirely supportive, it is important to exclude other differential diagnoses that will require specific treatment:

- cardiac
  - myocardial infarction
  - cardiomyopathy
  - heart failure secondary to volume overload
  - valvular disease
- respiratory
  - pulmonary edema secondary to volume overload
  - acute asthma
  - pulmonary embolus
- infectious
  - severe sepsis
  - chest
  - chorioamnionitis
  - endocarditis
- pregnancy complications
  - pre-eclampsia and eclampsia
  - HELLP syndrome (hemolysis, elevated liver enzymes, and low platelets)
  - ante- and postpartum hemorrhage
- others
  - anaphylaxis
  - air embolus
  - local anesthetic toxicity.

Investigations

Since AFE is a diagnosis of exclusion, investigations are necessary to exclude other differential diagnoses and to assess and monitor maternal and fetal well-being and response to treatment.

Routine observations are essential in the initial resuscitation of any unwell patient. Blood pressure, pulse, respiratory rate, and oxygen saturation should be monitored every 5 minutes. Temperature should also be taken to exclude sepsis.

Bloods tests are outlined in Table 40.1.

Table 40.1. Blood tests

Test	Utility
Full blood count	Hemoglobin, white cell count and platelet count
Coagulation screen	Presence and severity of any coagulopathy; in severe cases it may be obvious by direct observation of the blood loss that a coagulopathy is present
Urea and electrolytes and liver function tests	Renal or hepatic failure, helps to exclude a diagnosis of pre-eclampsia, HELLP, or acute fatty liver of pregnancy
Blood glucose	Excludes a diagnosis of hypoglycemia as a cause of collapse, although a bedside finger prick test is quicker
Others	C-reactive protein if sepsis is a concern; cardiac enzymes if a cardiac cause is suspected; tryptase, although its interpretation is difficult
Group and cross-match sample	To ensure cross-matched blood is available as soon as possible

Table 40.2 Presenting symptoms of amniotic fluid embolus

Investigation	Utility
Arterial blood gas, lactate	If oxygen saturations are low or there is concern about ventilation and acid–base status
Urine	Dipstick analysis; sepsis screening (ideally from a clean catch catheter sample)
Electrocardiography	Arrhythmias and any evidence of right or left heart strain; may help to exclude other cardiac causes for collapse such as myocardial infarction
Chest radiography	Pulmonary edema, infection, effusions, cardiomegaly; further images may be needed to assess response to treatment or to assess for development of complications such as the acute respiratory distress syndrome
Echocardiography	Cardiac function; to exclude a diagnosis of cardiomyopathy or endocarditis
Toxicity screen	If concern about maternal drug use or accidental administration of drugs
Ventilation/perfusion scan or CT pulmonary angiography	Exclude pulmonary embolus and assess ventilation; not suitable if the woman is unstable and unwell
Central venous pressure	Monitor fluid balance; provide a central access to deliver fluid and drugs
Pulmonary blood sample	Fetal debris within the pulmonary circulation

Fetal assessment should be made using cardiotocography when the woman is stable to allow decisions to made about delivery. However, decisions regarding delivery should be guided by the maternal condition and should always be made with maternal well-being as a primary concern.

Other investigations may be considered (Table 40.2).

Management

Management of AFE is a true multidisciplinary team effort. Obstetricians, midwives, anesthesiologists, neonatologists, critical care teams, and hematologists all play a vital role in caring for these women.

Early recognition of an unwell woman and timely resuscitative measures are the key to preventing mortality and morbidity.

Most AFE occurs on the labor ward around the time of delivery. However, intensive care is almost universally required and, if this is not readily available nearby, steps will need to be taken to secure this promptly following initial resuscitation.

Transfer to intensive care unit

Once the baby has been delivered or if the AFE occurred after delivery then when the woman is stable she will need immediate transfer to intensive care unit (level 3 supportive care). If she survives the initial phase of pulmonary hypertension, hypoxemia, and right heart failure, then she will require supportive care to deal with complications such as left ventricular failure, pulmonary edema, coagulopathy, and acute respiratory distress syndrome.

Clinical treatment

Aggressive resuscitation is the keystone to a good outcome for a woman and her fetus (Box 40.3). Initial management is supportive rather than specific. Basic resuscitation must be started immediately. Maximal initial oxygenation is required and, usually, early intubation and ventilation. An important step to consider as an integral part of the resuscitation of the mother is prompt delivery by cesarean section if the woman does not respond to cardiopulmonary resuscitation within 5 minutes. Prompt transfusion of fluids is necessary to replace blood loss. Vasopressors such as phenylephrine may help to restore aortic perfusion pressure [17].

As with any collapse, the early involvement of senior, experienced staff is critical, since the technical and practical aspects of resuscitation are more likely to be expertly performed by people who practice them regularly. A multidisciplinary approach involving obstetricians, anesthesiologists, intensivists, and hematologists carries the best prospect for the woman's survival. While the patient is being resuscitated, the team will have to investigate other causes of the collapse. The most useful diagnostic test to exclude a large segment of the differential diagnosis is a clotting screen. Clotting is often extremely abnormal even before the hemorrhage becomes apparent. If the patient is already hemorrhaging, abnormal clotting secondary to the hemorrhage needs to be considered.

Box 40.1. Aggressive resuscitation

Airway and breathing

The airway should be patent and secured. This may require intubation and ventilation; 100% oxygen should be administered. Effectiveness of oxygenation can be measured with oxygen saturations and arterial blood gases

Circulatory support

Two large intravenous lines should be inserted initially. Blood can be drawn from these for testing. Rapid intravenous fluids should be given (ideally warmed) or blood if this is felt to be necessary because of excess losses. Blood pressure needs to be maintained and drugs may be required such as inotropes and phenylephrine

Cardiopulmonary resuscitation

If cardiopulmonary resuscitation is required and the woman is still pregnant, this should be performed with a left lateral tilt or manual displacement of the gravid uterus to reduce aortocaval compression. If circulation does not return within 5 minutes, then perimortem cesarean section should be performed to empty the uterus

Coagulopathy

If hemorrhage is ongoing this needs to be treated. Uterine atony is treated with bimanual compression and drugs. Replacement of blood lost and clotting factors is also required

However, hemorrhage will not usually cause a coagulopathy by itself unless there is considerable blood loss and blood replacement.

If there are any signs of coagulopathy, such as blood in the urine or bleeding from the gums, the team should consider replacing clotting factor with fresh frozen plasma, cryoprecipitate, and platelets – even before massive blood loss is apparent and certainly before receiving the laboratory confirmation of coagulopathy. Indeed, cryoprecipitate may be of intrinsic value beyond its clotting factor components because it contains fibronectin, which helps the reticuloendothelial system to filter antigenic and toxic particulates [17].

It also is important to perform electrocardiography to look for signs of myocardial damage. However, AFE can cause bizarre cardiac rhythms, which may need specific treatment and can make interpretation difficult. Because myocardial suppression is more common, dopamine or other inotropes may be helpful. Early pulmonary artery catheterization has been recommended to guide therapy [7,17,18], helping to prevent the fluid overload that can worsen pulmonary edema and lead to adult respiratory distress syndrome. Most recently, less invasive techniques such as transesophageal echocardiography have been reported in helping the diagnosis and in guiding therapy for AFE. Arterial blood gases also may be of value, in addition to pulse oximetry, but will not differentiate causes specifically. In a patient who becomes stable, a ventilation/perfusion scan of the lungs may demonstrate defects. However, AFE can occlude the pulmonary vessels, so defects do not exclude it as a diagnosis.

If the fetal condition deteriorates suddenly, the team should consider coagulation studies and maternal pulse oximetry. These will be more appropriate if the fetus is unexpectedly severely acidotic. This is because fetal collapse may precede maternal collapse and additional maternal monitoring may identify early maternal deterioration.

A number of therapies have been used in managing AFE. In one case, AFE was thought to be in progress as air bubbles and vernix were seen in the left uterine vein at cesarean section [19]. The infundibulopelvic ligament and uterine arteries were ligated. Mild coagulopathy occurred but there were no other problems.

Various techniques of supporting cardiorespiratory function have been used in the acute phase of the condition. Cardiopulmonary bypass and open pulmonary artery thromboembolectomy produced a good outcome in one woman [20]. Extracorporeal membrane oxygenation and intra-aortic balloon counterpulsation have also been used successfully [21]. Inhaled prostacyclin has been used to dilate pulmonary vessels, and inhaled nitric oxide has been suggested but not documented in case reports [22,23]. Because the occurrence of AFE bears distinct similarities to anaphylaxis, Clark *et al.* [10] postulated that high-dose hydrocortisone (500 mg every 6 hours) may be appropriate, but no studies have yet examined this.

Because there is some "toxic" element to the effects of amniotic fluid, a number of reports have suggested that hemofiltration or plasma exchange may be effective in clearing the plasma and aiding recovery. In 1987, a report detailed a successful outcome after two exchange transfusions for a probable AFE following amniocentesis [24]. A report in 2001 suggested that

459

transfusing 1.5 times the patient's blood volume acted as an exchange transfusion [20]. When this "cleansing" process was achieved by continuous hemofiltration in one woman, clotting parameters improved dramatically [25]. This approach may be appropriate after the patient has been stabilized. However, since massive transfusion is a part of initial management when hemorrhage occurs, this may become a treatment by default.

All women who are critically unwell require urethral catheterization with hourly urine output documenting to monitor urine output and response to treatment. This forms part of the level 2 input/output charting.

Timing and mode of delivery

If a woman is still pregnant when AFE occurs, then fetal mortality is around 20–25%. Fetal morbidity is high with rates of hypoxic ischemic encephalopathy and cerebral palsy at about 50% if the baby was alive and still in utero at the time of the AFE [7]. If the woman suffers a cardiac arrest, then perimortem cesarean section should be undertaken within 5 minutes of commencing cardiopulmonary resuscitation in order to improve the effectiveness of maternal resuscitation by correcting diaphragmatic splintage and reducing oxygen requirements. If cardiopulmonary resuscitation is not required, then the baby needs to be delivered as quickly as possible after initial stabilization of the woman. This is invariably by cesarean section unless vaginal delivery is imminent or swiftly achievable by instrumental delivery. Once the baby has been delivered, it should be immediately assessed by the senior neonatology team. Since there is a significant risk of coagulopathy, cesarean section should be performed under general anesthesia.

Treatment of coagulopathy

Development of disseminated intravascular coagulation is almost synonymous with AFE. It can occur immediately after collapse or there can be a delay of several hours before coagulopathy develops. There is evidence from blood analysis of a consumptive coagulopathy that is exacerbated by bleeding postpartum, particularly from an atonic uterus.

Atonic postpartum hemorrhage should be treated using drugs and bimanual compression in the first instance. Drugs should be used in line with standard and any national guidance on management of postpartum hemorrhage. Intravenous oxytocin is used as a bolus and an infusion. Ergometrine, carboprost, and misoprostol can also be used. Since coagulopathy can be severe, early recourse to surgical management may be necessary or more appropriate if delivery has taken place by cesarean section. Hysterectomy to control bleeding is required in approximately 25% of patients [3].

Correction of the coagulopathy is required with clotting factors as well as transfusion of red blood cells to maintain blood volume. Cryoprecipitate, fresh frozen plasma, and platelets are all necessary and used routinely.

Recombinant factor VIIa has been used to treat hemorrhage in AFE patients even though it can combine with circulating tissue factor and form intravascular clots. It has been reported in a recent systematic review that patients with AFE and massive hemorrhage who were treated with recombinant factor VIIa had significantly worse outcomes than cohorts who did not receive it [26]. However, the review did not consider patients who did not require surgery. Nevertheless, recombinant factor VIIa should be used in patients with AFE only when the hemorrhage cannot be stopped by massive blood component replacement and following factor replacement.

Thromboprophylaxis

All women are at significant risk of venous thromboembolism in the postpartum period. Those who undergo cesarean section, laparotomy, or require admission to high dependency or intensive care units are at even higher risk. Blood transfusion and replacement of clotting factors, particularly factor VIIa, is a further risk factor. Women who have had AFE should, therefore, receive thromboprophylaxis postpartum.

Antiembolism "TED" stockings should be worn by all women provided there are no contraindications. Low-molecular-weight heparin prophylaxis should be administered as soon as the woman is stable, her coagulopathy has been corrected, and she is no longer at risk of hemorrhage. The role of thromboprophylaxis for 6 weeks postpartum is unclear in AFE, but risk factors should be assessed on an individual basis and a decision make at discharge from hospital.

Subsequent pregnancies

If a woman survives following AFE and retains her uterus, then future pregnancies are possible. There is no evidence to suggest that AFE will occur in subsequent pregnancies [4]. However, some women may be more sensitive to the effects of amniotic fluid within their circulation than others and so a subsequent AFE could never be excluded.

References

1. Tuffnell DJ, Hamilton S. Amniotic fluid embolism. *Obstet Gynaecol Reprod Med* 2008;**10**:1016–1020.

2. Dedhia JD, Mushambi MC. Amniotic fluid embolism. Continuing Education in Anaesthesia. *Crit CarePain* 2007;7:152–156.

3. Tuffnell DJ, Knight M, Plaat F. Amniotic fluid embolism: an update. *Anaesthesia* 2010;66:1–3.

4. Roberts CL, Algert CS, Knight M, *et al.* Amniotic fluid embolism in an Australian population-based cohort. *BJOG* 2010;**117**:1417–1421.

5. Knight M, Tuffnell DJ, Brocklehurst P, **et al.** Incidence and risk factors for amniotic fluid embolism. *Obstet Gynaecol* 2010;**115**:910–917.

6. Cantwell R, Clutton-Brock T, Cooper G, *et al.* Saving Mothers' Lives: Reviewing Maternal Deaths to make Motherhood Safer 2006–2008. The Eighth Report of the Confidential Enquiries into Maternal Deaths in the United Kingdom. *BJOG* 2011;**118**(Suppl 1):1–203.

7. Tuffnell DJ. United Kingdom Amniotic Fluid Embolism Register. *BJOG* 2005;**112**:1625–1629.

8. Kramer MS, Rouleau JR, Baskett TF, *et al.* Amniotic-fluid embolism and medical induction of labour: a retrospective, population-based cohort study. *Lancet* 2006;**368**:1444–1448.

9. Benson MD. Nonfatal amniotic fluid embolism. Three possible cases and a new clinical definition. *Arch Fam Med* 1993;2:989–994.

10. Clark SL, Hankins GD, Dudley DA, Dildy GA, Porter TF. Amniotic fluid embolism: analysis of the national registry. *Am J Obstet Gynecol* 1995;**172**:1158–1167.

11. Morgan M Amniotic fluid embolism. *Anaesthesia* 1979;34;20–32.

12. Department of Health, Welsh Office, Scottish Office Department of Health, Department of Health and Social Services, Northern Ireland. Why Mothers Die. *Report on Confidential Enquiries into Maternal Deaths in the United Kingdom, 1997–1999.* London: The Stationery Office, 2001.

13. Moore J. Amniotic fluid embolism: on the trail of an elusive diagnosis. *Lancet* 2006;**368**:1399–1401.

14. Garland IWC, Thompson WD. Diagnosis of amniotic fluid embolism using an antiserum to human keratin. *J Clin Pathol* 1983;**36**:625–627.

15. Kobayashi H, Ooi H, Hayakawa H, *et al.* Histological diagnosis of amniotic fluid embolism by monoclonal antibody TKH-2 that recognizes NeuAcalpha2-6GalNAc epitope. *Hum Pathol* 1997;**28**:428–433.

16. Kanayama N, Yamazaki T, Naruse H, *et al.* Determining zinc coproprophirin in maternal plasma. A new method for diagnosing amniotic fluid embolism. *Clin Chem* 1992;**38**:526–529.

17. Davies S. Amniotic fluid embolus: a review of the literature. *Can J Anaesth* 2001;**48**:88–98.

18. Burrows A, Khoo SK. The amniotic fluid embolism syndrome:10 years' experience at a major teaching hospital. *Aust N Z J Obstet Gynaecol* 1995;**35**:245–250.

19. Gogola J, Hankins GD Amniotic fluid embolism in progress: a management dilemma! *Am J Perinatol* 1998;**15**:491–493.

20. Esposito RA, Grossi EA, Coppa G, et al. Successful treatment of postpartum shock caused by amniotic fluid embolism with cardiopulmonary bypass and pulmonary artery thromboembolectomy. *Am J Obstet Gynecol* 1990;**163**:572–574.

21. Hsieh YY, Chang CC, Li PC, Tsai HD, Tsai CH. Successful application of extracorporeal membrane oxygenation and intra-aortic balloon counterpulsation as lifesaving therapy for a patient with amniotic fluid embolism. *Am J Obstet Gynecol* 2000;**183**:496–497.

22. Van Heerden PV, Webb SA, Hee G, Corkeron M, Thompson WR. Inhaled aerosolized prostacyclin as a selective pulmonary vasodilator for the treatment of severe hypoxaemia. *Anaesth Intensive Care* 1996;**24**:87–90.

23. Tanus-Santos JE, Moreno H Jr. Inhaled nitric oxide and amniotic fluid embolism. *Anesth Analg* 1999;**88**:691.

24. Dodgson J, Martin J, Boswell J, Goodall HB, Smith R. Probable amniotic fluid embolism precipitated by amniocentesis and treated by exchange transfusion. *Br Med J* 1987;**294**:1322–1323.

25. Kaneko Y, Ogihara T, Tajima H, Mochimaru F. Continuous hemodiafiltration for disseminated intravascular coagulation and shock due to amniotic fluid embolism: report of a dramatic response. *Intern Med* 2001;**40**:945–947.

26. Leighton B, Wall M, Lockart EM, et al. Use of recombinant factor VIIa in patients with amniotic fluid embolism: A systematic review of case reports. *Anesthesiology* 2011;**115**:1201–1208.

Maternal complications of fetal surgery

Jan Deprest and Kha M. Tran

Introduction

Fetal surgery is a relatively new and evolving field that lies at the intersection of many disciplines, such as obstetrics, pediatric surgery, anesthesiology, perinatology, neonatology, and radiology. Indications for fetal surgery are, in concept, similar to indications for adult or pediatric surgery. Primarily the goal is preventing fetal mortality, but recently an intervention for improving quality of life was added. This intervention is mid-gestation fetal surgery to close a myelomeningocele. This surgery will help the child by improving motor and sensory function and decreasing the need for ventriculoperitoneal shunting [1]. Another example is that of monochorionic twin pregnancy, which is complicated by the twin–twin transfusion syndrome and which threatens the life of both twins and also causes neurological morbidity in survivors [2]. Laser surgery can be undertaken to prevent both morbidity and mortality in these pregnancies. A fetus with a large airway tumor may not be compromised in utero, but life-threatening airway obstruction may occur at birth, and the fetal airway may need to be secured prior to birth to allow successful transition to neonatal life [3].

The diseases warranting fetal surgery affect quite a variety of fetal organ systems and may impair their normal development hence normal neonatal function. In a number of these conditions, the fetus may develop non-immune hydrops fetalis and may die. In some of these cases, the condition of the mother will "mirror" that of her sick fetus, and her life will also be threatened. Two classes of fetal surgical patient may require critical care. The first is the group of mothers who become critically ill as a result of the *fetal disease* processes, and the second is the group of mothers who require critical care and monitoring as a result of the *treatment* of the fetal disease processes.

Fetal disease necessitating therapy

Complicated multiple gestations

Two thirds of monozygotic or identical twins share a single placenta and are, therefore, monochorionic. These are at increased risk for complications compared with dichorionic twin pregnancies, whether they are mono- or dizygotic [4], the reason being that all monochorionic twins have intertwin vascular anastomoses. In unfavorable angioarchitecture, approximately 9% of monochorionic–diamniotic twins, and very rarely monochorionic–monoamniotic twins, will develop imbalanced blood flow between the fetuses. As a result, one twin will become hypovolemic, oliguric, and growth restricted, while the other twin becomes hypervolemic and polyuric. The smaller twin, therefore, appears with oligohydramnios or anhydramnios, and becomes "stuck" in a particular location because of the lack of amniotic fluid. The other twin will have polyhydramnios, and a number of them will also suffer from congestive heart failure. The polyhydramnios also causes maternal discomfort and/or preterm labor or rupture of the membranes. This condition is known as twin-to-twin transfusion syndrome.

Other feto-fetal transfusion syndromes are those monochorionic twins where one does not have a functional heart. This twin is, therefore, called an acardiac and acts as a parasite on the co-twin, causing additional and unnecessary workload and putting the normal twin at risk for high-output heart failure.

Neurological disease

The only neurological disease that has been shown to be helped by fetal therapy so far is myelomeningocele [1]. Although this is not a life-threatening condition, the

Maternal Critical Care: A Multidisciplinary Approach, ed. Marc Van de Velde, Helen Scholefield, and Lauren A. Plante. Published by Cambridge University Press. © Cambridge University Press 2013.

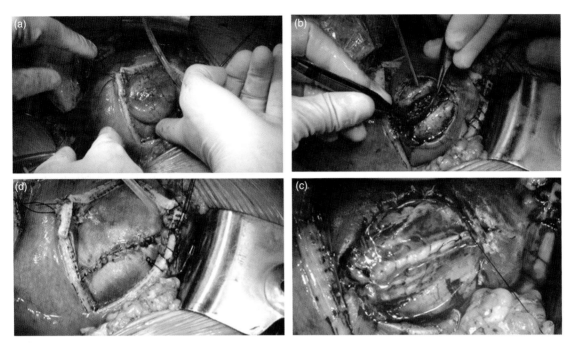

Figure 41.1. View of the different steps during fetal myelomeningocele repair with operators of both the Philadelphia and Leuven team. Through the hysterotomy, the lesion is exposed (a), the meninges (b) and the muscular layer (c) are closed, before finally closure of the fetal skin (d).

neonatal morbidity of this condition is significant. As most of these arise while the fetus is still in utero, in utero repair will avoid them. Prenatal closure of the myelomeningocele will protect the developing spinal cord from the neurotoxic environment of the amniotic fluid and direct trauma. This allows further growth and development of the spinal cord, which will allow improved neurological function. The associated herniation of the hindbrain through the foramen magnum resulting from abnormal cerebrospinal fluid drainage can be reversed, and the risk of hydrocephalus requiring ventriculoperitoneal shunting is decreased. Although endoscopic repair has been reported, the effectiveness of this operation is questionable, as recently demonstrated [5]. Fetal surgery to correct myelomeningocele, therefore, still requires maternal laparotomy and hysterotomy and while it is a procedure with proven fetal benefit [1], it exposes the mother to significant surgical and anesthetic risks (Figure 41.1). Even in uncomplicated cases, the postoperative management of these patients requires meticulous attention and close communication between members of the perioperative team.

Airway obstruction

Fetal airway obstruction can be intrinsic or extrinsic. Intrinsic airway obstruction typically arises from laryngeal cysts or webs, or iatrogenic tracheal occlusion for pulmonary hypoplasia or tracheal atresia; extrinsic obstruction is from tumors around the airway, such as lymphangiomas, teratomas, or other space-occupying lesions around the neck or oral cavities. In most cases, airway obstruction is not an issue until birth, as the placenta is the organ of fetal respiration, but in certain cases the fetal airway obstruction may be so complete that the life of the fetus is threatened. This is not intuitive, but the fetal airway must be patent enough to allow egress of fluid from the fetal lung into the amniotic space. If the fluid has no escape, the fetal lungs will experience massive hyperplasia, the diaphragms will evert and project into the abdomen, and the fetal lungs will compress on the heart and great vessels. The fetus is experiencing "tension hydrothorax," and the cardiac compression will result in heart failure, hydrops, and death [3,6]. Another side effect may be that the fetus cannot swallow normally so that polyhydramnios occurs, leading to preterm labor and/or ruptured membranes.

Lung lesions

The management of fetal lung tumors highlights the wide range of therapeutic options available and illustrates the fact that the pathophysiology and symptoms

463

of each patient must be considered when formulating a fetal treatment plan [7]. Tumors may be small or large, cystic or solid. Tumors may shrink or grow, and they may become so large that they impair development of the normal lung, and even become symptomatic (causing hydrops) at different stages of lung maturity. Small asymptomatic tumors will likely not require fetal therapy, but larger symptomatic tumors will require some fetal intervention. If a cystic tumor becomes symptomatic in mid-gestation with immature lungs, drainage with a one-time needle aspiration or placement of a chronic fetal thoracoamniotic shunt may be all that is required. Solid tumors may require maternal hysterotomy and fetal thoracotomy. The fetus is then replaced in the uterus to continue gestation, hopefully to term. If a solid tumor becomes symptomatic in late gestation, with mature lungs, ex utero intrapartum therapy (EXIT procedure) is indicated [8]. During the EXIT procedure, the lung tumor can be removed, and cardiac compression and mediastinal shift relieved immediately before the fetus is delivered.

The large lung tumor will no longer hamper neonatal resuscitation.

Congenital diaphragmatic hernia

While diaphragmatic hernia is not lethal in utero, the resulting pulmonary hypoplasia places neonates with this diagnosis at great risk of death and disability. Current fetal therapy focuses on fetal tracheal occlusion in the middle of gestation to promote lung growth. There is already considerable experience with percutaneous fetal endoluminal tracheal occlusion suggesting an increased survival rate (Figure 41.2). Trials are currently underway evaluating minimally invasive tracheal occlusion followed by relief of this occlusion several weeks later [9]. Obviously survivors will still undergo postnatal anatomical repair. The repair of the tracheal occlusion can be done in utero by needle puncture or second-look fetoscopy, or at the latest at the time of birth by an EXIT procedure.

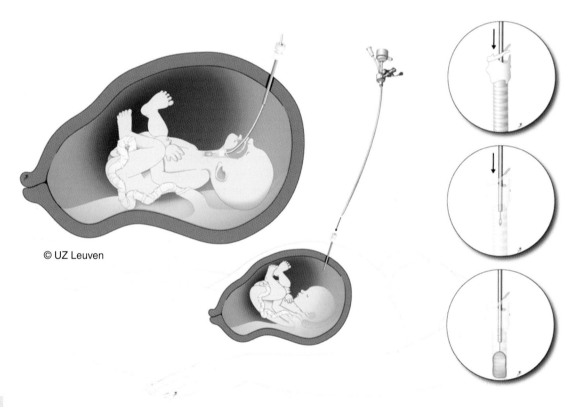

© UZ Leuven

Figure 41.2. Percutaneous approach for fetoscopic endoluminal tracheal occlusion and open fetal surgery, via laparotomy and hysterotomy, for fetal myelomeningocele repair.

Cardiac disease

Invasive treatment of fetal cardiac disease largely consists of catheter-based therapy to palliate the cardiac lesion until the fetus can be delivered and definitive therapy undertaken [10]. Diseases such as fetal aortic stenosis with evolving hypoplastic left heart syndrome, or fetal pulmonary valve atresia with evolving hypoplastic right heart, may be amenable to catheter-based fetal valvuloplasty. A fetus with hypoplastic left heart and an intact atrial septum may be helped with fetal atrial septostomy.

Renal disease

Fetal lower urinary tract obstruction, typically by posterior urethral valves, is challenging to treat [11]. The threat of this condition is double: neonates may die from pulmonary hypoplasia as a consequence of oligohydramnios or from renal failure. Fetal therapy has been shown to improve neonatal survival, but the ability to salvage renal function remains debated. Prenatal therapy involves decompression of the lower urinary tract, typically with a vesicoamniotic shunt placed percutaneously. Recently, diagnostic fetal cystoscopy with subsequent fulguration of fetal urethral valves has been introduced as a causal therapy, although experience remains scarce [12].

Sacrococcygeal teratoma

Sacrococcygeal teratoma are germ cell tumors that may grow rapidly and become more massive than the fetus itself. The tumors threaten the life of the fetus by causing high-output heart failure from a vascular steal phenomenon. Tumors may also rupture in utero and cause severe fetal anemia from hemorrhage. Definitive therapy is often not possible in utero, but if the tumor anatomy is favorable, then mid-gestation surgical debulking has successfully treated the high-output heart failure and allowed the mother to continue to carry the fetus to term [13].

Maternal mirror syndrome

Maternal mirror, or Ballantyne syndrome is the development of maternal edema along with fetoplacental hydrops. Other terms used to describe this syndrome are pseudotoxemia, triple edema (referring to the mother, placenta, and fetus), and maternal hydrops syndrome. While this does seem to be a rare complication of pregnancy, the true incidence of this process is difficult to estimate, given the literature consists mostly of case reports. Mirror syndrome can be associated with both immune and non-immune hydrops, but non-immune causes constitute the majority of reported cases [14]. The condition may be reversible, but when life threatening it may require early delivery of the fetus or termination of pregnancy.

Diagnosis

The clinical presentation of mirror syndrome is quite similar to if not the same as that of pre-eclampsia. Weight gain, elevations in blood pressure, proteinuria, oliguria, headache, visual changes, and increases in liver enzymes may all occur. One distinguishing factor associated more with mirror syndrome than pre-eclampsia seems to be hemodilution and mild anemia. Pulmonary edema occurred in 21% of reported cases [14].

Management

Stabilizing therapy for mirror syndrome should be supportive, but if fetal hydrops is diagnosed, then either treatment of the fetus to resolve the fetal hydrops or delivery of the fetus should be undertaken to avoid maternal complications of mirror syndrome. A brief overview of the types of treatment options available to the mother and fetus follows.

Types of fetal therapy

Fetal interventions may be classified into two broad categories, minimally invasive and open fetal interventions. Minimally invasive procedures typically involve the percutaneous insertion of small instruments, such as injection or radiofrequency ablation needles or fetoscopes with laser fibers, through the maternal abdominal wall and uterus into the amniotic fluid. These instruments may be guided by a combination of ultrasound and direct visualization. Minimally invasive interventions include laser surgery to ablate communicating vessels causing twin-to-twin transfusion syndrome, bipolar umbilical cord cautery or radiofrequency ablation to treat twin reversed arterial perfusion sequence, placement of shunts to decompress the fetal chest or bladder, cardiac valve ablation, and in utero cystoscopy. Minimally invasive surgery typically occurs between 18 and 24 weeks of gestation, but the clinical circumstances and the local legislation may result in some variation of this timing.

Open fetal interventions involve a maternal laparotomy, followed by a hysterotomy through which the surgeons gain direct access to the fetus. Only the necessary parts of the fetus are exposed for the surgical procedure, while the rest of the fetus is kept submerged in amniotic fluid, which is continually replaced by an infusion of warmed crystalloid. Compared with the minimally invasive interventions, these types of fetal intervention may occur at 22–37 weeks of gestation. A mid-gestation open intervention is undertaken if the fetus is showing signs of hydrops fetalis or if the mother is showing signs of mirror syndrome. Lung tumors and sacrococcygeal teratomas are two examples of fetal pathology that may result in hydrops, although by different mechanisms. The treatment of large lung lesions involves a fetal thoracotomy and resection of the diseased lung mass. Large fetal sacrococcygeal teratomas that are anatomically favorable and are causing heart failure may be debulked in mid-gestation.

The case of fetal myelomeningocele repair is unique in that it is the only mid-gestation surgery that is completely elective and not life saving. After mid-gestation fetal surgery is completed, the uterus and the maternal abdomen are closed. The hope is to deliver the fetus as close to term as possible via cesarean section.

Open fetal interventions may also occur much closer to term, when the fetal lungs are mature and the fetus has a condition that may not allow successful transition to extrauterine life. This type of open fetal intervention is often referred to as the EXIT procedure. The conditions that call for an EXIT procedure include the above list plus intrinsic or extrinsic airway obstruction from large airway teratomas or lymphangiomas, and intrinsic airway obstruction from laryngeal atresia, cysts, or webs. The last category of intrinsic airway obstruction has also been called congenital high airway obstruction syndrome.

The fetal airway must be secured to allow a successful transition to extrauterine life. This may be as simple as performing a direct laryngoscopy and intubating the fetus, or may be as complex as performing rigid bronchoscopy, tracheostomy, or retrograde wire intubations. Large lung tumors that did not cause hydrops in the middle of gestation may still cause physiological compromise and impair efforts of neonatal resuscitation. A thoracotomy to resect lung tumors causing mediastinal compression may be required. In contrast to a mid-gestation fetal procedure, where the fetus is replaced in the uterus at the completion of surgery, an EXIT procedure involves both completion of the fetal surgery and then delivery of the fetus.

Anesthetic management

Anesthetizing a mother for fetal interventions is unique for many reasons, one of which is the fact that the anesthesia team is caring for two patients simultaneously and the well-being of the fetus is dependent on the well-being of the mother. More detailed descriptions of the anesthetic management of both minimally invasive and open fetal surgical procedures can be found in other resources [15]. A brief treatment of this topic follows to provide a basis for understanding the critical care issues of these patients in the perioperative period. The goals of any anesthetic are maintaining the safety of the patient, while keeping the patient comfortable and facilitating the completion of whatever procedure needs to be done. The issues that must be integrated when the anesthesiologist formulates a plan include maternal and fetal physiology, specifics of the fetal pathophysiology, placental physiology and transport, and logistical details of the surgical procedure.

Many anesthetic techniques may be used for minimally invasive fetal interventions. The majority may be performed quite simply with local anesthetic infiltration and, when desired, administration of sedatives to the mother to ensure her comfort. Additionally, this may cause fetal sedation. The mother herself should not be excessively sedated as she is at greater risk for pulmonary aspiration of gastric contents. Neuraxial techniques such as spinal and epidural anesthesia may be performed, but given the small size of the instruments are not often warranted unless there is a real risk of performing a cesarean section for fetal distress. However, an epidural may also be used for postoperative analgesia and as a consequence may reduce the risk for preterm labor, and the need for tocolytics. Neuraxial techniques will also predispose to greater hemodynamic shifts, which may place fetuses with impaired placental perfusion at greater risk. General endotracheal anesthesia may be employed in selected cases where absolute uterine relaxation is needed, or when the mother cannot tolerate the sedation. General anesthesia also provides fetal anesthesia, its depth being dependent on the doses used. Standard maternal monitoring will suffice for these cases, including non-invasive blood pressure, 5-lead electrocardiogram, pulse oximetry, and temperature. Monitoring of inspired and expired gases and volatile anesthetic agents is obviously warranted in general endotracheal anesthesia.

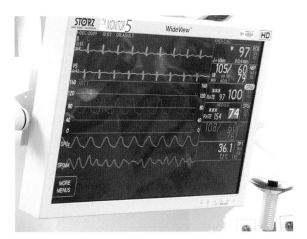

Figure 41.3. Physiological monitors during open fetal surgery. The waveforms from top to bottom include maternal 5-lead electrocardiogram, invasive arterial blood pressure, and pulse oximetry. The bottom waveform is from the fetal pulse oximeter. The numbers on the left include the following (from top to bottom): maternal heart rate, maternal non-invasive blood pressure, maternal oxygen saturation, fetal oxygen saturation, maternal invasive blood pressure, and maternal esophageal temperature.

Open fetal surgical procedures subject the mother to greater physiological stress than minimally invasive approaches, and so closer monitoring and tighter anesthetic control of the maternal and fetal physiology are warranted (Figure 41.3). The mother's safety is the highest priority, but she must be safely anesthetized with the goal of providing optimal conditions for fetal perfusion and well-being. Monitoring fetal well-being can be challenging; minimum monitoring includes intermittent fetal heart rate assessment by ultrasound. Continuous fetal pulse oximetry is often used in open fetal surgery and allows the team to continuously monitor both fetal heart rate and oxygen saturation. Fetal echocardiography can also be used, and rarely fetal blood gas analysis. To ensure fetal well-being, the team must ensure adequate fetal perfusion. The pieces of this puzzle include a patent umbilical cord, adequate amniotic fluid volume, intact uteroplacental interface, low uterine muscle tone, and adequate uterine blood flow and oxygen delivery. The anesthesia team can directly impact two of these factors: uterine smooth muscle tone and uterine blood flow. The other factors are under the care of the operating team.

High-dose volatile anesthetic or nitroglycerin administration both allow uterine relaxation; however, this relaxation comes at the expense of a decreased maternal blood pressure and increased risk of maternal bleeding. Uterine blood flow is directly proportional to the difference between uterine arterial and venous pressure and inversely proportional to the uterine vascular resistance. Ensuring adequate maternal arterial blood pressure will optimize blood flow to the uterus. This can be achieved by ensuring left uterine displacement, administration of vasopressors such as phenylephrine and ephedrine, and in some cases by optimizing cardiac preload with administration of intravenous crystalloid. Historically, mothers undergoing fetal surgery have had an increased incidence of pulmonary edema [16]. The causes of this are unclear, but factors released by the uterus, aggressive postoperative tocolysis with products that may cause pulmonary edema, and enthusiastic fluid loading may contribute. Experience with newer tocolytics, such as atosiban acetate (Tractocile), which may be less prone to causing pulmonary edema is at present lacking, in part because this drug is not registered worldwide. Mothers undergoing open mid-gestation surgery are typically restricted to 500 mL of intravenous crystalloid. This fluid restriction makes blood pressure management particularly challenging in the face of the high-dose volatile anesthetic agent. Since mothers undergoing EXIT procedure do not have as many problems with pulmonary edema, intravenous fluid administration can be more generous, and maintaining an adequate blood pressure is not as problematic. The EXIT procedure has been performed under epidural anesthesia with nitroglycerin as the sole agent used to provide uterine relaxation, but the fetal interventions have typically been brief [17]. The gravid uterus receives a large proportion of the maternal cardiac output, and even routine obstetric cases can be complicated by significant hemorrhage. With high-dose volatile anesthetic causing profound uterine relaxation, hemorrhage may be even more problematic. Fortunately, bleeding is rare, as special uterine stapling devices keep the edges of the hysterotomy from bleeding. Problems with the stapling device or bleeding from venous sinuses may still occur, typically when the hysterotomy is first made. Additionally, EXIT procedures may be complicated by bleeding after the fetus and placenta have been delivered, as it will take a longer period of time for the high doses of volatile anesthetic to be eliminated from the mother's body. The prolonged elimination of volatile anesthetic results in a slower increase of uterine tone and slower response to postdelivery uterotonics. Therefore, precautions have to be taken to have secondary uterotonics ready.

Postoperative management of fetal surgical patients

Minimally invasive surgery

Patients who have undergone minimally invasive fetal therapy typically do not require intensive monitoring or critical care decision making. Recovery from the anesthetic should be fairly brief and uncomplicated in most patients, as the anesthetics typically consist of light sedation combined with local anesthetic infiltration or a standard neuraxial anesthetic. As sedation medications may be quite variable, the recovery from sedation does deserve some mention. Many modern anesthetic medications (midazolam, remifentanil, propofol) are very short acting, but traditional sedation has often consisted of high doses of diazepam and morphine. Diazepam has quite a long half-life and its metabolites are also pharmacologically active. These patients should be monitored carefully for adequate oxygenation and ventilation in the postoperative period, as respiratory depression may persist for many hours after the procedure. Fluid shifts are not typically problematic. If a patient is given magnesium sulfate for tocolysis (which may be the local practice) at the end of the procedure, a typical anesthetic management would include restrictive administration of intravenous crystalloid to prevent pulmonary edema plus proactive observation for toxic side effects. Consequently, postoperative hypovolemia may ensue, and the patient's hemodynamics and urine output should be noted. Fluid boluses may be given judiciously. Depending on the invasiveness of the procedure, some patients are discharged after several hours of maternal and fetal observation, and some patients may stay overnight for observation.

Open mid-gestation surgery

Patients undergoing open mid-gestation fetal surgery require intensive postoperative monitoring and close collaboration between team members for medical decision making. The mother may be sick to begin with, as maternal mirror syndrome may be one of the reasons for performing the fetal intervention. Issues of note include recovering from a deep general anesthetic, postoperative analgesia, prevention of pulmonary edema, avoidance of significant hypovolemia or anemia, and tocolysis. A typical anesthetic for open mid-gestation surgery should provide intense uterine relaxation to optimize the surgical field and to minimize uterine vascular resistance and allow improved fetal perfusion. This intense uterine relaxation is often achieved by administering a high dose of a volatile inhalational anesthetic agent such as desflurane. The minimum alveolar concentration (of desflurane in a 25-year-old woman is 7.3%, and typical concentrations used in open fetal surgery can range from 12 to 16%. Although the volatile anesthetics are all quite short acting compared with many other medications, the high doses required may predispose patients to longer periods of sedation in the postoperative period.

The transverse incisions made for open fetal surgery are larger and more cephalad than the Pfannenstiel incision performed for a cesarean delivery. If the placenta has implanted on the anterior aspect of the uterine wall, the entire gravid uterus must be exteriorized so that the hysterotomy can be made on the posterior aspect of the uterus. While postoperative analgesia may certainly be achieved with intravenous opioid administration, continuous epidural infusion of local anesthetic with or without low-dose opioid provides more satisfactory analgesia without as much patient sedation. Given the high doses of volatile anesthetic administered, any measures to improve patient alertness will help with patient assessment. Some patients, however, will experience postoperative hypotension. This hypotension may or may not be a consequence of the epidural infusion. It also may or may not be symptomatic (maternal or fetal), and "treating the numbers" should be avoided. Other causes of hypotension, such as aortocaval compression, cardiac dysfunction, and hypovolemia, should obviously be excluded, but decreasing the epidural infusion rate is a frequently attempted maneuver aimed at increasing the maternal blood pressure.

Patients undergoing fetal surgery are at increased risk for developing pulmonary edema [16,18]. Oxygenation, ventilation, breath sounds, and work of breathing should be frequently assessed. Simple measures such as physiotherapy or supplemental oxygen via nasal cannula may be all that are needed, but advanced methods to assist with maternal oxygenation and ventilation should be available. Not all hypoxia is from pulmonary edema, and other causes such as atelectasis or pneumonia should also be considered. Intravenous fluid administration is quite restrictive in the perioperative period with the hopes of minimizing the incidence of maternal pulmonary edema, but this fluid restriction places the patients at risk for hypovolemia. Intraoperative infusion of vasopressors will allow adequate end-organ and fetal perfusion in the face of the relative hypovolemia caused by the high doses of volatile anesthetics. Postoperative vasopressor administration is rarely needed, but urine output must be closely monitored. Oliguria occurs commonly in these patients and should respond to small boluses of crystalloid. These boluses are given quite sparingly at the authors' institution. Central venous pressures have been used to guide fluid therapy in the past, but even in uncomplicated cases, central venous pressure is an imperfect surrogate for left ventricular filling pressure and volume. As this is the case, central venous pressure is virtually never monitored.

Bleeding is rare in these patients. If it is going to occur, the most likely time will be during the creation of the hysterotomy or with closure of the hysterotomy. When bleeding does occur, it is brisk, given the high percentage of cardiac output dedicated to the gravid uterus and the extraordinarily low uterine tone caused by administration of volatile anesthetic agents. Postoperative bleeding is quite rare but should be considered if unexplained, persistent, or worsening hypotension occurs.

Tocolytic regimens after open fetal surgery differ between various healthcare systems. Magnesium sulfate is used most commonly in the USA, whereas atosiban may be used more commonly in Europe. A bolus of 6 g magnesium sulfate followed by a 4 g/h infusion for several hours may result in varying degrees of magnesium toxicity. The patient must have frequent assessments of level of consciousness, respiration, hemodynamics, muscle strength, deep tendon reflexes, urine output, and serum levels of magnesium when this has been used. If magnesium levels are too high, administration of calcium gluconate or calcium chloride will antagonize the effects. Typically magnesium sulfate is used only briefly, and when further tocolytics will include nifedipine, this should not be started simultaneously.

The EXIT procedure

While the intraoperative management of a patient undergoing an EXIT procedure has many similarities with that of a patient undergoing open mid-gestation surgery, the postoperative patient transported to the recovery room has more in common with a postoperative patient after cesarean section patient than one after open mid-gestation fetal surgery. The incision will likely be the same type of incision as that used for open mid-gestation surgery. A postoperative epidural is likely to be in place. Intravenous fluid management will likely have been more similar to that for a cesarean delivery. Oxytocin will have been given. Secondary uterotonics may also have been administered, such as methylergonovine or prostaglandin $F_{2\alpha}$.

Maternal complications of fetal surgery

Intraoperative complications

Fetal surgery represents a significant undertaking for the mother, the fetus, and the whole family. Greater risk and more significant maternal complications will arise with more invasive procedures. The list of potential intraoperative anesthetic complications is the same as would occur during any anesthetic for any pregnant patient. These complications include, but are not limited to, lost maternal airway, pulmonary aspiration of gastric contents, pulmonary edema, bronchospasm, placental abruption with all its consequences, bleeding, hypotension, anaphylaxis, cardiac dysrhythmia, and local anesthetic toxicity. While amniotic fluid embolism is always a concern, no cases have yet been reported in the literature. Management of these intraoperative complications is standard and should be familiar to the anesthetic team involved in the care of pregnant patients.

Postoperative complications

A variety of maternal complications are reported after fetal surgery. Some of these occur in the immediate perioperative period and some do not present until subsequent pregnancies. Hemorrhage and pulmonary edema would be the most likely reasons to admit a mother to the intensive care unit. Hemorrhage is more likely during open fetal surgery but is also possible during minimally invasive surgery. It should be managed in the standard fashion, with close hemodynamic monitoring and measurement of hemoglobin concentrations, establishment of large-bore intravenous access, cross-matching of blood products, and transfusion as needed. Only rarely is bleeding uncontrollable. If this is the case, it might be necessary to proceed to hysterotomy and termination of pregnancy to empty the uterus. Placental abruption would be the most likely reason. Established obstetric hemorrhage protocols should be followed. Bleeding may occur during the initial fetal surgery [18] or may occur during the subsequent cesarean section for delivery of the child [1].

Pulmonary edema occurs in patients undergoing fetal surgery with more frequency and severity than in the general population, particularly where a maternal hysterotomy is required or mirror syndrome occurs. Rates of pulmonary edema as high as 27% have been reported from the earlier days of open fetal surgery [18]. These rates were associated with the use of multiple tocolytics, nitroglycerin, and liberal intravenous fluid administration [16,19]. Fortunately, however, the risk of developing pulmonary edema seems to be decreasing to rates as low as 6% [1]. This decrease likely reflects increased awareness of the risk of pulmonary edema, closer monitoring, restrictive intravenous fluid management, plus more frequent use of vasopressors and simplified tocolytic regimens.

Other complications may not necessitate maternal critical care in the traditional sense but do call for close observation of the mother and fetus. Preterm premature rupture of membranes occurs in mothers who undergo both minimally invasive surgery and, more frequently, open fetal surgery. Reported rates of iatrogenic membrane rupture range from 7 to 47% even in minimally invasive surgery [20]. Chorioamniotic membrane separation may also occur, and this increases the risk of premature rupture of the membranes, next to causing fetal distress [1]. The consequences of prolonged, preterm premature rupture of the membranes include oligohydramnios, increased risk of infection, preterm delivery, and placental abruption. Management of this complication may include bed rest and prophylactic administration of antibiotics. If prolonged bed rest is called for, thromboprophylaxis is an important consideration. Reported rates of preterm labor leading to delivery are similarly high, ranging from 12.9 to 32.9% [19]. Mean gestational age at delivery has been reported at approximately 30–32 weeks for a variety of open and minimally invasive interventions [18]. After myelomeningocele closure, only 21% of mothers carried the gestation to greater than 37 weeks, and mean gestational age at delivery was 34 weeks [1].

Myometrial wound healing and bleeding are important issues to highlight both in the pregnancy involved with the fetal surgery and in subsequent pregnancies. Partial or complete uterine dehiscence was found at delivery in 10% of the mothers participating in the Management of Myelomeningocele Study, and only 64% of these mothers had an intact, well-healed uterine scar. The exact relevance of these findings is uncertain; no clinical ruptures during pregnancy occurred. At the time of delivery, 9% of mothers who had fetal repair of myelomeningocele received a blood transfusion, compared with only 1% of mothers who were randomized to postnatal repair of the myelomeningocele. Surveys examining subsequent pregnancies have been sent to mothers who have previously undergone open fetal surgery, and have found rates of uterine dehiscence ranging from 12 to 14%, and rates of rupture ranging from 6 to 14% [21,22]. The rate of rupture is in the upper range to just above that of mothers who have had prior classical cesarean sections (6–9%) [21]. Bleeding is still an issue for subsequent pregnancies, with 6% of mothers responding to the survey experiencing excessive bleeding at the delivery [22].

Logistics of a comprehensive fetal surgery program

The range of fetal therapeutic procedures is wide, going from needle-based procedures, placement of shunts, and therapeutic applications of percutaneous fetoscopy, to procedures under general anesthesia via laparotomy and hysterotomy. Traditionally, open fetal surgery has never been much embraced in Europe, so training will be required in many places. As for any other complex surgical technique, one cannot expect to have similar outcomes from the beginning [23]. There are, at present, no guidelines; nor is there a consensus on which fetal surgical procedures should be offered regionally or how training should be structured and evaluated [24]. The US Agency for Healthcare Research and Quality has published a white paper on this and is expected to produce recommendations soon for the expertise and experience required for a center to operate and maintain competence. Two primary models of training are in use in the USA [25]. The first consists of experts traveling to teach at the candidate institution, and the second consists of the candidate team traveling to expert centers to learn from the experienced physicians and staff. The candidate team can then safely and effectively establish a program for open fetal surgeries, as well have return visits for further training or assistance. The learning process will be expedited by having a high-volume fetal surgery program, with an interdisciplinary board and team, and offering a variety of procedures (including EXIT experience) as well as having a large experimental program. In order to have a viable program, turnover should be sufficient to maintain proficiency both in diagnostic evaluation and in fetal surgery. Numbers for that are lacking at present.

Conclusions

Fetal surgery is a new and rapidly evolving field that holds promise for the treatment of diseases that can be either debilitating or life threatening to the fetus. The safety of the mother carrying that fetus must not be forgotten, as she is subjected to significant anesthetic and surgical risks while seeking to improve the welfare of her child. Many of these risks are similar to those encountered over the course of any anesthetic or pregnancy and can be treated in the same ways. Unique considerations, however, may arise when treating these patients, and they should be cared for in specialized centers with appropriate experience and infrastructure.

References

1. Adzick NS, Thom EA, Spong CY, *et al*. A randomized trial of prenatal versus postnatal repair of myelomeningocele. *N Engl J Med* 2011;**364**:993–1004.

2. Senat M-V, Deprest J, Boulvain M, *et al*. Endoscopic laser surgery versus serial amnioreduction for severe twin-to-twin transfusion syndrome. *N Engl J Med* 2004;**351**:136–144.

3. Liechty KW, Crombleholme TM, Flake AW, *et al*. Intrapartum airway management for giant fetal neck masses: the EXIT (ex utero intrapartum treatment) procedure. *Am J Obstet Gynecol* 1997;**177**:870–874.

4. Lewi L, Jani J, Deprest J. Invasive antenatal interventions in complicated multiple pregnancies. *Obstet Gynecol Clin North Am* 2005;**32**:105–126.

5. Verbeek RJ, Heep A, Maurits NM, *et al*. Fetal endoscopic myelomeningocele closure preserves segmental neurological function. *Dev Med Child Neurol* 2012;**54**:15–22.

6. Lim F-Y, Crombleholme TM, Hedrick HL, *et al*. Congenital high airway obstruction syndrome: natural history and management. *J Pediatr Surg* 2003;**38**:940–945.

7. Adzick NS, Flake AW, Crombleholme TM Management of congenital lung lesions. *Semin Pediatr Surg* 2003;**12**:10–16.

8. Hedrick HL, Flake AW, Crombleholme TM, *et al*. The ex utero intrapartum therapy procedure for high-risk fetal lung lesions. *J Pediatr Surg* 2005;**40**:1038–1043; discussion 1044.

9. DeKoninck P, Gratacos E, Van Mieghem T, *et al*. Results of fetal endoscopic tracheal occlusion for congenital diaphragmatic hernia and the set up of the randomized controlled TOTAL trial. *Early Hum Dev* 2011;**87**:619–624.

10. McElhinney DB, Tworetzky W, Lock JE. Current status of fetal cardiac intervention. *Circulation* 2010;**121**:1256–1263.

11. Cendron M, D'Alton ME, Crombleholme TM. Prenatal diagnosis and management of the fetus with hydronephrosis. *Semin Perinatol* 1994;**18**:163–181.

12. Ruano R. Fetal surgery for severe lower urinary tract obstruction. *Prenat Diagn* 2011;**31**:667–674.

13. Flake AW. Fetal sacrococcygeal teratoma. *Semin Pediatr Surg* 1993;**2**:113–120.

14. Braun T, Brauer M, Fuchs I, *et al*. Mirror syndrome: a systematic review of fetal associated conditions, maternal presentation and perinatal outcome. *Fetal Diagn Ther* 2010;**27**:191–203.

15. Tran KM. Anesthesia for fetal surgery. *Semin Fetal Neonatal Med* 2010;**15**:40–45.

16. DiFederico EM, Burlingame JM, Kilpatrick SJ, Harrison M, Matthay MA. Pulmonary edema in obstetric patients is rapidly resolved except in the presence of infection or of nitroglycerin tocolysis after open fetal surgery. *Am J Obstet Gynecol* 1998;**179**:925–933.

17. Clark KD, Viscomi CM, Lowell J, Chien EK. Nitroglycerin for relaxation to establish a fetal airway (EXIT procedure). *Obstet Gynecol* 2004;**103**:1113–1115.

18. Golombeck K, Ball RH, Lee H, *et al*. Maternal morbidity after maternal–fetal surgery. *Am J Obstet Gynecol* 2006;**194**:834–839.

19. Wu D, Ball RH. The maternal side of maternal–fetal surgery. *Clin Perinatol* 2009;**36**:247–253, viii.

20. Deprest J, Emonds M-P, Richter J, *et al*. Amniopatch for iatrogenic rupture of the fetal membranes. *Prenat Diagn* 2011;**31**:661–666.

21. Wilson RD, Johnson MP, Flake AW, *et al*. Reproductive outcomes after pregnancy complicated by maternal–fetal surgery. *Am J Obstet Gynecol* 2004;**191**:1430–1436.

22. Wilson RD, Lemerand K, Johnson MP, *et al*. Reproductive outcomes in subsequent pregnancies after a pregnancy complicated by open maternal–fetal surgery (1996–2007). *Am J Obstet Gynecol* 2010;**203**:209.e1–209e6.

23. Danzer E, Siegle J, D'Agostino JA, *et al*. Early neurodevelopmental outcome of infants with high-risk fetal lung lesions. *Fetal Diagn Ther* 2012;**31**:210–215.

24. Moise KJ, Johnson A, Carpenter RJ, Baschat AA, Platt LD. Fetal intervention: providing reasonable access to quality care. *Obstet Gynecol* 2009;**113**:408–410.

25. Walsh WF, Chescheir NC, Gillam-Krakauer M, *et al.*. *Maternal–fetal Surgical Procedures*. Rockville, MD: Agency for Healthcare Research and Quality, 2011.

Index

ketamine, 168, 201
kidney, *see* acute kidney injury in
    pregnancy; renal tract
Kleihauer–Betke test (rhesus), 360

labetalol, 307, 411
lactation
    establishing, 55–6
    medication considerations, 57
    postpartum changes in the breasts,
        55
    signs and symptoms of mastitis, 56–7
    suppressing, 56
    use of imaging contrast
        agents, 233
lamivudine, 384
lamotrigine, 154
latex allergy, 32, 167–8
leukemia, 317
levobupivacaine, 168
levosimendan, 165, 434
lipid intake in pregnancy, 204
lithium, 155
liver disease in pregnancy
    alcohol-induced liver injury, 386
    approach to diagnosis, 381–2
    autoimmune hepatitis, 385
    biochemical tests for, 379–81
    Budd–Chiari syndrome, 340, 385
    causes not related to pregnancy,
        383–6
    clinical assessment, 379
    diseases related to pregnancy, 382–3
    drug-induced liver injury, 386
    hepatic hemangioma, 340
    hepatic vein thrombosis, 385
    hepatitis viruses, 384
    hepatocellular adenomas and
        bleeding risk, 388
    herpes simplex virus hepatitis, 385
    hyperemesis gravidarum, 382
    imaging of the liver in pregnancy,
        381
    incidence, 379
    intrahepatic cholestasis of
        pregnancy, 382–3
    liver function tests, 379–81
    management of portal hypertension,
        386–8
    multidisciplinary approach, 389
    non-alcoholic fatty liver disease, 385
    portal vein thrombosis, 340
    pregnancy after liver transplantation,
        388
    spontaneous hepatic rupture,
        339–40
    Wilson disease, 386
    see also acute fatty liver of pregnancy
liver transplant
    in acute fatty liver of pregnancy, 425

living will, 68–70
local anesthetic toxicity, 298–8
    induced systemic toxicity, 138
local anesthetics
    allergic reactions to, 168
Loeys–Dietz syndrome, 261
long-chain 3-hydroxyacylcoenzyme A
    dehydrogenase (LCHAD)
    deficiency, 419
lopinavir, 154
lorazepam, 154
low birth weight, 204, 388
lung transplant recipients, 271–2
lupus nephritis, 304, 392
Lyme disease in pregnancy, 373

magnesium sulfate, 272, 411, 413–14
    toxicity, 134, 307
malaria during pregnancy
    clinical management, 369–70
    clinical manifestations, 368–9
    diagnosis, 369
    drug resistance in malaria parasites,
        370–1
    drug treatment, 370–1
    management of labor, 372
    mortality caused by, 367–8
    mosquitoes, 367
    need for more reporting on effects,
        376
    outcome, 372–3
    Plasmodium spp. infections,
        367–8
    prophylactic use of antimalarial
        drugs, 371–2
    treatment, 369–72
Managing Obstetric Emergencies and
    Trauma course, 140, 141, 442
Marfan syndrome, 251, 260–1
massive hemorrhage
    risk in placenta previa, 28–9
mastitis
    signs and symptoms, 56–7
maternal collapse
    approach to cardiac arrest in
        pregnancy, 141
    cardiopulmonary resuscitation,
        136–8
    causes, 134–5
    diagnostic evaluation, 138–9
    immediate considerations, 134
    improving management of, 140–1
    initial response, 135–6
    modified ACLS guidelines, 136–8
    perimortem cesarean delivery,
        139–40
    prediction of collapse or severe
        morbidity, 135
    see also early obstetric warning
        system, 135

maternal complications of fetal
    surgery, 469–70
maternal critical care
    admission criteria, 8–9, 11, 16
    advance directives, 68–70
    classification, 7–8
    clinical governance, 12–14
    definitions, 7–8, 16
    discharge criteria, 9, 11
    emergency simulation training for
        staff, 14
    ethical approach to decision making,
        68–70
    ethical aspects, 67–8
    family involvement in decision
        making, 73–4
    high dependency unit, 8
    ICU, 8, 10–11
    labor and delivery in ICU, 11–12
    levels of care, 7–8
    limits of, 67–8
    preventive ethics approach, 68–70
    quality of life issues, 67–8
    range of approaches to, 7
    record keeping, 14
    role of obstetric critical care, 8
    short- and long-term goals, 67–8
    transfer of the critically ill obstetric
        patient, 12
    trial of management, 68
    unit design and utilities, 9
    unit location, 9
    unit personnel, 9–10
maternal hydrops syndrome, 465
maternal mirror syndrome, 465
maternal morbidity
    causes of physical morbidity, 78
    cognitive impairment, 82–3
    delirium, 82–3
    depression in ICU survivors, 79,
        84–5
    disease-specific predictor
        (fullPIERS), 135
    epidemiology, 26–7
    follow-up after discharge, 85
    ICU-acquired weakness, 79
    non-physical morbidity, 79–83
    post-traumatic stress disorder, 82
    potential for further reduction, 37
    potential for prevention, 26–7
    prevalence, 1
    subsequent pregnancy, 83–5
    subsequent pregnancy case study, 85
    types of morbidity in ICU
        patients, 78
    see also maternal near miss
maternal mortality
    assessment and surveillance, 1
    definition (World Health
        Organization), 1

479

485